Applications of Nanotechnology in Biomedical Engineering

This book presents recent advancements in nanotechnology-based innovations in the biomedical sciences and engineering fields, including nanoimaging, nano-delivery of drugs and genes, antimicrobial and antiviral coatings, nano-nutraceuticals, and nano-cosmetics. It covers a wide range of topics, which include nanosensors, nano-based coatings, and wound healing, as well as scope for new research and development. It is a guide to the state-of-the-art nanotechnological advancements in medical image processing and disease detection.

Features are as follows:

- Covers industry-oriented applications of nanomaterials in the field of biomedical engineering
- Discusses development of nature-inspired nano-engineered nutraceuticals
- Reviews research on nano-coating to restrict biofilm formation and nosocomial infections
- Includes different aspects of both medical sciences and health sciences, ranging from medical imaging to cosmetics
- Explores micro-/nano-SMART devices for biomedical applications

This book is aimed at researchers and graduate students in biomedical engineering, nanotechnology, and related areas.

Applications of Nanotechnology in Biomedical Engineering

Edited by

Piyali Basak, Pratik Das, Suvendu Manna, and Tridib Kumar Sinha

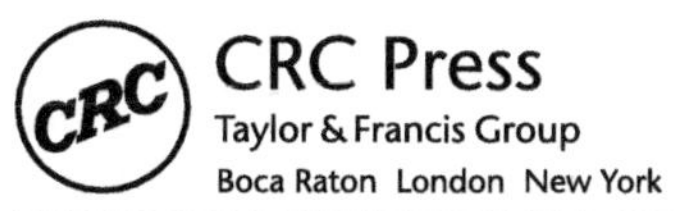

CRC Press is an imprint of the
Taylor & Francis Group, an **informa** business

First edition published 2025
by CRC Press
6000 Broken Sound Parkway NW, Suite 300, Boca Raton, FL 33487-2742

and by CRC Press
4 Park Square, Milton Park, Abingdon, Oxon, OX14 4RN

CRC Press is an imprint of Taylor & Francis Group, LLC

Library of Congress Cataloging-in-Publication Data
Names: Basak, Piyali, editor.
Title: Applications of nanotechnology in biomedical engineering /
edited by Piyali Basak, Pratik Das, Suvendu Manna, and Tridib Sinha.
Description: First edition. | Boca Raton, FL : CRC Press, 2025. |
Includes bibliographical references and index.
Identifiers: LCCN 2024033764 (print) | LCCN 2024033765 (ebook) |
ISBN 9781032485843 (hbk) | ISBN 9781032558721 (pbk) | ISBN 9781003432661 (ebk)
Subjects: LCSH: Nanomedicine. | Biomedical engineering.
Classification: LCC R857.N34 A673 2025 (print) | LCC R857.N34 (ebook) |
DDC 610.28–dc23/eng/20241001
LC record available at https://lccn.loc.gov/2024033764
LC ebook record available at https://lccn.loc.gov/2024033765

ISBN: 9781032485843 (hbk)
ISBN: 9781032558721 (pbk)
ISBN: 9781003432661 (ebk)

DOI: 10.1201/9781003432661

Typeset in Times
by codeMantra

Contents

Foreword

It gives me immense pleasure to write this foreword for *Applications of Nanotechnology in Biomedical Engineering.*

Nanotechnological innovations in biomedical sectors improve the properties of biomaterials many-fold. Since the last few decades, nanomaterials have been utilized in bioimaging to biomedicine. Sensing life-threatening diseases using nanomaterial-derived nano-sensors improves the understanding of disease prognoses and its mitigation pathways more accurately. Many of the metal nanoparticles have germicidal effects, and thus, they are being used for numerous medicinal applications as well. Due to these properties, many of them are also used in cosmetics.

This book presents a critical overview of the current nanotechnologies that are being utilized in biomedical applications. This book presents research, reviews, and case studies on the advancement in bioimaging, biosensing, drug and gene delivery, wound healing, nutraceuticals, and cosmetics through nanotechnological interventions. I would like to congratulate the entire editorial team members for conceptualizing such an emerging topic to discuss in their book and wish them all the success. I would also like to congratulate CRC Press for its foresight in planning this book and wish for its commercial success. I am sure that this book will be found in the literature of universities and research institutes and that researchers will enrich their knowledge. I wish for the success of the book.

Prof. Buddhadeb Sau
Vice Chancellor
Jadavpur University

Preface

Like other industrial sectors, the biomedical industries also flourished with the use of nanotechnological innovations. Every day some new nanomaterials are coming with new and improved properties. Some of them showed amazing biomedical properties. For example, silver nanoparticles are known to have high germicidal activities, whereas magnetic nanoparticles are being used for biomedical imaging and biosensing of diseases. Scientists are using such nanomaterials to coat over different surfaces to make them resistant to bacterial growth and restrict disease transmission. Most often, managing and healing wounds in immune-compromised patients is very difficult in medical industries. The surgical instruments, bandages, and cottons used for dressing wounds often are the major sources of cross-contamination. A complex of metal nanoparticles with bactericidal and virucidal effects could solve those issues. Tissue-specific drug delivery and gene delivery are also ambitious research currently ongoing where nanomaterial-driven materials are being developed for specific and direct delivery of drugs and genes. Many nanoparticles also showed therapeutic effects to some life-threatening diseases like cancer. The cosmetic industries are also experimenting with different nanoparticles to improve their products' properties.

This book provides our readers a comprehensive overview of the development on such research. Researchers, academicians, and industrial personnel share their research, reviews, and case studies in this book as book chapters on improvement in bioimaging, biosensing, wound healing, coating, and therapeutic and cosmetic application through direct and indirect nanotechnological intervention. The drawbacks, technical difficulties, and future research possibilities are also mentioned in most of the chapters.

We hope this book will be useful guidance to all those budding researchers who want to start research on this innovative topic. We would like to thank all of the contributing authors for associating with this project. We express deep sense of gratitude to Jadavpur University, Kolkata, and UPES, Dehradun, for allowing us to publish this book. We also would like to thank the Vice Chancellor, Pro-Vice Chancellor, and Registrar of both universities for their continuous support and motivation. We highly appreciate the efforts of all of our reviewers for their valuable time to voluntarily review the manuscripts and provide their comments and suggestions timely. We also would like to appreciate the efforts of CRC Press for accepting our proposal and publishing the book in a timely manner.

Dr. Piyali Basak

Mr. Pratik Das

Dr. Suvendu Manna

Dr. Tridib Kumar Sinha

Acknowledgments

We would like to extend our sincere gratitude to the following individuals and institutions whose support and guidance have been instrumental in the successful completion of the book, "Application of Nanotechnology in Biomedical Engineering." Firstly, we express our heartfelt thanks to the Dean of the Sustainability Cluster at UPES for their continuous encouragement and support throughout the research and writing process. We express our gratitude to the Vice Chancellor of UPES for his innovative leadership and dedication to fostering a conducive environment for academic research and excellence. A special acknowledgment goes to the Dean of FISLM at Jadavpur University for their valuable insights and contributions that enriched the content of this book. We would also like to express our sincere gratitude to the Vice Chancellor of Jadavpur University for his unconditional support and encouragement throughout this work. Additionally, we extend our gratitude to the Pro-Vice-Chancellor of Jadavpur University for their guidance and assistance in the development of this book. We are indebted to all the authors who dedicated their time and expertise to contribute valuable insights, making this collaborative effort possible. At last, we convey our appreciation to CRC Press for giving us the chance to share our knowledge and research through the publication of this book. This pursuit would not have been feasible without the collective exertions and backing of all individuals stated above, and we are genuinely appreciative for their input to this undertaking.

Editors

Dr. Piyali Basak is currently the Director of the School of Bioscience and Engineering at Jadavpur University, Kolkata, India. She authored more than 70 research and review articles in several international journals and several book chapters. Her research articles have reached 1,000 plus citations worldwide. She has obtained various research awards throughout her career. She is currently working on nano-biomaterials and polymer nanocomposites for various applications like drug delivery, wound healing, antimicrobial coatings over surgical instruments, and nanotherapeutics. She is also involved in works related to environmental studies, dye degradation, and natural product extract for therapeutic uses.

Mr. Pratik Das did his Masters of Engineering from the School of Bioscience and Engineering. Currently, he is pursuing his Ph.D. from Jadavpur University. He is working in the field of nanobiomaterials and their biomedical applications. He is currently continuing his research at the School of Bioscience and Engineering. He has authored or co-authored more than 17 international research and review articles in SCI and Scopus-indexed journals. His current research interests include green synthesis of silver nanoparticles, computational biology, biomaterials and their application in the biomedical industry, and synthesis and application of bio-derived carbon dots. His special interest involves the fabrication of wound-healing products.

Dr. Suvendu Manna did his Ph.D. from the Indian Institute of Technology, Kharagpur, in 2015. Currently, he is an assistant professor at the University of Petroleum and Energy Studies, Dehradun. He is an expert in biomaterials, wastewater remediation, environmental microbiology, and nanomaterial research. He has authored and co-authored 50 plus research and review articles published in SCI-indexed peer-reviewed journals. He edited six international books and wrote one reference book. He also serves as a reviewer for many reputed international journals.

Dr. Tridib Kumar Sinha is an assistant professor in the Department of Applied Sciences (Chemistry), University of Petroleum and Energy Studies, Dehradun, India. Priorly, he was a research professor (postdoc) in Gyeongsang National University (GNU), South Korea (2017–2021). He pursued his PhD from the Indian Institute of Technology (IIT), Kharagpur, in 2016. Before Ph.D., he was a research chemist (medicinal synthesis) in a contract research organization (2008–2010) in India. In brief, he is a materials chemist who designs and develops environmentally benign materials, particularly for sustainable energy and environment. He has published 45 plus research articles in SCI-indexed peer-reviewed journals.

Contributors

Jaideep Adhikari
School of Advanced Materials Green Energy and Sensor Systems
Indian Institute of Engineering Science and Technology
Shibpur, India

Kazi Asraf Ali
Department of Pharmaceutical Technology
Maulana Abul Kalam Azad University of Technology
Kolkata, India

M Tarik Arafat
Department of Biomedical Engineering
Bangladesh University of Engineering and Technology (BUET)
Dhaka, Bangladesh

Deepshikha Arora
Engineering Product Development
Singapore University of Technology and Design
Singapore, Singapore

Backiyalakshmi Gnanasekaran
Department of Biomedical Engineering
SRM Institute of Science and Technology
Kattankulathur, India

Somashree Bandyopadhaya
Department of Food Technology & Biochemical Engineering
Jadavpur University
Kolkata, India

Samiddha Banerjee
Department of Molecular Pathology
Suraksha Diagnostics
Kolkata, India

Ananya Barui
Centre for Healthcare Science and Technology
Indian Institute of Engineering, Science and Technology
Shibpur, India

Piyali Basak
School of Bioscience & Engineering
Jadavpur University
Kolkata, India

Soumyadeep Basu
School of Molecular Biosciences
College of Medical, Veterinary and Life Sciences, University of Glasgow
Glasgow, United Kingdom

Ajaya Kumar Behera
Department of Chemistry
Utkal University
Bhubaneswar, India

Debabrata Bera
Department of Food Technology & Biochemical Engineering
Jadavpur University,
Kolkata, India

Anu Bharti
Centre for Interdisciplinary Research and Innovation (CIDRI)
University of Petroleum and Energy Studies (UPES)
Dehradun, India

Seemesh Bhaskar
Department of Electrical and Computer Engineering
University of Illinois at Urbana-Champaign
Champaign, Illinois
Holonyak Micro and Nanotechnology Laboratory
Champaign, Illinois
Carl R. Woese Institute for Genomic Biology
Urbana, Illinois

Souptik Bhattacharya
Department of Food Technology
Guru Nanak Institute of Technology
Kolkata, India

Archisman Bhunia
Centre for Healthcare Science and Technology
Indian Institute of Engineering, Science and Technology
Shibpur, India

Amlan Bishal
Department of Pharmaceutical Technology
Maulana Abul Kalam Azad University of Technology
Kolkata, India
Bharat Technology
Howrah, India

Bikram Biswas
Department of Pharmaceutical Technology
Maulana Abul Kalam Azad University of Technology
Kolkata, India

Sreemoyee Chakraborty
Department of Food Technology & Biochemical Engineering
Jadavpur University
Kolkata, India

Kalyan Kumar Chattopadhyay
Thin Film and Nanoscience Lab, Department of Physics, School of Materials Science & Nanotechnology
Jadavpur University
Kolkata, India

Smarak Islam Chaudhury
Materials Research Centre
Indian Institute of Science
Bangalore, India

Sabyasachi Choudhuri
Department of Pharmaceutical Technology
Maulana Abul Kalam Azad University of Technology
Haringhata, India.

Bodhisatwa Das
Department of Biomedical Engineering
Indian Institute of Technology Ropar
Rupnagar, India

Narayan Chandra Das
Rubber Technology Centre
Indian Institute of Technology
Kharagpur, India

Piyali Das
Department of Biological Sciences, School of Life Science and Biotechnology
Adamas University
Kolkata, India

Subhankar Das
Biotechnology Unit
Mangalore University
Mangalore, India

Sudipto Das
Department of Pharmaceutical Technology
Maulana Abul Kalam Azad University of Technology
Haringhata, India

Sayamdipta Das Chowdhury
Department of Food Technology
Guru Nanak Institute of Technology
Kolkata, India

Nondita Datta
Department of Biomedical Engineering
Bangladesh University of Engineering and Technology (BUET)
Dhaka, Bangladesh

Suman Deb
Department Biological Sciences, School of Life Science and Biotechnology
Adamas University
Kolkata, India

Sayani Debnath
Department of Food Technology
Guru Nanak Institute of Technology
Kolkata, India

Shrestha Dutta
Department of Biotechnology
Amity Institute of Biotechnology, Amity University Kolkata
New Town, India

Rajdeep Ganguly
Centre for Healthcare Science and Technology
Indian Institute of Engineering, Science and Technology
Shibpur, India

Chandan Kumar Ghosh
School of Material Science and Nanotechnology
Jadavpur University
Kolkata, India

Manojit Ghosh
Department of Metallurgy and Materials
Engineering Indian Institute of Engineering Science and Technology
Shibpur, India

Shubhrima Ghosh
Trinity Translational Medicine Institute, School of Medicine
Trinity College Dublin
College Green, Ireland

Sreejita Ghosh
Maulana Abul Kalam Azad University of Technology
Kolkata, India
Department Biological Sciences, School of Life Science and Biotechnology
Adamas University
Kolkata, India

Pratik Gravit
Department of Biotechnology, School of Biosciences & Technology
Vellore Institute of Technology (VIT)
Vellore, India

Chowdhury Mobaswar Hossain
Department of Pharmaceutical Technology
Maulana Abul Kalam Azad University of Technology
Haringhata, India

Anh Igarashi
Graduate School of Engineering
Tohoku University
Sendai, Japan

Varnit Jain
Department of Metallurgy and Materials Engineering
Indian Institute of Engineering Science and Technology
Shibpur, India

Purvesh Kadam
Department of Biotechnology, School of Biosciences & Technology
Vellore Institute of Technology (VIT)
Vellore, India

Manjula Ishwara Kalyani
Department of Microbiology
Mangalore University
Mangalore, India

Mohit Kamboj
Department of Biomedical Engineering
Indian Institute of Technology Ropar
Rupnagar, India

Rohit Kapila
Materials Research Centre
Indian Institute of Science
Bangalore, India

Vivek Kaushik
Department of Microbiology
SOHST, UPES
Dehradun, India

Cansu Ilke Kuru-Sumer
Faculty of Science, Department of Biochemistry
Ege University
Izmir, Turkey
Buca Municipality Buca Science and Art Center
Izmir, Turkey

Likhith K
Department of Biomedical Engineering
Manipal Institute of Technology, Manipal Academy of Higher Education
Udupi, India

Nazmun Lyle
Dr. Ambedkar Institute of Pharmaceutical Science
Rourkela, India

Sourav Maji
Department of Pharmaceutical Technology
Maulana Abul Kalam Azad University of Technology
Kolkata, India

Suhasini Mallick
Department of Biotechnology
Maulana Abul Kalam Azad University of Technology
Simhat, India

Puja Mandal
Department of Pharmaceutical Technology
Maulana Abul Kalam Azad University of Technology
Haringhata, India

Suvendu Manna
Sustainability Cluster
SOAE, UPES
Dehradun, India

Tarun Mateti
Materials Research Centre
Indian Institute of Science
Bangalore, India

Ashish Mathur
Centre for Interdisciplinary Research and Innovation (CIDRI)
University of Petroleum and Energy Studies (UPES)
Dehradun, India

Afiya Mubasharah
Department of Biomedical Engineering
Bangladesh University of Engineering and Technology (BUET)
Dhaka, Bangladesh

Sampurna Mukherjee
School of Materials Science & Nanotechnology
Jadavpur University
Kolkata, India

Sagnik Nag
Department of Biotechnology, School of Biosciences & Technology
Vellore Institute of Technology (VIT)
Vellore, India

Aparajita Pal
Rubber Technology Centre
Indian Institute of Technology
Kharagpur, India

Samrat Paul
Department of Biotechnology
Brainware University
Kolkata, India

Nabarun Polley
Department of Biomedical Engineering
SRM Institute of Science and Technology
Kattankulathur, India

Sai Sathish Ramamurthy
6STAR Laboratory, Central Research Instruments Facility (CRIF), Department of Chemistry
Sri Sathya Sai Institute of Higher Learning
Anantapur, India

Rina Rani Ray
Maulana Abul Kalam Azad University of Technology
Kolkata, India
Materials Research Centre
Indian Institute of Science
Bangalore, India

S. Najes Riaz
School of Materials Science & Nanotechnology
Jadavpur University
Kolkata, India

Dipayan Roy
School of Materials Science & Nanotechnology
Jadavpur University
Kolkata, India

Lakshmishri Roy
Department of Food Technology
Techno Main Salt Lake
Kolkata, India

Souradeep Roy
Centre for Interdisciplinary Research and Innovation (CIDRI)
University of Petroleum and Energy Studies (UPES)
Dehradun, India

Aaishiki Saha
School of Materials Science & Nanotechnology
Jadavpur University
Kolkata, India

Prerona Saha
Department of Metallurgy and Materials Engineering
Indian Institute of Engineering Science and Technology
Shibpur, India

Gayatri Sahini
Department of Microbiology
SOHST, UPES
Dehradun, India

Sourav Sarkar
School of Materials Science & Nanotechnology
Jadavpur University
Kolkata, India

Moumita Shee
School of Nanoscience and Technology
Indian Institute of Technology
Kharagpur, India

Devendra Singh
Faculty of Biotechnology
Institute of Biosciences and Technology, Shri Ramswaroop Memorial University
Barabanki, India

Snekhalatha Umapathy
Department of Biomedical Engineering
SRM Institute of Science and Technology
Kattankulathur, India

Goutam Thakur
Department of Biomedical Engineering
Manipal Institute of Technology, Manipal Academy of Higher Education
Udupi,

Manas Thakur
School of Materials Science & Nanotechnology
Jadavpur University
Kolkata, India

Garima Tripathi
Department of Biotechnology, School of Biosciences & Technology
Vellore Institute of Technology (VIT)
Vellore, India

Fulden Ulucan-Karnak
Department of Medical Biochemistry
Ege University, Institute of Health Sciences
Izmir, Turkey

Sunil Kumar Verma
Faculty of Biotechnology
Institute of Biosciences and Technology, Shri Ramswaroop Memorial University
Barabanki, India

P. William
Department of Information Technology
Sanjivani College of Engineering, Savitribai Phule Pune University
Pune, India

Yanyu Xiong
Department of Electrical and Computer Engineering
University of Illinois at Urbana-Champaign
Champaign, Illinois
Holonyak Micro and Nanotechnology Laboratory
Champaign, Illinois

Pramod Yadav
Department of Biomedical Engineering
Indian Institute of Technology Ropar
Rupnagar, India

Yogeesh Nijalingappa
Department of Mathematics
Government First Grade College
Tumkur, India

1 Nanoparticles for Biomedical Imaging

History to Current Status

Afiya Mubasharah, Nondita Datta, and M Tarik Arafat

1.1 INTRODUCTION

Nanoparticles (NPs) are submicroscopic compounds ranging in size from 1 to 100 nm (Jeyaraj et al., 2019). Based on their attributes, they can be categorized into numerous groupings. The diverse groups include fullerenes, metal NPs, ceramic NPs, and polymeric NPs. NPs have unique physical and chemical properties owing to their nanoscale size and large surface area (Khan et al., 2019). Their optical properties, responsiveness, tenacity, and other characteristics depend on their morphological structure, size, and shape, which impart different hues due to visible spectrum absorption. Due to their characteristics, such as catalysis, imaging, medical applications, energy-based research, and environmental applications, they have numerous industrial and domestic uses.

Nanotechnology is currently being employed in the creation of innovative medical imaging systems that have the potential to benefit the medical field by providing more precise images of cellular processes. Current medical imaging techniques are being adapted to increase nanoscale capabilities and serve as contrast agents for tracing NPs introduced into the body. The necessity for early disease identification and diagnosis continues to drive the development of imaging technology and contrast agents. Developing non-toxic contrast agents with extended circulation period could remove impediments to quick and accurate imaging of tissue microstructures and lesion characterization, which is made possible via nanotechnology (Wallyn et al., 2019).

This chapter addresses nanoparticle-based contrast agents utilized in most biomedical imaging modalities, including X-ray, computed tomography (CT), magnetic resonance imaging (MRI), ultrasound (US), positron emission tomography (PET), and single-photon emission CT (SPECT). In addition, instances of its usefulness in each imaging modality substantiated by research are discussed. The chapter also provides an overview of the different types of NPs used for biomedical imaging, including metal NPs, magnetic NPs, and silica NPs. As contrast agents for imaging, NPs may substantially impact clinical practice. Nanomaterials permit the large-scale manufacturing of things with enhanced functionality at significantly lower costs, greener and cleaner manufacturing methods, and consequently

DOI: 10.1201/9781003432661-1

improving healthcare and reducing the environmental impact of manufacturing (Mashaghi et al., 2013). Overall, nanoparticle-based imaging agents offer unique advantages over traditional imaging techniques and have the potential to revolutionize the field of biomedical imaging.

1.2 HISTORICAL PERSPECTIVE OF USING NANOPARTICLES IN MEDICAL IMAGING

In the 4th century AD, a strange cup known as the "Lycurgus Cup" was made and its unusual optical characteristics baffled many. The cup looked green when light reflected off its surface, but it appeared red when light traveled through it. Scientists could not solve the mystery behind this odd phenomenon for many centuries. Michael Faraday was the first to investigate the metallic NPs in charge of the amazing optical characteristics of the Lycurgus Cup in 1857. He discovered that gold created strange hues when it was broken down to microscopic scales, which explained why the cup's color changed. In 1908, Gustav Mie expanded on Faraday's discoveries and showed that the optical characteristics of gold at microscopic length scales were very different from those of the bulk material. These findings provided light on the origins of the remarkable optical characteristics of the Lycurgus Cup and showed that NPs were used in ancient times long before they were completely known by current science (Bangham and Horne, 1964).

It was Richard Feynman who first proposed the idea of purposefully altering matter at the nanoscale in a 1959 talk at the American Physical Society (Mie, 1908). This lecture detailed a vision for altering and seeing objects on a small scale and how this will change many sectors as well as bring answers to many basic problems, especially in the context of understanding biology. Albert Hibbs is credited with giving the medical industry a glimpse into the future with his idea of "swallowing the surgeon," which would allow for the diagnosis to be made by little robots with access to the body inside to pinpoint the issue and fix it (Mie, 1908). Interestingly, the only papers in 1978 and 1979 that used the word "nanoparticle" also used the word "medicine." The term "nanoparticle" first appeared in scientific literature in 1978. An analysis of the 400 nm gelatin NPs' *in vivo* distribution was published in 1978. Nonetheless, nanoparticle research was being undertaken in the late 1960s and early 1970s using alternative terminology such as "nanopellet" or "nanocapsule" (MG et al. 2015). Surfaces could be imaged with atomic resolution in the early to mid-1980s thanks to the inventions of Binning and Rohrer, the scanning tunneling microscope (Binnig and Rohrer, 1986), and the atomic force microscope (Binnig et al., n.d), all of which were developed at International Business Machines Corporation (IBM). As a result of the imaging of atoms with a scanning tunneling microscope, nanotechnology was first realized in 1990, when xenon atoms were used to notably spell out IBM.

Targeted therapy, also known as "magic bullets," was first proposed in the early 1900s by Nobel Prize winner Paul Ehrlich. These treatments might be directed specifically at a given cellular target without damaging healthy tissue. This idea was then combined with nanotechnology to form the targeted nanoparticle concept.

The term "liposomes" for lipid-based NPs was coined by Alec Bangham in the 1960s while he was attempting to examine lipids using negative staining electron microscopy (EM) (Bangham and Horne, 1964). Over the years, there has been a significant increase in the field of nanoparticle research, with a significant percentage of that growth being devoted to the biomedical industry.

In time, the excitement and potential of nanotechnology would start to permeate the political sphere, leading to the establishment of the Interagency Working Group on Nanotechnology in 1998, which stimulated the launch of the National Nanotechnology Initiative in the United States in 2000. Around the world, similar programs would start, such as Canada's National Institute for Nanotechnology, which was established in 2001. Through multi-institutional collaboration, research, training, and characterization facilities, the National Cancer Institute of the United States' National Institute of Health established an alliance for nanotechnology in cancer in 2004. Many new advancements would be made possible by these financing booms, especially in the area of medicine.

1.3 USES OF NANOPARTICLES IN DIFFERENT IMAGING MODALITIES

Imaging technologies, such as X-ray, CT, MRI, and US, have revolutionized the diagnosis and treatment of disease. These technologies provide noninvasive visualization of the interior structures and functions of the body and facilitate the detection of disease. Many imaging modalities may have limited sensitivity, specificity, and spatial resolution in instances involving tiny lesions or early-stage diseases. NPs have emerged as a potential solution to these limitations. They can be used as contrast agents to enhance the signal-to-noise ratio (SNR) of an imaging modality or as drug transporters to assist the targeted delivery of medicine. Imaging modalities employ a variety of nanoparticle kinds, and researchers are continuously searching for better possibilities (Figure 1.1). This section will investigate the wide variety of NPs used in biological imaging techniques and their potential applications.

1.3.1 Uses of Nanoparticles in X-ray

Since the early stages of the development of X-ray imaging systems, poor native contrast between various soft tissues has led to the employment of exogenous contrast agents. Barium sulfate suspensions, which are mostly used for gastrointestinal (GI) tract imaging, and iodinated small molecules, which are primarily employed in various oral and intravascular applications, are the only two X-ray contrast agents that have received clinical approval. NPs have shown great potential for improving the sensitivity and specificity of X-ray imaging in a range of applications. Thus, the number of studies in this area has rapidly increased because scientists are more inclined to use NPs to enhance the quality of X-ray imaging (Figure 1.2). The ultrasmall size range (5 nm) of X-ray NP contrast agents has been specifically targeted in order to allow for quick clearance from the body, a crucial requirement for clinical approval.

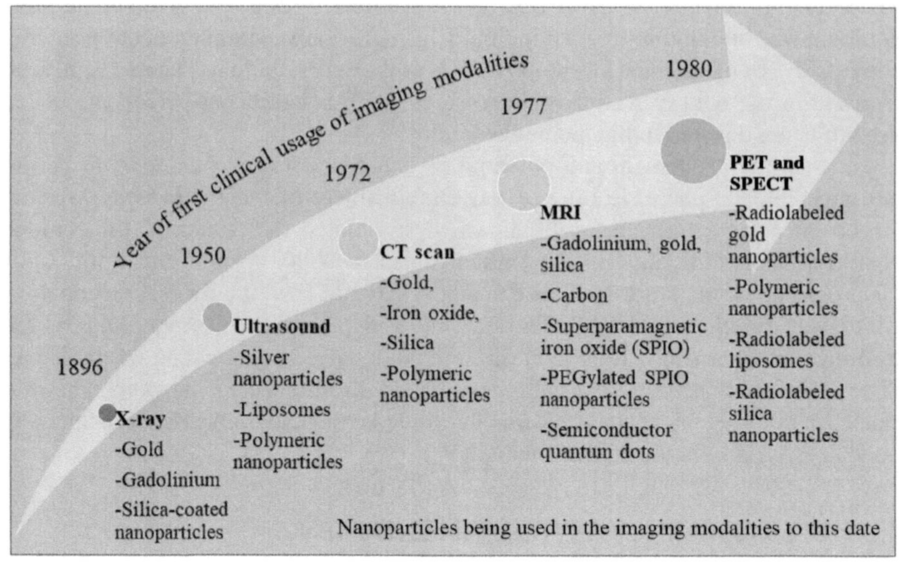

FIGURE 1.1 Evolving imaging modalities and different types of nanoparticle usage in the imaging techniques.

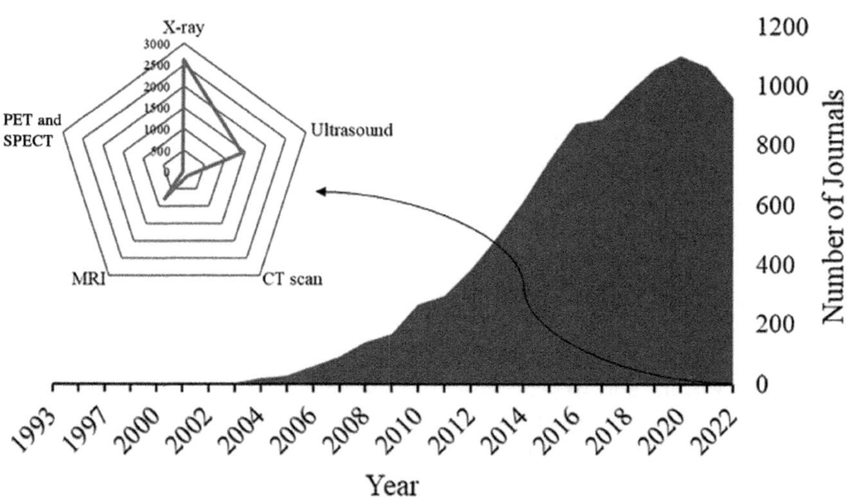

FIGURE 1.2 Research on nanoparticle inclusion in the field of biomedical imaging is increasing rapidly. In 2022, the highest number of studies was done on nanoparticle-based X-ray imaging techniques.

Additionally, they can be targeted passively or actively as contrast agents for disease imaging (Hsu et al., 2018). Furthermore, NP X-ray agents usually have the ability to simultaneously provide diagnostic and therapeutic benefits (Al Zaki et al., 2014).

The ability to provide excellent contrast for sophisticated X-ray imaging modalities such as spectral photon-counting computed tomography (SPCCT) and discrete element method (DEM) is the most crucial property of these NP agents, which have new chemical compositions (Karunamuni and Maidment, 2014).

The use of NPs in X-ray imaging dates back to the early 2000s, when researchers started using gold NPs to enhance the contrast of X-ray images of tumors in mice (Hainfeld et al., 2006). Heavy metal-based NPs are relevant for X-ray imaging applications in numerous preclinical studies; however, because the human body is unable to metabolize or transport these substances, sufficient (if not complete) clearance from the body is needed for their eventual clinical translation. Gold NPs with a core diameter of 1.9 nm were used to show for the first time that X-ray NP agents can be excreted through the kidneys. Since then, many other studies have investigated the use of NPs in X-ray imaging, including the development of techniques using gadolinium-based NPs (Alric et al., 2008; Bulte et al., 2001) and silica-coated gold NPs (Luke et al., 2013) to improve the visualization of cells and blood vessels in living organisms. Because of their better thermodynamic stability, optical characteristics, biocompatibility, and potential for bioconjugation, silica-coated gold NP has become a popular choice for photoacoustic contrast and therapeutic agents (Luke et al., 2013).

More recently, researchers have been exploring the use of NPs as a platform for targeted drug delivery in combination with X-ray imaging. For example, NPs made of iron oxide and calcium phosphate were used to deliver chemotherapy drugs to cancer cells while enhancing the contrast of X-ray images of the tumor (Zhao et al., 2022). In order to address the drawbacks of traditional drug delivery systems, X-ray contrasting NPs have recently attracted increasing interest for usage as carriers for nucleic acids and medicines, such as small interfering ribonucleic acid (siRNA) and chemotherapeutic medications. In a mouse model of Parkinson's disease, for instance, a polymer–AuNP complex was created as a gene-chemical co-delivery vehicle to treat dopaminergic neuron degeneration and enable drug delivery tracking. Upon entering particular sick cells, the complex was broken down in a reactive oxygen species (ROS)-rich milieu, releasing siRNA and curcumin to prevent synucelin-alpha (SNCA) aggregation and downregulate the SNCA gene. The mice's motor function and neurons both recovered as a result of the synergistic therapy. The liberated AuNP would assemble into gold clusters simultaneously and can be detected by the imaging modality.

1.3.2 Application of Different Nanoparticles as CT Scan Contrast Agent

CT scans can dramatically increase diagnostic accuracy, especially through using CT imaging with NPs. Instead of using conventional imaging methods, utilizing NPs as contrast agents can improve the visibility of soft tissue and make it simpler to locate tiny lesions, which contrasts with conventional imaging methods (Mahan and Doiron, 2018). NPs made of a wide variety of materials, such as gold, iron oxide, silica, and polymers, have been the primary focus of research into CT imaging in recent years (Luke et al., 2013).

CT contrast agents are divided into two groups. First, due to its extensive history in clinical imaging, iodine-based contrast agents are included. The second group of contrast agents is those made of metals, which are created into NPs utilizing different metals with high X-ray attenuation coefficients. Tantalum oxide, gold, and zirconium dioxide are some of the metals used in this group (Bonitatibus et al., 2010). The most prevalent example is gold NPs, employed as a contrast agent in CT imaging for translational research (Boote et al., 2010; Chien et al., 2012). Because of their high atomic number and strong X-ray attenuation, gold NPs have recently attracted much attention because they improve contrast in diagnostic imaging (Mahan and Doiron, 2018). Iron oxide NPs are another alternative being researched as a contrast agent in CT imaging. They can be used in MRI because of their influence on T2* relaxation and the ease with which they can be targeted through surface modifications (Shen et al., 2017).

In addition, NPs may be engineered to selectively target particular types of cells or tissues, enabling imaging that is very precise and highly specific in terms of disease-specific biomarkers. For example, Figure 1.3 represents gold NPs that were functionalized with a transmembrane protein named collagen-binding adhesion protein 35 (CNA35) to specifically target myocardial scar, making myocardial infarction visible in CT imaging. Thus, target-specific imaging technique paves the way for brand-new opportunities in illness diagnostics and therapy (Kim et al., 2007).

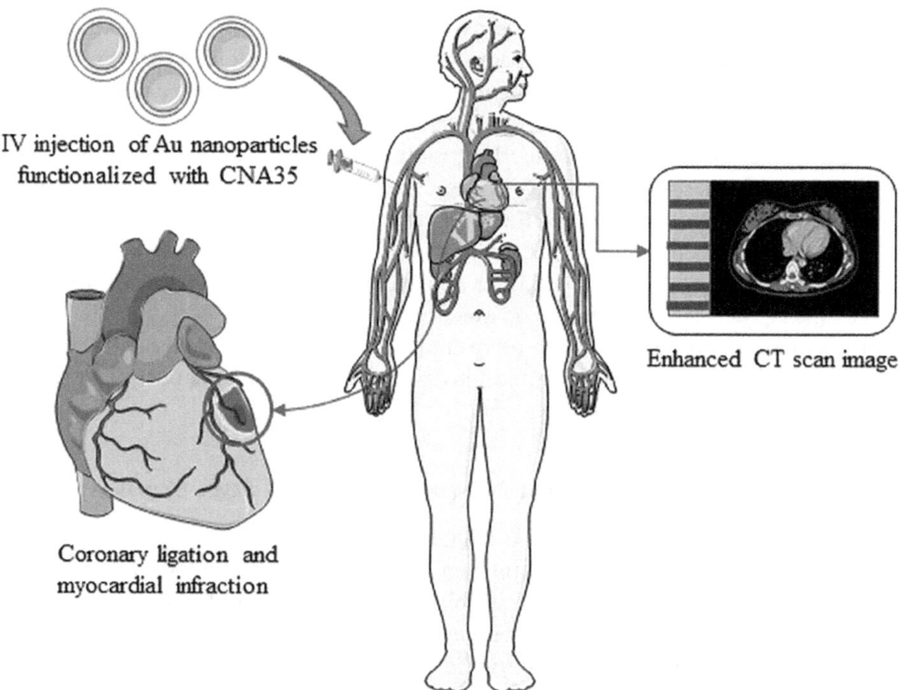

FIGURE 1.3 Molecular imaging NPs used during CT scan.

1.3.3 Application of Different Nanoparticles in MRI Technology

MRI provides clear images of the body's soft tissues. NPs of superparamagnetic iron oxide (SPIO), gadolinium, and carbon are commonly employed in MRI. These NPs can be utilized as contrast agents for better imaging clarity during MRI (Avasthi et al., 2020).

SPIO is a common type of NP employed in MRI. Because their very center is magnetized, they are highly reactive to magnetic fields. These NPs can be employed for imaging because macrophages transport them to the liver and spleen (Lin et al., 2012). SPIO NPs are more porous and remain in tumor tissue for longer, causing them to clump together. For this reason, they can be helpful in cancer imaging.

Iron oxide NPs can be employed as contrast agents in MRI along with SPIO NPs. Coating these NPs in dextran or polyethylene glycol (PEG) can increase their stability and biocompatibility. Iron oxide NPs can be functionalized for the selective imaging of diseased tissue using certain ligands (Shen et al., 2017).

Another type of NP utilized in MRI is gadolinium-based NPs. Because of their high magnetic moment, they are susceptible to magnetic fields. Gadolinium NPs are employed as contrast agents in MRI to enhance image clarity and aid in diagnosing medical conditions (Narmani et al., 2018). The enhanced ability of gadolinium-containing NPs to enter and persist within cells allows for their concentration in tissue and thus can be used in cancer imaging.

The optical and magnetic characteristics of copper NPs make them ideal for imaging applications (Perlman et al., 2015) and are ideal candidates for *in vivo* imaging because of their biocompatibility (Li et al., 2021). Carbon-based NPs used in MRI have a wide surface area and may be chemically functionalized for targeted imaging. They can be employed as contrast agents in MRI by being coated with biocompatible materials like PEG or chitosan (Liu et al., 2022), and ligands can be used to functionalize these NPs to target diseased cells.

Gold NPs are frequently used in biological applications as well because of their distinctive magnetic and optical characteristics. By incorporating gold NPs with other molecules, such as peptides or antibodies, contrast agents for MRI can be created (Şologan et al., 2019). The associated molecule identifies the target tissue and permits an MRI of the gold core.

Semiconductor quantum dots are light-producing NPs that are activated by lasers. Yet, these are also MRI contrast materials. They can be functionalized to increase their selectivity by using particular ligands (Gil et al., 2021). Biocompatible silica NPs have been the focus of various imaging and drug delivery investigations. As contrast agents in MRI, silica NPs containing paramagnetic ions, like manganese or gadolinium, can be utilized (Arkaban et al., 2023; Waters et al., 2022).

1.3.4 Uses of Nanomaterials in PET and SPECT

The molecular imaging method known as PET allows for the *in vivo* observation and tracking of molecular events. Several types of NPs have been researched for use in PET imaging. Due to their high X-ray attenuation and ability to accumulate radionuclides like 64Cu, radiolabeled gold NPs have been utilized to target the tumor's blood

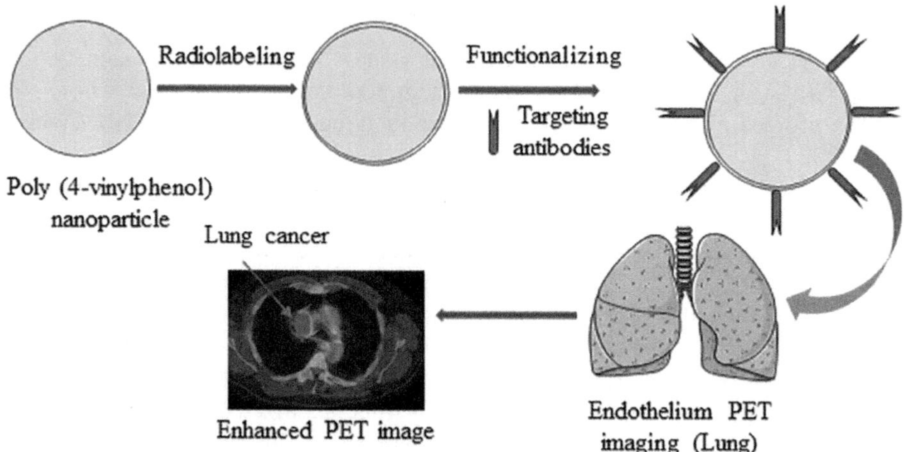

FIGURE 1.4 Nanoparticle usage for PET imaging.

supply (Jain et al., 2012). In a different study, polymeric NPs were used to deliver radiolabeled peptides to tumors for PET imaging (Mitchell et al., 2013). Figure 1.4 shows the usage of poly(4-vinylphenol) for endothelial tumor tissue PET imaging. Active targeting can be done through functionalizing the NPs with specific antibodies that will bind to the targeted site.

Using radiolabeled tracers, the molecular imaging technique known as SPECT can not only identify but also quantify *in vivo* molecular events. A variety of NP kinds have been employed in SPECT imaging research. Because they can concentrate in inflamed tissue, radiolabeled liposomes have been used to treat diseases like atherosclerosis and inflammation. Similar techniques have been used to detect bone metastases in breast cancer patients using radiolabeled silica NPs (Erdogan and Silindir, 2013).

Moreover, the imaging and monitoring of illnesses can be done with NPs. MRI can use magnetic NPs to provide high-resolution images of tissues and organs. By spotting changes in biomarkers or gene expression, NPs can potentially be used to track the development of diseases like cancer.

1.3.5 Uses of Nanomaterials in Ultrasound

US technology is a critical tool for diagnosis and therapy in the medical industry (Hu et al., 2022). As a result of technological advancements, using NPs in ultrasonography has given medical personnel new chances to improve patient outcomes. Employing contrast agents with NPs in ultrasonography is one of their most important applications. Gold and silver NPs, for example, can improve US image contrast and sensitivity, simplifying seeing and identifying disorders (Zeng et al., 2021). Microbubbles with a size between 1 and 8 μm make up the majority of currently marketed ultrasonography contrast agents (Hu et al., 2016), while the majority of US contrast NPs have a size of roughly 200 nm (Hu et al., 2016; Min et al., 2015).

In ultrasonography, NPs can be employed as therapeutic agents and medicine delivery systems. NPs can produce heat or mechanical forces that can destroy cancer cells or dangerous bacteria's cell membranes when exposed to ultrasonic frequencies. Sonodynamic therapy is the procedure and is being researched as a possible cancer and infection treatment. If exposed to ultrasonic vibrations, these particles can encapsulate medications and release them. Drug effectiveness can be increased, and negative effects can be minimized by administering medications specifically to target cells or tissues. Liposomes and polymeric NPs are examples of NPs being researched as potential drug delivery systems in ultrasonography (Li et al., 2020).

1.4 PRESENT-DAY NANOMATERIAL TECHNOLOGY FOR IMAGING APPLICATION

Nanoscale materials can aid in diagnosing, monitoring, and appropriately preventing additional consequences through specific therapeutic nanomedicine applications within medical biophysics. Due to tumor blood vessels' tendency to leak, which allows for their small size to allow for penetration and accumulation inside the tumor, NPs can detect cancer (Martelli and Chow, 2020; Siddique and Chow, 2020). In the past few decades, lanthanide luminescent nanomaterials have significantly advanced the field of biomedicine. This is mainly because rare earth luminescent materials have advantages over other luminescent materials, including stable photochemical properties, minimal photobleaching, and high fluorescence-to-noise ratios (Zhang et al., 2022).

Diagnostic imaging methods like X-ray, CT, US, and MRI are well-established and often employed in biochemical and medical research. However, only relatively late in the course of the disease can these tools analyze changes on the tissue's surface. Contrast and targeting agents based on nanotechnologies can enhance resolution and specificity by highlighting the diseased site at the tissue level. For example, gold NPs with a surface coating of a prostate-specific membrane antigen RNA aptamer had been found to have a higher CT density for prostate cancer cell imaging (D. Kim et al., 2010a). Moreover, MRI has demonstrated that lung cancers can be targeted by SPIO agents with nanoscale surfaces that have been coated with a high-affinity anti-epidermal growth factor receptor (EGFR) antibody (Wang et al., 2017). Gadolinium is a member of the rare earth element family, and thanks to its paramagnetic properties, it can provide brilliant pictures on T1-weighted imaging by shortening the longitudinal relaxation time (T1). The most popular positive MRI contrast material is gadolinium. It has been included in nanosized contrast agents, so they can play more potent functions due to the development of nanotechnology. Ferric oxide-based MRI contrast agents shorten the T2 relaxation time, which causes dark images on T2-weighted imaging and "negative" MRI contrast.

Nowadays, biomedical imaging applications use three different kinds of iron-based NPs. The first group is SPIO, which is where most of the research effort is concentrated. Magnetic iron oxide NPs comprise the second group of magnetic iron oxide nanoparticle (MION). MION has the ability to be a positive contrast agent when it is smaller than 5 nm, known as very small MION (extremely small MION (ES-MION)), and can be utilized as a negative contrast agent when it is greater than 10 nm (Strijkers et al., 2007). The last group is made up of cross-linked dextran-coated monocrystalline iron oxide (Högemann et al., 2002). Biomedical imaging applications that use ferric oxide MRI contrast chemicals include cancer diagnosis, lymph node identification, blood pool imaging, cell tracking, gene monitoring, and molecular imaging (Liu et al., 2011; Rahmer et al., 2013; Vilarino-Varela et al., 2008; Zhang et al., 2009).

Currently used for US imaging are three different NP contrast agents, each with a different composition. The first kind, the most frequently used substance in US contrast agents, uses gas (microbubbles) to produce significant sonic reflections. Some of these microbubbles include carbon dioxide, sulfur hexafluoride, nitrogen, and perfluorocarbon (van Rooij et al., 2015). The process is depicted in Figure 1.5. The micro- and nanobubbles accumulate at the site of tumor through the enhanced permeability and retention (EPR) effect. Though microbubbles can produce strong echo signals, they do not show extravasation due to their large size. Nanobubbles show effective distribution in the tumor tissue as well as extravasation. However, they cannot produce strong echo signals. Thus, a mixture of the particles can be a good choice for US imaging of the tumor tissue.

NPs in PET/SPECT are mainly employed for tumor identification. The EPR effect and particular receptor binding can be used to image tumors (Pressly et al., 2013). For instance, a multimodality platform comprising 64Cu-Fe-RGD-PEG-MNP can be used as an MRI imaging contrast agent, PET contrast agent, and photoacoustic contrast agent (Cheng, 2014).

Imaging resolution is still on a macroscopic scale, despite the widespread use of X-ray, CT, MRI, PET, SPECT, and US to find lesions. Regarding microscopic illness

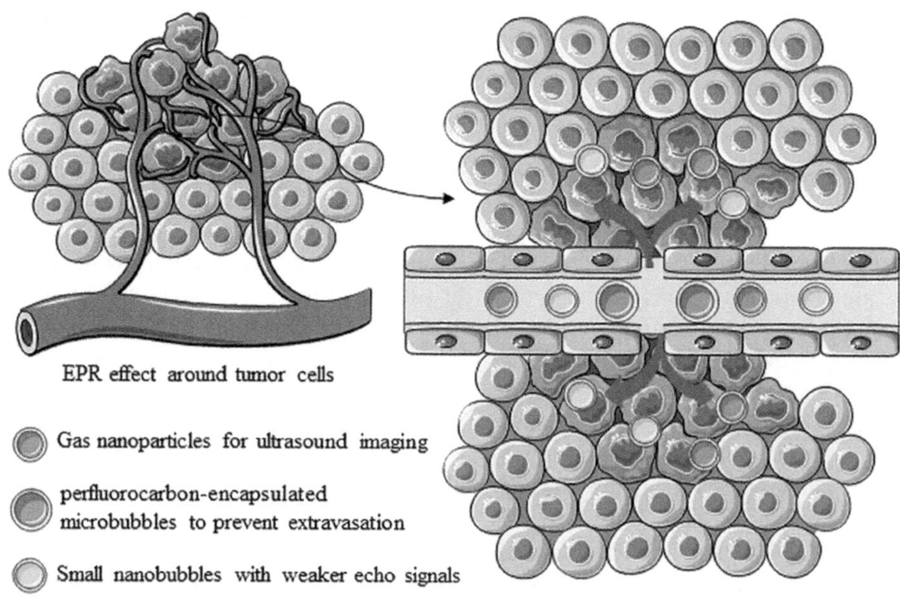

FIGURE 1.5 Ultrasound image enhancement using NPs.

diagnostics, fluorescence imaging technologies, particularly near-infrared (NIRF) imaging, can offer the best spatial resolution. Deeper tissue penetration and fewer non-specific tissue autofluorescences are two advantages NIRF has over visible light. A biocompatible platform with CT and fluorescence imaging capabilities is made up of fluorescein isothiocyanate (FI) linked to PEGylated gold NPs (Qin et al., 2014).

Peptides are one of the numerous substances that have been utilized to give selectivity, nevertheless, because of their long-term stability, target specificity, and speedy bloodstream clearance (Spicer et al., 2018; Zhang et al., 2018). They have been successfully exploited as new nanoprobes. Such peptides can be coupled with a range of imaging modalities thanks to their modular character, which has produced outstanding results in preclinical investigations and animal models. The next generation of bioimaging technology will still need to find a way to get beyond the image resolution constraint.

1.5 COMMERCIALLY AVAILABLE NANOPARTICLE-BASED CONTRAST AGENTS

In biomedical imaging, NP contrast agents are frequently utilized because they provide a number of benefits over conventional contrast agents. These substances, which are made up of tiny particles, are made to improve the contrast of the target tissue or organ during imaging. One of the key benefits of utilizing NP contrast agents is their capacity to target only particular tissues or cells, which can aid in the early diagnosis of sickness or injury. These substances can also be designed to have certain qualities including long circulation durations, biocompatibility, and the capacity to cross biological barriers like the blood–brain barrier (BBB). Table 1.1 lists the commercial contrast agents based on NPs that are utilized in biomedical imaging.

TABLE 1.1
Nanoparticles Contrast Agent Used in Biomedical Imaging

Imaging Modality	Nanoparticle Uses	Advantages	References
X-ray	Lipid-based structures (e.g., liposomes, emulsions, lipoproteins, or micelles), solid core-based NPs (e.g., metal, metal alloy, or metal salt), metal core-based NPs, and gold NPs	Lipid-based contrast agent NPs are generally considered to be biocompatible and have low toxicity, having a longer circulation time Gold NPs are biocompatible and non-toxic and can be engineered to target-specific tissues or cells in the body, which can improve the accuracy and sensitivity of X-ray imaging	Erdogan and Silindir (2013)
CT	Iron oxide NPs, gadolinium chelates, and gold NPs	These NPs can provide the desired circulation times, biodistribution, biological media solubility, and biocompatibility	Kim et al. (2017)

(Continued)

TABLE 1.1 (*Continued*)
Nanoparticles Contrast Agent Used in Biomedical Imaging

Imaging Modality	Nanoparticle Uses	Advantages	References
MRI	Iron oxide NPs or ferrites, and lanthanide metals	Lanthanide metal complexes provide positive contrast in T1-weighted images, while iron oxide NPs or ferrites provide negative contrast in T2-weighted images	Estelrich, Sánchez-Martín and Busquets, (2015); Yang et al. (2022)
US	Nanosized US contrast agents (nUCAs), silica-based NPs, and carbon-based NPs	Nanosized US contrast agents enhanced contrast, increased stability, and a better SNR	Zeng, Du and Chen (2021); Tarighatnia et al. (2022)
PET	Iron oxide NPs and radiolabeled NPs	Iron oxide NPs can increase probe biocompatibility and biodistribution while lengthening the blood half-life to achieve targeted target accumulation and non-toxicity	Forte et al. (2020)
SPECT	Radiolabeled polymer-based NPs and polymeric n-butyl-2-cyanoacrylate (PBCA) NPs	Polymeric n-butyl-2-cyanoacrylate (PBCA) NPs can boost BBB penetration, improve amyloid plaque retention, and accomplish targeted imaging and/or therapy	Erdogan and Silindir (2013)

1.6 FUTURE PROSPECTS

NPs play an essential part in the growth of the commercial sector of biomedical imaging. Undoubtedly, improvements in nanotechnology could lead to several innovations and new opportunities for the global economy. NPs could have a broader range of applications in the future. It is anticipated that nanotechnology will overcome the difficulty of creating high-resolution images. By improving the resolution of existing approaches, nanotechnology can move medical imaging to another level (Bulte and Modo, 2016). With the help of specially engineered nanoconstructs, this method increases the specificity of targeted imaging. Plasmonic nanostructures can demonstrate the field confinement effect, which is advantageous in numerous biological sensing and imaging applications (Kim et al., 2010b). This effect is locally magnified within a sub-diffraction-limited volume. The expanding cooperation between super-resolution imaging and plasmonics, as well as the various ways the two topics mutually benefit one another to advance our understanding of the nanoscale world in their review of the critical role of plasmonic NPs in the development of super-resolution imaging, was discussed in a previous study (Willets et al., 2017). This study shows how plasmonic NPs are being investigated as image contrast agents for super-resolution imaging and super-localization imaging and how these agents offer advantages like high photostability, distance-dependent spectral features, and a high SNR, but make it challenging to pinpoint certain NPs inside a diffraction-limited region. Plasmon-tailored excitation fields can be used to attain sub-diffraction-limited spatial resolution (Willets et al., 2017). The research supported the idea that limited excitation volumes or picture magnification can be produced using localized surface plasmons and surface plasmon polaritons.

The next generation of NPs will create a great revolution in the biomedical imaging field. Due to their intrinsic brightness, graphene quantum dots have been suggested for use in biological imaging. Nitrogen doping was what led to their incredibly active behavior in two-photon fluorescence imaging (Jing Lin et al., 2018). Moreover, graphene–semiconductor quantum dot composites were used in biological imaging (Zang et al., 2017). Lanthanide-doped NPs are becoming more and more common. It is currently being debated on up-converting NPs (Tsang et al., 2015), polymers, lanthanide-doped fluorides, oxides (Dong et al., 2015), and functionalized NPs (Han et al., 2016). Consideration is given to lanthanide ion-doped NPs for both their luminescence and their role in nuclear MRI (NMRI). They can also be employed as multimode contrast agents and infrared-emitting phosphors in luminescence imaging (Dong et al., 2015). By making imaging probes more effective at targeting specific molecules, recent nanobiotechnology developments have sped up molecular imaging development (Kim et al., 2018).

Luminescent bioprobes are one further instance of using nanomaterials for optical imaging and are strong analytical instruments (Mei et al., 2018). For usage in both light microscopy and EM, Shewring et al. (2017) described a small-molecule, multimodal Ir (III)-based probe. These findings support using Ir (III) complexes as probes since they offer superb picture contrast and quality for imaging with both luminescence and EM. Nano-bioimaging is the umbrella term for all of these correlative methods. Various imaging techniques can involve nanotechnology. For example, it was suggested that the fusion of the dynamic synergism of PET with nanotechnology might increase the sensitivity and quantitative nature of PET, which can assist in solving certain essential obstacles in the area (Goel et al., 2017). As a result, NPs can be considered the next generation of contrast agents and have certain extra qualities that produce supplemental functions, as for theragnostic applications, to get over the constraints of probes now used in the clinic. Notwithstanding concerns regarding what would happen if people consumed them, certain NP-based materials have been employed in humans, such as MRI with superparamagnetic iron oxide nanoparticles (SPIONs) as contrast agents. Because of their enormous potential as excellent probes due to their adaptability, NPs are now increasingly in demand for applications using human models in addition to having been found to be appropriate for investigations on animals.

Lesion characterization and quick, accurate imaging of tissue microstructures in biomedical imaging still present obstacles. However, it could be overcome by creating benign contrast agents with extended circulation time. NPs have shown targeting capability, enhanced signal intensity, and extended circulation duration both *in vivo* and *in vitro* in animal disease models, especially for cancer diagnostics and therapy. Single imaging modalities have improved in power thanks to nanotechnology, while multimodality imaging has shown substantial potential. It is still unclear exactly how harmful NPs become after metabolism. Depending on the underlying physiochemical characteristics of NPs, some components may cause harm to healthy cells. The freedom state, for instance, claims that rare earth metals from quantum dots are harmful. To fully comprehend the behavior of NPs in the future, more study is necessary, even though encapsulation and surface labeling have been investigated to limit harmful effects (Nastassja Lewinski et al., 2008). Currently, most nanocontrast compounds are still in the experimental stage. Clinical studies using nanocontrast materials are quite rare, despite the remarkable progress that has been accomplished. Improving targeted specificity while reducing toxicity should be the primary goal of ongoing NP research. Also, it is crucial to comprehend the precise pharmacokinetic profile of these drugs in humans and to increase translational potential by using suitable animal models. To produce NPs for biomedical imaging effectively, interdisciplinary teams of pharmacists, physicists, biologists, chemists, engineers, and physicians will be required. In spite of these challenges, NPs have great potential as innovative new imaging agents for a variety of clinical applications.

1.7 CONCLUSION

Diagnostic techniques, such as X-ray, ultrasonography, PET, SPECT, CT, and MRI, have become standard clinical tools by the start of the 21st century. Developing techniques like optical tomography and photoacoustic and fluorescence imaging have also started to appear in clinical settings. The development of hardware, new and quicker algorithms, complex picture acquisition, and improved processing software to boost diagnostic procedures and further increase resolution also evolved. Large-scale clinical studies with NPs have been completed after decades of study, which included challenges, such as limited *in vivo* stability, liver blockage, batch-to-batch variance, and valid issues that needed testing of each NP component. Recent advances in analytical chemistry, chemistry, molecular imaging, material science, cell biology, genome decoding, unraveling molecular pathways, and identifying various disease-specific biomarkers have led to a new generation of high-affinity NP-based contrast agents. The Food and Drug Administration (FDA) and other international regulatory organizations have approved several of these imaging agents. With the endorsement of regulatory organizations, we set out on a future full of opportunities where NP-based diagnostics will continue to alter lives and transform healthcare.

ACKNOWLEDGMENT

The project was supported by the Research and Innovation Centre for Science and Engineering (RISE), Bangladesh University of Engineering and Technology (BUET), under grant no. EU/RISE/2022-01-020/Centre-01.

The figures were partly generated using Servier Medical Art, provided by Servier, licensed under a Creative Commons Attribution 3.0 Unported license.

REFERENCES

AlZaki, A., Joh, D., Cheng, Z., De Barros, A.L.B., Kao, G., Dorsey, J., Tsourkas, A., 2014. Gold-loaded polymeric micelles for computed tomography-guided radiation therapy treatment and radiosensitization. *ACS Nano* 8(1), 104–112. https://doi.org/10.1021/nn405701q

Alric, C., Taleb, J., Le Duc, G., Mandon, C., Billotey, C., Le Meur-Herland, A., Brochard, T., Vocanson, F., Janier, M., Perriat, P., Roux, S., Tillement, O., 2008. Gadolinium chelate coated gold nanoparticles as contrast agents for both X-ray computed tomography and magnetic resonance imaging. *J Am Chem Soc* 130, 5908–5915. https://doi.org/10.1021/ja078176p

Arkaban, H., Jaberi, J., Bahramifar, A., Zolfaghari Emameh, R., Farnoosh, G., Arkaban, M., Taheri, R.A., 2023. Fabrication of Fe(III)-doped mesoporous silica nanoparticles as biocompatible and biodegradable theranostic system for Remdesivir delivery and MRI contrast agent. *Inorg Chem Commun* 150, 110398. https://doi.org/https://doi.org/10.1016/j.inoche.2023.110398

Avasthi, A., Caro, C., Pozo-Torres, E., Leal, M.P., García-Martín, M.L., 2020. Magnetic Nanoparticles as MRI Contrast Agents. *Top Curr Chem* 378, 40. https://doi.org/10.1007/s41061-020-00302-w

Bangham, A.D., Horne, R.W., 1964. Negative staining of phospholipids and their structural modification by surface-active agents as observed in the electron microscope. *J. Mol Biol* 8, 660–668. https://doi.org/10.1016/S0022-2836(64)80115-7

Binnig, G. and Rohrer, H., 1987. Scanning tunneling microscopy—from birth to adolescence. *Rev Mod Phys* 59(3), 615.

Binnig, G., Quate, C.F., Gerber, C., 1986. Atomic force microscope. *Phys Rev Lett* 56(9), 930.

Bonitatibus, P.J., Torres, A.S., Goddard, G.D., Fitzgerald, P.F., Kulkarni, A.M., 2010. Synthesis, characterization, and computed tomography imaging of a tantalum oxide nanoparticle imaging agent. *Chem Commun* 46. https://doi.org/10.1039/c0cc03302b

Boote, E., Fent, G., Kattumuri, V., Casteel, S., Katti, K., Chanda, N., Kannan, R., Katti, K., Churchill, R., 2010. Gold nanoparticle contrast in a phantom and juvenile swine. Models for molecular imaging of human organs using X-ray computed tomography. *Acad Radiol* 17. https://doi.org/10.1016/j.acra.2010.01.006

Bulte, J.W.M., Douglas, T., Witwer, B., Zhang, S.-C., Strable, E., Lewis, B.K., Zywicke, H., Miller, B., van Gelderen, P., Moskowitz, B.M., Duncan, I.D., Frank, J.A., 2001. Magnetodendrimers allow endosomal magnetic labeling and in vivo tracking of stem cells. *Nat Biotechnol* 19, 1141–1147. https://doi.org/10.1038/nbt1201-1141

Bulte, J.W.M., Modo, M.M.J., 2016. Nanoparticles as a technology platform for biomedical imaging, In: *Design and Applications of Nanoparticles in Biomedical Imaging*. https://doi.org/10.1007/978-3-319-42169-8_1

Cheng, K, 2014. Transferring biomarker into molecular probe: Melanin nanoparticle as a naturally active platform for multimodality imaging. *J Am Chem Soc* 136(43), 15185–15194.

Chien, C.C., Chen, H.H., Lai, S.F., Hwu, Y., Petibois, C., Yang, C.S., Chu, Y., Margaritondo, G., 2012. X-ray imaging of tumor growth in live mice by detecting gold-nanoparticle-loaded cells. *Sci Rep* 2. https://doi.org/10.1038/srep00610

Dong, H., Du, S.R., Zheng, X.Y., Lyu, G.M., Sun, L.D., Li, L.D., Zhang, P.Z., Zhang, C., Yan, C.H., 2015. Lanthanide nanoparticles: From design toward bioimaging and therapy. *Chem Rev*. https://doi.org/10.1021/acs.chemrev.5b00091

Erdogan, S., Silindir, M., 2013. Nanoparticulate Contrast Agents for CT, SPECT and PET Imaging, In: *Handbook of Nanobiomedical Research, Frontiers in Nanobiomedical Research*. World Scientific, pp. 47–76. https://doi.org/10.1142/9789814520652_0037

Estelrich, J., Sánchez-Martín, M.J., Busquets, M.A., 2015. Nanoparticles in magnetic resonance imaging: From simple to dual contrast agents. *Int J Nanomed* 10, 1727–1741. https://doi.org/10.2147/IJN.S76501

Forte, E., Fiorenza, D., Torino, E., Costagliola di Polidoro, A., Cavaliere, C., Netti, P.A., Salvatore, M., Aiello, M., 2020. Radiolabeled PET/MRI nanoparticles for tumor imaging', *J Clin Med* 9(1). https://doi.org/10.3390/jcm9010089

Gil, H.M., Price, T.W., Chelani, K., Bouillard, J.S.G., Calaminus, S.D.J., Stasiuk, G.J., 2021. NIR-quantum dots in biomedical imaging and their future. *iScience* 24, 102189. https://doi.org/10.1016/J.ISCI.2021.102189

Goel, S., England, C.G., Chen, F., Cai, W., 2017. Positron emission tomography and nanotechnology: A dynamic duo for cancer theranostics. *Adv Drug Deliv Rev*. https://doi.org/10.1016/j.addr.2016.08.001

Hainfeld, J.F., Slatkin, D.N., Focella, T.M., Smilowitz, H.M., 2006. Gold nanoparticles: A new X-ray contrast agent. *Br J Radiol* 79, 248–253. https://doi.org/10.1259/bjr/13169882

Han, G.M., Li, H., Huang, X.X., Kong, D.M., 2016. Simple synthesis of carboxyl-functionalized upconversion nanoparticles for biosensing and bioimaging applications. *Talanta* 147. https://doi.org/10.1016/j.talanta.2015.09.059

Högemann, D., Ntziachristos, V., Josephson, L., Weissleder, R., 2002. High throughput magnetic resonance imaging for evaluating targeted nanoparticle probes. *Bioconjug Chem* 13. https://doi.org/10.1021/bc015549h

Hsu, J.C., Naha, P.C., Lau, K.C., Chhour, P., Hastings, R., Moon, B.F., Stein, J.M., Witschey, W.R., McDonald, E.S., Maidment, A.D., Cormode, D.P., 2018. An all-in-one nanoparticle (AION) contrast agent for breast cancer screening with DEM-CT-MRI-NIRF imaging. *Nanoscale* 10(36), 17236–17248. https://doi.org/10.1039/c8nr03741h

Hu, C., Hou, B., Xie, S., 2022. Application of nanosonosensitizer materials in cancer sono-dynamic therapy. *RSC Adv* 12, 22722–22747. https://doi.org/10.1039/D2RA03786F

Hu, Y., Wang, Y., Jiang, J., Han, B., Zhang, S., Li, K., Ge, S., Liu, Y., 2016. Preparation and characterization of novel perfluorooctyl bromide nanoparticle as ultrasound contrast agent via layer-by-layer self-assembly for folate-receptor-mediated tumor imaging. *Biomed Res Int* 2016. https://doi.org/10.1155/2016/6381464

Jain, S., Hirst, D.G., O'Sullivan, J.M., 2012. Gold nanoparticles as novel agents for cancer therapy. *Br J Radiol* 85, 101–113. https://doi.org/10.1259/bjr/59448833

Jeyaraj, M., Gurunathan, S., Qasim, M., Kang, M.-H., Kim, J.-H., 2019. A comprehensive review on the synthesis, characterization, and biomedical application of platinum nanoparticles. *Nanomaterials* 9. https://doi.org/10.3390/nano9121719

Karunamuni, R., Maidment, A.D.A., 2014. Search for novel contrast materials in dual-energy x-ray breast imaging using theoretical modeling of contrast-to-noise ratio. *Phys Med Biol* 59(15), 4311–4324. https://doi.org/10.1088/0031-9155/59/15/4311

Khan, I., Saeed, K., Khan, I., 2019. Nanoparticles: Properties, applications and toxicities. *Arab J Chem* 12, 908–931. https://doi.org/10.1016/J.ARABJC.2017.05.011

Kim, D., Jeong, Y.Y., Jon, S., 2010a. A drug-loaded aptamer - gold nanoparticle bioconjugate for combined ct imaging and therapy of prostate cancer. *ACS Nano* 4. https://doi.org/10.1021/nn901877h

Kim, D., Kim, J., Park, Y. Il, Lee, N., Hyeon, T., 2018. Recent development of inorganic nanoparticles for biomedical imaging. *ACS Cent Sci* 4. https://doi.org/10.1021/acscentsci.7b00574

Kim, D., Park, S., Lee, J.H., Jeong, Y.Y., Jon, S., 2007. Antibiofouling polymer-coated gold nanoparticles as a contrast agent for in vivo X-ray computed tomography imaging. *J Am Chem Soc* 129, 7661–7665. https://doi.org/10.1021/ja071471p

Kim, J., Chhour, P., Hsu, J., Litt, H.I., Ferrari, V.A., Popovtzer, R., Cormode, D.P., 2017. Use of nanoparticle contrast agents for cell tracking with computed tomography. *Bioconjug Chem* 28(6), 1581–1597. https://doi.org/10.1021/acs.bioconjchem.7b00194

Kim, K., Oh, Y., Lee, W., Kim, D., 2010b. Plasmonics-based spatially activated light microscopy for super-resolution imaging of molecular fluorescence. *Opt Lett* 35. https://doi.org/10.1364/ol.35.003501

Krukemeyer, M.G., Krenn, V., Huebner, F., Wagner, W., Resch, R., 2015. History and possible uses of nanomedicine based on nanoparticles and nanotechnological progress. *J Nanomed Nanotechnol* 6, 336. https://doi.org/10.4172/2157-7439.1000336

Lewinski, N., Colvin, V., Drezek, R., 2008. Cytotoxicity of nanoparticles. *Small* 4(1), 26–49.

Li, L., Guan, Y., Xiong, H., Deng, T., Ji, Q., Xu, Z., Kang, Y., Pang, J., 2020. Fundamentals and applications of nanoparticles for ultrasound-based imaging and therapy. *Nano Select* 1, 263–284. https://doi.org/https://doi.org/10.1002/nano.202000035

Li, Y., Ye, F., Zhang, S., Ni, W., Wen, L., Qin, H., 2021. Carbon-coated magnetic nanoparticle dedicated to MRI/photoacoustic imaging of tumor in living mice. *Front Bioeng Biotechnol* 9, 800744.

Lin, C., Cai, S., Feng, J., 2012. Positive contrast imaging of SPIO nanoparticles. *J Nanomater* 2012, 734842. https://doi.org/10.1155/2012/734842

Lin, J., Huang, Y., Huang, P., 2018. Graphene-based nanomaterials in bioimaging. Sarmento, B, Neves JD (Eds) In: *Biomedical Applications of Functionalized Nanomaterials*, pp. 247–287, Elsevier, Netharlands.

Liu, G., Wang, Z., Lu, J., Xia, C., Gao, F., Gong, Q., Song, B., Zhao, X., Shuai, X., Chen, X., Ai, H., Gu, Z., 2011. Low molecular weight alkyl-polycation wrapped magnetite nanoparticle clusters as MRI probes for stem cell labeling and in vivo imaging. *Biomaterials* 32. https://doi.org/10.1016/j.biomaterials.2010.08.099

Liu, Z., Wang, K., Wang, T., Wang, Y., Ge, Y., 2022. Copper nanoparticles supported on polyethylene glycol-modified magnetic Fe3O4 nanoparticles: Its anti-human gastric cancer investigation. *Arab J Chem* 15, 103523. https://doi.org/https://doi.org/10.1016/j.arabjc.2021.103523

Luke, G.P., Bashyam, A., Homan, K.A., Makhija, S., Chen, Y.-S., Emelianov, S.Y., 2013. Silica-coated gold nanoplates as stable photoacoustic contrast agents for sentinel lymph node imaging. *Nanotechnology* 24, 455101. https://doi.org/10.1088/0957-4484/24/45/455101

Mahan, M.M., Doiron, A.L., 2018. Gold nanoparticles as X-ray, CT, and multimodal imaging contrast agents: Formulation, targeting, and methodology. *J Nanomater* 2018, 5837276. https://doi.org/10.1155/2018/5837276

Martelli, S., Chow, J.C.L., 2020. Dose enhancement for the flattening-filter-free and flattening-filter photon beams in nanoparticle-enhanced radiotherapy: A Monte Carlo phantom study. *Nanomaterials* 10. https://doi.org/10.3390/nano10040637

Mashaghi, S., Jadidi, T., Koenderink, G., Mashaghi, A., 2013. Lipid nanotechnology. *Int J Mol Sci* 14, 4242–4282. https://doi.org/10.3390/ijms14024242

Mei, J., Huang, Y., Tian, H., 2018. Progress and trends in AIE-based bioprobes: A brief overview. *ACS Appl Mater Interfaces*. https://doi.org/10.1021/acsami.7b14343

Mie, G., 1908. Beiträge zur Optik trüber Medien, speziell kolloidaler Metallösungen. *Ann Phys* 330, 377–445. https://doi.org/10.1002/andp.19083300302

Min, K.H., Min, H.S., Lee, H.J., Park, D.J., Yhee, J.Y., Kim, K., Kwon, I.C., Jeong, S.Y., Silvestre, O.F., Chen, X., Hwang, Y.S., Kim, E.C., Lee, S.C., 2015. PH-controlled gas-generating mineralized nanoparticles: A theranostic agent for ultrasound imaging and therapy of cancers. *ACS Nano* 9. https://doi.org/10.1021/nn506210a

Mitchell, N., Kalber, T.L., Cooper, M.S., Sunassee, K., Chalker, S.L., Shaw, K.P., Ordidge, K.L., Badar, A., Janes, S.M., Blower, P.J., Lythgoe, M.F., Hailes, H.C., Tabor, A.B., 2013. Incorporation of paramagnetic, fluorescent and PET/SPECT contrast agents into liposomes for multimodal imaging. *Biomaterials* 34, 1179–1192. https://doi.org/10.1016/j.biomaterials.2012.09.070

Narmani, A., Farhood, B., Haghi-Aminjan, H., Mortezazadeh, T., Aliasgharzadeh, A., Mohseni, M., Najafi, M., Abbasi, H., 2018. Gadolinium nanoparticles as diagnostic and therapeutic agents: Their delivery systems in magnetic resonance imaging and neutron capture therapy. *J Drug Deliv Sci Technol* 44, 457–466. https://doi.org/https://doi.org/10.1016/j.jddst.2018.01.011

Perlman, O., Weitz, I.S., Azhari, H., 2015. Copper oxide nanoparticles as contrast agents for MRI and ultrasound dual-modality imaging. *Phys Med Biol* 60, 5767–5783. https://doi.org/10.1088/0031-9155/60/15/5767

Pressly, E.D., Pierce, R.A., Connal, L.A., Hawker, C.J., Liu, Y., 2013. Nanoparticle PET/CT imaging of natriuretic peptide clearance receptor in prostate cancer. *Bioconjug Chem* 24. https://doi.org/10.1021/bc300473x

Qin, J., Peng, C., Zhao, B., Ye, K., Yuan, F., Peng, Z., Yang, X., Huang, L., Jiang, M., Zhao, Q. and Tang, G., 2014. Noninvasive detection of macrophages in atherosclerotic lesions by computed tomography enhanced with PEGylated gold nanoparticles. *Int J Nanomed* 9, 5575–5590.

Rahmer, J., Antonelli, A., Sfara, C., Tiemann, B., Gleich, B., Magnani, M., Weizenecker, J., Borgert, J., 2013. Nanoparticle encapsulation in red blood cells enables blood-pool magnetic particle imaging hours after injection. *Phys Med Biol* 58. https://doi.org/10.1088/0031-9155/58/12/3965

Shen, Z., Wu, A., Chen, X., 2017. Iron oxide nanoparticle based contrast agents for magnetic resonance imaging. *Mol Pharm* 14, 1352–1364. https://doi.org/10.1021/acs.molpharmaceut.6b00839

Shewring, J.R., Cankut, A.J., McKenzie, L.K., Crowston, B.J., Botchway, S.W., Weinstein, J.A., Edwards, E., Ward, M.D., 2017. Multimodal probes: Superresolution and transmission electron microscopy imaging of mitochondria, and oxygen mapping of cells, using small-molecule Ir(III) luminescent complexes. *Inorg Chem* 56. https://doi.org/10.1021/acs.inorgchem.7b02633

Siddique, S., Chow, J.C.L., 2020. Application of nanomaterials in biomedical imaging and cancer therapy. *Nanomaterials*. https://doi.org/10.3390/nano10091700

Şologan, M., Padelli, F., Giachetti, I., Aquino, D., Boccalon, M., Adami, G., Pengo, P., Pasquato, L., 2019. Functionalized gold nanoparticles as contrast agents for proton and dual proton/fluorine MRI. *Nanomaterials* 9. https://doi.org/10.3390/nano9060879

Spicer, C.D., Jumeaux, C., Gupta, B., Stevens, M.M., 2018. Peptide and protein nanoparticle conjugates: Versatile platforms for biomedical applications. *Chem Soc Rev*. https://doi.org/10.1039/c7cs00877e

Strijkers, G.J., M Mulder, W.J., F van Tilborg, G.A. and Nicolay, K., 2007. MRI contrast agents: Current status and future perspectives. *Anti-Cancer Agents Med Chem* 7(3), 291–305.

Tarighatnia, A., Fouladi, M.R., Nader, N.D., Aghanejad, A., Ghadiri, H., 2022. Recent trends of contrast agents in ultrasound imaging: A review of the classifications and applications. *Mater Adv* 3, 3726–3741. https://doi.org/10.1039/d1ma00969a

Tsang, M.K., Chan, C.F., Wong, K.L., Hao, J., 2015. Comparative studies of upconversion luminescence characteristics and cell bioimaging based on one-step synthesized upconversion nanoparticles capped with different functional groups. *J Lumin* 157. https://doi.org/10.1016/j.jlumin.2014.08.057

vanRooij, T., Daeichin, V., Skachkov, I., de Jong, N., Kooiman, K., 2015. Targeted ultrasound contrast agents for ultrasound molecular imaging and therapy. *Int J Hyperth*, 31, 90–106.

Vilarino-Varela, M.J., Taylor, A., Rockall, A.G., Reznek, R.H., Powell, M.E.B., 2008. A verification study of proposed pelvic lymph node localisation guidelines using nanoparticle-enhanced magnetic resonance imaging. *Radiother Oncol* 89. https://doi.org/10.1016/j.radonc.2008.07.023

Wallyn, J., Anton, N., Akram, S., Vandamme, T.F., 2019. Biomedical imaging: Principles, technologies, clinical aspects, contrast agents, limitations and future trends in nanomedicines. *Pharm Res* 36, 78. https://doi.org/10.1007/s11095-019-2608-5

Wang, Z., Qiao, R., Tang, N., Lu, Z., Wang, H., Zhang, Z., Xue, X., Huang, Z., Zhang, S., Zhang, G., Li, Y., 2017. Active targeting theranostic iron oxide nanoparticles for MRI and magnetic resonance-guided focused ultrasound ablation of lung cancer. *Biomaterials* 127. https://doi.org/10.1016/j.biomaterials.2017.02.037

Waters, M., Hopf, J., Tam, E., Wallace, S., Chang, J., Bennett, Z., Aquino, H., Roeder, R.K., Helquist, P., Stack, M.S., Nallathamby, P.D., 2022. Biocompatible, multi-mode, fluorescent, T_2 MRI contrast magnetoelectric-silica nanoparticles (MagSiNs), for on-demand doxorubicin delivery to metastatic cancer cells. *Pharmaceuticals* 15. https://doi.org/10.3390/ph15101216

Willets, K.A., Wilson, A.J., Sundaresan, V., Joshi, P.B., 2017. Super-resolution imaging and plasmonics. *Chem Rev*. https://doi.org/10.1021/acs.chemrev.6b00547

Yang, H., Wang, H., Wen, C., Bai, S., Wei, P., Xu, B., Xu, Y., Liang, C., Zhang, Y., Zhang, G., Wen, H., 2022. Effects of iron oxide nanoparticles as *T*2-MRI contrast agents on reproductive system in male mice. *J Nanobiotechnol* 20(1), 1–18. https://doi.org/10.1186/s12951-022-01291-2

Zang, Z., Zeng, X., Wang, M., Hu, W., Liu, C., Tang, X., 2017. Tunable photoluminescence of water-soluble AgInZnS–graphene oxide (GO) nanocomposites and their application in-vivo bioimaging. *Sens Actuators B Chem* 252. https://doi.org/10.1016/j.snb.2017.07.144

Zeng, F., Du, M., Chen, Z., 2021. Nanosized contrast agents in ultrasound molecular imaging. *Front Bioeng Biotechnol* 9(November), 1–7. https://doi.org/10.3389/fbioe.2021.758084

Zhang, P., Cui, Y., Anderson, C.F., Zhang, C., Li, Y., Wang, R., Cui, H., 2018. Peptide-based nanoprobes for molecular imaging and disease diagnostics. *Chem Soc Rev*. https://doi.org/10.1039/c7cs00793k

Zhang, Q., O'brien, S., Grimm, J., 2022. Biomedical applications of lanthanide nanomaterials, for imaging, sensing and therapy. *Nanotheranostics*. https://doi.org/10.7150/NTNO.65530

Zhang, Z., Mascheri, N., Dharmakumar, R., Fan, Z., Paunesku, T., Woloschak, G., Li, D., 2009. Superparamagnetic iron oxide nanoparticle-labeled cells as an effective vehicle for tracking the GFP gene marker using magnetic resonance imaging. *Cytotherapy* 11. https://doi.org/10.1080/14653240802420243

Zhao, J.-F., Zou, F.-L., Zhu, J.-F., Huang, C., Bu, F.-Q., Zhu, Z.-M., Yuan, R.-F., 2022. Nano-drug delivery system for pancreatic cancer: A visualization and bibliometric analysis. *Front Pharmacol* 13. https://doi.org/10.3389/fphar.2022.1025618

2 Characterization of Nanomaterials for Use in Medical Imaging

Manas Thakur, Aaishiki Saha*, Sampurna Mukherjee, S. Najes Riaz, Dipayan Roy, Kalyan Kumar Chattopadhyay, and Sourav Sarkar*

2.1 MNPS IN BIOMEDICAL APPLICATIONS

2.1.1 Introduction

The fusion of molecular biology, nanotechnology, and medicine has produced nanobiotechnology, a modern growing field of study that offers exciting opportunities to discover novel materials, processes, and phenomena. MNPs have received a lot of attention recently in the fields of medicine, pharmacology, and drug delivery systems. Using metallic particles heated by a magnetic field, Gilchrist et al. first treated lymphatic nodes and metastases in the 1950s [1]. Following that, MNPs were rapidly introduced in the fields of medication delivery and enzyme immobilization [2] and boosted the development of numerous new biotechnology applications. A variety of metals (pure or alloys) and metal oxides, which have magnetic properties, can be used to create MNPs. Due to their high spin magnetic moments, and low toxicity, MNPs are highly valued and investigated in the field of Biomedical sciences [3] (Figure 2.1).

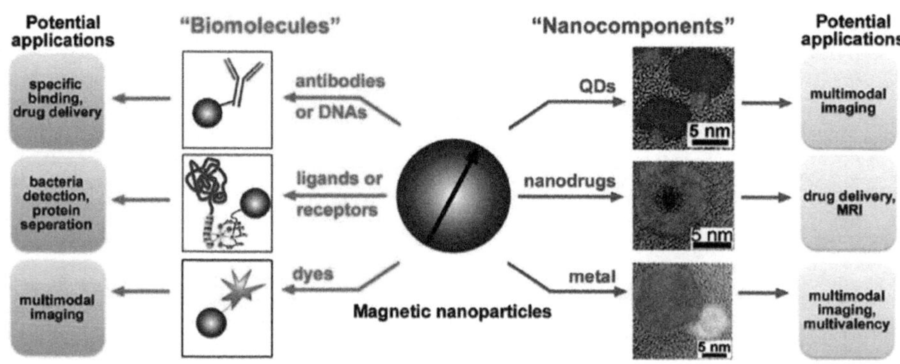

FIGURE 2.1 The schematic diagram of two usual methods of developing multifunctional MNPs and their prospective applications (reproduced with permission from [3]).

DOI: 10.1201/9781003432661-2

Though there are many MNPs, Iron oxide nanoparticles (IONPs) have received a lot of attention from researchers since they do not maintain any magnetization when the magnetic field is pulled out. Due to their ease of functionalization with polymers and other materials, IONPs (Fe_3O_4 and Fe_2O_3) have really been widely used for in vitro diagnosis [3]. Apart from iron oxide magnetic nanoparticles (IOMNPs), chitosan MNPs are highly considered for biomedical applications because of their unique courier type and non-toxic properties.

2.1.2 IOMNPs

2.1.2.1 Synthesis

Iron salt precipitation occurs when sodium nitrate/sodium hydroxide or ammonia is present, which results in the synthesis of IOMNPs. MNPs are modified using diluted sodium citrate, nitric acid, sodium alginate, or chemical stabilizers like polyvinyl pyrrolidone [4]. A blackish-brown precipitate will be obtained which is rinsed three times with de-ionized water and dried at room temperature [5].

From organo-metallic substances, including carbonyls, metal fatty acid salts, and metal acetylacetonates, thermal decomposition facilitates the synthesis of iron oxide nanoparticles (IONPs). The thermal decomposition process has been employed over the years to create metal oxide IONPs using two distinct approaches. Carbonyl metals are first thermally decayed, and then, the oxidation step is completed at a high temperature with the assistance of air or an oxidant [4–6].

For the synthesis of size-specific IONP, the hydrothermal method is used, and the reaction temperature ranges from 180°C to 220°C. The powder can be recovered immediately from the solution using the hydrothermal method, and the shape and size of the particle can be controlled by employing different precursor chemicals [6].

2.1.2.2 Characterization

From Figure 2.2, it can be seen that magnetic IONPs are made of mostly three layers:

1. The top layer, which includes functionalized proteins, doped metals, polymers, antibodies, tiny molecules, etc.,
2. The chemical substances in the shell layer differ from what makes up the primary component, and
3. The key chemical element, which is typically referred to as nanoparticles, is found in the core layer.

They have to be persistent in biological fluid mediums, biodegradable, biocompatible, and excretable from the body with low toxicity [7].

2.1.2.3 Applications

Due to their magnetic and plasmonic capabilities, IONPs are used for magnet-mediated targeted delivery, hyperthermia, and biological imaging of the needed biomolecules. IONPs serve as FDA-approved nanomedicine for a variety of diseases [5]. Moreover, they perform the function of contrasting agents *in vivo*. Nowadays,

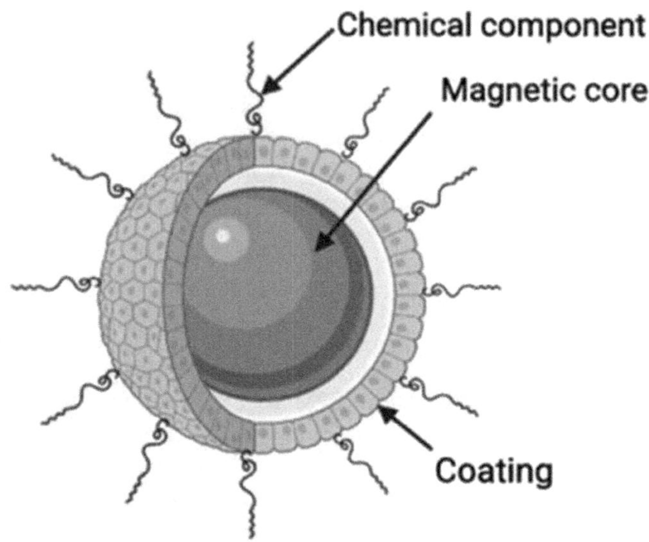

FIGURE 2.2 Different layers of IONPs (reproduced with permission from [5]).

photothermal therapy (PTT) and magnetic fluid hyperthermia (MFH) are the most performed techniques in cancer therapy. Basically, the working principle of MFH is dependent upon an external magnetic field controlling the MNPs in different directions; on the other hand, PTT is based on photo-absorbent agents absorbing light and converting it into heat [3,8]. Chan Ming-Hsien et al. produced an MFH process typically based on kaolinite-modified FePt nanoparticles with cetyltrimethylammonium bromide (CTAB) as visualized in Figure 2.3a. The nanocomposite showed potential for carrying the chemotherapeutic drug doxorubicin, and it might be helpful for magnetic resonance imaging (MRI)-guided targeting (Figure 2.3b) [9].

In addition to serving as contrasting substances in MRI, magnetic IONPs can be used to track a particular biomarker; cell; or organ in conditions, including stroke, cancer, aortic dysfunction, or brain dysfunction. Therefore, due to their complementary abilities for bioimaging and biomarker tracking, magnetic IONPs are seen as having several uses [4,5].

2.1.3 Chitosan MNPs

2.1.3.1 Synthesis

To synthesize chitosan MNPs with the ideal size, shape, stability, and biocompatibility, various methods of synthesis have been utilized. Compared to other approaches, the sol-gel process is more popular and has more industrial applications [10]. This technique can industrially create excellent nanoparticles of identical size because of their special qualities and traits. With this technique, metal and ceramic nanomaterials can be produced at temperatures between 70°C and 320°C. The excellent product purity, narrow particle size distribution, and creation of homogeneous nanostructure

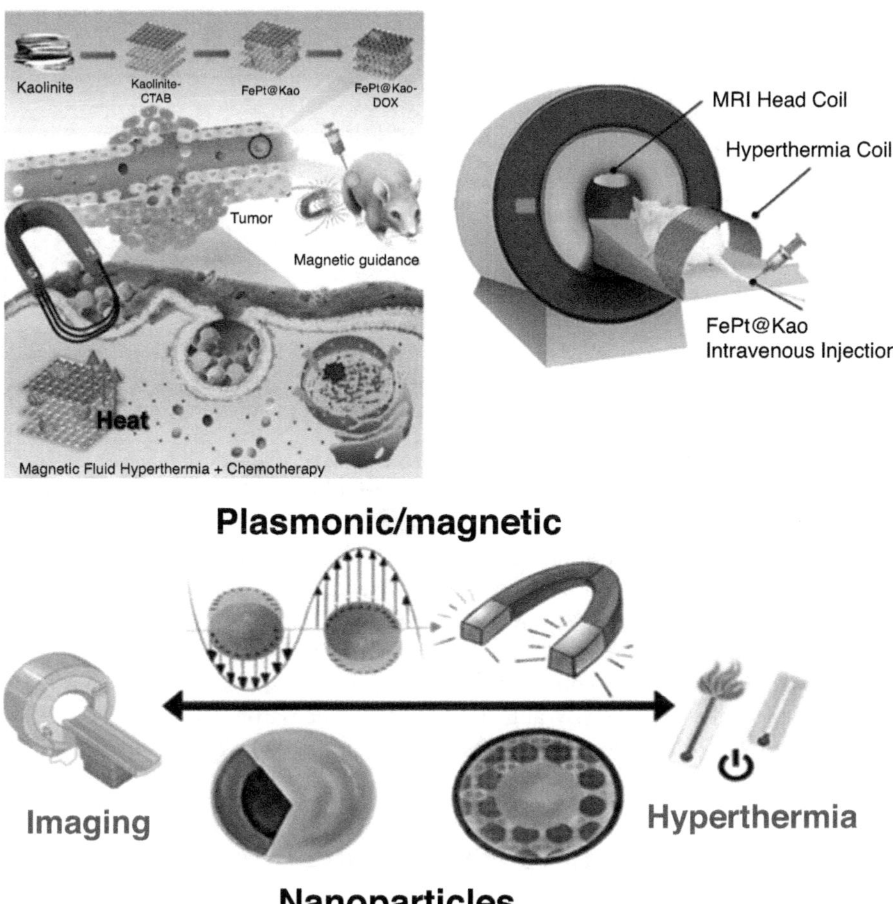

FIGURE 2.3 (a) Process of doxorubicin-loaded FePt nanoparticles combined with kaolinite modified with CTAB (FePt@Kao-Dox) (Reproduced with permission from [3]), (b) IONPs application as hyperthermia and imaging (reproduced with permission from [5]).

at low temperatures are the key benefits of the sol-gel technique [11–14]. Figure 2.4 shows a simple schematic of the sol-gel synthesis process to form aerogel, xerogel, and cryogel.

2.1.3.2 Applications

Due to the use of thermal activation therapy, hyperthermia is the most effective therapy for many diseases, including pulmonary challenges. MNPs, on the other hand, are the greatest choice for drug delivery systems like those deployed to treat lung cancer and cystic fibrosis because they have a greater capacity of being loaded and released into regulated areas [8]. MNPs' magnetic core and surface coating are frequently essential to the drug delivery system [9]. Due to the high ratio of surface to volume and improved biological and antibacterial characteristics, chitosan

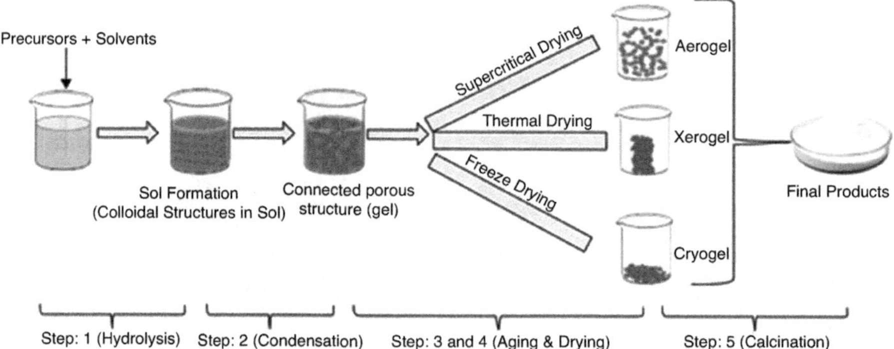

FIGURE 2.4 Sol-gel synthesis of chitosan (reproduced with permission from [10]).

nanoparticles have the potential to be a more effective drug delivery vehicle [15]. Chitosan-insulated IOMNPs that have been coated with phytic acid create thermally stable anticancer nanocomposites of phytic acid and chitosan iron oxide. Eun Hee Kim et al. showed superparamagnetic iron oxide (SPIO) microspheres wrapped in chitosan can enhance the contrast similar to the ferrofluid *in vitro* in MRI. The chitosan-encapsulated SPIO microspheres were injected into the blood vessels of the rabbit and MR contrast images of its kidneys were taken as shown in Figure 2.5 [16]. The chitosan nanoparticles synthesized with the sol-gel method can be used as a carrier polymer for drug delivery. Wang et al. showed successful loading of the chemotherapeutic agent 5-fluorouracil on chitosan-encapsulated IONPs and glutaraldehyde as crosslinking agent [17].

2.2 CQDS IN BIOIMAGING APPLICATIONS

2.2.1 Introduction

Noninvasive imaging of cells, tissues, and organs is essential for diagnosing and treating various diseases, including cancer. Over the past two decades, a significant amount of research has been conducted on various materials, such as quantum dots (QDs), for cell imaging [18–23]. Despite the apparent benefits of QDs in bioimaging, their usage is impeded by several notable limitations, with toxicity being the most critical concern. Semiconductor QDs are currently prevalent and are constrained by heavy metal constituents, such as cadmium, which have been extensively documented for their potential adverse effects on human health and the environment. The evidence indicates that QDs based on cadmium exhibit toxicity toward vertebrate systems even at low concentrations [24,25]. Additionally, risks may be associated with the bioaccumulation of these hazardous materials in organs and tissues [25,26]. Nanoscale silicon particles and, to a lesser extent, germanium particles have emerged as potentially viable alternatives for QDs, as suggested by several studies [27–30]. Notably, carbon, which belongs to the same group as silicon in the periodic table, has been found to offer a more efficient

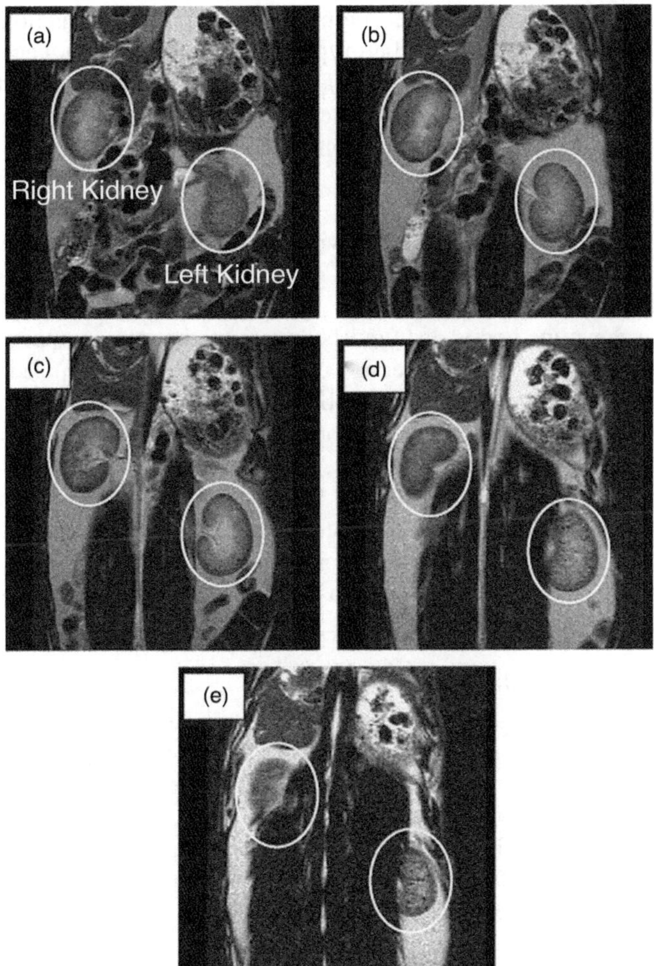

FIGURE 2.5 MR images of five slices of the kidneys: (a) Upper, (b) upper intermediate, (c) middle, (d) lower intermediate, (e) lower of Eun Hee Kim et al (reproduced with permission from [16]).

solution for creating substitutes for semiconductor QDs. This is due to the discovery of highly luminescent carbon-based materials [31–33]. CQDs or carbon dots (CDs) are a recent addition to the family of carbon nanomaterials [34,35]. The discovery of small carbogenic fluorescent nanoparticles by Xu et al. (2004) led to the emergence of a novel field of nanoparticle research with diverse applications [36]. CDs contain many chemical elements, such as carbon, oxygen, and hydrogen. Various supplementary components, such as nitrogen, sulfur, boron, etc., may be introduced via suitable synthesis techniques to modify the properties of CDs [37]. In addition, it should be noted that CDs exhibit favorable characteristics, such as high water solubility, minimal toxicity, ability to withstand photodegradation, and adjustable fluorescence properties. The presence of carboxyl functionality on the surface of those, as mentioned earlier, typically enhances their aqueous solubility. Functionalization with different chemical groups and surface passivation of CDs can be readily performed to modify their fluorescence characteristics, decrease their toxicity, and modify physical attributes [35,37].

2.2.1.1 Synthesis

Notably, many techniques have been devised for synthesizing CQDs within years, originating from diverse sources. These methods can be broadly categorized into two distinct synthesis strategies, namely "bottom-up" and "top-down" approaches [38]. The top-down method is distinguished from the bottom-up approach in that it involves the fragmentation or dispersion of carbonaceous macromolecules, such as graphite, nano-diamonds, carbon nanotubes, and activated carbon, into nano-sized CQDs. Conversely, the bottom-up method entails the polymerization and carbonization of small carbonaceous molecules, such as citric acid, glucose, and sucrose, through a series of chemical reactions [39]. The top-down approach involves arc discharge, laser ablation, chemical ablation, electrochemical ablation, and ultrasonic synthesis. In contrast, the hydrothermal method, microwave pyrolysis, thermal decomposition, templated routes, and plasma treatment are some of the bottom-up approach techniques.

2.2.1.1.1 Top-Down Approach

2.2.1.1.1.1 Chemical Ablation This controlled oxidation process converts small organic molecules into non-carbonaceous materials through carbonization by potent oxidizing acids. This method has some major drawbacks in severe conditions, so Travis-Sejdic and Peng worked through a simple facile process where carbohydrates were first dehydrated with sulfuric acid. The then-obtained carbonaceous structures were broken into CQDs after treatment with nitric acid, and finally, surface stabilization was done by amine-terminated compounds to enhance their photoluminescence properties [40].

2.2.1.1.1.2 Electrochemical Ablation The method of synthesizing CQDs from a carbon precursor mass under standard temperature and pressure conditions has been extensively reported. Zhang and his co-workers prepared CQDs using a traditional three-electrode system, and the obtained CQDs did not need any surface passivation or purification treatment. The size of the CQDs can be controlled by varying the potential, and thus, high CQDs can be processed from different small molecular alcohols [41–43] (Figure 2.6).

2.2.1.1.1.3 Ultrasonic Synthesis In the synthesis process, the ultrasonic waves' vigorous energy creates alternative high and low pressures in the liquid to create vacuum bubbles. These vacuum bubbles help in de-agglomeration and hydrodynamic shear force, which assists in breaking down large carbon materials into CQDs. This method shows low crystallinity, good dispersion, surface rich functional groups in CQDs [42,46].

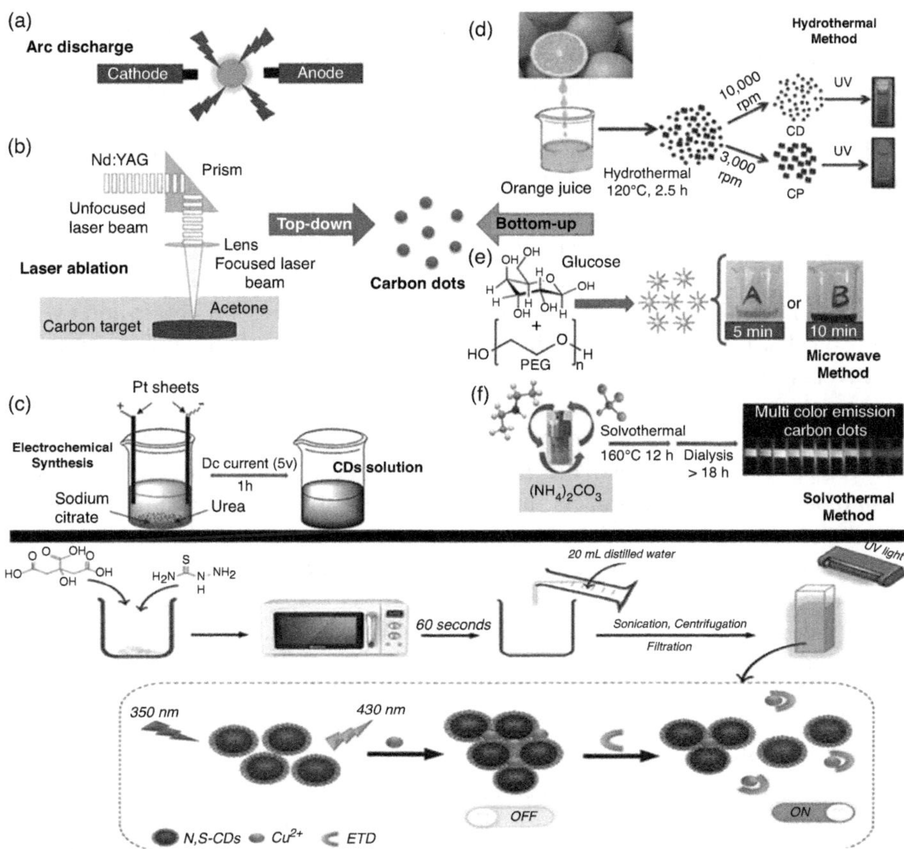

FIGURE 2.6 (i) Synthesis of CDs. Top-down approaches: (a) arc discharge, (b) laser ablation, (c) electrochemical synthesis [44]. Bottom-up approaches: (d) hydrothermal method, (e) microwave treatment, (f) solvothermal method [45]. (ii) Synthesis of nitrogen and sulfur co-doped carbon dots (N, S-CDs) and strategy for Cu^{2+} and Explosives trace detector (ETD) detection by microwave pyrolysis technique [39].

2.2.1.1.2 Bottom-Up Approach

2.2.1.1.2.1 Hydrothermal Synthesis Hydrothermal treatment or hydrothermal carbonization (HTC): This is the most common, affordable, environmentally friendly, non-toxic way of producing carbon-based nanomaterials of nearly uniform size with high luminescence. Various methods like chitosan, proteins, and glucose have been used to synthesize CQD by HTC. These precursors combine under high boiling points and pressure in a closed system to form carbon cores and grow in CQDs. Qi et al. (2019) used an easy hydrothermal process to create effective CQDs from rice and glycine as carbon and nitrogen sources. Using these CQDs as probe, it was possible to detect tetracycline (TC) drugs and Fe^{3+} with remarkable accuracy [42,47].

2.2.1.1.2.2 Microwave Pyrolysis A highly favored method utilizing the bottom-up approach involves a synthesis procedure characterized by its rapidity, efficiency, and time-saving properties. This method employs a diverse range of electromagnetic waves, ranging from 300 MHz to 300 GHz, to impart substantial energy that facilitates the breakdown of chemical bonds within the substrate. Liu et al. generated highly radiant CQDs through the utilization of citric acid and multiple amine compounds in the process of microwave pyrolysis [42]. Jaiswal et al. synthesized green luminescent CQDs using diethylene glycol (DEG) as a precursor. The resulting CQDs exhibited remarkable water dispersibility and clarity. The researchers Liu et al. determined that their findings indicated the successful absorption by glioma C6 cells, thereby rendering them a viable option for utilization in bioimaging endeavors [46,48].

2.2.1.1.2.3 Thermal Decomposition The process under consideration is a cost-effective and user friendly technique that can be executed without the requirement of any solvent. The process involves the application of external heat to facilitate the carbonization and dehydration of organic materials, ultimately leading to the formation of CQDs. Jia et al. produced fluorescent CQDs possessing desirable properties, such as biocompatibility, aqueous dispersibility, pH, excitation, polarity-dependent luminescence, and up-conversion fluorescence characteristics through the low-temperature heating of ascorbic acid in an aqueous medium. [46,49,50].

2.2.1.2 Application

Due to their impressive fluorescence properties, easily modified surface functional groups, biocompatibility, and low toxicity, CQDs are collectively used in cancer cells for in vitro imaging. He et al administered these fluorescent CQDs (synthesized by citric acid and ethylenediamine) at the HeLa tumor site tissues in mice, which showed [Figure 2.7(i)] excellent imaging capability and tumor uptake [45,51]. Zheng et al. also injected oxaliplatin-conjugated highly luminescent CQDs in mice. They observed a gradient intensity pattern [Figure 2.7(i)] that suggested the biodistribution of these CQDs to other organs and elimination from the body system [45,52]. Zhao and his group also prepared some functionalized CQDs, which also displayed organ visualization [Figure 2.7(i)] through bioimaging [45,53]. Recently Bao et al. prepared near-infrared CQDs, which showed effective accumulation at the tumor site (Figure 2.7(i)), further attributed to the enhanced permeability and retention (EPR) effect [45]. Globally, brain cancers contribute a major part of mortality rates. Zheng et al. successfully attributed a novel Carbon quantum dots-Aspartic acid (CQD-ASP) that suggested free penetrating ability across the blood-brain-barrier (BBB), confirming the precise accumulation of these CQDs in the glioma region of the brain through imaging, Figure 2.7(ii) [54,55]. Graphene carbon nitride CQDs (GCNCQDs) are an emerging fluorescence probe that showed some prospective results of cell nucleus bioimaging [Figure 2.7(iii)] experiments [54,56].

According to their distinctive attributes, colloidal quantum dots (CLQDs) have garnered significant attention as promising contenders for cancer imaging applications. The effectiveness of utilizing colloidal quantum dots (CQDs) has been demonstrated

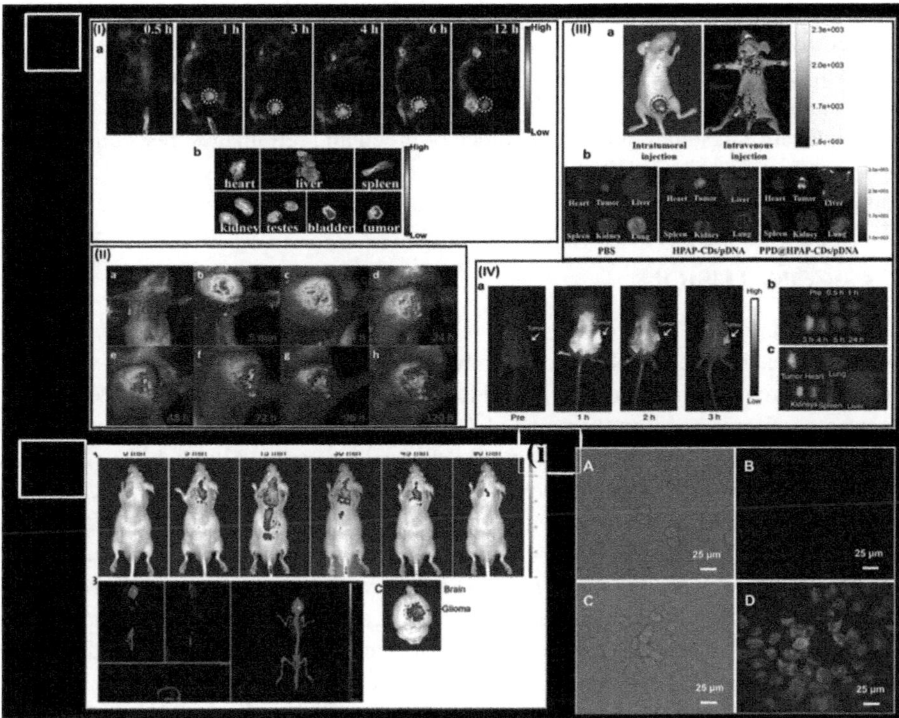

FIGURE 2.7 (i) In vivo imaging and biodistribution [45], (ii) In vivo and ex vivo fluorescence images of CD-ASP-injected C6 glioma-containing mice [45], (iii) Images of HeLa cells taken in the absence (A and B) and presence (C and D) of GCNQDs under bright field (A and C) and at an excitation wavelength of 488 nm (B and D) with 50 μg/mL of GCNQDs. Microwave synthesis of green fluorescent graphitic carbon nitride QDs for vitro bioimaging [54].

in the field of *in vitro* cell and tissue imaging, utilizing both one- and two-photon excitations. The utilization of CQDs for *in vivo* imaging is restricted due to their absorption wavelength being situated in the ultraviolet region. The issue has emerged as a significant subject of discussion in chemistry and its associated disciplines. Various strategies have been explored to overcome this challenge to transform CQDs into potential candidates for imaging and diagnosis, particularly for target-specific imaging. The utilization of zebrafish in biological and biochemical research has been extensive [57].

In their study, Kang et al. utilized zebrafish as a model organism to investigate CQDs' toxicity, *in vivo* system damage, transport, and biocompatibility [58]. The validation of multicolor *in vivo* fluorescence imaging utilizing CQDs as a probe shows brightfield and multicolor fluorescence images of embryos subjected to soaking with CQDs. The fluorescence images reveal varying affinities of CQDs to the yolk and inner mass of embryos, as evidenced by different brightness levels between these tissues. Consequently, introducing CQDs into embryos was achieved through immersion, whereby they could traverse the chorion and germ ring and ultimately accumulate within the yolk sac due to their diminutive dimensions. The intensity of fluorescence images of embryos exhibits a positive correlation with the concentration of CQDs. Conversely, the brightfield images of embryos do not indicate any discernible variation concerning each other. The utilization of ultraviolet light irradiation resulted in the observation of a blue fluorescence image of embryos. In contrast, using blue and green light irradiation resulted in the observance of green and red images, respectively. The fluorescence of CQDs facilitates the visualization of their spatial arrangement within zebrafish embryos, confirming the feasibility of CQDs as viable imaging agent.

2.3 CONCLUSION

Magnetic nanoparticles exhibit a range of properties that make them highly versatile and applicable in diverse fields, including but not limited to medicine, sensing, imaging, and environmental remediation. It is widely recognized that the nanoparticles exhibit an average diameter within the range of 1–100 nm, rendering them appropriate for utilization in targeted gene delivery to a particular cell or organ. Although the coating of IONPs has demonstrated notable benefits, certain discrepancies have been documented in scholarly literature. Prior research has indicated that the application of D-mannose or poly-L-lysine as coatings for IONPs did not effectively mitigate their toxicity in murine neural stem cells. The utilization of chitosan nanoparticles exhibits considerable promise in drug delivery through various routes, such as gastrointestinal, nasal, and pulmonary. Thus far, chitosan has exhibited minimal or negligible toxicity in animal models and no documentation of significant unfavorable outcomes in healthy human participants exists. However, there is a dearth of clinical data on the subject. On the other hand, CQDs are being widely investigated in bioimaging. Because of their water solubility, luminescence property, semiconducting band gap, and non-toxic nature, CQDs have been used as biomarkers and contrast agents in the imaging of biomolecules.

NOTE

* Both authors contributed equally to the writing of this manuscript.

REFERENCES

1. Gilchrist, R.K., Medal, R., Shorey, W.D., Hanselman, R.C., Parrott, J.C. and Taylor, C.B., 1957. Selective inductive heating of lymph nodes. *Annals of Surgery*, *146*(4), p. 596.
2. Vaghari, H., Jafarizadeh-Malmiri, H., Mohammadlou, M., Berenjian, A., Anarjan, N., Jafari, N. and Nasiri, S., 2016. Application of magnetic nanoparticles in smart enzyme immobilization. *Biotechnology Letters*, *38*, pp. 223–233.
3. Materón, E.M., Miyazaki, C.M., Carr, O., Joshi, N., Picciani, P.H., Dalmaschio, C.J., Davis, F. and Shimizu, F.M., 2021. Magnetic nanoparticles in biomedical applications: A review. *Applied Surface Science Advances*, *6*, p. 100163.
4. Ali, A., Shah, T., Ullah, R., Zhou, P., Guo, M., Ovais, M., Tan, Z. and Rui, Y., 2021. Review on recent progress in magnetic nanoparticles: Synthesis, characterization, and diverse applications. *Frontiers in chemistry*, *9*, p. 629054.
5. Gambhir, R.P., Rohiwal, S.S. and Tiwari, A.P., 2022. Multifunctional surface functionalized magnetic iron oxide nanoparticles for biomedical applications: A review. *Applied Surface Science Advances*, *11*, p. 100303.

6. Kermanian, M., Naghibi, M. and Sadighian, S., 2020. One-pot hydrothermal synthesis of a magnetic hydroxyapatite nanocomposite for MR imaging and pH-Sensitive drug delivery applications. *Heliyon*, *6*(9), p. e04928.
7. Dasari, A., Xue, J. and Deb, S., 2022. Magnetic nanoparticles in bone tissue engineering. *Nanomaterials*, *12*(5), p. 757.
8. Zhang, X. and Zhang, Y., 2021. Experimental study on enhanced heat transfer and flow performance of magnetic nanofluids under alternating magnetic field. *International Journal of Thermal Sciences*, *164*, p. 106897.
9. Chan, M.H., Hsieh, M.R., Liu, R.S., Wei, D.H. and Hsiao, M., 2019. Magnetically guided theranostics: Optimizing magnetic resonance imaging with sandwich-like kaolinite-based iron/platinum nanoparticles for magnetic fluid hyperthermia and chemotherapy. *Chemistry of Materials*, *32*(2), pp. 697–708.
10. Bokov, D., Turki Jalil, A., Chupradit, S., Suksatan, W., Javed Ansari, M., Shewael, I.H., Valiev, G.H. and Kianfar, E., 2021. Nanomaterial by sol-gel method: Synthesis and application. *Advances in Materials Science and Engineering*, 2021, pp. 1–21.
11. Li, B., Wang, X., Yan, M. and Li, L., 2003. Preparation and characterization of nano-TiO2 powder. *Materials Chemistry and Physics*, *78*(1), pp. 184–188.
12. Vijayalakshmi, R. and Rajendran, V., 2012. Synthesis and characterization of nano-TiO_2 via different methods. *Archives of Applied Science Research*, *4*(2), pp. 1183–1190.
13. Jaroenworaluck, A., Sunsaneeyametha, W., Kosachan, N. and Stevens, R., 2006. Characteristics of silica-coated TiO2 and its UV absorption for sunscreen cosmetic applications. *Surface and Interface Analysis: An International Journal Devoted to the Development and Application of Techniques for the Analysis of Surfaces, Interfaces and Thin Films*, *38*(4), pp. 473–477.
14. Verma, R., Mantri, B. and Kumar Srivastava, A., 2015. Shape control synthesis, characterizations, mechanisms and optical properties of larg scaled metal oxide nanostructures of ZnO and TiO2. *Advanced Materials Letters*, *6*(4), pp. 324–333.
15. Lucena, G.N., dos Santos, C.C., Pinto, G.C., Amantéa, B.E., Piazza, R.D., Jafelicci Júnior, M. and Marques, R.F.C., 2020. Surface engineering of magnetic nanoparticles for hyperthermia and drug delivery. *Medical Devices & Sensors*, *3*(6), p. e10100.
16. Kim, E.H., Ahn, Y. and Lee, H.S., 2007. Biomedical applications of superparamagnetic iron oxide nanoparticles encapsulated within chitosan. *Journal of Alloys and Compounds*, *434*, pp. 633–636.
17. Arami, H., Stephen, Z., Veiseh, O. and Zhang, M., 2011. Chitosan-coated iron oxide nanoparticles for molecular imaging and drug delivery. In: Jayakumar, R., Prabaharan, M., Muzzarelli, R. (eds), *Chitosan for Biomaterials I*, Advances in Polymer Science, vol 243, pp. 163–184, Springer, Berlin, Heidelberg.
18. Cherukula, K., Manickavasagam Lekshmi, K., Uthaman, S., Cho, K., Cho, C.S. and Park, I.K., 2016. Multifunctional inorganic nanoparticles: Recent progress in thermal therapy and imaging. *Nanomaterials*, 6(4), p. 76.
19. Cattaneo, A.G., Gornati, R., Sabbioni, E., Chiriva-Internati, M., Cobos, E., Jenkins, M.R. and Bernardini, G., 2010. Nanotechnology and human health: Risks and benefits. *Journal of Applied Toxicology*, *30*(8), pp. 730–744.
20. Gutiérrez Millán, C., Colino Gandarillas, C.I., Sayalero Marinero, M.L. and Lanao, J.M., 2012. Cell-based drug-delivery platforms. *Therapeutic Delivery*, *3*(1), pp. 25–41.
21. Hola, K., Zhang, Y., Wang, Y., Giannelis, E.P., Zboril, R. and Rogach, A.L., 2014. Carbon dots—Emerging light emitters for bioimaging, cancer therapy and optoelectronics. *Nano Today*, *9*(5), pp. 590–603.
22. G Nair, B., Hanna Varghese, S., Nair, R., Yoshida, Y., Maekawa, T. and Sakthi Kumar, D., 2011. Nanotechnology platforms; an innovative approach to brain tumor therapy. *Medicinal Chemistry*, *7*(5), pp. 488–503.

23. Orive, G., Ali, O.A., Anitua, E., Pedraz, J.L. and Emerich, D.F., 2010. Biomaterial-based technologies for brain anti-cancer therapeutics and imaging. *Biochimica et Biophysica Acta (BBA)-Reviews on Cancer, 1806*(1), pp. 96–107.
24. Poliandri, A.H., Cabilla, J.P., Velardez, M.O., Bodo, C.C. and Duvilanski, B.H., 2003. Cadmium induces apoptosis in anterior pituitary cells that can be reversed by treatment with antioxidants. *Toxicology and Applied Pharmacology, 190*(1), pp. 17–24.
25. Hardman, R., 2006. A toxicologic review of quantum dots: Toxicity depends on physicochemical and environmental factors. *Environmental Health Perspectives, 114*(2), pp. 165–172.
26. Thévenod, F., 2003. Nephrotoxicity and the proximal tubule. *Nephron Physiology, 93*(4), pp. p87–p93.
27. Holmes, J.D., Ziegler, K.J., Doty, R.C. and Pell, L.E., 2001. Johnston KP and Korgel BA. *Journal of the American Chemical Society*, 2001, p. 123.
28. Kang, Z., Liu, Y. and Lee, S.T., 2011. Small-sized silicon nanoparticles: New nanolights and nanocatalysts. *Nanoscale, 3*(3), pp. 777–791.
29. Prabakar, S., Shiohara, A., Hanada, S., Fujioka, K., Yamamoto, K. and Tilley, R.D., 2010. Size controlled synthesis of germanium nanocrystals by hydride reducing agents and their biological applications. *Chemistry of Materials, 22*(2), pp. 482–486.
30. Lambert, T.N., Andrews, N.L., Gerung, H., Boyle, T.J., Oliver, J.M., Wilson, B.S. and Han, S.M., 2007. Water-soluble germanium (0) nanocrystals: Cell recognition and near-infrared photothermal conversion properties. *Small, 3*(4), pp. 691–699.
31. Sun, Y.P., Zhou, B., Lin, Y., Wang, W., Fernando, K.A., Pathak, P., Meziani, M.J., Harruff, B.A., Wang, X., Wang, H., Luo, P.G., Yang, H., Kose, M.E., Chen, B., Veca, L.M. and Xie, S.Y., 2006. Quantum-sized carbon dots for bright and colorful photoluminescence. *Journal of the American Chemical Society*, 128, p. 7756.
32. (a) Kim, S., Hwang, S.W., Kim, M.K., Shin, D.Y., Shin, D.H., Kim, C.O., Yang, S.B., Park, J.H., Hwang, E., Choi, S.H. and Ko, G., 2012. Anomalous behaviors of visible luminescence from graphene quantum dots: Interplay between size and shape. ACS Nano, 6, 8203; (b) Cao, L., Wang, X., Meziani, M.J., Lu, F., Wang, H., Luo, P.G., Lin, Y., Harruff, B.A., Veca, L.M., Murray, D. and Xie, S.Y., 2007. Carbon dots for multiphoton bioimaging. *Journal of the American Chemical Society*, 129, pp. 11318–11319.
33. Yang, J., Shang, Y., Hannigan, M. P., Zhu, R., Wang, Q. G., Qin, C. and Xie, M., 2021. Collocated speciation of PM2.5 using tandem quartz filters in northern Nanjing, China: Sampling artifacts and measurement uncertainty. *Atmospheric Environment*, 246, p. 118066.
34. Mitchell, M., 2014. New nanoparticles bring cheaper, lighter solar cells outdoors. *Rdmag.com. Retrieved*, pp. 08–24.
35. Hola, K., Zhang, Y., Wang, Y., Giannelis, E.P., Zboril, R. and Rogach, A.L., 2014. Carbon dots—Emerging light emitters for bioimaging, cancer therapy and optoelectronics. *Nano Today, 9*(5), pp. 590–603.
36. Xu, X.Y., Ray, R., Gu, Y.L., Plohehn, H.J., Gearhart, L., Rocker, K. and Scripens, W.A., 2015. Photoelectric analysis and purification of fluorescent carbon nanotubes. *Journal of the American Chemical Society, 126*(40), pp. 12736–12737.
37. Jaleel, J.A. and Pramod, K., 2018. Artful and multifaceted applications of carbon dot in biomedicine. *Journal of Controlled Release, 269*, pp. 302–321.
38. Wang, B., Cai, H., Waterhouse, G.I., Qu, X., Yang, B. and Lu, S., 2022. Carbon dots in bioimaging, biosensing and therapeutics: A comprehensive review. *Small Science, 2*(6), p. 2200012.
39. Luo, P.G., Sahu, S., Yang, S.T., Sonkar, S.K., Wang, J., Wang, H., LeCroy, G.E., Cao, L. and Sun, Y.P., 2013. Carbon "quantum" dots for optical bioimaging. *Journal of Materials Chemistry B, 1*(16), pp. 2116–2127.
40. Peng, H. and Travas-Sejdic, J., 2009. Simple aqueous solution route to luminescent carbogenic dots from carbohydrates. *Chemistry of Materials, 21*(23), pp. 5563–5565.

41. Molaei, M.J., 2019. Carbon quantum dots and their biomedical and therapeutic applications: A review. *RSC Advances*, *9*(12), pp. 6460–6481.
42. Azam, N., Najabat Ali, M. and Javaid Khan, T., 2021. Carbon quantum dots for biomedical applications: Review and analysis. *Frontiers in Materials*, *8*, p. 700403.
43. Rong, M., Feng, Y., Wang, Y. and Chen, X., 2017. One-pot solid phase pyrolysis synthesis of nitrogen-doped carbon dots for Fe^{3+} sensing and bioimaging. *Sensors and Actuators B: Chemical*, *245*, pp. 868–874.
44. Hou, Y., Lu, Q., Deng, J., Li, H. and Zhang, Y., 2015. One-pot electrochemical synthesis of functionalized fluorescent carbon dots and their selective sensing for mercury ion. *Analytica Chimica Acta*, *866*, pp. 69–74.
45. Jana, P. and Dev, A., 2022. Carbon quantum dots: A promising nanocarrier for bioimaging and drug delivery in cancer. *Materials Today Communications*, *32*, p. 104068.
46. Rahmandoust, M. and Ayatollahi, M.R. eds., 2019. *Nanomaterials for Advanced Biological Applications* (Vol. 104). Springer, Switzerland AG.
47. Zhang, Q., Song, K., Zhao, J., Kong, X., Sun, Y., Liu, X., Zhang, Y., Zeng, Q. and Zhang, H., 2009. Hexanedioic acid mediated surface–ligand-exchange process for transferring NaYF4: Yb/Er (or Yb/Tm) up-converting nanoparticles from hydrophobic to hydrophilic. *Journal of Colloid and Interface Science*, *336*(1), pp. 171–175.
48. Jaiswal, A., Ghosh, S.S. and Chattopadhyay, A., 2012. One step synthesis of C-dots by microwave mediated caramelization of poly (ethylene glycol). *Chemical Communications*, *48*(3), pp. 407–409.
49. Jia, X., Li, J. and Wang, E., 2012. One-pot green synthesis of optically pH-sensitive carbon dots with upconversion luminescence. *Nanoscale*, *4*(18), pp. 5572–5575.
50. Li, J.Y., Liu, Y., Shu, Q.W., Liang, J.M., Zhang, F., Chen, X.P., Deng, X.Y., Swihart, M.T. and Tan, K.J., 2017. One-pot hydrothermal synthesis of carbon dots with efficient up-and down-converted photoluminescence for the sensitive detection of morin in a dual-readout assay. *Langmuir*, *33*(4), pp. 1043–1050.
51. He, H., Wang, X., Feng, Z., Cheng, T., Sun, X., Sun, Y., Xia, Y., Wang, S., Wang, J. and Zhang, X., 2015. Rapid microwave-assisted synthesis of ultra-bright fluorescent carbon dots for live cell staining, cell-specific targeting and in vivo imaging. *Journal of Materials Chemistry B*, *3*(24), pp. 4786–4789.
52. Zheng, M., Liu, S., Li, J., Qu, D., Zhao, H., Guan, X., Hu, X., Xie, Z., Jing, X. and Sun, Z., 2014. Integrating oxaliplatin with highly luminescent carbon dots: An unprecedented theranostic agent for personalized medicine. *Advanced Materials*, *26*(21), pp. 3554–3560.
53. Zhao, H., Duan, J., Xiao, Y., Tang, G., Wu, C., Zhang, Y., Liu, Z. and Xue, W., 2018. Microenvironment-driven cascaded responsive hybrid carbon dots as a multifunctional theranostic nano platform for imaging-traceable gene precise delivery. *Chemistry of Materials*, *30*(10), pp. 3438–3453.
54. Miao, X., Yan, X., Qu, D., Li, D., Tao, F.F. and Sun, Z., 2017. Red emissive sulfur, nitrogen codoped carbon dots and their application in ion detection and theraonostics. *ACS Applied Materials & Interfaces*, *9*(22), pp. 18549–18556.
55. Agarwal, S., Sane, R., Oberoi, R., Ohlfest, J.R. and Elmquist, W.F., 2011. Delivery of molecularly targeted therapy to malignant glioma, a disease of the whole brain. *Expert Reviews in Molecular Medicine*, *13*, p. e17.
56. Chen, B., Li, F., Li, S., Weng, W., Guo, H., Guo, T., Zhang, X., Chen, Y., Huang, T., Hong, X. and You, S., 2013. Large-scale synthesis of photoluminescent carbon nanodots and their application for bioimaging. *Nanoscale*, *5*(5), pp. 1967–1971.
57. Deniz Koç, N. and Yüce, R., 2012. A light-and electron microscopic study of primordial germ cells in the zebra fish (*Danio rerio*). *Biological Research*, *45*(4), pp. 331–336.
58. Kang, Y.F., Li, Y.H., Fang, Y.W., Xu, Y., Wei, X.M. and Yin, X.B., 2015. Carbon quantum dots for zebrafish fluorescence imaging. *Scientific Reports*, *5*(1), p. 11835.

3 Drug Delivery and Medical Imaging Using Nanotechnology

Sunil Kumar Verma and Devendra Singh

3.1 INTRODUCTION

Nanoscience refers to the investigation of the one-of-a-kind characteristics that are exhibited by substances that range in size from 1 to 100 nanometers (nm), and nanotechnology refers to the utilization of this type of research in order to produce or alter novel objects. NM can be created thanks to advances in technology that allow structures to be manipulated on an atomic scale (Belkin et al., 2015; Drexler, 1992). NM have recently attracted a lot of attention as a result of the growing demand for controlling desired molecules that are present in both the human body as well as the surroundings (Kumar et al., 2022b; Mohanty et al., 2017; Swamy and Rao, 2011). This nanomaterial is made up of NPs, each of which is smaller than 100 nm in at least one of its dimensions. The term "nanotechnology" refers to the study of extremely small materials, specifically those with dimensions of one sub-nanometer or several hundred nanometers (Kumar and Verma, 2022; Rodrigues et al., 2016). Information from many different fields, for instance, chemistry, physics, electronics, biology, computer science, agriculture, engineering, and so on, is required for the precise synthesis as well as tuning of the properties of NM (Das et al., 2022; Rodrigues et al., 2016; Singh et al., 2022a; Singh and Singh, 2022). This can pave the way for the development of new as well as multifunctional nanotechnologies.

The fascinating nanomaterial properties have attracted the scientific/researchers all over the world toward their application in multiple fields, like medicine, the food industry, transportation, and information technology, among others (Allhoff, 2010). It is anticipated that the strategic application of NM will improve the electronic devices' (biomolecular) performance, resulting in higher sensitivities as well as lower detection limits. Nanotechnologies have a major impact in nearly all sectors of industry as well as areas of society due to the fact that they offer products that are i) safer as well as cleaner, ii) better built, iii) durable, and iv) smarter for fields such as agriculture, communications, medicine, and other sectors (Das et al., 2022). In general, there are two distinct types of nanomaterial applications that can be found in common consumer goods. To begin, nanomaterial can be combined with or added to an already prevailing product to enhance the objects' complete performance by lending several of the exceptional properties that NM possess. In any other case, this

 DOI: 10.1201/9781003432661-3

nanomaterial, like nanocrystals as well as NPs, could be used directly to create powerful and advanced devices as a result of the unique properties that they possess. The advantages offered by NM have the potential to have an impact on the foreseeable future of virtually all industrial sectors (Kumar et al., 2022a; Sim and Wong, 2021; Singh et al., 2022b).

Numerous commonplace products, such as sunscreen, cosmetics, athletic equipment, tires, and electronic devices, make use of NM in ways that are beneficial to the products (Sim and Wong, 2021). In addition, the advent of nanotechnologies has caused a revolution in the medical field, particularly in the fields of imaging, drug delivery, and diagnostic procedures.

3.1.1 Different Kinds of NPs

To this day, a number of NPs and NM have been researched and found to be safe for use in clinical settings. The following paragraphs will go over some of the more common kinds of NPs. Figure 3.1 shows the systematic representation of different kinds of NPs.

3.1.2 Liposomes

Liposomes are vesicles that take the shape of spheres and are composed of lipid bilayers. Their particle sizes range from 30 nm to some microns. The aqueous phase of a liposome can be used to incorporate therapeutic agents that are hydrophilic, and the liposomal membrane layer can be used to incorporate agents that are hydrophobic. Liposomes are adaptable; their surface properties can be improved with polymers, proteins, and/or antibodies. This makes it possible for liposomes to incorporate macromolecular drugs, such as nucleic acids and crystalline metals (Lombardo et al., 2019). The first nanomedicine to be approved by the FDA for the treatment of cancer (breast) is called Doxil. This medication has been shown to increase the effective concentration of the drug in malignant effusions without necessitating an increase in the total dose (Katsuki et al., 2017; Lombardo et al., 2019).

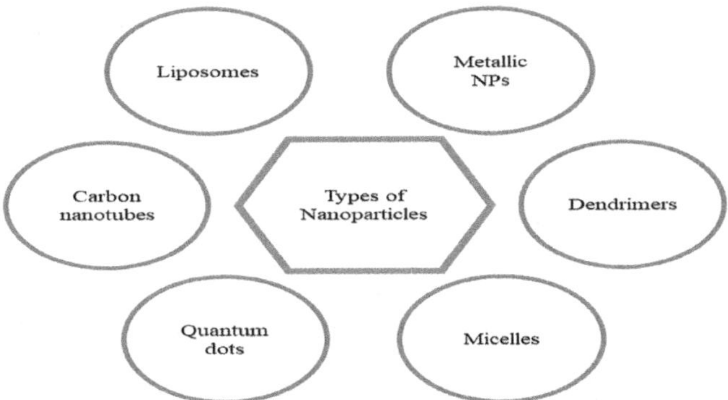

FIGURE 3.1 Shows the systematic representation of different types of NPs.

3.1.3 Carbon Nanotubes

The molecules known as carbon nanotubes have the shape of cylinders and are made up of rolled-up sheets of graphene (Kumar and Verma, 2022). It can have a single wall or multiple walls, or it can be composed of a few nanotubes that are linked concentrically to one another (Nune et al., 2009; Rezaei et al., 2019; Shi Kam et al., 2004). As drug carriers, carbon nanotubes have the potential to achieve significantly high loading capacities due to the high external surface area of the nanotubes. Additionally, as a result of their one-of-a-kind optical, mechanical, and electronic properties, carbon tubes have proven to be useful as biological sensors as well as imaging contrast agents (Shi Kam et al., 2004).

3.1.4 Quantum Dots

Quantum dots, also known as QDs, are tiny semiconductor nanocrystals that emit fluorescent light and range in size from one to one hundred nm. Because of their possible potential, they can be used in several biomedical applications like cellular imaging as well as drug delivery (Nune et al., 2009; Probst et al., 2013). QDs have a shell-core arrangement, with the core structure characteristically consisting of elements from the II-VI group and/or III-V group of the periodic table (Han et al., 2019). The shell structure is made up of electrons and holes. QDs have been utilized in the medical imaging field due to their distinct optical properties and sizes, as well as their high brightness and stability (Probst et al., 2013).

3.1.5 Metallic NPs

These NPs include gold as well as ferric oxide NPs. NPs of iron/ferric oxide are made up of a magnetic core that is 4–5 nm in size, as well as hydrophilic polymers like polyethylene glycol (PEG) or dextran (Nune et al., 2009). On the other side, gold NPs are made up of an Au atom core that is enclosed by negatively charged reactive groups. These NPs have the ability to be functionalized by the addition of a monolayer of external moieties that act as ligands for targeting (Nune et al., 2009), laser treatment (Morgan et al., 2005), imaging agents (Acharya and Sahoo, 2011), vehicles for drug delivery, as well as optical biosensors (Morgan et al., 2005), and they are some of the many applications where metallic NPs are used (Rezaei et al., 2019).

3.1.6 Dendrimers

They are the macromolecules with functional groups around them on their surface. They are made up of branched repetitive units that spread out from a central core (Lombardo et al., 2019; Morgan et al., 2005). These groups could have cationic, neutral, or anionic terminals, and also, they are able to transform not only the overall structure but also the chemical as well as physical properties of the molecule. Dendrimers are exceptionally bioavailable and biodegradable due to the fact that curative agents can be encapsulated within the dendrimer's interior space or attached to the dendrimer's surface groups. It has been demonstrated that conjugates of dendrimers with saccharides or peptides exhibit enhanced stability as well as solubility upon absorption of curative drugs in addition to enhanced antimicrobial, anti-prion, and antiviral properties (Tiriveedhi et al., 2011). Dendriplexes are polyamidoamine dendrimer–DNA complexes examined as potential gene delivery vectors. These complexes hold potential in terms of helping successive gene expression, improving the efficacy of the drug and drug target delivery (Palmerston Mendes et al., 2017). Because of their malleable properties, dendrimers show great promise as potential particulate systems for use in biomedical applications (Nune et al., 2009), particularly in imaging and drug delivery.

3.1.7 Micelles

Micelles are a type of amphiphilic surfactant molecules that are made up of lipids as well as other amphiphilic molecules. Due to the fact that they spontaneously accumulate as well as self-assemble onto circular vesicles in aqueous environments, micelles can be employed to contain hydrophobic medicinal substances (Katsuki et al., 2017; Kumar et al., 2022b). These micelles have a hydrophobic core as well as a hydrophilic monolayer (outer). Because of their one-of-a-kind characteristics, micelles are able to improve the solubility of hydrophobic drugs, which in turn leads to an increase in bioavailability. Micelles have a diameter that ranges from 10 to 100 nm. Micelles can be utilized in a variety of contexts, including as agents for the delivery of drugs, contrast agents, imaging agents, as well as curative agents (Katsuki et al., 2017; Kumar et al., 2022b).

3.2 CONFINEMENT AT THE QUANTUM LEVEL

In the field of quantum mechanics (QMs), the individual radius of an electron is referred to as the radius of Bohr exciton (BE). Because the radius of electron mobility in bulk semiconductor materials is known to be greater than the radius of BE mobility, the mobility of electrons in these materials is not disturbed or confined in any way. If the particle size is so small that it cannot be compared to the electron wavelength, then the quantum confinement effect will occur (Sumanth Kumar et al., 2018). When the particles of a material are reduced to a size that is comparable to the radius of BE or smaller, the mobility of the electrons in the material is restricted. The phenomenon known as “quantum confinement” of electron–hole pairs occurs as a result of the electrons and holes being packed into increasingly smaller particles. The term “confinement” refers to the process of limiting the motion of electrons that are otherwise moving randomly to particular energy levels (discreteness). If the dimensions of a particle are on the nanoscale, then the confining dimensions will cause the energy levels to be discrete. As a result, the material band gap or the energy gap will be increased or widened. Due to the quantum confinement effect, the excitonic transition energy, blue shift in the absorption, and luminescence band gap energy all increase when the size of a particle approaches the BE radius (Bera et al., 2010; Ramalingam et al., 2020). Figure 3.2 represents the characteristics of synthesized NPs.

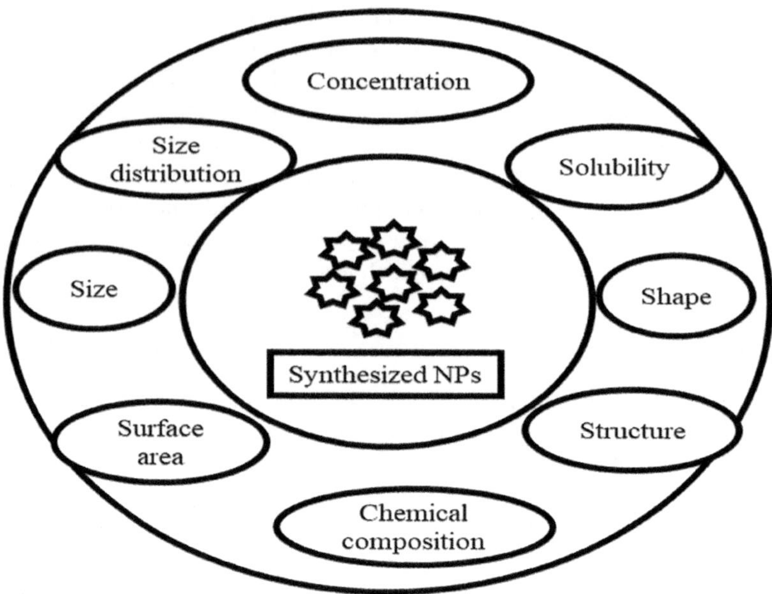

FIGURE 3.2 Denotes the different characteristics of synthesized NPs.

3.3 SURFACE AREA

Assume that a cube with dimensions of 1cm × 1cm × 1cm is cut into several equal pieces, with each piece resulting in a cube with dimensions of 0.1mm × 0.1mm × 0.1mm. If we were to cut the cube into smaller cubes, the volume of each of the smaller cubes would be equal to that of the original cube (Rezaei et al., 2019). The area of the surface of each cube is one hundred times larger than the area of the surface of the cube with which we began. When compared to the surface area of the initial cube, the area of the surfaces will increase 10 million times if additional cubes with dimensions of 1mm × 1mm × 1 mm are cut from the original cube. Because of this, the ratio of surface area to volume in nanomaterial is extremely high. This makes it possible for NM to interact with their surroundings or other materials in a more profound way than is possible with bulk materials. The interior atoms of a material are much more coordinated than the surface atoms because there are more bonds between them, which results in the interior atoms being stable. The atoms at the corners and edges have less coordination than the atoms in the interior, which results in the corners and edges having less stability (Das et al., 2022; Singh et al., 2022a). The surface of a nanomaterial can become extremely reactive when the dimensions of the material are on the nanoscale. This can result in extraordinary catalytic and absorbance activity.

3.4 NANOMATERIAL SYNTHESIS

Producing nanomaterials in their various forms like nanoclusters, colloidal particles, thin films, nanopowders, nanorods, nanotubes, nanowires, and so on can be accomplished through the use of a variety of different methods (Verma et al., 2023). The traditional approaches, with some adjustments made, can be used to successfully obtain nanomaterial (Mani et al., 2017; Nune et al., 2009). For the purpose of preparing NM, a variety of methods, including chemical, physical, hybrid, and biological ones, have been developed. The nanomaterial type or material of interest, like 0D, 1D, or 2D as well as the sizes of the NM and the quantity that is desired, all play a role in the choice of synthesis technique (Mani et al., 2017; Nune et al., 2009).

3.4.1 Bottom-Up Approach

This approach involves the miniaturization of material elements at the atomic level, which is then followed by the process of self-assembly, which ultimately results in creating the nanostructures. Nanostructured materials make up the fundamental unit of a better structure that is assembled through the process of self-assembly (Singh et al., 2022a). Both the quantum dots formation during epitaxial growth as well as the NPs formation from colloidal dispersal have been accomplished with the help of this technique. This strategy results in fewer flaws and a more consistent chemical makeup than alternative methods (Singh et al., 2022a). Figure 3.3 describes the bottom-up approaches used for the synthesis of nanomaterial.

3.4.2 Top-Down Approach

This approach is characterized by the fact that the large structure (macroscopic) can be controlled from the outside during the processing of the desired nanostructures. This strategy utilizes techniques, such as ball milling. The existence of defectiveness in the structure surface is one of the most significant drawbacks of utilizing this method. Because of the high aspect ratio, surface defects in this method have the potential to have an effect on both the surface as well as physical properties of NPs (Kumar and Verma, 2022; Singh et al., 2022a). Figure 3.4 describes the top-down approaches used for the synthesis of NM.

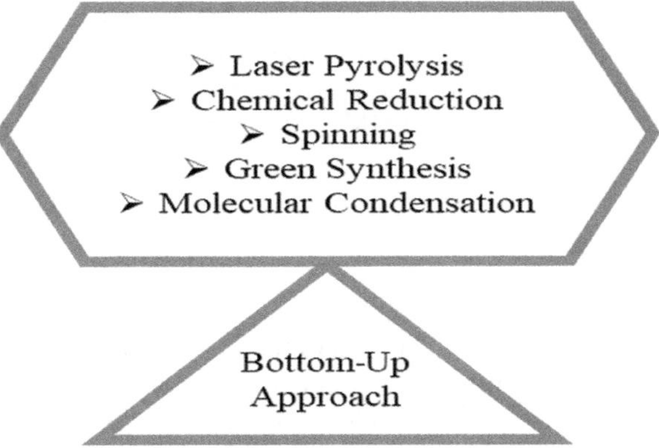

FIGURE 3.3 The bottom-up approaches used for the nanomaterial synthesis.

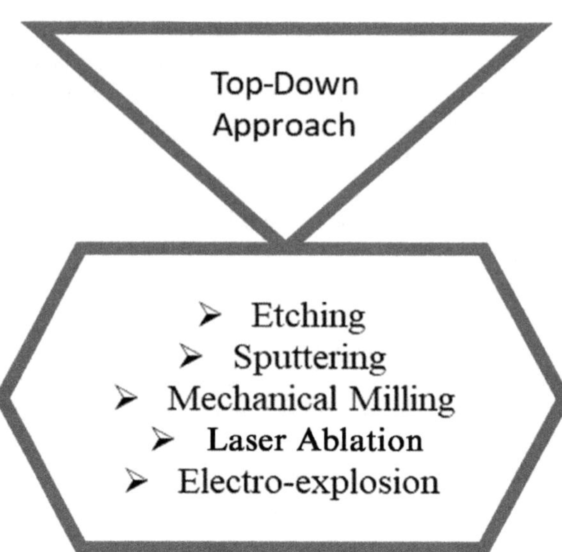

FIGURE 3.4 The top-down approaches used for the nanomaterial synthesis.

3.5 NANOTECHNOLOGY'S SEVERAL POTENTIAL APPLICATIONS

NM are currently being investigated for potential applications in a variety of fields, including chemistry, medicine, biomedicine, and physics, with the end goal of developing miniature versions of existing devices (Sim and Wong, 2021). As a result of the fact that all biological systems are excellent examples of the principles of nanotechnology, the possibility of NM's applications in the fields of biomedical science is among the significant areas that are gathering momentum. Due to the fact that the size of nanomaterial is comparable to that of biological materials, such as nucleotides, enzymes, proteins, and antibodies, which makes their use in therapeutic applications more feasible, it has been predicted that NMs will have a tremendous impact on medicine, biotechnology, as well as biology. The unusual properties of NMs, i.e., tuning property in optical emission, their large surface area, magnetic as well as electrical properties, and so on, can be used in bioengineering in a variety of applications ranging from biosensors to drug delivery. These applications can be realized from the extraordinary properties of NMs (Kumar et al., 2022a; Singh et al., 2022a) as mentioned in Figure 3.5.

3.6 BIOSENSORS

Biosensors are useful to check the pollution in the water, soil, air, and other mediums; toxic components in foods; biohazardous microbes; as well as biomolecules in medical diagnostics to fulfill the need for selective, fast, and sensitive equipment (Nie et al., 2014). Because of their rapid analysis, low cost, inherent simplicity, as well as miniaturization, and their easy handling, these biosensors have a huge potential thanks to their many advantages. It is hypothesized that biosensors will find use

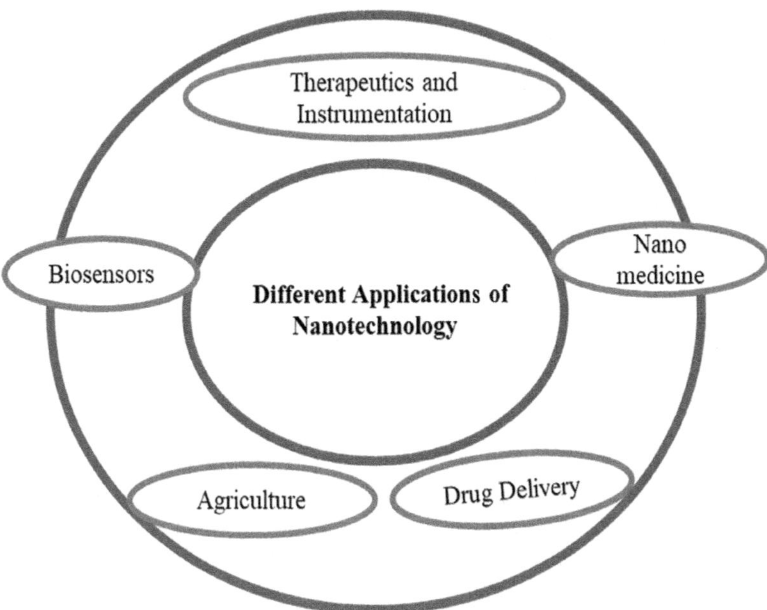

FIGURE 3.5 A diagrammatic sketch representing the different nanotechnology applications.

in a variety of fields, including health care, military, controlling industrial processes, food control, environmental monitoring, as well as microbiology (including the study of bacteria and viruses, among other topics). Various researchers and scientists have come up with their own definitions of the term "bio-sensor" (Nie et al., 2014).

An analytical electronic device known as a biosensor is one that generates an electronic signal through interactions between a receptor and an analyte target. A bioreceptor, also known as a biologically derived sensing element, is the primary component of a biosensor (Zhang et al., 2009). A bioreceptor is a component that is integrated into or closely linked to a physicochemical transducer. The production of a digital electronic signal by a biosensor, which is directly proportional to the concentration of the biomolecule targeted, is the primary objective of this type of sensor. As per the definition provided by the IUPAC, "a biosensor is a self-contained integrated device that is capable of providing specific quantitative or semi-quantitative analytical information using a biological recognition element (receptor) which is in direct spatial contact with a transducer element" (Parveen et al., 2012; Zhang et al., 2009). In 1962, Clark and Lyons were the first people to successfully fabricate an electrochemical biosensor. In order to determine the concentration of glucose, they immobilized molecules [glucose oxidase (GOD) enzyme] on the surface of an oxygen electrode (Parveen et al., 2012). Glucose is reduced to gluconic acid in the presence of GOD, which results in the release of two electrons and two protons and the conversion of glucose to gluconic acid (oxidized). Again, hydrogen peroxide and GOD are the products of a reaction involving electrons, protons, oxygen, and reduced GOD (oxidized). The amount of glucose can be used to determine whether or not there is a correlation between increased hydrogen peroxide and decreased oxygen content (Nie et al., 2014).

The desired analytes can be recognized by bioreceptor molecules found in a typical biosensor. These bioreceptor molecules can take the form of enzymes, oligonucleotides, cells, antibodies, and so on. The interaction of bioreceptor molecules with target analytes triggers the activation of a transducer, which then transforms a biochemical signal into an electrical signal. This is an essential component of the detection system. The strength of the signal that is produced can be proportional to the analyte concentration of interest either directly or inversely. Electric potential, electric current, the intensity as well as phase of electromagnetic radiations, viscosity, temperature, impedance, conductance, as well as mass are some instances of the elements that could make up a transducer (Nie et al., 2014).

With the assistance of a microcontroller, the output signal that is produced by a transducer can be converted into a digital format by a signal-conditioning circuit and then displayed in real time on a liquid crystal display monitor. Biosensors can be broken down into three different generations. Oxygen is a prerequisite for the operation of the first generation of biosensors, which includes the electrode that was proposed by Clark in 1962 (Singh et al., 2022b; Singh and Singh, 2022). In this scenario, the product that is produced as a result of the reaction has the potential to diffuse to the transducer, which will result in a signal (electrical). The biosensors of the second generation do not need oxygen to function, but they do require a particular mediator to be placed in between the reaction and the transducer in order to improve the response signal. The response signal can be caused by the reaction itself in biosensors of the third generation, meaning that a mediator is no longer directly involved in the process. Any intermediate electron transfer (ET) reactions with redox species are ruled out when direct ET occurs between the electrode and biomolecules.

3.7 IMAGING AND DIAGNOSIS FACILITATED BY NANOTECHNOLOGY

The process of diagnosing a disease is one of the most important steps involved in providing medical care. In order to reduce the number of instances of a 'false negative,' it is essential that all diagnoses be completed rapidly while maintaining accuracy and specificity. In vivo imaging is a method that does not require the patient to go through surgery in order to diagnose any signs or symptoms that may be present within the patient's living tissues (Medina et al., 2007). Utilizing biological markers that are able to detect variations in the tissues at the cellular level is one of the previous improvements that have been made to diagnostic imaging techniques. The use of a biological marker as an early detection tool has as its primary purpose: the diagnosis of disease or the identification of symptoms (Ratner and Bryant, 2004). It is important to note that several high-precision molecular imaging agents will be developed with the help of nanotechnology. Imaging is essential not only for the purpose of diagnosis but also for the research of controlled drug release, the assessment of drug circulation inside the human body, and the close checking of the development of a remedy. Imaging plays a role in all of these areas. The possibility of observing the drug's distribution throughout the human body as well as releasing the medicine as needed both contribute to the possibility of reducing the potential toxicity of drugs (Sakiyama-Elbert and Hubbell, 2001).

3.8 UTILIZATION OF NANOTECHNOLOGY IN THE DELIVERY OF DRUGS

In clinical practice, treatment involves administering drugs to a designated target area (Tian et al., 2017). In the event that an internal path for the distribution of drugs is not feasible, alternative therapeutic approaches, like surgical procedures as well as radiotherapy, may be utilized instead. In the fight against disease, these approaches are frequently interchanged with one another or used in tandem. The purpose of treatment is to permanently and selectively eliminate the tumors or other causes of illness. This must be done in order for the treatment to be considered successful (Ochekpe et al., 2009). Nanotechnology is making a significant role in this field through the development of novel methods for the delivery of drugs; some of these methods have been demonstrated to be effective in a clinical environment and are currently being utilized in clinical practice (Singh et al., 2022b; Singh and Singh, 2022). For instance, the drug doxorubicin, which has a high level of toxicity, can be directly delivered to tumor cells through the use of liposomes (Doxil) without having an effect on the heart or the kidneys. In addition, the chemotherapeutic treatment of metastatic breast cancers often involves the use of paclitaxel, which has been combined with polymeric methoxy poly(ethylene glycol)-poly(lactide) (mPEG-PLA) micelles under the brand name Genexol-PM (Lombardo et al., 2019; Ochekpe et al., 2009). The improved *in vivo* distribution, pharmacokinetic properties that are favorable, and evasion of the reticuloendothelial system are all factors that have contributed to the success of nanotechnologies in the field of drug delivery (Ochekpe et al., 2009).

Control over the drug release and the ability to precisely target the drug's destination are both essential components of the ideal drug delivery system. By selectively targeting and destroying cancerous or harmful cells, it is possible to significantly reduce the severity of side effects while also ensuring the efficacy of the drug. In addition to this, controlled drug release is an effective method for minimizing the negative effects of drug use (Jain et al., 2009). Nanoparticle drug delivery systems have a number of advantages, including reduced irritant reactions and enhanced body penetration, thanks to their diminutive size. These advantages make intravenous administration, as well as other delivery methods, possible. These techniques have led to favorable outcomes, including enhanced bioavailability of the drug, targeted drug distribution to the specific site, as well as low-solubility medication uptake (Jain et al., 2011; Kakani et al., 2003).

3.9 DIAGNOSTIC IMAGING

Imaging methods that have been around for a long time and are reliable include X-ray, computed tomography, ultrasound, nuclear medicine, as well as MRI. These imaging methods are utilized extensively in therapeutic as well as biochemical research

(Hachani et al., 2017). Nevertheless, these methods may only examine the changes on the surface of tissue relatively late in the disease progression, despite the fact that they may be improved via the use of targeting as well as contrast agents based on the use of nanotechnologies, which can improve the specificity as well as resolution by indicating the site of disease at the cellular level (Kolouchova et al., 2018). The majority of contrast agents used in modern medical imaging are small molecules, and because of their rapid metabolism and non-specific distribution, they have the potential to cause toxic side effects that are unfavorable and undesirable (Mitchell et al., 2021). The most significant contribution that nanotechnologies have made to the realm of medicine is in this particular area. They accomplish this by strengthening existing contrast agents for virtually all imaging methods. This is made possible by the fact that NMs display lower toxicity, as well as retention effects, and improved permeability in tissues. Bio-distribution, cellular uptake, blood circulation half-life, tissue penetration, as well as targeting are all significantly impacted by the NPs' size (Lanone and Boczkowski, 2006; Wickline and Lanza, 2003).

There are some restrictions placed on the utilization of NPs in X-ray imaging. It is necessary to transport several numbers of heavy atoms into the specific target location without triggering any toxic chemical reactions in order to achieve the desired enhancement of contrast. This can be accomplished by using surface atoms that are stable and unreactive, such as silver (Ag) as well as gold (Au). Because of this, Au nanoshells have attracted a lot of attention due to the fact that they are relatively nontoxic (Mani et al., 2017). Heavy metal NPs with a dielectric core that is encased in Au shells have been recommended as one of the greatest promising materials for optical imaging in several diseases. Au nanoshells are made up of heavy metal NPs (Choi et al., 2007). Gold nanoshells have a low cost, are risk-free because of their noninvasive nature, and have the potential to provide high-resolution imaging. The unified response (electronic) of the metal to the light that results in active optical absorption is present in both gold nanoshells and gold colloids, which is one of the physical characteristics that gold nanoshells and gold colloids share (Abbasi et al., 2017; Choi et al., 2007). Researchers use gold nanoshells extensively as contrast agents in the Optical Coherence Tomography (OCT) of a diseased cell. This is due to the fact that the optical resonance of Au nanoshells can be accurately adjusted over a wide range of frequencies, containing the near-infrared, which is a region of the spectrum in which tissue transmissivity is on the higher side (Abbasi et al., 2017). Understanding and predicting the effects of these NM when they are introduced into biological systems will require a substantial amount of additional research and pre-clinical testing.

3.10 UTILIZATION OF NANOTECHNOLOGIES IN THE TREATMENT OF CARDIOVASCULAR CONDITIONS

Another area that could potentially benefit from utilizing the properties of NPs is that of cardiovascular diseases. Because more people are leading sedentary lifestyles, cardiovascular diseases have become the leading cause of death worldwide. The incidence of these diseases is also rising at an alarming rate (McGill et al., 2008). Stroke, hypertension, and conditions in which blood flow is restricted or blocked in a particular region are all examples of common cardiovascular diseases that can affect multiple people at the same time. These diseases account for the majority of cases of extended incapacity as well as fatalities (Kumar et al., 2022a, b; McGill et al., 2008). New potential medical as well as diagnostic approaches for the management of cardiac diseases can be opened up through the use of nanotechnologies.

The majority of the threat factors for cardiovascular diseases, like smoking, hypertension, hypercholesterolemia, diabetes mellitus, and homocystinuria, are related to impaired production of nitric oxide (NO) by endothelial cells. It has been established that the first step in the development of atherosclerosis is dysfunction in endothelial function. The supply of NO has been improved using gold and silica NPs, which have been developed for possible application in the treatment of cardiovascular diseases, which are characterized by low NO bioavailability (Balaji et al., 2009; Deshpande et al., 2008, 2016). It has been demonstrated that systemic delivery of the 17-E-loaded Cys-Arg-Glu-Lys-Ala (CREKA) peptide-modified nano emulsion system lowers levels of pathogenic precursors to early atherosclerosis. This is accomplished by reducing the size of the atherosclerotic lesion, lowering the circulating plasma lipids levels, and lowering the expression of genes of inflammatory markers that are related to the infection. In addition, it has been demonstrated that new preparations of block copolymer micelles that are designed using propylene sulfide as well as PEG can suppress the pro-inflammatory cytokines levels, and these formulations have shown tremendous potential for the atherosclerosis management (Deshpande et al., 2016; Wu et al., 2018).

It has been demonstrated that administering a drug inside liposomes is an efficient method for preventing platelet aggregation, as well as atherosclerosis and thrombosis. PGE-1, also known as prostaglandin E-1, has a wide variety of pharmacological effects, such as platelet aggregation inhibition, leukocyte adhesion, as well as vasodilation, and then, it also has an anti-inflammatory effect. These are just some of its properties. Clinical trials (phase III) for treating various cardiovascular diseases, along with restenosis followed by angioplasty, are currently being conducted using liposomal drug delivery of PGE-1 (Liprostin) (Bulbake et al., 2017). The use of liposomes containing the thrombolytic medication urokinase has also been studied; urokinase-encapsulated cyclic arginylglycylaspartic acid (cRGD) peptide liposomes can specifically attach to a glycoprotein IIb/IIIa (GPIIb/IIIa) receptor, increasing their thrombolytic potency by almost four-fold (Bulbake et al., 2017).

Conventional thrombolytic drugs have the potential to see improvements in their efficacy and effectiveness through the use of innovative nano-therapeutic approaches. Because of the high fluid shear strains that are present within blood vessels, it is possible for medications to be selectively directed to blockage (vascular) sites by utilizing mechanical activation inside the blood vessels. Interestingly, the results of *in vitro* as well as *in vivo* analysis have been promising, which validates this method for usage in blood clots lysis, requiring a significantly lower quantity of thrombolytic medication than is typically required (Deshpande et al., 2008, 2016; Wu et al., 2018). Dendrimers are an application of this technology that serve as an example. In order to facilitate the delivery of therapeutic agents in the treatment of a number of diseases, dendrimers have been utilized. An alternate medication delivery mechanism has been created by successfully attaching dendrimers to plasminogen activator (PA). This allows for the concentration of the complex (dendrimer-PA) to be fine-tuned throughout the course of disease treatment by adjusting the dilution proportions of each part of the complex in varying amounts (Najlah et al., 2007). One additional possible use for NPs is in the prevention of hemorrhaging, which is a serious risk associated with the use of thrombolytic drugs. Targeted thrombolysis with PA is bound to the polyacrylic acid (PAA) coated NPs, which reduces the amount of bleeding that occurs inside the brain and increases the drug's capacity to remain at the location where it was intended to be used (Ference et al., 2017; Katsuki et al., 2017; Kumar et al., 2022b). Incorporating nanotechnologies has helped reduce the adverse effects of medications while, at the same time, allowing for lower doses of those medications to be used in the treatment of cardiovascular diseases.

3.11 NANOTECHNOLOGY'S STRUGGLES AND OPPORTUNITIES

Soon after the nanostructures in the earliest meteorites were discovered, there was a surge of interest in the field of NM. In 1857, Michael Faraday was the first person to report successfully synthesizing gold NPs. 1940 marked the beginning of the synthesis and commercialization of fumed silica NPs in the United States of America. At a meeting of American Physical Society in 1959 that was held at Caltech, an American physicist named Richard Feynman made the statement, "there is plenty of room at the bottom," which served as an inspiration for the development of nanotechnology (Iavicoli et al., 2014). In the year 1960, metallic nano powders were created specifically for use in magnetic recording tapes. A Japanese researcher coined the term "nanotechnology" during a conference that took place in 1974 (Iavicoli et al., 2014). He was attempting to explain the process of semiconductor thin-film deposition as well as ion beam milling, both of which showed a specific control on the nanometer scale. He defined "nanotechnology" as the process of dividing and deforming materials on the scale of a single atom or molecule, which he said was the essence of the term. Granqvist and Buhrman published their method for producing nanocrystals using inert gas evaporation in 1976. This was the first time that nano crystals had been created. In 1981, Eric Drexler published his first article (a research paper) on the topic of nanotechnology. He was the first person to use the term "nanotechnology." The concept that Eric Drexler had in mind is commonly referred to as "molecular manufacturing" or "molecular nanotechnology" (Cheng et al., 2016). In the early 1980s, the field of nanotechnology was given a push forward, thanks to the invention of two significant pieces of machinery, namely the scanning tunneling microscope and cluster science. The subsequent developments led to the discovery of fullerenes in the year 1985, and a few years later, it was reported that "carbon nanotubes" had been synthesized. Fullerenes were discovered as a result of these developments (Palmerston Mendes et al., 2017; Patra et al., 2018).

The term "nanomaterial" refers to a group of substances that each has at least one dimension that is either 1–100 nm or less than 100 nm. One nanometer is equal to one-millionth of a millimeter, which is approximately one hundred thousand times smaller than the diameter of a human hair. There are naturally occurring instances of certain NM. NM have the potential to be engineered for a variety of applications, and they are already being utilized in a variety of commercial products and processes. NM are distinguished by the presence of characteristics that have not been seen before.

3.12 CONCLUSION

Because they serve as a foundation for developments in the biotechnology, medicinal, and pharmaceutical industries, nanotechnologies have, without a shadow of a doubt, made a contribution to an improvement in the standard of living of patients. They have also made the processes involved in healthcare more manageable from therapeutic to diagnosis interventions and monitoring of follow-up care. With the final goal of creating medical practices that are more individualized, cost-effective, as well as secure, there is a persistent thrust to make as well as develop novel NPs to improve the diagnosis as well as treatments of disease in a manner that is accurate, targeted, long-lasting, and potent. Researchers have conducted an extensive investigation into the potential applications of NMs in biosensor technology for the point-of-care settings. The use of NMs in biosensors results in significant improvements to the characteristics of the biosensors like selectivity, rapid response, sensitivity, as well as cost. Utilizing appropriate NM while mitigating the risk of any adverse effects is essential to realizing the full potential of nanotechnology. As is the case with the approval of any other product, new nano-based products must first undergo risk assessments before they can be used in clinical and commercial settings. This is done with the goal of reducing the number of potential dangers to both human health and the natural environment. To determine the viability and safety of their use over the long term with a greater degree of precision, a comprehensive life cycle analysis is required.

REFERENCES

Abbasi, A., Park, K., Bose, A., Bothun, G.D., 2017. Near-Infrared Responsive Gold–Layersome Nanoshells. *Langmuir* 33, 5321–5327. https://doi.org/10.1021/acs.langmuir.7b01273

Acharya, S., Sahoo, S.K., 2011. PLGA Nanoparticles Containing Various Anticancer Agents and Tumour Delivery by EPR Effect. *Adv. Drug Deliv. Rev.* 63, 170–183. https://doi.org/10.1016/j.addr.2010.10.008

Allhoff, F., 2010. *What is Nanotechnology and Why Does It Matter?: From Science to Ethics.* Wiley-Blackwell, Hoboken, NJ.

Balaji, D.S., Basavaraja, S., Deshpande, R., Mahesh, D.B., Prabhakar, B.K., Venkataraman, A., 2009. Extracellular Biosynthesis of Functionalized Silver Nanoparticles by Strains of *Cladosporium cladosporioides* Fungus. *Colloids Surf. B Biointerfaces* 68, 88–92. https://doi.org/10.1016/j.colsurfb.2008.09.022

Belkin, A., Hubler, A., Bezryadin, A., 2015. Self-Assembled Wiggling Nano-Structures and the Principle of Maximum Entropy Production. *Sci. Rep.* 5, 8323. https://doi.org/10.1038/srep08323

Bera, D., Qian, L., Tseng, T.-K., Holloway, P.H., 2010. Quantum Dots and Their Multimodal Applications: A Review. *Materials* 3, 2260–2345. https://doi.org/10.3390/ma3042260

Bulbake, U., Doppalapudi, S., Kommineni, N., Khan, W., 2017. Liposomal Formulations in Clinical Use: An Updated Review. *Pharmaceutics* 9, 12. https://doi.org/10.3390/pharmaceutics9020012

Cheng, H.N., Doemeny, L.J., Geraci, C.L., Grob Schmidt, D., 2016. Nanotechnology Overview: Opportunities and Challenges, in: Cheng, H. N., Doemeny, L., Geraci, C. L., Grob Schmidt, D. (Eds.), *ACS Symposium Series.* American Chemical Society, Washington, DC, pp. 1–12. https://doi.org/10.1021/bk-2016-1220.ch001

Choi, M.-R., Stanton-Maxey, K.J., Stanley, J.K., Levin, C.S., Bardhan, R., Akin, D., Badve, S., Sturgis, J., Robinson, J.P., Bashir, R., Halas, N.J., Clare, S.E., 2007. A Cellular Trojan Horse for Delivery of Therapeutic Nanoparticles into Tumors. *Nano Lett.* 7, 3759–3765. https://doi.org/10.1021/nl072209h

Das, R., Deb, P., Pandey, H., Shyam, P., Singh, D., 2022. Botanical Synthesis of Silver Nanoparticles (AgNPs) and Its Antifungal Effect against *Alternaria porri* Causing Purple Blotch of Onion: An *in vitro* and Natural Epiphytic Study. *J. Agric. Food Res.* 10, 100390. https://doi.org/10.1016/j.jafr.2022.100390

Deshpande, A.D., Harris-Hayes, M., Schootman, M., 2008. Epidemiology of Diabetes and Diabetes-Related Complications. *Phys. Ther.* 88, 1254–1264. https://doi.org/10.2522/ptj.20080020

Deshpande, D., Kethireddy, S., Janero, D.R., Amiji, M.M., 2016. Therapeutic Efficacy of an ω-3-Fatty Acid-Containing 17-β Estradiol Nano-Delivery System against Experimental Atherosclerosis. *PLoS One* 11, e0147337. https://doi.org/10.1371/journal.pone.0147337

Drexler, K.E., 1992. Nanosystems: Molecular Machinery, Manufacturing, and Computation | Wiley [WWW Document]. Wiley.com. URL https://www.wiley.com/en-us/Nanosystems%3A+Molecular+Machinery%2C+Manufacturing%2C+and+Computation-p-9780471575184 (accessed 12.26.22).

Ference, B.A., Ginsberg, H.N., Graham, I., Ray, K.K., Packard, C.J., Bruckert, E., Hegele, R.A., Krauss, R.M., Raal, F.J., Schunkert, H., Watts, G.F., Borén, J., Fazio, S., Horton, J.D., Masana, L., Nicholls, S.J., Nordestgaard, B.G., van de Sluis, B., Taskinen, M.-R., Tokgözoğlu, L., Landmesser, U., Laufs, U., Wiklund, O., Stock, J.K., Chapman, M.J., Catapano, A.L., 2017. Low-Density Lipoproteins Cause Atherosclerotic Cardiovascular Disease. 1. Evidence from Genetic, Epidemiologic, and Clinical Studies. A Consensus Statement from the European Atherosclerosis Society Consensus Panel. *Eur. Heart J.* 38, 2459–2472. https://doi.org/10.1093/eurheartj/ehx144

Hachani, R., Birchall, M.A., Lowdell, M.W., Kasparis, G., Tung, L.D., Manshian, B.B., Soenen, S.J., Gsell, W., Himmelreich, U., Gharagouzloo, C.A., Sridhar, S., Thanh, N.T.K., 2017. Assessing Cell-Nanoparticle Interactions by High Content Imaging of Biocompatible Iron Oxide Nanoparticles as Potential Contrast Agents for Magnetic Resonance Imaging. *Sci. Rep.* 7, 7850. https://doi.org/10.1038/s41598-017-08092-w

Han, X., Xu, K., Taratula, O., Farsad, K., 2019. Applications of Nanoparticles in Biomedical Imaging. *Nanoscale* 11, 799–819. https://doi.org/10.1039/c8nr07769j

Iavicoli, I., Leso, V., Ricciardi, W., Hodson, L.L., Hoover, M.D., 2014. Opportunities and Challenges of Nanotechnology in the Green Economy. *Environ. Health Glob. Access Sci. Source* 13, 78. https://doi.org/10.1186/1476-069X-13-78

Jain, D., Daima, H.K., Kachhwaha, S., Kothari, S.L., 2009. Synthesis of Plant-Mediated Silver Nanoparticles Using Papaya Fruit Extract and Evaluation of their Anti Microbial Activities. *Dig. J. Nanomater. Biostructures* 4(3), 557–563.

Jain, N., Bhargava, A., Majumdar, S., Tarafdar, J.C., Panwar, J., 2011. Extracellular Biosynthesis and Characterization of Silver Nanoparticles Using *Aspergillus flavus* NJP08: A Mechanism Perspective. *Nanoscale* 3, 635–641. https://doi.org/10.1039/c0nr00656d

Kakani, V.G., Reddy, K.R., Zhao, D., Sailaja, K., 2003. Field Crop Responses to Ultraviolet-B Radiation: A Review. *Agric. For. Meteorol.* 120, 191–218. https://doi.org/10.1016/j.agrformet.2003.08.015

Katsuki, S., Matoba, T., Koga, J., Nakano, K., Egashira, K., 2017. Anti-Inflammatory Nanomedicine for Cardiovascular Disease. *Front. Cardiovasc. Med.* 4, 87. https://doi.org/10.3389/fcvm.2017.00087

Kolouchova, K., Sedlacek, O., Jirak, D., Babuka, D., Blahut, J., Kotek, J., Vit, M., Trousil, J., Konefał, R., Janouskova, O., Podhorska, B., Slouf, M., Hruby, M., 2018. Self-Assembled Thermoresponsive Polymeric Nanogels for 19 F MR Imaging. *Biomacromolecules* 19, 3515–3524. https://doi.org/10.1021/acs.biomac.8b00812

Kumar, P., Rai, S., Verma, S.K., Prakash, P.S., Chitara, D., 2022a. Classification, Mode of Action and Uses of Various Immunomodulators, in: Kesharwani, R. K., Keservani, R. K., Sharma, A. K. (Eds.), *Immunomodulators and Human Health*. Springer Nature Singapore, Singapore, pp. 3–38. https://doi.org/10.1007/978-981-16-6379-6_1

Kumar, P., Verma, S.K., 2022. Entrepreneurial Opportunities in Bioenergy, in: Rathoure, A. K., Khade, S. M. (Eds.), *Advances in Environmental Engineering and Green Technologies*. IGI Global, pp. 32–43. https://doi.org/10.4018/978-1-6684-5269-1.ch003

Kumar, P., Verma, S.K., Rai, S., Prakash, P.S., Chitara, D., 2022b. Role of Homocysteine Metabolism in Cardiovascular Diseases, in: Dubey, G.P., Misra, K., Kesharwani, R.K., Ojha, R.P. (Eds.), *Homocysteine Metabolism in Health and Disease*. Springer Nature Singapore, Singapore, pp. 257–276. https://doi.org/10.1007/978-981-16-6867-8_14

Lanone, S., Boczkowski, J., 2006. Biomedical Applications and Potential Health Risks of Nanomaterials: Molecular Mechanisms. *Curr. Mol. Med.* 6, 651–663. https://doi.org/10.2174/156652406778195026

Lombardo, D., Kiselev, M.A., Caccamo, M.T., 2019. Smart Nanoparticles for Drug Delivery Application: Development of Versatile Nanocarrier Platforms in Biotechnology and Nanomedicine. *J. Nanomater.* 2019, 3702518. https://doi.org/10.1155/2019/3702518

Mani, P., Sharma, H., Gautam, A., Singh, T., Verma, S., Hussain, R., 2017. Hydroxyapatite (HA) Attenuate TiO2 Toxicity in Bio-System Triggering *E. coli* and Mouse Bone Marrow Mono-Nuclear Cells (BMMNC's). *Int. J. Life Sci. Pharma Res.* 7, 46–57.

McGill, H.C., McMahan, C.A., Gidding, S.S., 2008. Preventing Heart Disease in the 21st century: Implications of the Pathobiological Determinants of Atherosclerosis in Youth (PDAY) Study. *Circulation* 117, 1216–1227. https://doi.org/10.1161/CIRCULATIONAHA.107.717033

Medina, C., Santos-Martinez, M.J., Radomski, A., Corrigan, O.I., Radomski, M.W., 2007. Nanoparticles: Pharmacological and Toxicological Significance: Nanoparticles. *Br. J. Pharmacol.* 150, 552–558. https://doi.org/10.1038/sj.bjp.0707130

Mitchell, M.J., Billingsley, M.M., Haley, R.M., Wechsler, M.E., Peppas, N.A., Langer, R., 2021. Engineering Precision Nanoparticles for Drug Delivery. *Nat. Rev. Drug Discov.* 20, 101–124. https://doi.org/10.1038/s41573-020-0090-8

Mohanty, S.K., Swamy, M.K., Sinniah, U.R., Anuradha, M., 2017. *Leptadenia reticulata* (Retz.) Wight & Arn. (Jivanti): Botanical, Agronomical, Phytochemical, Pharmacological, and Biotechnological Aspects. *Molecules* 22, 1019. https://doi.org/10.3390/molecules22061019

Morgan, M.T., Carnahan, M.A., Finkelstein, S., Prata, C.A.H., Degoricija, L., Lee, S.J., Grinstaff, M.W., 2005. Dendritic Supramolecular Assemblies for Drug Delivery. *Chem. Commun.* 4309–4311. https://doi.org/10.1039/B502411K

Najlah, M., Freeman, S., Attwood, D., D'Emanuele, A., 2007. In Vitro Evaluation of Dendrimer Prodrugs for Oral Drug Delivery. *Int. J. Pharm.* 336, 183–190. https://doi.org/10.1016/j.ijpharm.2006.11.047

Nie, L., Liu, F., Ma, P., Xiao, X., 2014. Applications of Gold Nanoparticles in Optical Biosensors. *J. Biomed. Nanotechnol.* 10, 2700–2721. https://doi.org/10.1166/jbn.2014.1987

Nune, S.K., Gunda, P., Thallapally, P.K., Lin, Y.-Y., Forrest, M.L., Berkland, C.J., 2009. Nanoparticles for Biomedical Imaging. *Expert Opin. Drug Deliv.* 6, 1175–1194. https://doi.org/10.1517/17425240903229031

Ochekpe, N.A., Olorunfemi, P.O., Ngwuluka, N.C., 2009. Nanotechnology and Drug Delivery Part 1: Background and Applications. *Trop. J. Pharm. Res.* 8. https://doi.org/10.4314/tjpr.v8i3.44546

Palmerston Mendes, L., Pan, J., Torchilin, V.P., 2017. Dendrimers as Nanocarriers for Nucleic Acid and Drug Delivery in Cancer Therapy. *Molecules* 22, 1401. https://doi.org/10.3390/molecules22091401

Parveen, S., Misra, R., Sahoo, S.K., 2012. Nanoparticles: A Boon to Drug Delivery, Therapeutics, Diagnostics and Imaging. *Nanomed. Nanotechnol. Biol. Med.* 8, 147–166. https://doi.org/10.1016/j.nano.2011.05.016

Patra, J.K., Das, G., Fraceto, L.F., Campos, E.V.R., Rodriguez-Torres, M. del P., Acosta-Torres, L.S., Diaz-Torres, L.A., Grillo, R., Swamy, M.K., Sharma, S., Habtemariam, S., Shin, H.-S., 2018. Nano Based Drug Delivery Systems: Recent Developments and Future Prospects. *J. Nanobiotechnol.* 16, 71. https://doi.org/10.1186/s12951-018-0392-8

Probst, C.E., Zrazhevskiy, P., Bagalkot, V., Gao, X., 2013. Quantum Dots as a Platform for Nanoparticle Drug Delivery Vehicle Design. *Adv. Drug Deliv. Rev.* 65, 703–718. https://doi.org/10.1016/j.addr.2012.09.036

Ramalingam, G., Kathirgamanathan, P., Ravi, G., Elangovan, T., Kumar, B.A., Manivannan, N., Kasinathan, K., Ramalingam, G., Kathirgamanathan, P., Ravi, G., Elangovan, T., Kumar, B.A., Manivannan, N., Kasinathan, K., 2020. *Quantum Confinement Effect of 2D Nanomaterials, Quantum Dots - Fundamental and Applications*. IntechOpen. https://doi.org/10.5772/intechopen.90140

Ratner, B.D., Bryant, S.J., 2004. Biomaterials: Where We Have Been and Where We Are Going. *Annu. Rev. Biomed. Eng.* 6, 41–75. https://doi.org/10.1146/annurev.bioeng.6.040803.140027

Rezaei, R., Safaei, M., Mozaffari, H.R., Moradpoor, H., Karami, S., Golshah, A., Salimi, B., Karami, H., 2019. The Role of Nanomaterials in the Treatment of Diseases and Their Effects on the Immune System. *Open Access Maced. J. Med. Sci.* 7, 1884–1890. https://pmc.ncbi.nlm.nih.gov/articles/PMC6614262/

Rodrigues, T., Reker, D., Schneider, P., Schneider, G., 2016. Counting on Natural Products for Drug Design. *Nat. Chem.* 8, 531–541. https://doi.org/10.1038/nchem.2479

Sakiyama-Elbert, S., Hubbell, J., 2001. Functional Biomaterials: Design of Novel Biomaterials. *Annu. Rev. Mater. Res.* 31, 183–201. https://doi.org/10.1146/annurev.matsci.31.1.183

Shi Kam, N.W., Jessop, T.C., Wender, P.A., Dai, H., 2004. Nanotube Molecular Transporters: Internalization of Carbon Nanotube−Protein Conjugates into Mammalian Cells. *J. Am. Chem. Soc.* 126, 6850–6851. https://doi.org/10.1021/ja0486059

Sim, S., Wong, N., 2021. Nanotechnology and Its Use in Imaging and Drug Delivery (Review). *Biomed. Rep.* 14, 42. https://doi.org/10.3892/br.2021.1418

Singh, D., Pandey, H., Shrivastava, N.K., Das, R., Singh, V., 2022a. Green Synthesized Gold and Silver Nanoparticles for Antimicrobial Applications, in: Baskar, C., Ramakrishna, S., Daniela La Rosa, A. (Eds.), *Encyclopedia of Green Materials*. Springer Nature Singapore, Singapore, pp. 1–12. https://doi.org/10.1007/978-981-16-4921-9_254-1

Singh, V., Pandey, H., Misra, V., Tiwari, V., Srivastava, P., Singh, D., 2022b. Hypolipidemic Effect of [6]-Gingerol-Loaded Eudragit Polymeric Nanoparticles in High-Fat Diet-Induced Rats and Gamma Scintigraphy Evaluation of Gastric-Retention Time. *J. Appl. Pharm. Sci.* 156–163. https://doi.org/10.7324/JAPS.2022.120615

Singh, Virendra & Pandey, Himanshu & Misra, Vatsala & Singh, Devendra. (2022). Biocompatible Herbal Polymeric Nano-formulation of [6]-Gingerol: Development, Optimisation, and Characterization. *Ecology, Environment and Conservation.* 1473–1477. https://doi.org/10.53550/EEC.2022.v28i03.052.

Sumanth Kumar, D., Jai Kumar, B., Mahesh, H.M., 2018. *Quantum Nanostructures (QDs): An Overview*. Elsevier, pp. 59–88. https://doi.org/10.1016/B978-0-08-101975-7.00003-8

Swamy, K.N., Rao, S.S.R., 2011. Effect of Brassinosteroids on the Performance of Coleus (*Coleus forskohlii*). *J. Herbs Spices Med. Plants* 17, 12–20. https://doi.org/10.1080/10496475.2011.556985

Tian, T., Zhang, T., Zhou, T., Lin, S., Shi, S., Lin, Y., 2017. Synthesis of an Ethyleneimine/Tetrahedral DNA Nanostructure Complex and Its Potential Application as a Multi-Functional Delivery Vehicle. *Nanoscale* 9, 18402–18412. https://doi.org/10.1039/C7NR07130B

Tiriveedhi, V., Kitchens, K.M., Nevels, K.J., Ghandehari, H., Butko, P., 2011. Kinetic Analysis of the Interaction between Poly(Amidoamine) Dendrimers and Model Lipid Membranes. *Biochim. Biophys. Acta BBA - Biomembr.* 1808, 209–218. https://doi.org/10.1016/j.bbamem.2010.08.017

Verma, S.K., Dubey, D.A., Verma, R.K., 2023. Recent Advancements in Skin Tissue Engineering in the Application of Nanotechnology. *Res. J. Biotechnol.* 18, 127–136. https://doi.org/10.25303/1802rjbt1270136

Wickline, S.A., Lanza, G.M., 2003. Nanotechnology for Molecular Imaging and Targeted Therapy. *Circulation* 107, 1092–1095. https://doi.org/10.1161/01.CIR.0000059651.17045.77

Wu, T., Chen, X., Wang, Y., Xiao, H., Peng, Y., Lin, L., Xia, W., Long, M., Tao, J., Shuai, X., 2018. Aortic Plaque-Targeted Andrographolide Delivery with Oxidation-Sensitive Micelle Effectively Treats Atherosclerosis via Simultaneous ROS Capture and Anti-Inflammation. *Nanomed. Nanotechnol. Biol. Med.* 14, 2215–2226. https://doi.org/10.1016/j.nano.2018.06.010

Zhang, X., Guo, Q., Cui, D., 2009. Recent Advances in Nanotechnology Applied to Biosensors. *Sensors* 9, 1033–1053. https://doi.org/10.3390/s90201033

4 Synthesis, Characterization, and Application of Nanomaterials in Cancer Theranostics

Samiddha Banerjee, Piyali Das, and Suman Deb

4.1 INTRODUCTION

Cancer is still one of the most lethal diseases in the world near the completion of the second decade of the 21st century. Cancer is a serious life-threatening disease despite the vast array of chemotherapeutic drugs and therapeutic strategies that are employed in treatment procedures. The anticancer treatments that have evolved over the years, such as radiation, chemotherapy, and tumor removal surgery, have not been able to completely eradicate the illness. Besides that, conventional anticancer therapies have serious adverse reactions and can affect the patient's life (Davis et al., 2008; García-Pinel et al., 2019). The major causes behind the lack of effective cancer diagnosis and therapy include biological hurdles such as genetic abnormalities, blood–brain barriers (BBBs), and endothelial cell barriers. The fundamental challenges in converting any anticancer strategy into a therapeutic platform are the pharmacological hurdles, such as restricted biodistribution, perfusion, toxic effects, absorption, and functional impairment.

Early diagnosis, tailored drug delivery, drug discovery, and effective anticancer therapy are all possible with the application of nanotechnology-based techniques and nanomaterials in cancer treatment (Amendola and Meneghetti, 2009). For instance, gold nanoparticles (AuNPs) have been widely used as drug transportation systems for treating prostate and breast malignancies. Due to its dependable qualities, such as its ability to scatter and capture light as well as transform optical energy into heat, AuNPs are taken into consideration. The entire capability of nanomaterials in cancer, however, may be constrained by the recently discovered nanotoxicity of several kinds of nanomaterials, which may encourage off-target reactions and bioaccumulation of metal-based NPs. In order to apply diverse types of NPs with the convenience of detection and focused treatment, it is necessary to create and optimize smart ways to reduce their hazardous effects.

DOI: 10.1201/9781003432661-4

Nanotechnology has created a huge impact in today's world. The unique physical and chemical characteristics of NPs have led to their application in different fields, especially in cancer therapeutics. Nanodrugs are of great valuation to scientists as a tool for cancer therapy. Due to the shape, size, diameter, and other physical properties of NPs, they are being used in cancer theragnostics like chemotherapy, radiation therapy, and photothermal therapy as well. Nanomaterials demonstrate great importance for imaging and diagnosis of cancer since they exhibit good cellular uptake, prolonged circulation time, and site specificity as a drug carrier for targeted drug delivery. Moreover, having a higher surface area, i.e., a high surface-to-volume ratio, nanomaterials can load numerous drugs that can be delivered to the target; they possess enhanced permeability and huge retention effect. Hence, nanomaterial-based therapeutics are responsible for greater anticancer efficacy by reducing several other side effects. Nanotechnology is now widely used to diagnose and treat a wide range of illnesses, including several deadly ones like cardiovascular disease, cancer, diabetes, many bacterial infections, and also neurodegenerative diseases. The conventional therapeutic strategies give rise to several limitations due to which different research groups have focused on developing nanoscale agents, including liposomal NPs, metal NPs, viral NPs, protein NPs, and lipid NPs (García-Pinel et al., 2019). It is important to note that the smaller size of NPs, simplicity in fabrication, improved drug loading (due to the high surface-to-volume ratio), easy penetration capabilities, and improved retention inside the target tissue have significantly improved the diagnostics and therapeutics of various cancers.

Blended or complex platforms of hybrid nanostructures (HNCs) are the focus of advanced nanomedicine. Smart medicines can carry out fully regulated or on-demand therapies, diagnostics, and therapeutic surveillance by transporting and discharging chemotherapeutic agents and pharmaceuticals in response to external inputs (Tillotson et al., 2001). The characteristics of smart materials are transformed in the new stage of nanomedicine, promising better safety and excellent therapeutic outcomes in tailored cancer therapy over standard nanomedicine.

Physicians develop cancer treatment regimens based on the volume, phase, region, and severity of the malignant tumor. Cancer is treated with surgery, radiation, and chemotherapy, either individually or in conjunction with radiotherapy + chemotherapy programs. In pre-clinical circumstances, existing nanomedicines are typically employed as a monotherapy alternative. As a result, it is challenging to obtain high treatment efficacy throughout the advanced trials since monotherapies have only produced extremely few results in terms of utility and client classification. Hence, using nanotheranostics in improved nanomedicine offers various benefits: (i) effective vascular perfusion and permeability to drugs are provided by nanotheranostics; (ii) enhanced efficiency of HNC surface properties benefit from multicargo packing; (iii) physical energy selectively provided more payloads to the tumor microenvironment (TME); (iv) designed multimodality of nanomedicine response to remote triggers that are locally applied; and (v) this site-specific peripheral sensation provokes restricted chemotaxis. These components incorporate anticancer nanomedicine that is extremely innovative and powerful in targeted therapeutics. Thus, it is necessary to create and improve creative techniques to lessen the hazardous effects of various nanomaterial types so that the nanomaterials can be used conveniently for diagnostics and tailored distribution (Altissimo, 2010; Whitesides et al., 2001). This theory asserts that a number of nanomaterial-based cancer-targeting drugs have been developed by utilizing the features of the TME. Yet, there are still chances for further research into the susceptibility of nanotherapy to the TME, which may lead to advancements in palliative care in addition to diagnostics and treatment.

In this review, various nanomaterials, their characterization, synthesis, and application in cancer therapy are discussed. Types of NPs like lipid-based NPs (LBNPs), carbon-based NPs, metal-based NPs, polymer-based NPs, and dendrimers are highlighted in the study.

4.2 CHARACTERIZATION OF DIFFERENT TYPES OF NANOPARTICLES

4.2.1 Liposomes or Lipid-Based Nanoparticles

Liposomes are composed of natural or synthetic lipids and are used to encapsulate hydrophilic or hydrophobic drugs. They are capable of protecting drugs from degradation, increasing drug bioavailability, and targeting drugs to specific cells or tissues. LBNP importance lies in breast cancer therapy (García-Pinel et al., 2019).

LBNPs and liposomes both have pros and cons based on the specific application. Liposomes have a lower drug loading capacity, whereas LBNPs have a higher drug loading capacity (Table 4.1).

TABLE 4.1
Different Types of Nanoparticles

Types of Nanoparticles	Method of Synthesis	Application in Cancer Theranostics	References
Liposomes or LBNPs	Vapor deposition	Breast cancer	García-Pinel et al. (2019)
Polymer-based NPs and micelles	Electrochemical deposition	Tissue engineering, imaging and medication delivery, and solid tumors	Davis et al. (2008)
Dendrimers	Electrochemical deposition	Drug administration, imaging, and sensing	Mattheolabakis et al. (2012)
Metallic and magnetic NPs	Bottom-up method	Magnetic data storage, biomedical imaging, and drug delivery	
Metal oxide-based NPs	Bottom-up method	Electronics, catalysis, energy, and healthcare	Ealia and Saravanakumar (2017)

4.2.2 Polymer-Based Nanoparticles and Micelles

These are extended chains of polymer units that repeat. In order to create nanoscale particles with certain size and shape, polymer-based NPs are often created by synthesizing and altering polymers. They have a wide range of uses, including tissue engineering, imaging, and medication delivery. These particles have the benefit of being relatively small in size in comparison with other medications, which makes it very simple to target solid tumors (Davis et al., 2008).

Micelles, on the other hand, are self-assembling structures composed of amphiphilic polymers, which have both hydrophilic and hydrophobic components. In aqueous solutions, amphiphilic polymers can spontaneously form micelles with a hydrophobic core and a hydrophilic shell. Micelles can be used for drug delivery, as they can solubilize hydrophobic drugs and improve their bioavailability.

4.2.3 Dendrimers

These are highly branched, nanoscale macromolecules with a unique structure that consists of a central core, multiple branches (called dendrons), and a shell of functional end groups (Mattheolabakis et al., 2012). Drug administration, imaging, and sensing are just a few of the uses for dendrimers, which have a lot of special qualities. The size and shape of dendrimers allow for specific targeting and delivery of drugs or other agents. These are synthesized from biocompatible materials, which can reduce toxicity and improve biocompatibility for in vivo applications.

4.2.4 Carbon-Based Nanoparticles

Fullerenes, carbon nanotubes, graphene and its derivatives, graphene oxides, nano-diamonds, and carbon-based quantum dots are examples of carbon-based NPs.

4.2.5 Metallic and Magnetic Nanoparticles

Metallic NPs are particles made of metals that range in size from 1 to 100 nanometers (nm). Due to their small size and high surface area-to-volume ratio, they possess special qualities such as enhanced reactivity, optical characteristics, and mechanical properties. The combination of metallic and magnetic NPs has led to the development of a new class of materials known as magnetic metallic NPs. These materials have unique properties that can be exploited in various applications, such as magnetic data storage, biomedical imaging, and drug delivery.

4.2.6 Inorganic Nanoparticles

Non-carbon-based NPs are referred to as inorganic NPs, which are classified as those made of metal or metal oxide.

4.2.7 Metal-Based Nanoparticles

Metal-based NPs refer to NPs that are composed of one or more metals. These particles can be synthesized using a variety of methods, such as chemical reduction, electrochemical deposition, and laser ablation. AuNPs are used in imaging and diagnostic applications, as well as in drug delivery systems. Platinum NPs have catalytic properties and are used in chemical reactions. Silver NPs have antibacterial properties and are used in wound dressings and medical devices.

4.2.8 Metal Oxide-Based Nanoparticles

These NPs have unique properties due to their high surface area-to-volume ratio, which makes them appealing for a variety of applications. Some common metal oxide NPs include titanium dioxide (TiO_2) NPs, zinc oxide (ZnO) NPs, iron oxide (Fe_2O_3) NPs, aluminum oxide (Al_2O_3) NPs, and cerium oxide (CeO_2) NPs. There are numerous uses for metal oxide NPs in industries like electronics, catalysis, energy, and healthcare (Ealia and Saravanakumar, 2017).

A number of distinctive nanodrugs have been identified, researched, and are currently undergoing clinical practice. Free pharmaceuticals will now assist in the eradication of many forms of carcinoma as further advancements in research lead to the dominance of nanomedicine over current treatment alternatives (Markman et al., 2013).

4.3 SYNTHESIS

4.3.1 Bottom-Up Method

The size and shape of the final NPs are determined by the chemical reaction circumstances. This is the process of creating nanomaterials from individual atoms and molecules in which they are mixed to generate nanoscale structures. The following are the various sorts of bottom-up methods.

4.3.1.1 Sol–Gel Method

To create a gel, metal alkoxides or metal salts are hydrolyzed and condensed (Sivasamy, 2013), which is then dried and calcined to obtain the desired NPs. To restore the crystallinity of the NPs, heat treatment is given during the intermediate synthesis (Rane et al., 2018). The final product is, however, determined by the hydrolysis and the condensation process. The advantage of this method is that it produces NPs with uniform shape and structure in the presence of a ligand in a pure form, as a result of which a high amount of impurities are accumulated from its byproducts (Tillotson et al., 2001).

4.3.1.2 Vapor Deposition

This method involves the reaction of vapor-phase precursors on a substrate to deposit thin films or NPs (Bhaviripudi et al., 2007). With the help of this technique, metal vapors that progressively form thin films, alloy coatings, and reactive oxygen, nitrogen, and methane are produced and transmitted via a vacuum chamber. The thin film forms as a result of metal ion vapors leaving the condensed phase and then returning to it (Venables et al., 1984). Due to the inert atmosphere when the metal vapors are condensed and as a result of thermal treatment, nanocomposites are obtained (Abegunde et al., 2019). The advantage of this method is that few inorganic and organic materials are used compared to other procedures, and hence, it is an eco-friendly process, and the disadvantage is that it is a complex procedure with a low yield of material, and also, it is cost-ineffective (Mattox, 2002).

4.3.1.3 Electrochemical Deposition

This method involves the electrochemical reduction of metal ions in a solution to deposit NPs on a substrate.

4.3.1.4 Hydrothermal Synthesis

This involves the reaction of metal salts or precursors in a high-pressure, high-temperature water-based solution to form NPs.

4.3.1.5 Self-Assembly

According to this technique, molecular building blocks spontaneously transform into NPs through noncovalent interactions like hydrogen bonds and van der Waals forces (Figure 4.1).

4.3.2 Top-Down Method

The top-down or destructive process involves breaking down large materials into little particles. Here are some significant top-down techniques.

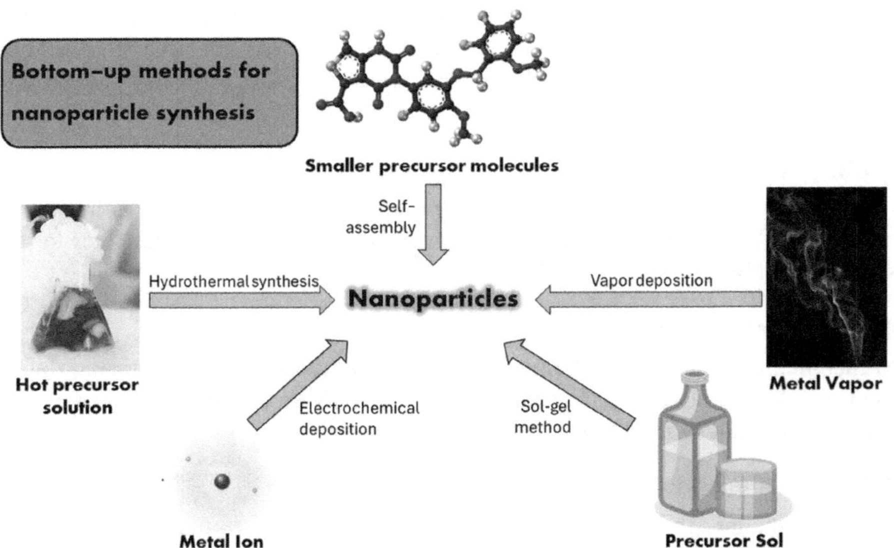

FIGURE 4.1 Bottom-up methods for NP synthesis.

4.3.2.1 Milling

This involves the use of high-energy mechanical forces to break down the bulk material into smaller particles by placing the materials in a closed container in bulk. The material is usually placed in a ball mill or a planetary mill and is exposed to excessive mechanical forces (Yadav et al., 2012). By using the reactive ball mining technique, the materials are ground into tiny NPs throughout this process (Sun et al., 2009). Fine nanotubes are obtained. The advantages of the milling methods include the following: (i) fine powders and churned nanotubes are obtained and (ii) corrosive materials are ground and milled, and the disadvantages of the method are as follows: (i) it is a time-consuming method and (ii) it increased the risk of contamination due to the attrition of the balls (Delogu et al., 2017).

4.3.2.2 Lithography

This includes the usage of laser beams to cut out small patterns in a thin film of material. The patterns are used as templates for the production of NPs (Amendola and Meneghetti, 2009; Hulteen et al., 1999). There are several different lithography techniques including ultraviolet (UV) lithography, photolithography, e-beam lithography, soft lithography, and scanning lithography (Pimpin and Srituravanich, 2012). Photolithography is a light-dependent technique where an image is formed in a silicon wafer medium on a projected light (Paik et al., 2020). In the case of UV lithography, a specific type of wavelength is used where submicron level of pattern occurs. The disadvantage of this technique is the free radical production during the entire procedure as a result of which deoxyribonucleic acid (DNA) damage might occur in the process of photo-initiation (Sha et al., 2001). E-beam lithography uses scanning electron beam to pattern the surface without the usage of a mask (Altissimo, 2010). An elastomeric stamp is used in soft lithography to deposit ink on a substrate. The benefits of these techniques are low cost and great throughput (Whitesides et al., 2001). Scanning probe lithography modifies the surface with atomic resolution. It can produce features of any shape, size, geometry pattern, and nonplanar surfaces.

4.3.2.3 Etching

Chemical reactions are used in this case to remove selected material from the surface of a huge bulk of material. The resulting structures can be used as templates for the synthesis of NPs (Kühnel et al., 2018).

4.3.2.4 Electrospinning

In this method, a polymer solution is drawn into a fine jet by the application of an electric field and the tiny jet then hardens into a fiber. Various mechanical and chemical processes can be used to separate the fiber into NPs.

4.3.2.5 Thermal Decomposition

Heat that shatters the molecular bonds in a substance causes thermal decomposition, which is an endothermic chemical breakdown. The decomposition temperature is the precise temperature at which an element begins to chemically break down.

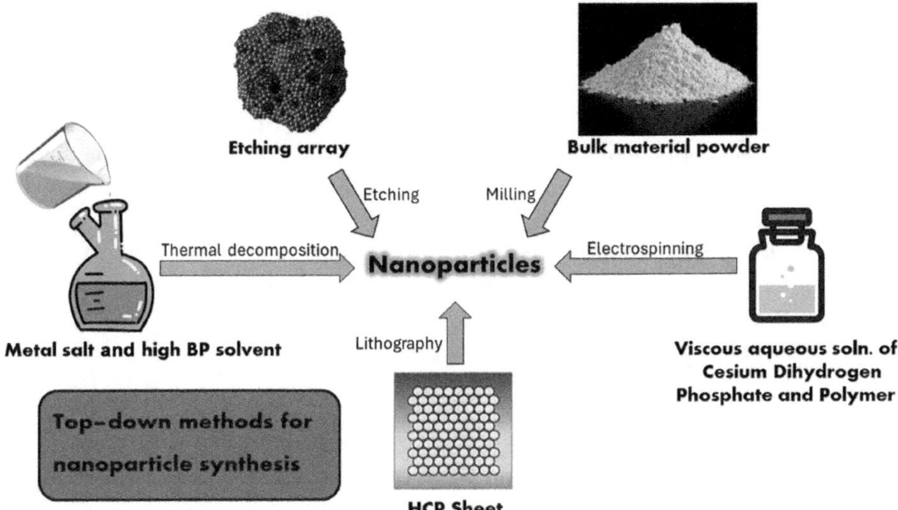

FIGURE 4.2 Top-down methods for NP synthesis.

By breaking down the metal at particular temperatures and experiencing a chemical reaction that results in byproducts, the NPs are created. This technique produces metal and metal oxide-based NPs (Figure 4.2).

4.4 NANOMEDICINES IN CANCER THERANOSTICS

Nanomedicines have shown great potential in cancer theragnostics, which refers to the combination of diagnosis and therapy. NPs can be engineered to carry drugs or contrast agents, and they can also be designed to target specific cancer cells or tissues.

The use of nanomedicines in cancer theragnostics has benefits since they can improve the delivery of therapeutic drugs to tumor cells while causing the least amount of harm to healthy tissues. This is accomplished by taking advantage of the enhanced permeability and retention (EPR) effect, which explains how tumor leaky blood arteries and ineffective lymphatic drainage cause NPs to collect there.

Nanomedicines can be utilized for imaging, in addition to drug delivery. To improve the sensitivity and specificity of imaging modalities like magnetic resonance imaging (MRI), computed tomography (CT), and positron emission tomography (PET), for instance, NPs can be labeled with contrast agents.

Another important application of nanomedicines in cancer theragnostics is their ability to monitor treatment response. By incorporating imaging agents or sensors into the NPs, it is possible to track the distribution and effectiveness of therapeutic agents over time.

Overall, nanomedicines have the potential to revolutionize cancer diagnosis and treatment by providing targeted and personalized therapies with enhanced efficacy and reduced side effects. However, more research is needed to fully realize their potential and address potential safety concerns.

4.5 BIOLOGICALLY INSPIRED NANOPARTICLES IN CANCER THERANOSTICS

Cancer being a threat to human life had some conventional treatment systems, like surgeries, chemotherapy, and radiation therapies. Tumor-specific antigens, which are expressed by cancer cells, are then designated as targets for monoclonal antibody-based therapies, which were later developed with improved findings and knowledge (Vigneron et al., 2013). In addition to all these progresses in the field of cancer, biologically inspired NPs have gained significant attention in the field of cancer theragnostics. These NPs are designed to mimic biological structures found in nature, such as viruses or lipoproteins, to improve their interactions with cancer cells and to enhance their therapeutic efficacy.

4.5.1 Liposomes

One example of a biologically inspired NP is the liposome. Liposomes are synthetic vesicles that can encapsulate drugs or other therapeutic agents and can be modified to target specific cancer cells. Additionally, liposomes can be created to release their contents in reaction to environmental cues like pH or temperature changes enabling the delivery of specific drugs to the cancer cells (Wang et al., 2008).

4.5.2 Abraxane

The appeal of protein-based NPs is due to their abundance in nature. The Food and Drug Administration (FDA) has approved Abraxane (albumin-bound paclitaxel) as a vehicle for delivering imaging and anticancer medicines to TME (Rosenberg et al., 1990). Patients using this Abraxane have displayed greater improvements with very little toxicity (Gradishar, 2006).

4.5.3 Virus-Like Particles (VLPs)

Another example is VLPs, which are nanoscale structures that mimic the structure of viruses but are non-infectious. VLPs can be used to deliver therapeutic agents, such as drugs or vaccines, to cancer cells, and can also be modified to target specific types of cancer cells.

4.5.4 Phyto-Based Metallic Nanoparticles

Common medical imaging techniques include CT, MRI, PET, and ultrasound, which are having an issue to get a precise and specific problem after diagnosis. Moreover, the expense issue of these procedures leads to an exploration of novel strategies to fight against cancer. Reduction in drug effectiveness, lack of dissemination, and absorbance properties of pharmaceuticals have prone to discover new techniques and methods to deliver a better treatment. Gold, iron, and silver NPs are synthesized in a natural way since the light emitted scatters more prominently than the molecules in a striking manner to induce a better imaging quality. The synthesis of plant phyto-based NPs is comparatively economical and is produced on a large scale. Different biomolecules in plant extracts such as amino acids, enzymes, vitamins, polysaccharides, proteins, and organic acids are combined with different metallic NPs to form an environment-friendly complex (Gulia et al., 2022). Reports have shown that plants like *Arabidopsis halleri* and *Thlaspi caerulescens* detoxify harmful metals (Celia et al., 2013). Several parts of the plants like stem, root, and leaves are widely used for green NP synthesis due to their capability of producing high-quality phytochemicals.

4.5.5 Quantum Dots

Biologically inspired NPs are used therapeutically for cancer imaging as well as diagnosis. For instance, imaging agents like quantum dots, which are fluorescent semi-conductor nanocrystals, can be utilized to see cancer cells in real time. For MRI, other imaging agents such as iron oxide NPs can be employed to find malignant areas (Madamsetty et al., 2019).

Overall, biologically inspired NPs show significant potential for enhancing the efficacy and accuracy of cancer theragnostics, and future development of more potent and precise cancer therapies is anticipated as a result of current research in this field (Table 4.2).

TABLE 4.2
Biologically Inspired Nanoparticles

Biologically Inspired Nanoparticle	Advantages	Uses	References
Liposome	• Can encapsulate desired molecules • Can be modified for targeted delivery • Can be designed to release contents on specific cues	Targeted drug delivery to specific cancer cells	Wang et al. (2008)
Abraxane	• Abundance • Less toxicity	Delivering imaging and anticancer drugs to TME	Gradishar, (2006); Rosenberg et al. (1990)
VLPs	Targeted delivery like viruses but non-infectious	Modified to target specific cancer cells to deliver therapeutic agents	
Quantum dots	Fluorescent, semi-conductor nanocrystals	See cancer cells in real time	Madamsetty et al. (2019)
Phyto-based metallic NPs like Au, Ag, and Fe	• Detoxified • Prominent light scattering.	Inducing better quality imaging	Celia et al., (2013); Gulia et al. (2022)

4.6 FUTURE PROSPECTS AND CONCLUSION

NPs proved great advancement in cancer theragnostics, which is the solution of diagnosis and treatment under one platform. Several future prospects are there that might assure a better therapeutic effect in the field of cancer. Targeted delivery of NPs is of great importance since it leaves other cells unharmed. This targeted delivery can improve the effectiveness of chemotherapy while reducing side effects. NPs can also be used in imaging techniques such as MRI, CT, and PET. These particles can accumulate in tumors, making them more visible in scans. The targeting can be done by virtue of specific properties these NPs owe, such as the ability to turn themselves on or off based on different stimuli such as the presence of enzymes or chemical molecules that are specifically upregulated in cancer tissues, which provide control over the time and amount of medication implemented by using external stimuli.

Moreover, they can be loaded with multiple drugs, allowing for combination therapy. This approach can be particularly effective in treating drug-resistant tumors. NPs can be designed and used as personalized medicine to respond to specific biomarkers associated with certain types of cancer, where treatment is tailored to the individual patient. Overall, the future of NPs in cancer theragnostics looks promising. As researchers continue to develop and refine these technologies, they have the potential to improve cancer treatment and patient outcomes.

Future research in the area of cancer diagnosis, imaging, and cancer therapy will be guided by nanomaterial-based cancer therapy. It is clear that these medications will soon be licensed and developed through clinical studies. NPs in the form of nanomedicines reduce collateral damage and have minimal side effects. Recent discoveries and advancements in nanotheragnostics have high outputs in the detection and screening of cancer cells and biomarkers.

The main aim is to get maximum information regarding the type of cancer, produce more and more diagnostic information at early detection, and reduce the time frame for diagnosis also. Moreover, tailoring a hybrid treatment using nanodelivery systems containing the drugs of interest and detection molecules that identify specific cancer biomarkers would allow to treat the disease more efficiently by monitoring when a therapeutic agent reaches its highest tolerable concentration in a TME to prevent over-treatment, which may lead to undesirable effects, while also making sure to avoid under-treatment that would not even completely treat the tumor.

Despite all these benefits, it has proven difficult to successfully translate the medicinal potential of nanomaterials into clinical trials. Most critically, nothing is known about the health danger that NPs bring to the human body and their toxicity. The biocompatibility of the clinically approved nanodrugs can only be attained by modifying nanomaterials with membranes or other biomaterials. Because the metal NPs, quantum dots, and other nanomaterials are not biodegradable, their ability to persist in the body after delivery increases their cytotoxicity. Therefore, the NPs must be biodegradable and biocompatible in order to have superior clinical utility. The use of NPs that possess some therapeutic abilities themselves is also one possible direction to look toward while assessing future directions in the nanotheragnostic field, and with properties of NPs such as wave-particle duality, NPs can really revolutionize cancer treatment using nanomedicine.

With the potential of easing the way for better cancer detection, management, and therapy, clinical nanotechnology has begun to merge diagnosis and treatment. More crucially, the diversity and biocompatibility offer prospects for multifunctionalization and the development of smart particles allowing for the systematic use of a single platform to identify tumors, treat them, track treatment responses, and direct therapy. A nanomaterial-based combination of therapeutic and diagnostic applications enables an integrated approach to patient management.

REFERENCES

Abegunde, O.O., Akinlabi, E.T., Oladijo, O.P., Akinlabi, S., Ude, A.U., Abegunde, O.O., Akinlabi, E.T., Oladijo, O.P., Akinlabi, S., Ude, A.U., 2019. Overview of thin film deposition techniques. *AIMS Mater. Sci.* 6, 174–199. https://doi.org/10.3934/matersci.2019.2.174

Altissimo, M., 2010. E-beam lithography for micro-nanofabrication. *Biomicrofluidics* 4, 026503. https://doi.org/10.1063/1.3437589

Amendola, V., Meneghetti, M., 2009. Laser ablation synthesis in solution and size manipulation of noble metal nanoparticles. *Phys. Chem. Chem. Phys.* 11, 3805–3821. https://doi.org/10.1039/B900654K

Bhaviripudi, S., Mile, E., Steiner, S.A., Zare, A.T., Dresselhaus, M.S., Belcher, A.M., Kong, J., 2007. CVD synthesis of single-walled carbon nanotubes from gold nanoparticle catalysts. *J. Am. Chem. Soc.* 129, 1516–1517. https://doi.org/10.1021/ja0673332

Celia, C., Trapasso, E., Locatelli, M., Navarra, M., Ventura, C.A., Wolfram, J., Carafa, M., Morittu, V.M., Britti, D., Di Marzio, L., Paolino, D., 2013. Anticancer activity of liposomal bergamot essential oil (BEO) on human neuroblastoma cells. *Colloids Surf. B Biointerfaces* 112, 548–553. https://doi.org/10.1016/j.colsurfb.2013.09.017

Davis, M.E., Chen, Z.G., Shin, D.M., 2008. Nanoparticle therapeutics: An emerging treatment modality for cancer. *Nat. Rev. Drug Discov.* 7, 771–782. https://doi.org/10.1038/nrd2614

Delogu, F., Gorrasi, G., Sorrentino, A., 2017. Fabrication of polymer nanocomposites via ball milling: Present status and future perspectives. *Prog. Mater. Sci.* 86, 75–126. https://doi.org/10.1016/j.pmatsci.2017.01.003

Ealia, S.A.M., Saravanakumar, M.P., 2017. A review on the classification, characterisation, synthesis of nanoparticles and their application. *IOP Conf. Ser.: Mater. Sci. Eng.* 263, 032019. https://doi.org/10.1088/1757-899X/263/3/032019

García-Pinel, B., Porras-Alcalá, C., Ortega-Rodríguez, A., Sarabia, F., Prados, J., Melguizo, C., López-Romero, J.M., 2019. Lipid-based nanoparticles: Application and recent advances in cancer treatment. *Nanomaterials* 9, 638. https://doi.org/10.3390/nano9040638

Gradishar, W.J., 2006. Albumin-bound paclitaxel: A next-generation taxane. *Expert. Opin. Pharmacother.* 7, 1041–1053. https://doi.org/10.1517/14656566.7.8.1041

Gulia, K., James, A., Pandey, S., Dev, K., Kumar, D., Sourirajan, A., 2022. Bio-inspired smart nanoparticles in enhanced cancer theranostics and targeted drug delivery. *J. Funct. Biomater.* 13, 207. https://doi.org/10.3390/jfb13040207

Hulteen, J.C., Treichel, D.A., Smith, M.T., Duval, M.L., Jensen, T.R., Van Duyne, R.P., 1999. Nanosphere lithography: Size-tunable silver nanoparticle and surface cluster arrays. *J. Phys. Chem. B* 103, 3854–3863. https://doi.org/10.1021/jp9904771

Kühnel, M., Fröhlich, T., Füßl, R., Hoffmann, M., Manske, E., Rangelow, I.W., Reger, J., Schäffel, C., Sinzinger, S., Zöllner, J.-P., 2018. Towards alternative 3D nanofabrication in macroscopic working volumes. *Meas. Sci. Technol.* 29, 114002. https://doi.org/10.1088/1361-6501/aadb57

Madamsetty, V.S., Mukherjee, A., Mukherjee, S., 2019. Recent trends of the bio-inspired nanoparticles in cancer theranostics. *Front. Pharmacol.* 10, 1264.

Markman, J.L., Rekechenetskiy, A., Holler, E., Ljubimova, J.Y., 2013. Nanomedicine therapeutic approaches to overcome cancer drug resistance. *Adv. Drug Deliv. Rev.* 65, 1866–1879. https://doi.org/10.1016/j.addr.2013.09.019

Mattheolabakis, G., Rigas, B., Constantinides, P.P., 2012. Nanodelivery strategies in cancer chemotherapy: Biological rationale and pharmaceutical perspectives. *Nanomedicine* 7, 1577–1590. https://doi.org/10.2217/nnm.12.128

Mattox, D.M., 2002. Physical vapor deposition (PVD) processes. *Metal Fin.* 100, 394–408. https://doi.org/10.1016/S0026-0576(02)82043-8

Paik, S., Kim, G., Chang, S., Lee, S., Jin, D., Jeong, K.-Y., Lee, I.S., Lee, Jekwan, Moon, H., Lee, Jaejun, Chang, K., Choi, S.S., Moon, J., Jung, S., Kang, S., Lee, W., Choi, H.-J., Choi, H., Kim, H.J., Lee, J.-H., Cheon, J., Kim, M., Myoung, J., Park, H.- G., Shim, W., 2020. Near-field sub-diffraction photolithography with an elastomeric photomask. *Nat. Commun.* 11, 805. https://doi.org/10.1038/s41467-020-14439-1

Pimpin, A., Srituravanich, W., 2012. Review on micro- and nanolithography techniques and their applications. *Eng. J.* 16, 37–56. https://doi.org/10.4186/ej.2012.16.1.37

Rane, A.V., Kanny, K., Abitha, V.K., Thomas, S., 2018. Methods for synthesis of nanoparticles and fabrication of nanocomposites, in: Mohan Bhagyaraj, S., Oluwafemi, O. S., Kalarikkal, N., Thomas, S. (Eds.), *Synthesis of Inorganic Nanomaterials, Micro and Nano Technologies*. Woodhead Publishing, pp. 121–139. https://doi.org/10.1016/B978-0-08-101975-7.00005-1

Rosenberg, S.A., Aebersold, P., Cornetta, K., Kasid, A., Morgan, R.A., Moen, R., Karson, E.M., Lotze, M.T., Yang, J.C., Topalian, S.L., 1990. Gene transfer into humans--immunotherapy of patients with advanced melanoma, using tumor-infiltrating lymphocytes modified by retroviral gene transduction. *N. Engl. J. Med.* 323, 570–578. https://doi.org/10.1056/NEJM199008303230904

Sha, D.Y., Hsieh, L., Chen, K., 2001. Wafer rework strategies at the photolithography stage. *Int. J. Ind. Eng.: Theory. Appl. Pract.* 8, 122–130.

Sivasamy, R., 2013. Sol-gel synthesis and characterization of nanoparticles. *J. Nanosci.* 2013. https://doi.org/10.1155/2013/929321

Sun, J.F., Wang, M.Z., Zhao, Y.C., Li, X.P., Liang, B.Y., 2009. Synthesis of titanium nitride powders by reactive ball milling of titanium and urea. *J. Alloys Compd.* 482, L29–L31. https://doi.org/10.1016/j.jallcom.2009.04.043

Tillotson, T.M., Gash, A.E., Simpson, R.L., Hrubesh, L.W., Satcher, J.H., Poco, J.F., 2001. Nanostructured energetic materials using sol–gel methodologies. *J. Non-Cryst. Solids* 285, 338–345. https://doi.org/10.1016/S0022-3093(01)00477-X

Venables, J.A., Spiller, G.D.T., Hanbucken, M., 1984. Nucleation and growth of thin films. *Rep. Prog. Phys.* 47, 399. https://doi.org/10.1088/0034-4885/47/4/002

Vigneron, N., Stroobant, V., Van den Eynde, B.J., van der Bruggen, P., 2013. Database of T cell-defined human tumor antigens: The 2013 update. *Cancer Immun.* 13, 15.

Wang, X., Yang, L., Chen, Z.G., Shin, D.M., 2008. Application of nanotechnology in cancer therapy and imaging. *CA Cancer J. Clin.* 58, 97–110. https://doi.org/10.3322/CA.2007.0003

Whitesides, G.M., Ostuni, E., Takayama, S., Jiang, X., Ingber, D.E., 2001. Soft lithography in biology and biochemistry. *Annu. Rev. Biomed. Eng.* 3, 335–373. https://doi.org/10.1146/annurev.bioeng.3.1.335

Yadav, T.P., Yadav, R.M., Singh, D.P., 2012. Mechanical milling: A top down approach for the synthesis of nanomaterials and nanocomposites. *Nanosci. Nanotechnol.* 2, 22–48.

5 Quantum Dots
The Next Generation Candidate for Biomedical Imaging

Tarun Mateti, Rohit Kapila, Smarak Islam Chaudhury, Likhith K, and Goutam Thakur

5.1 INTRODUCTION

In today's fast-changing world—where people innovate using sophisticated techniques—quantum dots emerge as versatile materials that find applications in various domains. These are nanoparticles of a semiconducting material and are unlike their bulk counterpart. They are typically made of elements from groups II–VI of the periodic table and display size-dependent optical and electronic properties. The term "quantum" originates from the Latin word "quantus," which means "how much" or "how great," whereas the word "dots" refers to the small size of these particles: like the size of twinkling stars scattered across the night sky (Norman, Mirin and Bowers, 2021)!

Modern technology has utilized quantum dots to design products and techniques superior to those previously possible with traditional materials. A few exciting applications (Figure 5.1) are mentioned below:

1. Quantum dot light-emitting diodes (LEDs) have been developed for televisions, smartphones, and monitors that improve color, brightness, and energy efficiency, resulting in more vibrant and lifelike images with a broader color gamut and improved performance over traditional and organic LEDs (Bourzac, 2013; Liu et al., 2020; Kortlever et al., 2022).
2. Quantum dots are critical in advancing solar energy harvesting: they can be integrated into solar cells to improve their efficiency by broadening the absorption spectrum and reducing thermalization loss (Sun et al., 2018; Fu et al., 2022; Huang et al., 2023b). Research on quantum dot-based solar cells suggests the potential to surpass the Shockley–Queisser limit, which is the maximum theoretical efficiency for conventional solar cells (Böhm et al., 2015; Ehrler et al., 2020; Chi et al., 2022).
3. Quantum dots have applications in environmental monitoring (Niu et al., 2018; Wei et al., 2018; Kurniawan et al., 2022), food analysis (Nemati et al., 2018; Hu et al., 2020; Carneiro et al., 2021), and medical diagnostics

DOI: 10.1201/9781003432661-5

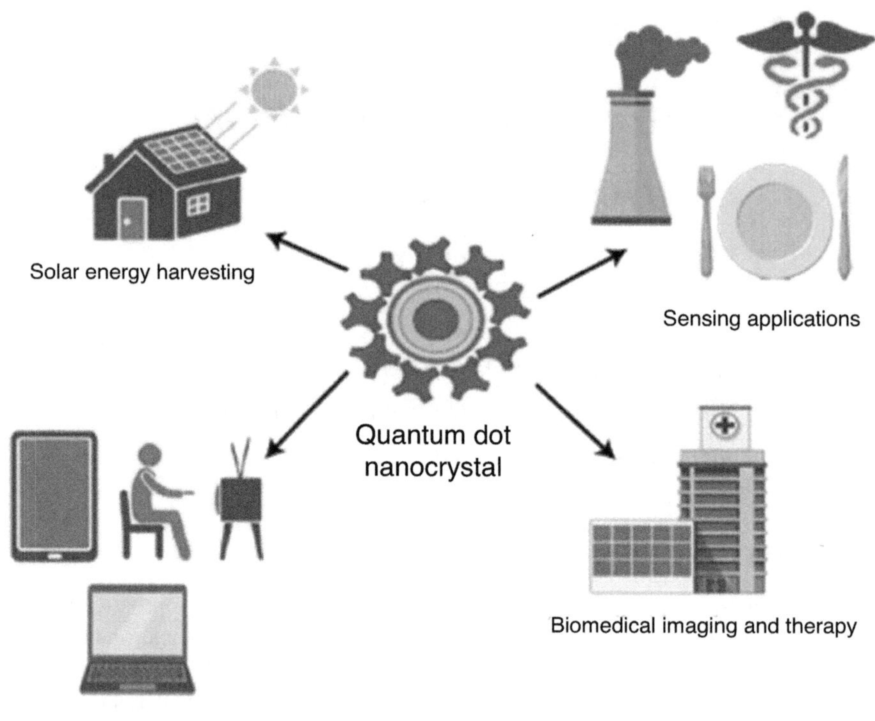

FIGURE 5.1 Applications of quantum dots in modern technology.

(Han et al., 2001; Sukhanova et al., 2012; Safardoust-Hojaghan et al., 2017), where they can detect various chemical and biological substances due to their unique optical properties and sensitivity to environmental changes.

4. Quantum dots can be used as carriers to precisely deliver therapeutic agents to specific cells or tissues, which helps reduce side effects and improve treatment efficacy (Cai et al., 2016; Samimi, Ardestani and Dorkoosh, 2021; Huang et al., 2023a).
5. Quantum dots have been employed in cancer therapy to selectively target and destroy tumor cells while minimizing damage to healthy tissues (Moasses Ghafary et al., 2022; Murali et al., 2022; Rahmani et al., 2022).
6. Quantum dots can help develop more powerful and efficient quantum processors capable of solving problems currently intractable for classical computers (Ruffino et al., 2021; Kriekouki et al., 2022; Seidler et al., 2022).

Recently, there has been a growing interest in using quantum dots for biomedical imaging. Quantum dots can be used as fluorescent markers for cellular and molecular processes (Cao et al., 2022; Zhang et al., 2022; Linghu et al., 2023) and for image and multiplexed labeling (Panagiotopoulou et al., 2016; Shellaiah et al., 2022; Tsuboi and Jin, 2022). As a result, quantum dots have revolutionized *in vitro* and *in vivo* imaging by improving visualizing capabilities and analyzing biological and cellular processes, which this chapter describes in detail.

However, potential environmental and health impacts are associated with using quantum dots. Some quantum dots contain toxic elements such as cadmium, which can pose environmental and human health risks if not properly managed (Chen et al., 2012). To mitigate these concerns, researchers are actively developing less toxic alternatives, such as indium-based (Jalali et al., 2022) or carbon-based (Sun et al., 2020) quantum dots. Also, many quantum dots are synthesized using hydrophobic ligands (Peng and Peng, 2001) and are not inherently water-soluble, which poses challenges for their application in biological systems where water solubility is critical for effective interaction with cells and tissues.

This chapter provides an overview of the types and associated characteristics of quantum dots, their synthesis techniques, their use in biomedical imaging, and their drawbacks. Quantum dots hold immense potential in modern technology, with applications across various fields. While there are challenges to overcome, ongoing research and development are expected to lead to discoveries and breakthroughs, further expanding the potential uses and benefits of these remarkable nanoscale particles.

5.2 A GLIMPSE THROUGH HISTORY: FROM FEYNMAN TO THE DISCOVERY OF QUANTUM DOTS

On December 29, 1959, the American physicist Richard Feynman lectured, "There's Plenty of Room at the Bottom," at an American Physical Society meeting at the California Institute of Technology (Caltech). In his lecture, Feynman discussed the potential of controlling individual atoms and exploring the uncharted territories of the atomic level. Feynman posed two critical questions during his lecture: Why cannot we write the entire 24 volumes of the Encyclopedia Britannica on the head of a pin? And, what would happen if we could arrange atoms one by one (Feynman, 2018)? These questions sparked the imagination and inspired researchers worldwide.

However—contrary to popular belief—it did not lead to the conceptual beginnings of the field of nanotechnology; beginning in the 1980s, nanotechnology advocates cited the lecture to establish the scientific credibility of their work. As measured by citations in the scientific literature, the numerous published versions of Feynman's lecture had a negligible impact in the 20 years following its initial publication and not much more impact in the decade following the invention of the scanning tunneling microscope in 1981 (Toumey, 2008). In the early 1990s, there was an increased interest in Feynman's lecture, which is likely because the term "nanotechnology" gained serious attention just prior to that time, following its use by Eric Drexler in his book, "Engines of Creation: The Coming Era of Nanotechnology" in 1986 (Drexler, 1987) and in a cover article titled "Nanotechnology" published later that year in a scientific magazine (Drexler, no date).

Around the same time as Feynman's lecture, the demand for more powerful electronic devices grew: the research focused on continually shrinking the size of transistors and other components, increasing their performance, reducing power consumption, and lowering manufacturing costs—the birth of the semiconductor revolution (Alferov, 2013)! This quest of the semiconductor industry had fortunately intersected with the ideas of

Feynman. In a conference in 1979, the Japanese scientist Norio Taniguchi was the first to use the term "nano-technology" to describe semiconductor processes exhibiting characteristic control on the order of a nanometer (Taniguchi, 1974). However, the term was not used again until 1986 when Eric Drexler coined "nanotechnology" in his book, which deterministically explored the concept of handling individual atoms and molecules.

In modern times, physicists use colored glasses—so-called Schott glasses—as optical filters, and it was well understood that the optical properties of these glasses activated by halogens are determined by "colloidal particles" dispersed in a glass matrix. Intriguingly, the preparation protocols for these glasses derive in part from ancient alchemical texts: add such-and-such compounds to the glass melt, reduce the melt to such-and-such a temperature, and then reheat it and maintain it at such-and-such a temperature for a specific amount of time—these methods were entirely empirical! In 1979, Ekimov began working at the S. I. Vavilov State Optical Institute, equipped with the technology necessary for Schott glass growth. Ekimov wanted to investigate the fundamental physicochemical mechanisms responsible for various colors in semiconductor-activated glasses by ascertaining the colloidal particles' structure, chemical composition, and synthesis mechanism. He decided to test the effect of a specific compound on the activation of glass, as opposed to the traditional methods. Experiments were conducted with glasses activated by CuCl, CuBr, CdS, and CdSe. Ekimov initially struggled with CdS and CdSe-activated glasses, but success came with studying glasses activated by CuCl—the first quantum dots synthesized in a glass matrix in 1981 (Efros and Brus, 2021)!

Surprisingly, the first quantum dots synthesized in a colloidal suspension (Figure 5.2) were accidental! In 1983, Louis Brus was studying CdS aqueous colloids

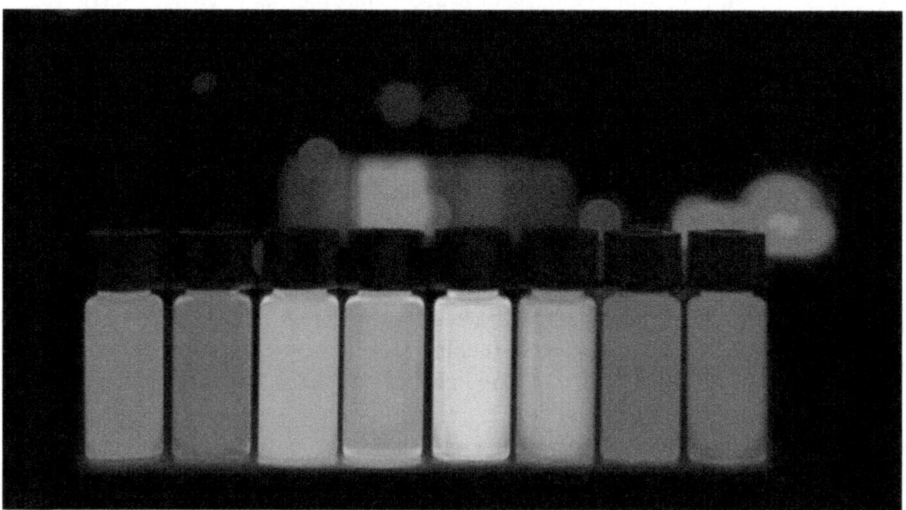

FIGURE 5.2 Colloidal suspension quantum dots of various sizes exhibiting different fluorescence properties (Commons, no date). [This figure is reproduced from Wikimedia Commons, where it has been uploaded by Antipoff. The content is licensed under CC BY-SA 3.0, and we declare that no changes have been made to the figure by us. Also, the licensor does not endorse us or our use of the figure.]

when he observed something peculiar: the CdS properties sometimes changed with aging. He suspected that the observed change was a "size" effect, and to confirm this idea, he made smaller CdS and found that the property changes intensified (Efros and Brus, 2021)—reporting the first quantum dot colloidal suspension.

In the years following the discovery of quantum dot colloidal suspensions, the field of quantum dot research has seen remarkable growth and diversification. By developing new synthesis techniques, quantum dot types, and surface modification strategies, and exploring innovative applications, researchers have unlocked the potential of these unique nanoscale materials across a wide range of disciplines.

5.3 TYPES AND CHARACTERISTICS OF QUANTUM DOTS

5.3.1 Core-Type Quantum Dots

Core-type quantum dots (Figure 5.3) typically comprise single semiconducting materials with uniform internal compositions, such as chalcogenides (selenides, sulfides, or tellurides) of metals like cadmium, lead, or zinc. A few examples are CdSe, CdTe, and InP. Core-type quantum dots emit high amounts of light due to their small size and ability to convert much of the absorbed energy into emitting light, making them suitable for devices such as LEDs, solar cells, and sensors (Ca et al., 2019).

5.3.2 Core–Shell-Type Quantum Dots

Core–shell-type quantum dots (Figure 5.3) have a shell(s) or small region(s) of another semiconducting material around them. Such shells increase the amount of emitted light by minimizing the number of processes that can cause absorbed energy to be released in ways other than emitting light. Also, such particles are more robust to processing conditions for various applications (Dorfs and Eychmüller, 2006; Rao, Müller and Cheetham, 2006; Smith and Nie, 2009).

5.3.3 Alloyed-Type Quantum Dots

Alloyed-type quantum dots (Figure 5.3) offer an alternative method to tune properties without changing the particle size: by changing the composition and internal structure. These are formed by alloying together two semiconductor materials,

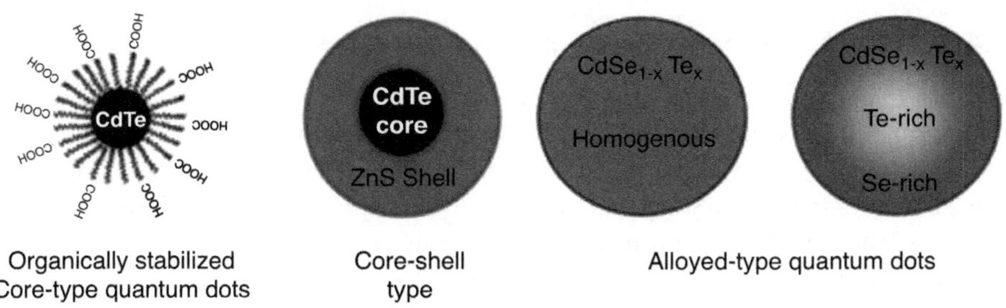

FIGURE 5.3 Various types of quantum dots (Munasinghe et al., 2019) [Open access].

which exhibit properties distinct from their bulk counterparts and those of their parent semiconductors. Thus, alloyed-type quantum dots possess novel and additional properties besides those that emerge due to size effects (Vastola, Zhang and Shenoy, 2012).

5.4 SYNTHESIS METHODS OF QUANTUM DOTS

5.4.1 Micellar Synthesis

Micellar synthesis (Figure 5.4) is a widely employed method for preparing quantum dots due to its simplicity, versatility, and ability to produce quantum dots emitting high amounts of light. In this process, the precursors are dissolved in a solvent, with surfactant molecules and phospholipid molecules with polyethylene glycol and amine headgroups to improve biocompatibility and bioconjugation (Fan et al., 2005). In contrast, the surfactant molecules act as stabilizing agents to prevent the aggregation of the particles. The solution is then heated to a specific temperature, allowing micelles to form small clusters of surfactant molecules that encapsulate the precursors. These micelles act as a reaction chamber, where the precursors can react and form quantum dots in a controlled manner. This method allows precise control of the size and shape of the resulting quantum dots by adjusting the temperature, surfactant concentration, and reaction time.

5.4.2 Hydrothermal Synthesis

In the hydrothermal synthesis process (Figure 5.5), the precursors are dissolved in a solvent and placed in a sealed vessel with a high-pressure water source known as a hydrothermal reactor. The mixture is then heated for a few hours to a high temperature and pressure, typically above the solvent's boiling point. Under these conditions, the precursors react with the solvent and form quantum dots in a controlled manner. The high pressure and temperature allow for the growth of uniform and high-quality quantum dots with small sizes. The reaction time and temperature can also be controlled to tune the size and shape of the quantum dots. It is a simple and low-cost method that can produce a wide range of materials and compositions, including semiconductors and metal-based quantum dots (Aboulaich et al., 2012; Liu, Ji and Tan, 2013; Zhu et al., 2013).

5.4.3 Hot Injection Method/Organometallic Synthesis

The hot injection method (Figure 5.6) involves injecting a precursor solution into a high-temperature surfactant and coordinating solvent solution, where the precursor is typically made up of metal salts and organic ligands. The high temperature of the solvent allows the precursor ions to react and form quantum dots, allowing precise control of the size and composition. It is widely used because of its efficiency, reproducibility, and versatility, and it can also be used to produce core–shell quantum dots (Murray, Norris and Bawendi, 1993).

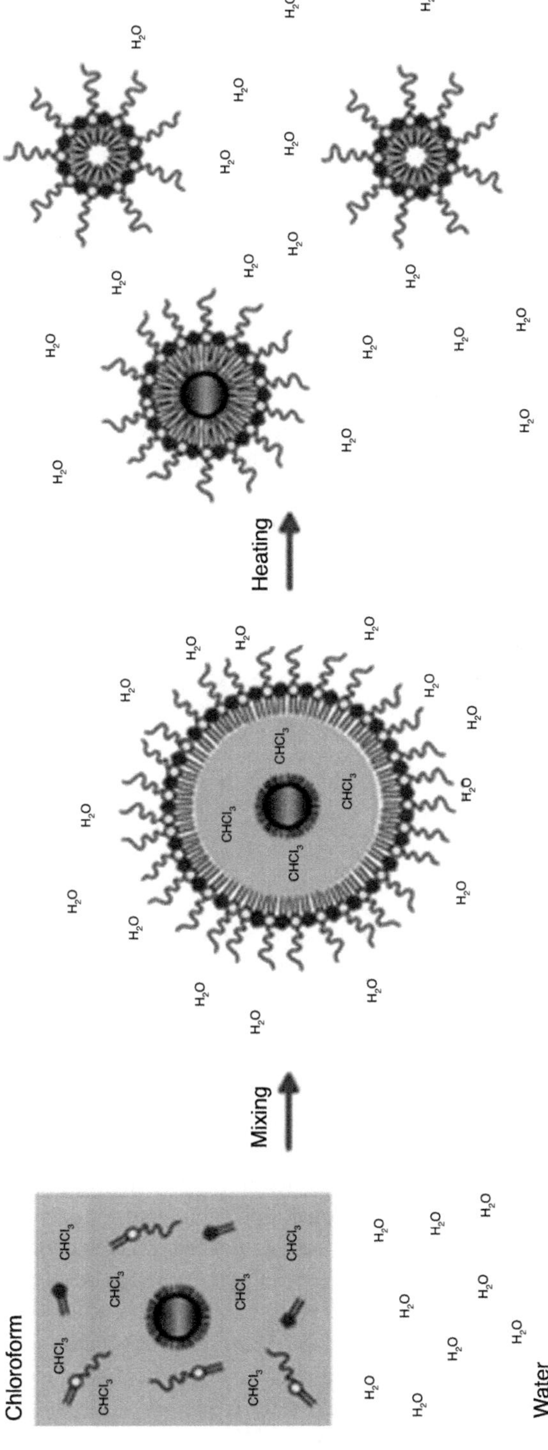

FIGURE 5.4 Schematic representation of the micellar synthesis of quantum dots with a paramagnetic micellar coating. Quantum dots and lipids in chloroform are slowly infused in hot water that, via chloroform-in-water emulsions, swiftly form micelles when chloroform evaporates, some of which have a quantum dot core. (Mulder et al., 2010) [Open access].

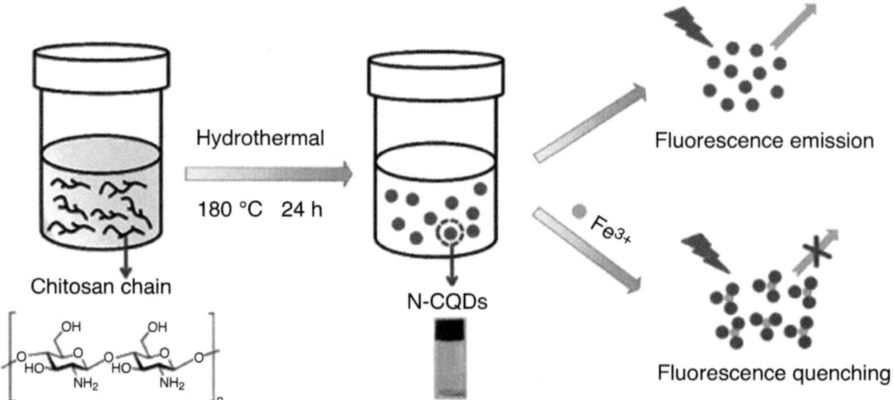

FIGURE 5.5 Schematic of the hydrothermal method used to prepare highly luminescent nitrogen-doped carbon quantum dots (N-CQDs) with chitosan (Zhao et al., 2019) [Open access].

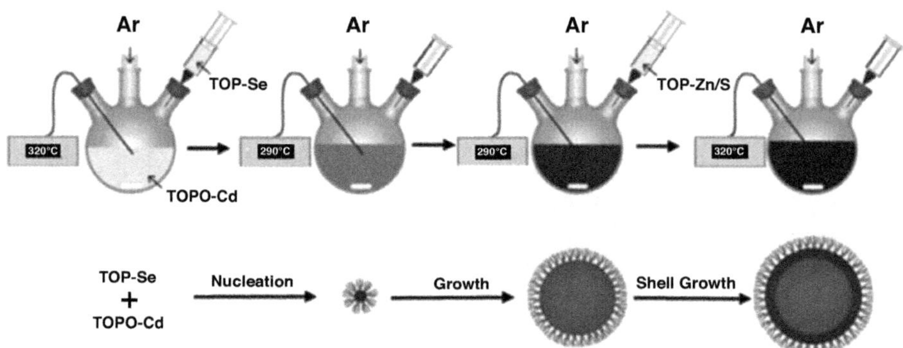

FIGURE 5.6 Hot injection synthesis of CdSe (where trioctylphosphine (TOP) and TOP oxide (TOPO)) (Mohamed et al., 2021) [Open access].

5.4.4 Electrochemical Synthesis

The electrochemical synthesis method (Figure 5.7) involves using an electrochemical cell consisting of an anode and a cathode immersed in an electrolyte solution. The anode and cathode are connected to an external power source, which controls the electron transfer rate. Quantum dots are formed by reducing metal ions at the cathode, and their size and shape can be controlled by adjusting the voltage, current density, and reaction time. This method offers several advantages over other synthesis methods, including high purity, small particle sizes, and ease of post-synthesis modifications. A significant advantage of electrochemical synthesis is that it can produce large quantities of quantum dots. Furthermore, using non-toxic and low-cost precursors, such as metal salts and organic compounds, makes electrochemical synthesis a sustainable and environmentally friendly method (Gopalakrishnan et al., 2015; Ahirwar, Mallick and Bahadur, 2017).

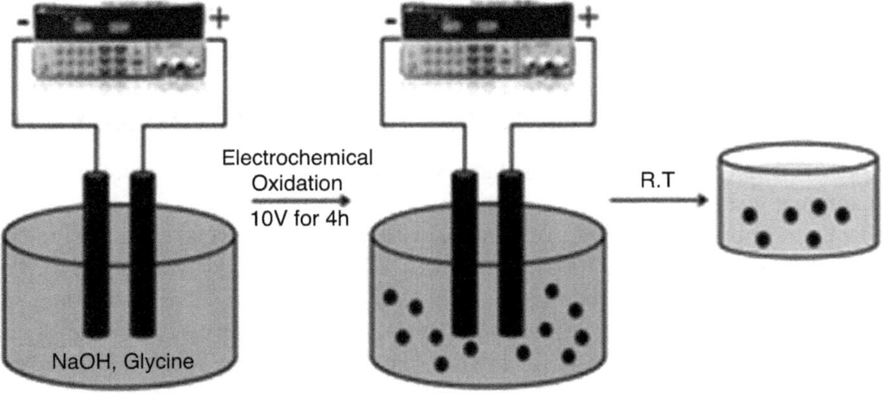

FIGURE 5.7 Synthesis of glycine functionalized graphene quantum dots based on the direct exfoliation and oxidation from graphite rods (Fu, Liu and Zhi, 2018) [Open access].

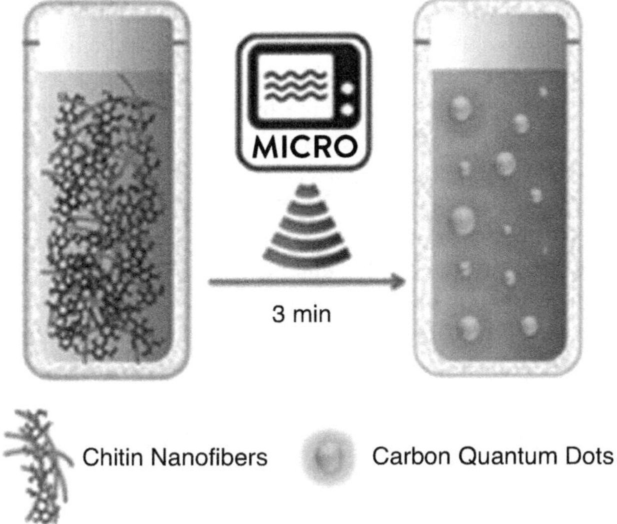

FIGURE 5.8 Schematic of the process of microwave-assisted synthesis of carbon quantum dots from chitin nanofibers (Pan et al., 2020) [Open access].

5.4.5 Microwave Synthesis

The microwave method (Figure 5.8) involves using a microwave reactor, which generates electromagnetic waves that induce the heating of the reaction mixture. The metal precursors and the reducing agent are mixed in a suitable solvent, and the mixture is irradiated with microwaves to induce the formation of quantum dots. The size and shape of the quantum dots can be controlled by adjusting the reaction conditions, such as the power of the microwave, the reaction time, and the concentration of the precursors while using surfactants or capping agents to control the surface chemistry and stability. The technique can also be easily scaled up to produce large quantities of quantum dots (Singh et al., 2019).

5.5 TOXICITY AND FUNCTIONALIZATION OF QUANTUM DOTS

Safety and biocompatibility are the factors that must be considered before employing quantum dots in biological applications. Exposure to quantum dots may have adverse effects on human health, but the fundamental cause–effect relationship is unclear (Derfus, Chan and Bhatia, 2004). The toxicity of quantum dots is influenced by their inherent physicochemical properties, such as their size, charge, concentration, surfactants, functional groups, and environmental conditions (Derfus, Chan and Bhatia, 2004; Hardman, 2006; Pan et al., 2007). Surface coating and core–shell structures are considered practical solutions for eliminating quantum dot toxicity resulting from releasing heavy metal ions (Dabbousi et al., 1997; Selvan, 2010).

Functionalization of quantum dots is needed to tailor their properties for specific applications. For quantum dots to be utilized in biological applications, they must be water-soluble. One way to achieve this is directly synthesizing quantum dots in an aqueous solution with hydrophilic surfactants. The second involves exchanging the pre-existing ligand with another ligand to alter the surface chemistry of the quantum dots, making them more compatible with specific solvents or biological environments. This makes the quantum dots more hydrophilic, allowing them to be more easily dispersed in water-based solutions (Bilan et al., 2015). It also improves its biocompatibility, and in some cases, it can enhance the performance of quantum dots (Tian et al., 2014; Ghanbari et al., 2021). Another concern is the possible leaching of toxic metals from the quantum dot core, such as cadmium or lead. However, functionalization can help stabilize the quantum dot surface and reduce the potential for metal leaching. Functionalized quantum dots have been shown to be less toxic than unmodified quantum dots (Gidwani et al., 2021), likely due to their improved biocompatibility and reduced tendency to aggregate.

5.6 QUANTUM DOTS: THE NEXT BIG THING IN BIOMEDICAL IMAGING

Clinical applications employ various imaging techniques, such as magnetic resonance imaging, computed tomography, positron emission tomography, single-photon emission computed tomography, and ultrasound. These have distinct benefits and drawbacks: for example, magnetic resonance imaging can generate high-resolution anatomical and functional images with exceptional tissue penetration; however, it lacks image contrast. Positron emission tomography is highly sensitive, but its resolution is limited (Judenhofer et al., 2008). Most of these imaging techniques require expensive and large machines to produce images and have scanning periods ranging from minutes to hours, along with lengthy image reconstruction times (Alkhybari et al., 2018).

Fluorescence imaging is an alternative technique for real-time imaging with high contrast and resolution (Zhang et al., 2019a; Huang et al., 2019). However, for the biological implications of fluorophores and their use in imaging, these probes must exhibit specific characteristics: they must be sensitive to their intended target, non-toxic to the organism, emit high amounts of light, and possess photostability. These characteristics will help visualize the probe's distribution and localization at a reasonable depth within the tissue. Existing fluorescent materials include small organic pigments, metal complexes (e.g., Ir, Ru, and Ln), fluorescent proteins, polymers, and nanoparticles. Unfortunately, these are detrimental in biological applications (Hemmer et al., 2016).

Quantum dots, one of the most promising pre-clinical materials, can substitute fluorescent substances. Its compact size, exceptional light-emitting properties in aqueous solutions, excellent photostability, and biocompatibility are its primary advantages over conventional molecular dyes and other materials (Resch-Genger et al., 2008) and permit developing of novel therapeutic applications with enhanced properties (Samia, Chen and Burda, 2003). As quantum dots offer unparalleled sensitivity and specificity, they become indispensable disease detection, monitoring, and treatment tools.

5.6.1 *In vitro* Imaging

In vitro imaging allows visualizing and studying biological processes at the cellular and molecular levels. Quantum dots are suitable fluorescent instruments for *in vitro* imaging applications due to their exceptional optical properties, which can be used to label various biological targets, such as proteins, deoxyribonucleic acid (DNA), and cellular membranes, to enable real-time monitoring of biological processes.

5.6.1.1 Protein Labeling

Quantum dots have been extensively utilized for protein labeling, as they can be conjugated with various biomolecules, such as antibodies, peptides, and aptamers, to enable targeted imaging and detection of proteins of interest (Wang et al., 2015). These have also been used to image intracellular proteins such as actin, tubulin, and histones to facilitate the study of living cells (Katrukha et al., 2017).

Using quantum dots in protein labeling has also led to significant advances in fluorescence microscopy, particularly in single-molecule tracking and super-resolution imaging techniques. The enhanced photostability of quantum dots allows for long-term tracking of individual proteins in live cells and provides insights into protein dynamics and interactions (Huang et al., 2008).

5.6.1.2 DNA Labeling

Quantum dots can be used for DNA labeling by conjugating with DNA-binding molecules, such as intercalating pigments or peptides and enabling real-time DNA visualization (Zhang et al., 2019b). These have also been utilized to image chromosomal DNA, allowing for the visualization of chromosome organization and dynamics in living cells (Dubertret et al., 2002).

Quantum dots have been utilized to label specific DNA sequences within cells and tissue samples by conjugating them to peptide nucleic acid probes. This approach, known as quantum dot-fluorescence *in situ* hybridization, offers improved photostability and signal brightness compared to traditional organic fluorophore techniques. Also, DNA-based biosensors can be used to detect specific target molecules, such as metal ions, small molecules, and proteins (Zhang et al., 2005).

5.6.1.3 Cellular Membrane Labeling

Quantum dots can label cellular membranes by conjugating them with lipids, such as phospholipids or cholesterol, to enable real-time imaging of cellular membranes (Mandal and Jana, 2017). These have been utilized for imaging subcellular structures, such as mitochondria and lysosomes, for understanding cellular processes such as apoptosis and autophagy (Unnikrishnan et al., 2020).

Quantum dots can help track lipids crucial in various cellular processes, including signal transduction and membrane trafficking (Gao et al., 2004). They have also been employed to study membrane protein interactions and dynamics (Jares-Erijman and Jovin, 2006).

The unique optical properties of quantum dots have enabled their use in super-resolution microscopy techniques, such as stochastic optical reconstruction microscopy and photoactivated localization microscopy, which rely on the precise localization of individual fluorophores to achieve resolution beyond the diffraction limit (Huang et al., 2008). These techniques can provide high-resolution images of membrane structures and molecular interactions by labeling cell membrane components with quantum dots.

5.6.2 *In vivo* Imaging

One of the critical advantages of quantum dots for *in vivo* imaging is their greater luminosity and photostability compared to conventional organic dyes, making them appropriate for long-term imaging research and enabling the detection of minor signal intensity variations over time (Wu et al., 2002).

5.6.2.1 Cell Imaging

Quantum dots can precisely target cells or subcellular structures by being functionalized with biomolecules like peptides, antibodies, or aptamers. Cancer cell research is one of the most promising uses of quantum dot-based cellular imaging: labeling cancer cells with quantum dots helps identify cancer cells *in vivo* and monitor tumor growth (Wang et al., 2015).

In addition to imaging cancer cells, quantum dots can identify and monitor stem cells *in vivo*, allowing the study of stem cell differentiation and migration (Srivastava and Bulte, 2014). These have also been used to mark immune cells (Byers and Hitchman, 2011), neurons, and glial cells, allowing *in vivo* monitoring of immunological and neural networks (Zhang et al., 2019c).

Quantum dots have been employed in live-cell imaging to study various dynamic cellular processes, such as endocytosis, exocytosis, and intracellular trafficking. For instance, quantum dots conjugated to epidermal growth factor help visualize and track receptors in live cells (Lidke et al., 2004). This approach allowed the real-time observation of receptor trafficking and endocytic pathways, providing new insights into cell membrane dynamics and molecular interactions.

Quantum dots have also been used in fixed-cell imaging to label and visualize cellular structures and components, such as the cytoskeleton, organelles, and nucleic acids (Dahan et al., 2003). For example, quantum dots conjugated to phalloidin—a toxin that specifically binds to F-actin, a key spine component—help visualize the actin cytoskeleton in fixed cells (Courty et al., 2006). This approach enabled high-resolution imaging of actin filaments and their organization within the cell. In conjunction with stochastic optical reconstruction microscopy, quantum dots can achieve super-resolution imaging of multiple cellular targets, including microtubules, mitochondria, and the Golgi apparatus (Howarth et al., 2008).

Quantum dots have also been employed in multiplexed imaging, allowing the simultaneous visualization of multiple cellular components within a single sample. Researchers can image multiple cellular structures and processes in parallel by conjugating quantum dots of different sizes and emission wavelengths to distinct target-specific probes (Xing et al., 2007).

5.6.2.2 Tissue Imaging

The study of cellular processes and the diagnosis of diseases rely heavily on tissue imaging. Quantum dots have emerged as a promising instrument for tissue imaging due to their unique optical properties, including high luminosity, photostability, and tunable emission spectra. Their small dimensions—one of their key advantages—allow rapid diffusion and distribution throughout the body and can be conjugated with targeting ligands, such as antibodies, peptides, and aptamers, to target specific cells and tissues, such as cancer (K. Iyer, He and M. Amiji, 2012).

Quantum dots have been employed in tissue imaging by conjugating them to tissue-specific probes like antibodies and peptides or small molecules targeting specific tissue structures or biomolecules (Smith et al., 2008). Also, quantum dots have been successfully applied in *in vivo* and *ex vivo* tissue imaging to visualize tissue organization, molecular interactions, and dynamic processes in various tissue types.

Quantum dots are also used to image vascular structures and tissue blood vessels. Quantum dots coated with polyethylene glycol and conjugated to the vascular targeting peptides could be used for *in vivo* imaging of tumor angiogenesis as they help visualize tumor vasculature, providing insights into tumor growth and progression (Ballou et al., 2004).

Moreover, neuroscience has applied quantum dots to imaging neural tissue structures and processes by conjugating them to a nerve growth factor to visualize and track the growth factor's transport in live neurons. This approach provided new insights into the nervous system's neuronal signaling and axonal transport mechanisms (Michalet et al., 2005).

5.7 CONCLUSION AND PROSPECTS

In recent years, significant progress has been made in creating new kinds of quantum dots for biological applications. Advancements in optical detection and biosensing suggest quantum dots are prosperous in biological imaging, especially in fluorescence tracking experiments that could improve our understanding of cellular events. The development of quantum dot-based nanocomposites, which could serve as *in vitro*, *in vivo*, and potential therapeutic agents, is an additional up-and-coming area. However, several critical issues and problems must be deciphered, addressed, and resolved before scaling up the approaches for producing multimodal nanocomposites.

Quantum dots have several intriguing properties that make them clinically useful. Quantum dots showed promise in bioimaging, suggesting they could replace contrast dyes and radioactive isotopes in human diagnostic imaging. They can also be modified with specific ligands or coupled to specific antibodies to control their accumulation in desired tissues/organs after intravenous delivery, enabling high-efficiency and biosafety tissue imaging compared to conventional probes. However, it is necessary to address a few critical factors to enhance their clinical translatability:

1. Eco-friendly, aqueous solvent-based, or biotechnology-based synthetic methods should be adopted to reduce environmental risks, enhance scalability, and omit unnecessary post-synthetic modifications, thereby reducing the system's complexity and production cost.
2. Functional coating with intelligent materials such as pH-responsive polymers and biomaterials should be encouraged to enhance stability and scalability.
3. Synthesis using heavy metals should be eliminated to reduce biosafety risks associated with the accumulation of heavy metals in the body.
4. A balance between the body retention and clearance ability of quantum dots should be achieved by manipulating particle size, charge, and surface properties to ensure that the administered quantum dots remain in the body for sufficient time to exert their intended application while ensuring their clearance to avoid toxicity risks.
5. Establishing experimental protocols for the various applications is necessary to expand their utilization compared to traditional alternatives.
6. Despite significant progress and the potential of quantum dot-based nanomaterials, the overwhelming majority can only be used for fundamental research or remain of academic interest owing to their potential toxicity and stringent regulations in *in vivo* applications. The modes of toxicity must be verified and investigated, and novel procedures must be developed to reduce their risk factors.
7. Lastly, the cost of producing biocompatible quantum dots should be minimized. This will necessitate readily scalable and trustworthy techniques, access to inexpensive non-hazardous precursors, low-energy approaches, eco-friendly solvents, and low-cost processing technologies and facilities.

We anticipate significant advancements in fundamental research and quantum dots' practical applications. The synthesis of novel materials with unusual structures and properties is a limitless frontier and will continue to produce surprises in the upcoming future.

REFERENCES

Aboulaich, A. et al. (2012) 'One-pot noninjection route to CdS quantum dots via hydrothermal synthesis', *ACS Applied Materials and Interfaces*, 4(5), pp. 2561–2569. doi: 10.1021/AM300232Z/SUPPL_FILE/AM300232Z_SI_001.PDF.

Ahirwar, S., Mallick, S. and Bahadur, D. (2017) 'Electrochemical method to prepare graphene quantum dots and graphene oxide quantum dots', *ACS Omega*, 2(11), pp. 8343–8353. doi: 10.1021/ACSOMEGA.7B01539/ASSET/IMAGES/LARGE/AO-2017-01539G_0005.JPEG.

Alferov, Z. I. (2013) 'The semiconductor revolution in the 20th century', *Russian Chemical Reviews*, 82(7), pp. 587–596. doi: 10.1070/RC2013V082N07ABEH004403/XML.

Alkhybari, E. M. et al. (2018) 'Determining and updating PET/CT and SPECT/CT diagnostic reference levels: A systematic review', *Radiation Protection Dosimetry*, 182(4), pp. 532–545. doi: 10.1093/RPD/NCY113.

Ballou, B. et al. (2004) 'Noninvasive imaging of quantum dots in mice', *Bioconjugate Chemistry*, 15(1), pp. 79–86. doi: 10.1021/BC034153Y/SUPPL_FILE/BC034153YSI20040109_033449.PDF.

Bilan, R. et al. (2015) 'Quantum dot surface chemistry and functionalization for cell targeting and imaging', *Bioconjugate Chemistry*, 26(4), pp. 609–624. doi: 10.1021/ACS.BIOCONJCHEM.5B00069/ASSET/IMAGES/LARGE/BC-2015-00069M_0006.JPEG.

Böhm, M. L. et al. (2015) 'Lead telluride quantum dot solar cells displaying external quantum efficiencies exceeding 120%', *Nano Letters*, 15(12), pp. 7987–7993. doi: 10.1021/ACS.NANOLETT.5B03161/ASSET/IMAGES/LARGE/NL-2015-031618_0004.JPEG.

Bourzac, K. (2013) 'Quantum dots go on display', *Nature*, 493(7432), p. 283. doi: 10.1038/493283A.

Byers, R. J. and Hitchman, E. R. (2011) 'Quantum dots brighten biological imaging', *Progress in Histochemistry and Cytochemistry*, 45(4), pp. 201–237. doi: 10.1016/J.PROGHI.2010.11.001.

Ca, N. X. et al. (2019) 'Photoluminescence properties of CdTe/CdTeSe/CdSe core/alloyed/shell type-II quantum dots', *Journal of Alloys and Compounds*, 787, pp. 823–830. doi: 10.1016/J.JALLCOM.2019.02.139.

Cai, X. et al. (2016) 'PH-sensitive ZnO quantum dots-doxorubicin nanoparticles for lung cancer targeted drug delivery', *ACS Applied Materials and Interfaces*, 8(34), pp. 22442–22450. doi: 10.1021/ACSAMI.6B04933/ASSET/IMAGES/LARGE/AM-2016-049336_0007.JPEG.

Cao, Y. et al. (2022) 'Dual-color quantum dot-loaded nanoparticles based lateral flow biosensor for the simultaneous detection of gastric cancer markers in a single test line', *Analytica Chimica Acta*, 1218, p. 339998. doi: 10.1016/J.ACA.2022.339998.

Carneiro, S. V. et al. (2021) 'Highly sensitive sensing of food additives based on fluorescent carbon quantum dots', *Journal of Photochemistry and Photobiology A: Chemistry*, 411, p. 113198. doi: 10.1016/J.JPHOTOCHEM.2021.113198.

Chen, N. et al. (2012) 'The cytotoxicity of cadmium-based quantum dots', *Biomaterials*, 33(5), pp. 1238–1244. doi: 10.1016/J.BIOMATERIALS.2011.10.070.

Chi, W. et al. (2022) 'Performance improvement of perovskite solar cells by interactions between nano-sized quantum dots and perovskite', *Advanced Functional Materials*, 32(28), p. 2200029. doi: 10.1002/ADFM.202200029.

Commons, W. (no date) *File:Quantum Dots with emission maxima in a 10-nm step are being produced at PlasmaChem in a kg scale.jpg*. Available at: https://en.m.wikipedia.org/wiki/File:Quantum_Dots_with_emission_maxima_in_a_10-nm_step_are_being_produced_at_PlasmaChem_in_a_kg_scale.jpg (Accessed: 17 April 2023).

Courty, S. et al. (2006) 'Tracking individual kinesin motors in living cells using single quantum-dot imaging', *Nano Letters*, 6(7), pp. 1491–1495. doi: 10.1021/NL060921T/SUPPL_FILE/NL060921TSI20060425_064605.PDF.

Dabbousi, B. O. et al. (1997) '(CdSe)ZnS core-shell quantum dots: Synthesis and characterization of a size series of highly luminescent nanocrystallites', *Journal of Physical Chemistry B*, 101(46), pp. 9463–9475. doi: 10.1021/JP971091Y/ASSET/IMAGES/LARGE/JP971091YF00016.JPEG.

Dahan, M. et al. (2003) 'Diffusion dynamics of glycine receptors revealed by single-quantum dot tracking', *Science*, 302(5644), pp. 442–445. doi: 10.1126/SCIENCE.1088525/SUPPL_FILE/DAHAN.SOM.PDF.

Derfus, A. M., Chan, W. C. W. and Bhatia, S. N. (2004) 'Probing the cytotoxicity of semiconductor quantum dots', *Nano Letters*, 4(1), pp. 11–18. doi: 10.1021/NL0347334/SUPPL_FILE/NL0347334SI20030903_032807.PDF.

Dorfs, D. and Eychmüller, A. (2006) 'Multishell semiconductor nanocrystals', *Zeitschrift fur Physikalische Chemie*, 220(12), pp. 1539–1552. doi: 10.1524/ZPCH.2006.220.12.1539/MACHINEREADABLECITATION/RIS.

Drexler, E. (1987) *Engines of creation: The coming era of nanotechnology*. Anchor Doubleday, New York City.

Drexler, E. (no date) *The promise that launched the field of nanotechnology*. Available at: https://web.archive.org/web/20110714075738/https://metamodern.com/2009/12/15/when-a-million-readers-first-encountered-nanotechnology/ (Accessed: 16 April 2023).

Dubertret, B. et al. (2002) 'In vivo imaging of quantum dots encapsulated in phospholipid micelles', *Science*, 298(5599), pp. 1759–1762. doi: 10.1126/SCIENCE.1077194/SUPPL_FILE/DUBERTRET.SOM.PDF.

Efros, A. L. and Brus, L. E. (2021) 'Nanocrystal quantum dots: From discovery to modern development', *ACS Nano*, 15(4), pp. 6192–6210. doi: 10.1021/ACSNANO.1C01399/ASSET/IMAGES/LARGE/NN1C01399_0009.JPEG.

Ehrler, B. et al. (2020) 'Photovoltaics reaching for the shockley-queisser limit', *ACS Energy Letters*, 5(9), pp. 3029–3033. doi: 10.1021/ACSENERGYLETT.0C01790/ASSET/IMAGES/MEDIUM/NZ0C01790_M002.GIF.

Fan, H. et al. (2005) 'Surfactant-assisted synthesis of water-soluble and biocompatible semiconductor quantum dot micelles', *Nano Letters*, 5(4), pp. 645–648. doi: 10.1021/NL050017L/SUPPL_FILE/NL050017LSI20050104_114415.PDF.

Feynman, R. (2018) 'There's plenty of room at the bottom', In *Feynman and computation*. CRC Press, Boca Raton, pp. 63–76.

Fu, H. et al. (2022) 'Quantum dot hybridization of piezoelectric polymer films for non-transfer integration of flexible biomechanical energy harvesters', *ACS Applied Materials and Interfaces*, 14(26), pp. 29934–29944. doi: 10.1021/ACSAMI.2C07297/ASSET/IMAGES/LARGE/AM2C07297_0008.JPEG.

Fu, Y., Liu, R. and Zhi, J. (2018) 'Facile synthesis of graphene quantum dots based on electrochemical method and their application for specific Fe3+ detection', *Advanced Materials Letters*, 9(9), pp. 614–618. doi: 10.5185/AMLETT.2018.2052.

Gao, X. et al. (2004) 'In vivo cancer targeting and imaging with semiconductor quantum dots', *Nature Biotechnology*, 22(8), pp. 969–976. doi: 10.1038/nbt994.

Ghanbari, N. et al. (2021) 'Tryptophan-functionalized graphene quantum dots with enhanced curcumin loading capacity and pH-sensitive release', *Journal of Drug Delivery Science and Technology*, 61, p. 102137. doi: 10.1016/J.JDDST.2020.102137.

Gidwani, B. et al. (2021) 'Quantum dots: Prospectives, toxicity, advances and applications', *Journal of Drug Delivery Science and Technology*, 61, p. 102308. doi: 10.1016/J.JDDST.2020.102308.

Gopalakrishnan, D. et al. (2015) 'Electrochemical synthesis of luminescent MoS2 quantum dots', *Chemical Communications*, 51(29), pp. 6293–6296. doi: 10.1039/C4CC09826A.

Han, M. et al. (2001) 'Quantum-dot-tagged microbeads for multiplexed optical coding of biomolecules', *Nature Biotechnology*, 19(7), pp. 631–635. doi: 10.1038/90228.

Hardman, R. (2006) 'A toxicologic review of quantum dots: Toxicity depends on physicochemical and environmental factors', *Environmental Health Perspectives*, 114(2), pp. 165–172. doi: 10.1289/EHP.8284.

Hemmer, E. et al. (2016) 'Exploiting the biological windows: Current perspectives on fluorescent bioprobes emitting above 1000 nm', *Nanoscale Horizons*, 1(3), pp. 168–184. doi: 10.1039/C5NH00073D.

Howarth, M. et al. (2008) 'Monovalent, reduced-size quantum dots for imaging receptors on living cells', *Nature Methods*, 5(5), pp. 397–399. doi: 10.1038/nmeth.1206.

Hu, Q. et al. (2020) 'An ultra-selective fluorescence method with enhanced sensitivity for the determination of manganese (VII) in food stuffs using carbon quantum dots as nanoprobe', *Journal of Food Composition and Analysis*, 88, p. 103447. doi: 10.1016/J.JFCA.2020.103447.

Huang, B. et al. (2008) 'Three-dimensional super-resolution imaging by stochastic optical reconstruction microscopy', *Science*, 319(5864), pp. 810–813. doi: 10.1126/SCIENCE.1153529/SUPPL_FILE/HUANG.SOM.PDF.

Huang, J. et al. (2019) 'Renal-clearable molecular semiconductor for second near-infrared fluorescence imaging of kidney dysfunction', *Angewandte Chemie International Edition*, 58(42), pp. 15120–15127. doi: 10.1002/ANIE.201909560.

Huang, K. et al. (2023a) 'MMP9-responsive graphene oxide quantum dot-based nano-in-micro drug delivery system for combinatorial therapy of choroidal neovascularization', *Small*, p. 2207335. doi: 10.1002/SMLL.202207335.

Huang, K. et al. (2023b) 'Perovskite-quantum dot hybrid solar cells: A multi-win strategy for high performance and stability', *Journal of Materials Chemistry A*, 11(9), pp. 4487–4509. doi: 10.1039/D2TA09434G.

Jalali, H. B. et al. (2022) 'Past, present and future of indium phosphide quantum dots', *Nano Research*, 15(5), pp. 4468–4489. doi: 10.1007/S12274-021-4038-Z.

Jares-Erijman, E. A. and Jovin, T. M. (2006) 'Imaging molecular interactions in living cells by FRET microscopy', *Current Opinion in Chemical Biology*, 10(5), pp. 409–416. doi: 10.1016/J.CBPA.2006.08.021.

Judenhofer, M. S. et al. (2008) 'Simultaneous PET-MRI: A new approach for functional and morphological imaging', *Nature Medicine*, 14(4), pp. 459–465. doi: 10.1038/nm1700.

K. Iyer, A., He, J. and M. Amiji, M. (2012) 'Image-guided nanosystems for targeted delivery in cancer therapy', *Current Medicinal Chemistry*, 19(19), pp. 3230–3240. doi: 10.2174/092986712800784685.

Katrukha, E. A. et al. (2017) 'Probing cytoskeletal modulation of passive and active intracellular dynamics using nanobody-functionalized quantum dots', *Nature Communications*, 8(1), pp. 1–8. doi: 10.1038/ncomms14772.

Kortlever, R. et al. (2022) 'Industry outlook of perovskite quantum dots for display applications', *Nature Nanotechnology*, 17(8), pp. 813–816. doi: 10.1038/s41565-022-01163-8.

Kriekouki, I. et al. (2022) 'Interpretation of 28 nm FD-SOI quantum dot transport data taken at 1.4 K using 3D quantum TCAD simulations', *Solid-State Electronics*, 194, p. 108355. doi: 10.1016/J.SSE.2022.108355.

Kurniawan, D. et al. (2022) 'Plasma nanoengineering of bioresource-derived graphene quantum dots as ultrasensitive environmental nanoprobes', *ACS Applied Materials and Interfaces*, 14(46), pp. 52289–52300. doi: 10.1021/ACSAMI.2C15251/ASSET/IMAGES/LARGE/AM2C15251_0007.JPEG.

Lidke, D. S. et al. (2004) 'Quantum dot ligands provide new insights into erbB/HER receptor–mediated signal transduction', *Nature Biotechnology*, 22(2), pp. 198–203. doi: 10.1038/nbt929.

Linghu, X. et al. (2023) 'Fluorescence immunoassay based on magnetic separation and ZnCdSe/ZnS quantum dots as a signal marker for intelligent detection of sesame allergen in foods', *Talanta*, 256, p. 124323. doi: 10.1016/J.TALANTA.2023.124323.

Liu, C., Ji, Y. and Tan, T. (2013) 'One-pot hydrothermal synthesis of water-dispersible ZnS quantum dots modified with mercaptoacetic acid', *Journal of Alloys and Compounds*, 570, pp. 23–27. doi: 10.1016/J.JALLCOM.2013.03.118.

Liu, Z. et al. (2020) 'Micro-light-emitting diodes with quantum dots in display technology', *Light: Science & Applications*, 9(1), pp. 1–23. doi: 10.1038/s41377-020-0268-1.

Mandal, S. and Jana, N. R. (2017) 'Quantum dot-based designed nanoprobe for imaging lipid droplet', *Journal of Physical Chemistry C*, 121(42), pp. 23727–23735. doi: 10.1021/ACS.JPCC.7B07571/SUPPL_FILE/JP7B07571_LIVESLIDES.MP4.

Michalet, X. et al. (2005) 'Quantum dots for live cells, in vivo imaging, and diagnostics', *Science*, 307(5709), pp. 538–544. doi: 10.1126/SCIENCE.1104274/SUPPL_FILE/MICHALET.SOM.PDF.

Moasses Ghafary, S. et al. (2022) 'Design and preparation of a theranostic peptideticle for targeted cancer therapy: Peptide-based codelivery of doxorubicin/curcumin and graphene quantum dots', *Nanomedicine: Nanotechnology, Biology and Medicine*, 42, p. 102544. doi: 10.1016/J.NANO.2022.102544.

Mohamed, W. A. A. et al. (2021) 'Quantum dots synthetization and future prospect applications', *Nanotechnology Reviews*, 10(1), pp. 1926–1940. doi: 10.1515/NTREV-2021–0118/ASSET/GRAPHIC/J_NTREV-2021–0118_FIG_013.JPG.

Mulder, W. J. M. et al. (2010) 'Quantum dots for multimodal molecular imaging of angiogenesis', *Angiogenesis*, 13(2), pp. 131–134. doi: 10.1007/S10456-010-9177-X/FIGURES/3.

Munasinghe, E. et al. (2019) 'Magnetic and quantum dot nanoparticles for drug delivery and diagnostic systems', *Colloid Science in Pharmaceutical Nanotechnology*. doi: 10.5772/INTECHOPEN.88611.

Murali, G. et al. (2022) 'Hematoporphyrin photosensitizer-linked carbon quantum dots for photodynamic therapy of cancer cells', *ACS Applied Nano Materials*, 5(3), pp. 4376–4385. doi: 10.1021/ACSANM.2C00443/ASSET/IMAGES/LARGE/AN2C00443_0009.JPEG.

Murray, Cb., Norris, D. J. and Bawendi, M. G. (1993) 'Synthesis and characterization of nearly monodisperse CdE (E= sulfur, selenium, tellurium) semiconductor nanocrystallites', *Journal of the American Chemical Society*, 115(19), pp. 8706–8715.

Nemati, F. et al. (2018) 'Sensitive recognition of ethion in food samples using turn-on fluorescence N and S co-doped graphene quantum dots', *Analytical Methods*, 10(15), pp. 1760–1766. doi: 10.1039/C7AY02850D.

Niu, X. et al. (2018) 'A "turn-on" fluorescence sensor for Pb2+ detection based on graphene quantum dots and gold nanoparticles', *Sensors and Actuators B: Chemical*, 255, pp. 1577–1581. doi: 10.1016/J.SNB.2017.08.167.

Norman, J. C., Mirin, R. P. and Bowers, J. E. (2021) 'Quantum dot lasers—history and future prospects', *Journal of Vacuum Science & Technology A: Vacuum, Surfaces, and Films*, 39(2), p. 020802. doi: 10.1116/6.0000768.

Pan, M. et al. (2020) 'Fluorescent carbon quantum dots—synthesis, functionalization and sensing application in food analysis', *Nanomaterials*, 10(5), p. 930. doi: 10.3390/NANO10050930.

Pan, Y. et al. (2007) 'Size-dependent cytotoxicity of gold nanoparticles', *Small*, 3(11), pp. 1941–1949. doi: 10.1002/SMLL.200700378.

Panagiotopoulou, M. et al. (2016) 'Molecularly imprinted polymer coated quantum dots for multiplexed cell targeting and imaging', *Angewandte Chemie*, 128(29), pp. 8384–8388. doi: 10.1002/ANGE.201601122.

Peng, Z. A. and Peng, X. (2001) 'Formation of high-quality CdTe, CdSe, and CdS nanocrystals using CdO as precursor', *Journal of the American Chemical Society*, 123(1), pp. 183–184. doi: 10.1021/JA003633M/ASSET/JA003633M.FP.PNG_V03.

Rahmani, E. et al. (2022) 'Preparation of a pH-responsive chitosan-montmorillonite-nitrogen-doped carbon quantum dots nanocarrier for attenuating doxorubicin limitations in cancer therapy', *Engineering in Life Sciences*, 22(10), pp. 634–649. doi: 10.1002/ELSC.202200016.

Rao, C. N. R., Müller, A. and Cheetham, A. K. (2006) *The chemistry of nanomaterials: Synthesis, properties and applications*. John Wiley & Sons., Weinheim.

Resch-Genger, U. et al. (2008) 'Quantum dots versus organic dyes as fluorescent labels', *Nature Methods*, 5(9), pp. 763–775. doi: 10.1038/nmeth.1248.

Ruffino, A. et al. (2021) 'A cryo-CMOS chip that integrates silicon quantum dots and multiplexed dispersive readout electronics', *Nature Electronics*, 5(1), pp. 53–59. doi: 10.1038/s41928-021-00687-6.

Safardoust-Hojaghan, H. et al. (2017) 'Preparation of highly luminescent nitrogen doped graphene quantum dots and their application as a probe for detection of *Staphylococcus aureus* and *E. coli*', *Journal of Molecular Liquids*, 241, pp. 1114–1119. doi: 10.1016/J.MOLLIQ.2017.06.106.

Samia, A. C. S., Chen, X. and Burda, C. (2003) 'Semiconductor quantum dots for photodynamic therapy', *Journal of the American Chemical Society*, 125(51), pp. 15736–15737. doi: 10.1021/JA0386905/SUPPL_FILE/JA0386905SI20031114_115000.PDF.

Samimi, S., Ardestani, M. S. and Dorkoosh, F. A. (2021) 'Preparation of carbon quantum dots-quinic acid for drug delivery of gemcitabine to breast cancer cells', *Journal of Drug Delivery Science and Technology*, 61, p. 102287. doi: 10.1016/J.JDDST.2020.102287.

Seidler, I. et al. (2022) 'Conveyor-mode single-electron shuttling in Si/SiGe for a scalable quantum computing architecture', *npj Quantum Information*, 8(1), pp. 1–7. doi: 10.1038/s41534-022-00615-2.

Selvan, S. T. (2010) 'Silica-coated quantum dots and magnetic nanoparticles for bioimaging applications (mini-review)', *Biointerphases*, 5(3), p. FA110. doi: 10.1116/1.3516492.

Shellaiah, M. et al. (2022) 'Methylammonium tin tribromide quantum dots for heavy metal ion detection and cellular imaging', *ACS Applied Nano Materials*, 5(2), pp. 2859–2874. doi: 10.1021/ACSANM.2C00028/ASSET/IMAGES/LARGE/AN2C00028_0008.JPEG.

Singh, R. K. et al. (2019) 'Progress in microwave-assisted synthesis of quantum dots (graphene/carbon/semiconducting) for bioapplications: A review', *Materials Today Chemistry*, 12, pp. 282–314. doi: 10.1016/J.MTCHEM.2019.03.001.

Smith, A. M. et al. (2008) 'Bioconjugated quantum dots for in vivo molecular and cellular imaging', *Advanced Drug Delivery Reviews*, 60(11), pp. 1226–1240. doi: 10.1016/J.ADDR.2008.03.015.

Smith, A. M. and Nie, S. (2009) 'Next-generation quantum dots', *Nature Biotechnology*, 27(8), pp. 732–733. doi: 10.1038/nbt0809-732.

Srivastava, A. K. and Bulte, J. W. M. (2014) 'Seeing stem cells at work in vivo', *Stem Cell Reviews and Reports*, 10(1), pp. 127–144. doi: 10.1007/S12015-013-9468-X/FIGURES/6.

Sukhanova, A. et al. (2012) 'Oriented conjugates of single-domain antibodies and quantum dots: Toward a new generation of ultrasmall diagnostic nanoprobes', *Nanomedicine: Nanotechnology, Biology and Medicine*, 8(4), pp. 516–525. doi: 10.1016/J.NANO.2011.07.007.

Sun, B. et al. (2018) 'Multibandgap quantum dot ensembles for solar-matched infrared energy harvesting', *Nature Communications*, 9(1), pp. 1–7. doi: 10.1038/s41467-018-06342-7.

Sun, Y. et al. (2020) 'Recent development of carbon quantum dots: Biological toxicity, antibacterial properties and application in foods', *Food Reviews International*, 38(7), pp. 1513–1532. doi: 10.1080/87559129.2020.1818255.

Taniguchi, N. (1974) 'On the basic concept of nanotechnology', In *Proceeding of the ICPE.*

Tian, R. et al. (2014) 'Tailoring surface groups of carbon quantum dots to improve photoluminescence behaviors', *Applied Surface Science*, 301, pp. 156–160. doi: 10.1016/J.APSUSC.2014.02.028.

Toumey, C. P. (2008) 'Reading Feynman into nanotechnology: A text for a new science', *Techné: Research in Philosophy and Technology*, 12(3), pp. 133–168.

Tsuboi, S. and Jin, T. (2022) 'In vitro and in vivo fluorescence imaging of antibody-drug conjugate-induced tumor apoptosis using annexin V-EGFP conjugated quantum dots', *ACS Omega*, 7(2), pp. 2105–2113. doi: 10.1021/ACSOMEGA.1C05636/ASSET/IMAGES/LARGE/AO1C05636_0009.JPEG.

Unnikrishnan, B. et al. (2020) 'Fluorescent carbon dots for selective labeling of subcellular organelles', *ACS Omega*, 5(20), pp. 11248–11261. doi: 10.1021/ACSOMEGA.9B04301/ASSET/IMAGES/LARGE/AO9B04301_0008.JPEG.

Vastola, G., Zhang, Y. W. and Shenoy, V. B. (2012) 'Experiments and modeling of alloying in self-assembled quantum dots', *Current Opinion in Solid State and Materials Science*, 16(2), pp. 64–70. doi: 10.1016/J.COSSMS.2011.10.004.

Wang, L. W. et al. (2015) 'Quantum dots-based tissue and in vivo imaging in breast cancer researches: Current status and future perspectives', *Breast Cancer Research and Treatment*, 151(1), pp. 7–17. doi: 10.1007/S10549-015-3363-X/TABLES/2.

Wei, J. et al. (2018) 'One-pot synthesis of N, S co-doped photoluminescent carbon quantum dots for Hg2+ ion detection', *New Carbon Materials*, 33(4), pp. 333–340. doi: 10.1016/S1872–5805(18)60343-9.

Wu, X. et al. (2002) 'Immunofluorescent labeling of cancer marker Her2 and other cellular targets with semiconductor quantum dots', *Nature Biotechnology*, 21(1), pp. 41–46. doi: 10.1038/nbt764.

Xing, Y. et al. (2007) 'Bioconjugated quantum dots for multiplexed and quantitative immunohistochemistry', *Nature Protocols*, 2(5), pp. 1152–1165. doi: 10.1038/nprot.2007.107.

Zhang, A. et al. (2019a) 'Carbon-gold hybrid nanoprobes for real-time imaging, photothermal/photodynamic and nanozyme oxidative therapy', *Theranostics*, 9(12), pp. 3443–3458. doi: 10.7150/THNO.33266.

Zhang, C. Y. et al. (2005) 'Single-quantum-dot-based DNA nanosensor', *Nature Materials*, 4(11), pp. 826–831. doi: 10.1038/nmat1508.

Zhang, L. J. et al. (2019b) 'Quantum dot based biotracking and biodetection', *Analytical Chemistry*, 91(1), pp. 532–547. doi: 10.1021/ACS.ANALCHEM.8B04721/ASSET/IMAGES/LARGE/AC-2018–047214_0010.JPEG.

Zhang, M. et al. (2019c) 'Quantum dot cellular uptake and toxicity in the developing brain: Implications for use as imaging probes', *Nanoscale Advances*, 1(9), pp. 3424–3442. doi: 10.1039/C9NA00334G.

Zhang, Q. et al. (2022) 'SARS-CoV-2 detection using quantum dot fluorescence immunochromatography combined with isothermal amplification and CRISPR/Cas13a', *Biosensors and Bioelectronics*, 202, p. 113978. doi: 10.1016/J.BIOS.2022.113978.

Zhao, L. et al. (2019) 'Facile synthesis of nitrogen-doped carbon quantum dots with chitosan for fluorescent detection of Fe^{3+}', *Polymers*, 11(11), p. 1731. doi: 10.3390/POLYM11111731.

Zhu, Y. et al. (2013) 'One-pot preparation of highly fluorescent cadmium telluride/cadmium sulfide quantum dots under neutral-pH condition for biological applications', *Journal of Colloid and Interface Science*, 390(1), pp. 3–10. doi: 10.1016/J.JCIS.2012.08.003.

6 Nanotechnology in Biosensing

The Future of Disease Diagnosis

Nabarun Polley, Backiyalakshmi Gnanasekaran, and Snekhalatha Umapathy

6.1 INTRODUCTION

The history of disease diagnosis can be traced back to ancient times when people used observation and experience to identify symptoms of various illnesses. In the Middle Ages, medical examination started to become a part of the routine where the diagnosis of illness by doctors included a combination of observation, experience, and examination. The development of the microscope in the seventeenth century revolutionized disease diagnosis by enabling doctors and researchers to pinpoint microbes and analyze cellular and tissue architecture. As a result, more efficient and precise diagnostic methods, like blood tests and tissue biopsies, became a part of diagnostic routines. In fact, we are in constant need of a more efficient way of diagnosis and prognosis of diseases in order to improve the quality of life, in general. The conventional way of diagnosis includes symptomatic signatures of the body to indicate a glimpse of the health condition. A better understanding of health conditions can be achieved by identifying and monitoring biomarkers for specific health conditions (Sesay, Tervo and Tikkanen, 2018) instead of symptomatic signatures only. The definition of biomarkers varies from field to field; however, in the context of biosensing, biomarkers are a physiological or molecular indicator that may provide a quantifiable biological or physiological medical diagnostic glimpse. For instance, blood levels of C-reactive protein (CRP) are a useful biomarker for tracking inflammation in the body (Ding et al., 2013) or cholesterol level in the blood for the assessment of cardiovascular disease (Albert, 2011). There are known biomarkers used to diagnose heart failure (Sarhene et al., 2019), cancer (Henry and Hayes, 2012), and multiple sclerosis (Ziemssen, Akgün and Brück, 2019), and they are an active field of research to identify biomarkers for different health conditions. It is worth mentioning that there could be more than one biomarker for a specific health condition (Aronson and Ferner, 2017; Califf, 2018). Often, monitoring biomarkers is easier and cheaper to perform than conventional testing (Aronson, 2005). For instance, in order to determine the risk of heart disease, determining the level of cholesterol in the blood is

DOI: 10.1201/9781003432661-6

easier than investigating the plaque formation in the arteries of the heart invasively (Sesay, Tervo and Tikkanen, 2018).

Biomarkers are traditionally detected by biochemical tests, where tests are performed in laboratory conditions. These tests are often time-consuming, require specialized equipment and trained personnel, and may not be sensitive or specific enough for certain applications. The gold standard to detect and quantify biomarkers including antibodies, antigens, proteins, deoxyribonucleic acid (DNA), glycoproteins, and hormones with high sensitivity and specificity is called enzyme-linked immunosorbent assays (ELISAs). The high sensitivity and specificity are achieved by complexing antibodies and antigens for detection. However, ELISA is performed by trained personnel and has a significant time gap between sample collection and conclusion drawn-out of the test. This is where the biosensor comes into play. Biosensors do not require a laboratory setting for testing and trained personnel to perform the test. Biosensors are also faster and more sensitive, with the ability to detect analytes in real time. There are three main components of a biosensor, namely biorecognition molecule (recognizes the specific analyte (biomarker) of interest), transducers (which convert the recognition event into measurable signal), and internal electronics (to convert the measurable signal into understandable values). Since the biological recognition molecule is an integral part of the biosensor, it is possible to perform chemical-free test for live monitoring of the biorecognition event.

The concept of biosensor was proposed by Professor Leland C. Clark (Clark Jr. and Lyons, 1962; Mascini, 2006) back in 1962. He proposed an electrode-based system for continuous monitoring of pH, pO_2, and pCO_2 during cardiovascular surgery (Clark Jr. and Lyons, 1962). A subsequent study by Updike and Hicks in 1967 described a similar device for the rapid and quantitative determination of glucose (Updike and Hicks, 1967). The first commercial device for measuring glucose in diluted blood was introduced to the market by Yellow Springs Instrument Company (Ohio, USA) in 1974 (Turner, Karube and Wilson, 1987). Over the years, the requirement of sensitive, faster, cheaper, easy-to-use, portable biosensors became the motivation of developing new biosensors and biosensing strategies. One major demand from the healthcare industry is the requirement of a tool for screening at early stage prognosis of a patient for quick and effective treatments (Ashley and Sun, 2018).

At the early stage of disease, most biomarkers are present at very low concentrations (below pg/mL) (Altug et al., 2022); hence, the sensitivity of the biosensor becomes crucial. In this regard, the continuous innovation in nanotechnology comes along the way toward the improvement of the biosensor sensitivity among other benefits. Thanks to the humongous change in surface-to-volume ratio compared to its bulk counterpart, it is capable of detecting biomolecules at the single molecular level (Zijlstra, Paulo and Orrit, 2012). Further advances in microfabrication and nanotechnology have allowed for the development of more complex and sensitive biosensors. For the detection of a wide range of biomolecules, including glucose, lactate, cholesterol, and DNA, utilizing nanotechnology for biosensing application has been commercialized or is on the verge of commercialization. Currently, there are more than 500 companies across the globe involved in the field of biosensors and bioelectronics (Shukla and Suneetha, 2017). Diagnostic concepts like point-of-care (POC), wearable, and multiplexed biosensors are the key to future diagnostics. It will enable providing health care in a personalized manner by early detection, continuous monitoring, and treatment of health conditions. Before we deep dive into the topic, let's have a look at what to expect from the book.

The essence of different types of biosensing strategies, different types of nanomaterials, and their corresponding biosensing applications are presented in this chapter. You will get a sense of how the biosensing field has developed in the past, where we are today, and what are the major thrust areas expected to flourish in the future. For new researchers and students who wish to work in the field, this chapter will be useful. It is expected to benefit individuals currently working in this field.

Key learnings are as follows:

- Different types of biosensors.
- Parameters for the performance evaluation of a biosensor.
- Common types of nanomaterials used are biosensing applications.
- Application of nanotechnology in biosensing strategies.
- Future thrust areas of nanotechnology-based biosensing applications.

6.2 BIOSENSORS: DEFINITION, STRUCTURE, CATEGORIES, AND CHARACTERISTICS

According to the International Union of Pure and Applied Chemistry (IUPAC), "a device that uses specific biochemical reactions mediated by isolated enzymes, immunosystems, tissues, organelles or whole cells to detect chemical compounds usually by electrical, thermal or optical signals" are called biosensors (Nagel, Dellweg and Gierasch, 1992). Biorecognition molecule being an integral part of the sensor, chemical-free live detection of analytes (biomarker molecules) can be monitored. In the following sections, the components, categories, and characteristics have been described.

6.2.1 Structure and Components

There are three main primary components of biosensors. Those are biorecognition element, transducer, and internal electronics. Additional components may vary based on application and sensor type.

Biorecognition element: Also known as biorecognition molecule or bioreceptor or ligand (more generalized) are biological molecules that selectively recognize the analyte molecule of interest (biomarker) from a sample (a concoction of molecules). Biorecognition molecule normally undergoes a binding event upon recognition of analyte molecule (biomarker) with specificity. Binding between antigen and antibody is the most specific of all types, and due to their high specificity, the binding event is often called the "lock-and-key" mechanism. Based on requirement, biorecognition molecule could be any one or combination but not limited to enzyme, DNA, ribonucleic acid (RNA), antibody, antigen, aptamers, and peptides (Davis and Altintas, 2018).

Transducer: The binding event between the biorecognition molecule and analyte is converted into some form of measurable signal by the transducer. The generated signal is normally proportional to the number of binding events took place. The signal could be in any form of change in terms of potential, conductivity, light intensity, color, refractive index, mass, frequency, temperature, etc.

Internal electronics: The measurable signal is converted into some understandable values by the internal electronics. The obtained value may be presented on a display or expressed in levels or simply by positive or negative indication.

6.2.2 Categories of Biosensors

Biosensors come in different shapes and sizes with applications ranging from pathogen detection to pH measurement. They can be categorized by mainly three possible ways: (i) the biorecognition element in use, (ii) the transduction strategy, or (iii) the intended application of the biosensor. Based on biorecognition element, they can be categorized as enzyme, antibody, antigen, DNA and RNA, aptamers, peptide, and polymer-based biosensor. Detailed discussion on categories based on biorecognition element and application will be exhaustive, and it is recommended to go through existing literature (Mohanty and Kougianos, 2006; Kaur, Sharma and Kumar, 2022; Naresh and Lee, 2021; Bhalla et al., 2016) to have a comprehensive view on this topic. Based on the transduction strategy, the biosensors can be normally categorized into four sections: (i) electrochemical (EC), (ii) optical, (iii) piezoelectric, and (iv) calorimetric. It is still an evolving field, and there are sensors based on other transaction strategies available, e.g., electronic biosensor (Presnova et al., 2017) and acoustic biosensor (Fogel, Limson and Seshia, 2016).

6.2.2.1 Electrochemical

Biosensors based on the EC transduction strategy are the most successful ones (Maruccio and Narang, 2022). The concept of EC biosensors originates from the already existing electroanalytical methods in analytical chemistry to determine the properties of a chemical substance. This type of biosensor consists of electrodes, and change in current and/or voltage is monitored as the transduction strategy. For electrodes modified with bioreceptors when interacting with an analyte, the EC properties of the medium are altered, which can further be correlated with the concentration of the analyte.

The electroanalytical methods cyclic voltammetry, amperometry, and impedance spectroscopy are frequently utilized in EC biosensors. Cyclic voltammetry is a method that assesses how the electrode reacts in terms of current when a changing voltage is applied to it, revealing details on the redox processes taking place at the electrode surface. Impedance spectroscopy examines the resistance and capacitance of the electrode–electrolyte interface, whereas amperometry measures the current generated by a redox reaction at a certain applied voltage.

The first EC biosensor was developed by Leland C. Clark Jr. and Champ Lyons in 1962 (Clark Jr. and Lyons, 1962), which is an amperometric biosensor and utilized an oxygen electrode and the enzyme glucose oxidase to detect glucose in blood samples.

For applications like POC diagnostics or patient care at the bedside, where size with ease of use and affordability are key, electrical biosensors offer the most potential. Advances in microfabrication and nanotechnology have enabled the development of highly sensitive and selective biosensors that can detect a wide range of analytes with high accuracy and specificity (Molinero-Fernandez, Lopez and Escarpa, 2020).

6.2.2.2 Optical Biosensors

Optical biosensors translate the recombination of biorecognition molecule and biomarker in terms of any one or combination of the properties of light, i.e., intensity, wavelength, optical path, bandwidth, phase, and polarization. Conventional optical detection techniques rely on the direct interaction of the target analytes with light. The analyte concentration is further linked with the absorbance or fluorescence signal. However, most target analytes, particularly smaller ones (enzymes, proteins, and DNA), don't exhibit much absorbance or fluorescence. In addition, the concentration required to create a detectable signal is much below the relevant detection range of a conventional detection device (typically in the ppm or ppb range). In order to bypass the issue, some well-known compounds that have a high extinction coefficient (for absorbance) or a high quantum yield (for fluorescence) are attached chemically to target analytes. This action is referred to as labeling. This method is the foundation of the ELISA, the gold standard of biochemical testing. Testing performed by ELISA needs costly equipment and several preparatory processes (therefore higher cost). This is where nanotechnology comes into play to overcome most of the issues. The category of sensing strategy dealing with the optical behavior of nanostructures (mostly metal) is called plasmonic biosensing. It is possible to identify tiny compounds down to the single-molecule level without labeling processes (Zijlstra, Paulo and Orrit, 2012). Furthermore, plasmonic sensing makes it feasible to access binding or reaction kinetics in real time, which is not attainable with traditional methods. The narrow volume of the sensing zone, which is restricted to a small location near the surface of the nanostructured plasmonic material, is another benefit of plasmonic sensing.

According to the definition, a plasmonic sensor is a particular class of sensors that investigates the use of light interaction with plasmonic nanostructures, which are often metallic, as a transduction method. Different sorts of plasmonic characteristics can be examined for sensing in a wide range of plasmonic sensors, depending on their geometric configuration. The so-called localized surface plasmon resonance (LSPR) is demonstrated using plasmonic nanoparticles. The LSPR can be directly activated by light and can identify molecules that are a few nanometers away from the plasmonic surface. The propagating SPR (PSPR) in thin gold films, on the other hand, can only be indirectly activated by prism coupling. In this instance, there is a considerable increase in the detection volume above the plasmonic surface. Metallic films can exhibit both LSPR and PSPR if they have periodic "voids," known as plasmonic nanohole array (Quint and Pacholski, 2009). Surface-enhanced Raman scattering (SERS), surface-enhanced infrared absorption spectroscopy (SEIRA), and surface-enhanced fluorescence (SEF) are other ways that plasmonic nanostructures are being exploited for biosensing purposes. Gold (Au), silver (Ag), aluminum (Al), and copper (Cu) are most often considered for fabricating plasmonic sensors.

It is worth mentioning that other novel materials like graphene also show plasmonic properties with promising biosensing applications.

6.2.2.3 Piezoelectric Effect

The piezoelectric effect is the ability of some materials to generate an electric charge in response to mechanical stress or strain. This phenomenon happens as a result of the material's crystal lattice structure being deformed by mechanical stress, which in turn results in an electric polarization. On the other hand, if an electric field is provided to the material, it deforms or vibrates mechanically. The mechanical vibration of the crystals results in a natural frequency of the material. Any change in mass as low as in sub-nanogram range will result in a change in the natural frequency of the crystal, exactly what is utilized for biosensing application. A piezoelectric crystal modified with biorecognition element undergoes a natural frequency vibration; whenever the analyte undergoes recombination with biorecognition element, the frequency changes and is utilized as the transduction strategy. Due to the natural vibration of the piezoelectric crystals, an acoustic wave is generated. Based on the nature of propagation of the acoustic wave, it can be classified as bulk acoustic wave (BAW) or surface acoustic wave (SAW) (Nagraik et al., 2021). The majority of the available sensors is based on BAW phenomena. One main advantage of the piezoelectric detection strategy is its high dynamic range compared to other detection strategies. Application of piezoelectric biosensors can be observed from the detection of prostate cancer, and the detection of single-point mutation on a p53 gene has been reported in the literature (Altintas and Masdor, 2018). The major disadvantages of piezoelectric biosensors are their environmental factors and contaminants, which have already been addressed by the incorporation of microfluidic-based piezoelectric detection strategy.

6.2.2.4 Calorimetric Biosensors

The characteristics of biological reactions based on absorption (endothermic) or release of heat energy (exothermic) are monitored as the transduction strategy for calorimetric biosensors (Xie et al., 1993). Despite several reports based on this strategy, there are several shortcomings of calorimetric strategy. There is no clear way to distinguish between specific and non-specific heat changes, which limits the use of calorimetric devices. This is due to the relatively drawn-out experimental procedures and lack of specificity in temperature measurement. However, some of these shortcomings were overcome by the development of the enzyme thermistor based on flow injection analysis in conjunction with an immobilized biocatalyst and heat-sensing element (Naresh and Lee, 2021).

6.2.3 Characteristics of a Biosensor

The performance of biosensors is assessed based on parameters like sensitivity, selectivity, specificity, stability, detection limit or limit of detection, reproducibility, response time, range, linearity, resolution, response time, hysteresis, and shelf life (Bhalla et al., 2016; Gupta, Shrivastav and Usha, 2017; Tetyana, Morgan Shumbula and Njengele-Tetyana, 2021). Though the parameters may sound intuitive, quantification of the same is often challenging, especially when comparing sensor performance across two different transduction strategies. Parameters mentioned above are for the assessment of biosensors intended for lab usage. When it is required to have biosensors for POC applications, which is exactly where we are moving, a few additional parameters add to the lists like portability, affordability, sampling, environmental dependency, and ease of use. Most of the requirements of a "good" biosensor can be fulfilled by incorporating nanotechnology into the biosensing strategy.

6.3 NANOTECHNOLOGY IN BIOSENSING

Nanotechnology is the branch of science that deals with materials of nanoscale between 1 and 100 nm in size. The material that has at least one of its dimensions in the nanoscale range is called nanomaterials. The concept of nanotechnology started even before the term has been coined as such when physics Nobel Laureate Richard Feynman in his famous talk for the American Physical Society at California Institute of Technology quoted, "There is Plenty of Room at the Bottom." He conferred that anything is possible to build by manipulating atoms and molecules at the atomic level and making a new material. From there, the nanoscience concept has expanded and opened new doors for research. When a material reduces from its bulk form to nanoscale, the associated properties of the material change, thereby enabling it to be used in a wide range of applications. These nanomaterials acquire unique optical, electronic, and magnetic properties of their own due to the reduction in size compared to their bulk counterparts. One of the main reasons for these distinctive properties is their high surface area-to-volume ratio. Due to this, nanotechnology has been used in different applications like pharmaceuticals, cosmetics, energy, textiles, environment, and health care (diagnostics and therapeutics). Due to the following reasons, nanomaterials play a significant role in transduction strategies.

Increased surface area: Nanomaterials have a high surface area-to-volume ratio, which allows them to interact efficiently with biomolecules, increasing the sensitivity of the biosensor. These are the following reasons why nanomaterials are chosen for biosensing applications (Figure 6.1).

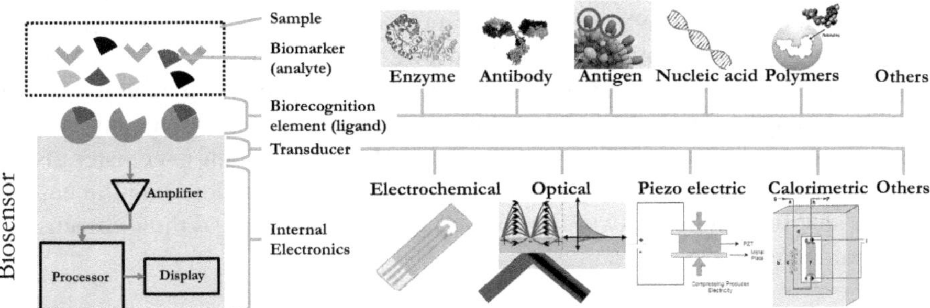

FIGURE 6.1 Schematic representation of a common biosensor with three main components biorecognition element (ligand), transducer, and internal electronics. Common types of biosensors categorized based on the use of biorecognition elements and transduction strategies are presented.

Amplification of signals: Nanomaterials can amplify signals generated during the biosensing process, enabling the detection of low-concentration biomolecules that are challenging to detect using conventional techniques.

Selective detection: Nanomaterials can be functionalized with specific ligands, such as antibodies, aptamers, or enzymes, which can selectively bind to target biomolecules. This functionalization process can be tailored to optimize the detection of a particular biomolecule, improving the sensitivity and specificity of the biosensor.

Optical properties: Some nanomaterials exhibit unique optical properties that can be exploited for biosensing applications. For example, gold nanoparticles (AuNPs) exhibit strong SPR that can be used to detect changes in the refractive index of the surrounding medium.

Miniaturization: Nanomaterials enable the miniaturization of biosensing devices, which can be integrated into portable or handheld devices for on-site or POC testing.

In the upcoming sections, we will discuss the classifications of nanomaterials, their properties, and applications in the medical field.

Types of nanomaterials:

Nanomaterials are primarily classified based on their dimensions into four major types : (i) zero-dimensional, (ii) one-dimensional, (iii) two-dimensional, and (iv) three-dimensional.

Nanomaterials can also be classified based on the composition of materials into three categories: (i) organic nanomaterials, (i) inorganic nanomaterials, and (iii) hybrid nanomaterials (Figure 6.2).

Each of these nanomaterials can be synthesized by different methods, and the properties of these materials also vary based on their synthesis methods and their shape (Figure 6.3).

6.3.1 Carbon-Based Nanomaterials

Carbon nanomaterials are extensively used in many applications due to their distinctive physical and chemical properties. Carbon is the most abundant element on the earth, and it makes up everything from living to non-living things. It has four valence electrons that help in forming covalent bonds with other elements. This covalent bond leads to the formation of long chains of carbon. Thus, carbon can be present in different molecular forms called carbon allotropes such as graphite and diamond. This unique nature of carbon helps in synthesizing different carbon nanomaterials like zero-dimensional carbon nanoparticles, fullerenes and carbon dots, one-dimensional carbon nanotubes (CNTs), two-dimensional graphene sheets, and three-dimensional nanodiamonds.

6.3.1.1 Fullerenes

Fullerenes, otherwise known as buckyballs, are an allotrope of carbon made of 60 carbon atoms. It was officially identified in 1985 by Harold Kroto from the University of Sussex and Robert Curl and Richard Smalley from Rice University (Kroto et al., 1985).

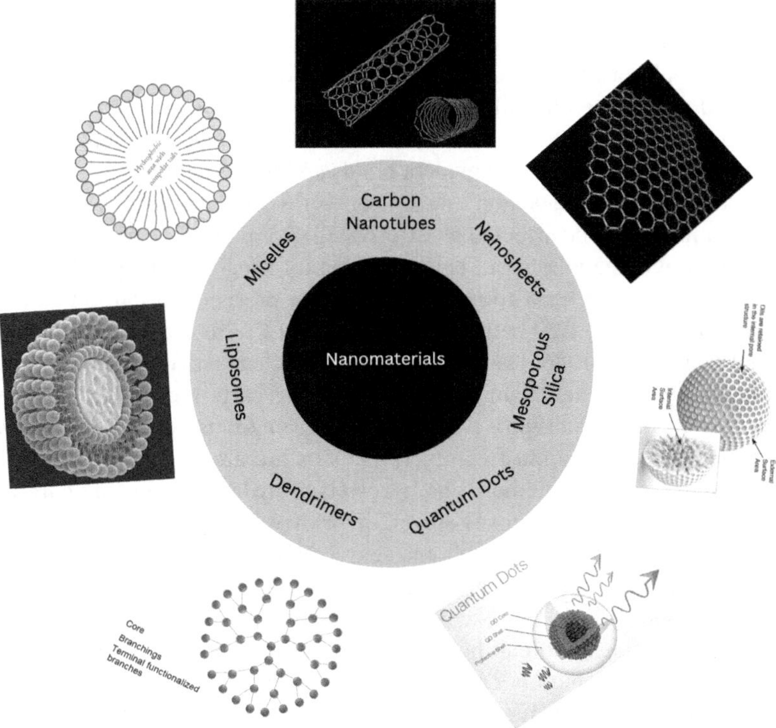

FIGURE 6.2 Illustration of different types of nanomaterials utilized in biosensing applications namely carbon nanotubes, nanosheets, mesoporous silica, quantum dots, dendrimers, liposomes, and micelles.

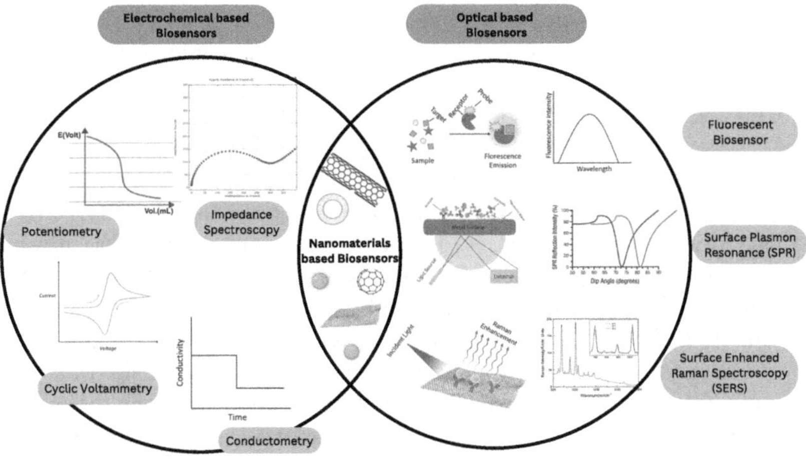

FIGURE 6.3 Utilization of nanomaterials for biosensing applications based on the two most common transduction strategies; electrochemical biosensors, and optical biosensors.

It was previously discovered by different scientists like Eiji Osawa in 1970 from Japan, RW Henson from the United Kingdom, and a group of scientists from Russia in 1973 (Shanbogh and Sundaram, 2015). But these discoveries were not properly acknowledged due to the unavailability of proper scientific evidence. As fullerenes are made up of 60 carbon atoms, it is also called as C60. Each carbon atom is linked with three other carbon atoms by covalent bonds and forms a hollow spherical shape with 12 pentagon and 20 hexagon faces. Due to this molecular formation, C60 is highly stable and cannot be affected by external environment. The formula for fullerene is $C_{n,}$ where n is the number of carbon atoms forming the buckyballs. Different forms of fullerenes have been formed based on the presence of carbon atoms like C20, C70, and C80, with C20 being the smallest. But C60 is the mostly synthesized and studied material. In 1985, Harold et al. and his colleagues first discovered fullerenes in the sooty waste left behind after vaporizing carbon in a helium or argon environment (Kroto et al., 1985). After that, many methods have been followed to produce fullerenes, and the most common methods are arc discharge method, laser ablation, plasma discharge method, and pyrolysis of hydrocarbon using carbon precursors. C-atoms found in fullerenes are sp2-hybridized carbon atoms in closed, hollow cages, and they exhibit a hydrophobic characteristic, and as their size increases, their solubility declines (Speranza, 2021). Due to these hybridization characteristics and their topology, C60 has excellent chemical reactivity with other materials, has good EC properties, and can be functionalized with many numbers of materials. These extensive EC and optical properties along with their highly stable hollow cage-like structure make them an excellent candidate for drug delivery and in vivo diagnostic applications. As fullerenes are hydrophobic, they are required to be functionalized before using in in vivo applications.

After proper functionalization, fullerenes can be used as a photosensitizer in photodynamic therapy (PDT) for cancer applications and as an antimicrobial agent for pathogenic cell death (Bakry et al., 2007). Photosensitizer is a material that upon irradiation with an ultraviolet (UV) or visible light source gets excited and produces reactive oxygen species and singlet oxygen, which in turn kills cancer cells and pathogenic cells. This process is known as photodynamic therapy. C60 upon photon irradiation transfers from the ground state to the excited state and produces singlet C60 and then further excited to triplet state 3C60. Further, this C60 in triplet state reacts with the molecular oxygen to produce singlet oxygen 1O2, which is highly reactive and responsible for molecular cell death. To be used in biological applications, fullerenes have to be functionalized properly to specifically affect the tumor and pathogenic cells. In order to improve the cytotoxicity of C60, it was conjugated with antisense oligonucleotide sequence that specifically targets its DNA or RNA counterparts for the required cell death (Jensen, Wilson and Schuster, 1996; Yamakoshi et al., 1996). As fullerenes are hydrophobic, they were conjugated covalently with N-vinylpyrrolidone through polymerization to improve the water-soluble property of C60. It has shown high water solubility compared to any other methods that have been introduced so far (Iwamoto and Yamakoshi, 2006). In another work, malonic acid C60 tris-adduct and dendritic C60 mono-adduct's cytotoxicity were evaluated on Jurkat cells. It has been shown that dendritic C60 mono-adduct derivative reduced the cell growth up to 19% upon 2-week incubation compared to malonic acid C60 tris-adduct derivative. But photo-cytotoxic effects of C60 malonic acid tris-adduct were found to be effective compared to the mono-adduct derivative of C60 upon irradiation with UV light. The cytotoxicity mainly depends on damage to the cell membrane and the dosage of UV light. From this, it was concluded that the two different derivatives of C60 react distinctively with the cell membranes producing separate cytotoxic effects (Rancan et al., 2002).

Metallofullerenes are fullerenes that carry metal atoms inside the caged structure of C60 for diagnostic applications. Compared to metal chelates, endofullerenes or metallofullerenes have high stability in in vivo condition and do not release the captured metal atom. Thus, they help in X-ray, magnetic resonance imaging (MRI), and radiopharmaceuticals as contrast agents (Bakry et al., 2007). 99mTc@C60 and 99mTc@C70 were the first radio-endofullerenes developed to detect minute levels of analytes in vitro by encapsulating radionuclide (Karam, Mitch and Coursey, 1997). This caging of radionuclide inside the carbon chamber helps in easy and stable transport through the biological systems. When labeled with proper antibody, the radio-endofullerenes can easily transport to the targeted site inside the body. These cage-like structures of fullerenes along with their low toxicity make them a suitable candidate for drug and gene delivery. Promising medical applications are now emerging from the direct targeting of fullerene and its derivatives to biological targets. The distinctive chemical and physical characteristics of the fullerene, notably their photodynamic capabilities, are what have attracted such interest to them (Bakry et al., 2007).

6.3.1.2 Carbon Nanotubes

In 1991, Japanese scientist Sumio Lijima accidentally discovered multiwalled CNTs on the soot material obtained in the burning of graphite rods. Then, after 2 years and many experiments later, in 1993, single-walled CNTs (SWCNTs) were discovered by lijima's research group (Iijima, 1991). But it turns out that since 1952, researchers have continuously recorded the presence of multiwalled CNTs (MWCNTs). LV Radushkevich and VM Lukyanovich were the ones who first discovered CNTs and published a paper on the same in the Journal of Physical Chemistry of Russia in 1952 (Manikandan et al., 2021). After the discovery of SWCNT in 1993, experiments were developed to synthesize large number of SWCNTs for application in different fields. CNTs are made by rolling up graphene sheets in a way to make a hollow cylindrical shape. The directions or chirality in which the graphene sheets are rolled determines the different characteristics and properties of CNT. Based on the number of graphene sheets used for CNT, it is divided into SWCNTs and MWCNTs (Lozano-Castelló et al., 2013). SWCNTs are made of single graphene sheet with smaller diameter of 0.6–2.4 nm, and MWCNTs are made of many graphene sheets from 2 to 50 numbers with an outer diameter of 2.5 to 100 nm and an inner diameter of 1.5–15 nm (Wang, 2005; Lozano-Castelló et al., 2013). Just like fullerenes, CNTs have hexagonal arrays of carbon atoms, which makes them have a strong affinity toward other molecules. CNTs are mainly synthesized by arc discharge, laser ablation/vaporization, and carbon vapor deposition (CVD) (Karfa et al., 2019). Among these methods, CVD is the most widely used technique, where CNT is produced under high temperature and pressure using carbon precursor (Colomer et al., 2000). Arc discharge is the basic method, where CNTs are formed on the cathode when current passes through two graphite rods (Awasthi, Srivastava and Srivastava, 2005). MWCNTs are often produced by laser vaporization of graphite in a silica tube-lined, high-temperature furnace; however, SWCNTs can also be produced if catalytic metal nanoparticles are used. Just by adjusting the experimental conditions of CNT synthesis, a wide variety of CNTs with different sizes and properties can be developed. Due to their high stability, better mechanical and electrical properties, and biocompatibility, CNTs have been used in a wide array of biomedical applications including sensing, tissue regeneration, and drug delivery. CNT hexagonal atom formation like fullerenes makes them easily bind with different drugs and biological molecules like protein, DNA, antibody, and antigen, and their hollow tube-like structure helps in carrying drugs to different target sites in the body smoothly without losing the drug molecule (Lamberti et al., 2015). For targeted drug delivery, drugs can either be encapsulated inside the tube or attached to the surface of the tube. Compared to surface binding where the drug is released in the fluid even before entering into the cell, in encapsulation the drugs are released specifically to the site (Lamberti et al., 2014). SWCNTs coated with chitosan (CHI) were used as a novel drug delivery system (DDS) for the controlled loading and release of the anticancer medication doxorubicin (DOX) (Ji et al., 2012). It was found to be effectively killing the HCC SMMC-7721 cell lines and inhibiting the growth of tumor cells in mice. Due to the intact transfer of drugs and other biological molecules into the human body, CNTs have been used for gene (DNA) delivery applications (He et al., 2013). The first DNA delivery using CNTs as a vehicle was reported by Pantarotto and coworkers (Pantarotto et al., 2004). Due to their better electronic property and high conductivity, CNTs have been used for glucose sensor by coupling with glucose oxidase enzyme to increase the sensitivity and specificity of the biosensor (Wang, 2005; Usui et al., 2012; Digge, Moon and Gattani, 2012). CNTs are also used for the detection of organophosphate pesticides by immobilizing acetylcholine esterase on the CNT surface in the EC method. Apart from these applications, CNTs are also used for pharmacological studies, as an antioxidant and immunotherapy (He et al., 2013).

6.3.1.3 Metallic Nanoparticles

The most commonly used metal and metal oxide-based nanoparticles are Au, silver (Ag), and iron oxide nanoparticles. These metal nanoparticles are synthesized by metal precursors and are made of only one element (Kaushik et al., 2019). Metal-based nanoparticles can be synthesized by different methods including physical vapor deposition, chemical vapor deposition, solvothermal, hydrothermal, sol–gel, spray pyrolysis, microwave-assisted, and green synthesis (bio-assisted) (Jamkhande et al., 2019). Biomedical application of metallic nanoparticles is mainly due to their high stability and excellent optical and electronic properties. As the size of the nanoparticles reduces, structure, shape, and properties of the material change.

AuNPs show a deep red color compared to gold particles. As size increases, the color changes to yellow due to their LSPR. AuNPs have been used for many biomedical applications due to their inert, biocompatible, and low-toxic effect inside the body (Hammami et al., 2021). Depending on the level of aggregation, the optical characteristics of AuNPs can alter. This property can be used in biosensor and colorimetric immunoassays (Altintas, 2018). A smartphone colorimetric-based rapid detection of cysteine was demonstrated using β-cyclodextrin (β-CD) functionalized AuNPs. β-CD AuNP aggregation upon reaction with Cys produces low SPR band intensity (Rajamanikandan, Lakshmi and Ilanchelian, 2020). A colorimetric-based detection of pathogens using a plasmonic immunoassay was developed using a cysteine-loaded liposome with AuNPs. When in contact with any pathogens, cysteine-loaded nanoliposomes open and lead to the aggregation of AuNPs, which in turn leads to the visual color change from red to dark blue (Bui, Ahmed and Abbas, 2015).

Similar to AuNPs, silver nanoparticles exhibit LSPR absorption, which results in a range of colored solutions based on the size of the nanoparticles. The optical properties of silver nanoparticles can vary based on their size, shape, degree of aggregation, and other factors, just like they can with AuNPs. Silver nanoparticles are most commonly used as antibacterial agents due to their excellent antimicrobial properties. These nanoparticles can be synthesized by different methods like evaporation, condensation, laser ablation, microemulsion, UV-initiated photoreduction, and microwave-assisted synthesis (Abou El-Nour et al., 2010; Altintas, 2018). AgNP instability in bacterially rich settings poses a unique challenge to their usage as antimicrobials, which reduces or eliminates their anti-pathogenic action. Numerous inorganic, organic (Chien et al., 2018), synthetic, natural (Muhammad et al., 2016), biotic, and abiotic materials were utilized as capping agents to increase the stability of AgNPs in solution (Burduşel et al., 2018). Pathogenic drug resistance is an alarming and emerging phenomenon that poses a huge concern for the global healthcare system. AgNPs are therefore strong candidates for the creation of new, powerful, and biocompatible nanostructured materials for innovative antibacterial applications based on nanotechnology (Burduşel et al., 2018; Premkumar et al., 2018). Excellent bactericidal property of silver nanoparticles disrupts the cell wall by penetrating into the cell and damaging the structure and leads to cell death (Yan et al., 2018). Due to the inherent antibacterial and anti-inflammatory properties of metallic nanoparticles, AgNPs have been effectively exploited to design and produce superior wound and burn dressings. Plenty of research has been going on in fabricating and commercializing nanosilver-based products for better antimicrobial applications. Silver nanoparticles are also used for drug delivery, dental applications like implant coating and antibacterial mouthwash, anticancer drug, and wound healing (Burduşel et al., 2018).

6.3.1.4 Quantum Dots

Quantum dots (QDs) were first identified by Rosetti and coworkers in their work on quantum size effects of CdS particle in the year 1983 (Rossetti, Nakahara and Brus, 1983). Later in the year 1993, a group of QDs (CdS, CdSe, and CdTe) were synthesized with the size range of 1–12 nm (Murray, Noms and Bawendi', 1993). QDs are core–shell semiconductor nanoparticles typically in the size range of 1–10 nm with a wide range of optical and electronic properties due to their quantum confinement. Quantum confinement is a phenomenon where the diameter of the particle is less than the de Broglie wavelength of electrons in which energy confinement depends on physical dimensions of the particle (Ramalingam et al., 2020). Due to these unique characteristics, QDs have excellent optical properties. When QDs are exposed to a light source, electron from the ground state moved to the higher energy level and creates a hole in the valence band. Then, after some time the excited electron moved to the ground state (hole) by releasing energy in the form of photon. This process of light emission is called photoluminescence, and the color of the photon emission depends on the size of the QDs. QDs have better quantum yields and have shown good photostability compared to other organic dyes (Altintas, 2018). After the initial discovery, QDs have been synthesized by different methods such as sol–gel, micro-emulsion, hydrothermal, arc discharge, X-ray lithography, e-beam lithography, and hot injection (Altintas, 2018; Maxwell et al., 2020). The hydrothermal method is mostly used for the synthesis of inorganic QDs especially carbon QDs. The most commonly synthesized and studied QDs are cadmium-based QDs, and nowadays, carbon-based QDs have been emerging.

By manipulating the size of QDs, the optical and electronic properties can be changed and this helps in using QDs in different applications including medical diagnostics and therapeutics. QDs have featured broad excitation spectra, narrow emission spectra, and significant Stokes shifts when compared to typical chemical dyes and luminous proteins. Additionally, QDs have better optical qualities, such as high intensity, wide optical fluorescence spectrum range, and high stability over photobleaching (Smith et al., 2008; Wagner et al., 2019). QDs have a broad range of spectra from UV to infrared in electromagnetic spectrum. Due to this wide range of spectrum, QDs can penetrate deep into the biological tissues and do not interfere with autofluorescence (Resch-Genger et al., 2008; Li et al., 2014). Due to these optical properties, QDs can be used as photosensitizers for PDT applications. Samia et al. synthesized phthalocyanine photosensitizers bonded to CdSe QDs for photodynamic-based cancer therapy (Samia, Chen and Burda, 2003). Photosensitizer gets activated between 550 and 600 nm, and QDs get activated between 400 and 500 nm. Thus, the synthesized phthalocyanine (Pc4)-based CdSe QDs can be activated between 400 and 650 nm. This enables them to use in deep tissue photodynamic therapy-based cancer applications (Samia, Chen and Burda, 2003; Uprety and Abrahamse, 2022). It was the first study that used QDs for PDT applications other than imaging. As a result, numerous research studies have been published on using metallic QDs for PDT applications, particularly those with a CdSe core (Uprety and Abrahamse, 2022). Further, this deep tissue penetration property by near infrared (NIR) can also be used in in vivo medical imaging. Li et al. developed a Ag2S QD-based fluorescent probe in the NIR-II window of 1,000–1,350 for the imaging of lymphatic and vascular systems (Li et al., 2014). Comparatively, the NIR-II window is better than NIR-I because it can produce clearer imaging than is possible in NIR-I, mainly because the higher wavelengths have significantly lower photon scattering, absorbance, and tissue autofluorescence (Wang and Zhang, 2014). A next-generation NIR-II QDs with deep tissue penetration, excellent spatial imaging resolution, multi-color imaging, and quick acquisition for a range of in vivo imaging applications was recently reported by Bruns et al. In this study, a range of indium/arsenide QDs without heavy metals were created and are reported to have a narrow and size-tunable emission and a much greater quantum yield (up to 30%) compared to other reported works. QDs enable more accurate diagnostic tools and fluoroimmunoassays, multiplexed imaging, dual imaging and therapeutic platforms, real time in vivo imaging, and monitoring of single cells and biological components. The design and development of

QDs have improved dramatically during the last 10 years due to the vastly increased interest in inorganic particles (Wagner et al., 2019).

6.4 CURRENT DIAGNOSTIC APPLICATIONS

6.4.1 Label-Free Diagnostic Devices

Label-free biosensors (LFBs) make use of biological receptors to detect the analyzed substances directly from the sample. This modern LFB has the advantages of simplified pattern analysis, rapid response time, low-cost portability, reduced consumption of solvents, multiplexing, detection of small molecules, etc. There are several different types of label-free biosensors such as optical, EC, microwave, and mass-based (Figure 6.4).

6.4.1.1 Optical Label-Free Biosensors

The optical biosensors perform direct detection of targeted biomolecules under the study. The electron interaction with electromagnetic wave is used for representing the light wave propagation. The photodetector detects the absorption and reflection of light wave as it propagates to the analyte. Advanced technologies in LFB aid in the innovation of modern technologies such as SPR (Golichenari et al., 2018; Kimuda et al., 2018; Zhang et al., 2019), interferometry, fiber optics (Polley et al., 2019, 2022), and Raman spectroscopy (Serebrennikova et al., 2021). SPR consists of monochromatic and polarized light sources, a prism made up of glass material, a metal film

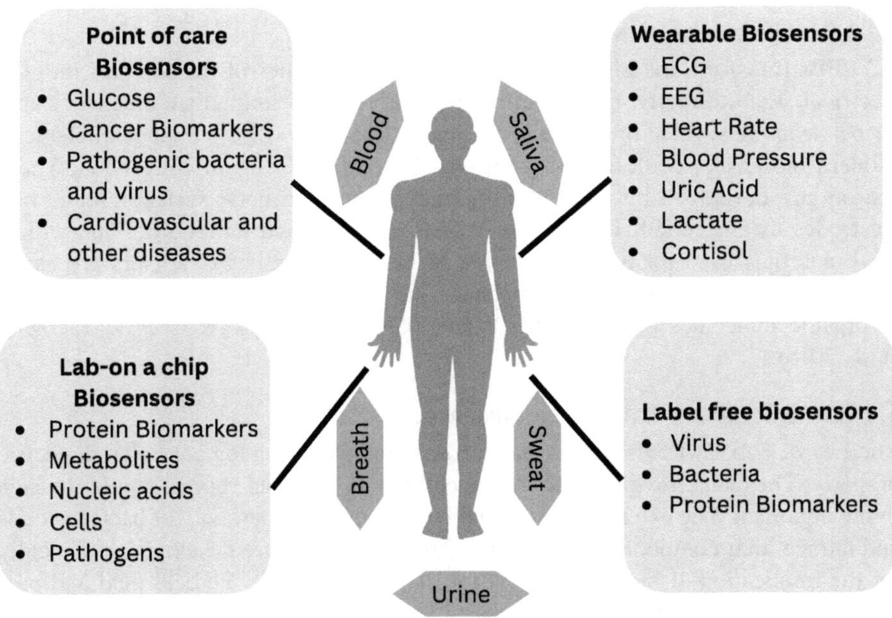

FIGURE 6.4 Schematic representation of different types of invasive and non-invasive biosensors for the detection of various biomarkers.

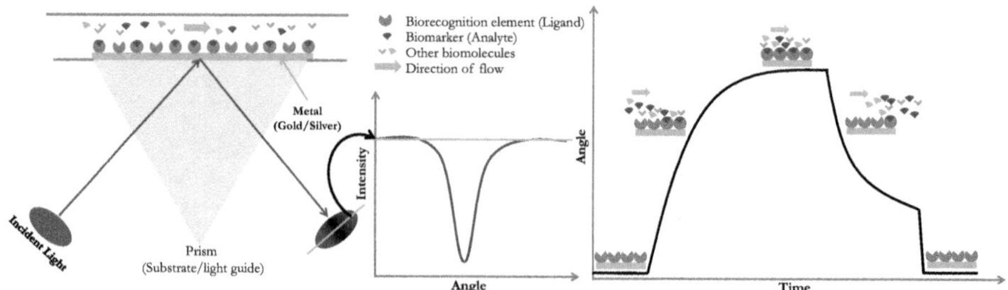

FIGURE 6.5 Working of the propagating surface plasmon-based biosensor also known as SPR biosensor. A part of the light energy couples through the metal (gold/silver) layer with the electrons in the metal surface at a certain angle of incidence, causing the electrons to move as a result of excitation. Consequently, light intensity drops at a certain angle, which changes with the change in the refractive index of the exact vicinity of the metal layer. This correlation between change in refractive index and angle is utilized for biosensing applications. With the specific interaction between the ligand and analyte the local refractive index changes and hence the angle.

on prism, and a photodetector. The light ray falls on the prism base and causes total internal reflection followed by a damped wave received by the metal layer, which propagates from the prism. The biological molecules in SPR-based biosensor are detected based on changes in the reflected beam angle/intensity/wavelength during the experimental process (Figure 6.5).

6.4.1.2 Electrochemical Label-Free Biosensors

EC LFBs transform the biological and chemical properties of the samples into the electrical signal directly. EC detection is mainly due to immediate electron transfer between the surface of the electrode and active center of the biological element. Modern biosensors could detect pathogens based on EC signal conversion. These sensors are developed by incorporating changes on the metal surface and carbon electrodes using recognizing agents such as enzymes and antibodies. The widely used materials used for the construction of bioelectrodes in EC sensors are nanostructured metal oxides, CNTs, graphene, and self-organizing monolayers (SAMs) of organic molecules (Campuzano, Yáñez-Sedeño and Pingarrón, 2017; Teengam et al., 2018).

6.4.1.3 Microwave Label-Free Biosensors

Microwave (MiW) LFBs are based on the principle of biological cell's dielectric property. The dielectric properties of the cell are distinct and very particular to each living organism. The external electric field influences the coercivity of bacterial cells and intracellular components of bacteria. The MiW LFBs are developed specifically for the implication of biological agent for diagnostics in the medical field and protection of environment and safety. Oberoi et al. built MiW-based biosensor for the identification and detection of 1–2 colony-forming units (CFUs) of *E coli.* in water molecules (Oberoi, Daya and Tirumalai, 2012).

6.4.2 Point-of-Care Diagnostic Devices

POC diagnostic devices are user-friendly, application-specific, rapid, robust, and easily affordable to developing countries like India. Early detection of coronary heart disease has been detected by Cholestech LDX analysis developed by Abbot India Ltd. (*Cholestech LDX™ Analyzer*, no date). Advanced diagnostic devices such as nanotechnology-based biosensor have been used as ultra-sensitive POC devices for the detection of many types of cancer. For the detection of carcinoembryonic antigen, a highly susceptible paper-based biosensor was designed by Kumar et al. using polymer and reduced graphene oxide (RGO) composite (Kumar et al., 2015).

Dengue virus was detected based on DNA hybridization technique using electrospun nanofibers (Tripathy et al., 2017). Borse et al. developed a lateral flow immunoassay (LFIA)-based POC test for detecting orthopedic implant-related infections (Borse and Srivastava, 2019a). A double antibody sandwich technique was used in the LFIA test using fluorescent cadmium telluride QDs (Borse and Srivastava, 2019b). LFIA strips have been designed that can scan the fluorescence signal using a portable fluorescence reader.

EC biosensors were developed by Mandal et al. to detect the α-amylase in human serum (Mandal et al., 2019). Choudhary et al. (2016) developed an EC-based immunosensor to detect the oral cancer marker CD 59 in a non-invasive method. A recent study illustrated that a paper-based method to detect the nucleic acid in COVID-19 using loop-mediated isothermal amplification (LAMP) in combination with smartphones has potential POC diagnostic devices (Udugama et al., 2020; Xiang et al., 2020; Yang et al., 2020).

During COVID-19, the National Institute of Virology (NIV), Pune, has innovated an ELISA kit, which has been approved by the Indian Council of Medical Research (ICMR) for the diagnosis of COVID-19 at home. They performed technology transfer to a global healthcare company named Zydus Cadila and were involved in the mass production of kits in association with ICMR and the kit as COVID Kavach ELISA (Kumar et al., 2021).

6.4.3 Wearable Diagnostic Devices

Wearable diagnostic devices monitor different physiological parameters for diagnosing various diseases. Wearable devices are categorized into three broad areas such as non-invasive skin-based wearables, microfluidic-based wearable devices, and wearables for drug delivery.

6.4.3.1 Non-Invasive Skin-Based Wearable Devices

Wearable devices based on skin type are used for monitoring the physiological variables and treatment of different diseases such as cardiovascular disease (CVD) and neuromuscular diseases. The two types of skin-based wearable devices are textile and epidermal-based healthcare wearable devices (HWDs).

Textile-based wearable devices embed the sensors in the cloth material and are generally used for sensing the parameters such as temperature, respiration rate, and heart rate. Recently, numerous textile-based wearable biosensors have become viable platforms for personalized health care, fitness monitoring, and pre-diagnostics, thanks to the rapid technical advancement in materials engineering and device integration (Shi et al., 2023).

6.4.3.2 Tattoo-Based HWD

Epidermal tattoo-based biosensors are developed as a possible extension of the wearable sensor in order to improve wearability (He et al., 2021). The tattoo-based biosensor is closely attached or embedded into the skip for the detection of biomarkers. Monitoring biomarkers including glucose level (Bandodkar et al., 2015), pH, and uric acid has been reported in the contemporary literature and in an active field of research (Smith, Li and Tse, 2023).

6.4.4 Lab-on-a-Chip Devices

Earlier in 1990, micro-total analysis systems (MTASs) were developed to perform biochemical tests with less volume of samples in a miniaturized system. Later on, microfluidics has emerged, which employs structures in microscales to test very low volume of fluids. Integrating all the laboratory tests on a single chip called lab-on-a-chip (LOC) has been ongoing research work worldwide. LOC has advantages of automation, low cost, low volume of samples to test, portability, multiplexing, etc. Based on the type of biomarker and operating principle of the LOC, detection principles are used, which may be optical or electrical detection (D. Chin, Linder and K. Sia, 2007).

6.4.4.1 Continuous Flow Microfluidics

Continuous flow microfluidics are single-phase fluid flow that is controlled inside microfluidic channels. Initially, continuous flow microfluidics are constructed using a glass. A delicate structure is being formed by glass layer stuck with another glass piece forming micro-meter scale. One of the examples of continuous flow microfluidics used for disease diagnosis is the Agilent on-chip capillary electrophoresis system. It consists of a bench-top analyzer and separate cartridges for DNA, RNA, and protein. The system consists of channels constructed using glass and bonded to a plastic housing. The plastic housing contains wells for keeping sample solution, etc. The samples are run by the process of electroosmosis through a microfluidic channel. Then, the separation of DNA, RNA, and protein is attained, which is imaged using laser-induced fluorescence unit and displayed as electropherograms (Song et al., 2019).

6.4.4.2 Paper-Based LOC

Paper-based LOC devices have gained significant attention due to their ease of use, extremely low cost per test, and possibility of mass production (Noviana et al., 2021). Paper is comprised of cellulose fibers creating a porous structure. As paper is cheap, lightweight, and biodegradable, it can be used as a transport medium and can be changed by chemicals, which are well suitable for applications in the medical field. The applicability of the paper-based LOC has been improved by the incorporation of nanomaterials, and numerous diagnostic applications have been reported (Ge et al., 2014).

6.5 FUTURE OF DISEASE DIAGNOSIS

The global forecast for biosensor market is expected to reach USD 36.7 billion by 2026 (*Biosensors Market Size, Share, Industry Trends, Companies, Growth Analysis -2032*) with a compound rate of 7.5%. It simply indicates that a significant number of companies (more than 500 (Shukla and Suneetha, 2017)) work in this market. Considering nanotechnology, there are more than 2,400 companies worldwide working in the field of nanotechnology research and development according to the National Institute of Standards and Technology (NIST) database, although the precise number of companies working with the incorporation of nanotechnology into biosensing is not so clear. Nanotechnology in biosensing is an active field of research, and we expect to see more and more of these commercial sensors with highly sensitive and specific detection of biomarkers. Based on the current trends of research and commercial demand, it is expected to have a major thrust in the following direction.

Multiplexed biosensing: Performance of a standard biosensor is based on the detection of single biomarker corresponding to specific diseases. Often, there are multiple biomarkers associated with some health conditions. Since we are targeting a single biomarker, it might lead to false conclusions. However, instead of one if we aim for multiple biomarkers at once (multiplexed sensing) the accuracy of the result will increase and we will have a better understanding of the health condition in general. On the same note, the detection of multiple biomarkers simultaneously (indicating different health conditions) can improve the accuracy of diagnosis and enable earlier detection of diseases. We expected to see a lot of development in this direction, which is called multiplex biosensing.

Personalized medicine: Healthcare professionals may customize drug doses and treatment plans to meet the unique needs of each patient by using biosensors to monitor multiple biomarkers in a patient's body in real time, accurately, and non-invasively. Biosensors can give personalized predictions and insights into a patient's health condition and treatment outcomes by continually monitoring these indicators, enabling more accurate and successful therapies that are catered to each person's requirements. Because of the integration and interrelationship of several technologies involved in nanodiagnostics, those who conduct these tests or devise new tests will be taking a more active part in decision-making in future healthcare systems.

Rapid point-of-care testing: A significant portion of the market size of biosensor is shared by POC biosensors followed by wearable biosensors. Because of miniaturization possibilities, nanotechnology in biosensing is playing a major role in POC diagnostics and it is going to change the diagnostic systems all together in the upcoming years. Due to the reduced wait time between sample collection and diagnostic conclusion compared to conventional diagnostic procedures, it is expected to replace conventional diagnostic testing eventually.

Early disease diagnosis: One major advantage of utilizing nanotechnology in biosensing is their significant enhancement of sensitivity. Sensitivity reaching single molecular level is reported enabling genetic diagnostics to become a reality. With further improvement in both nanotechnology and electronic/optic instrumentation, early detection of diseases like cancer and heart disease is going to be a reality in the upcoming years.

Wearable biosensors: In general, wearable technology is getting popular by days due to awareness of health in public. The boundary of parameters is not limited to heart rate or respiration rate, SpO_2, and electrocardiogram (ECG) only, and the detection of live glucose monitoring throughout the day is a reality now (Purohit et al., 2022). However, nanotechnology-based biosensors are compatible with a variety of platforms, including smartphones and wearable technology, enabling remote monitoring and real-time data analysis. Better illness management and individualized treatment choices may result from this.

Biosensor-integrated organs-on-a-chip: Microfluidic integration into biosensing is revolutionizing health care by decentralizing laboratory tests. Continuing the trend, the next big revolution already underway in the field of drug discovery is the incorporation of biosensing into the organs-on-a-chip (OoC) concept. OoC refers to the replication of essential organ function in a micro-physiological environment, i.e., in microfluidic chips. These models hold great promise for unraveling the biological mechanisms underpinning morphogenetic and pathogenetic processes as well as for examining cellular mechanisms that are crucial for the advancement of the drug screening process possibly by replacing animal testing in the drug development process. The requirement of on-chip monitoring of essential parameters for OoC can be fulfilled by utilizing nanotechnology-based biosensing strategies.

6.6 CONCLUSION

Nanotechnology in biosensing presents a highly promising avenue for the future of disease diagnosis. The ability to design highly sensitive and specific biosensors at the nanoscale enables the detection of disease biomarkers with unprecedented accuracy and efficiency. Nanotechnology-based biosensors have the potential to revolutionize medical diagnostics by facilitating earlier disease detection, multiplexed sensing, personalized treatment, and improved patient outcomes. However, there are still challenges that need to be addressed in the development and implementation of nanotechnology-based biosensors, such as improving their stability, reproducibility, and affordability. Continued investment in research and development in this field will be critical to realizing the full potential of nanotechnology-based biosensing for disease diagnosis. Considering the current interest of market and research, it is safe to say that the future of disease diagnosis utilizing nanotechnology for biosensing is bright.

REFERENCES

Abou El-Nour, K.M.M. et al. (2010) 'Synthesis and applications of silver nanoparticles', *Arabian Journal of Chemistry*, 3(3), pp. 135–140. Available at: https://doi.org/10.1016/j.arabjc.2010.04.008.

Albert, M.A. (2011) 'Biomarkers and heart disease', *Journal of Clinical Sleep Medicine : JCSM : Official Publication of the American Academy of Sleep Medicine*, 7(5 Suppl), pp. S9–S11. Available at: https://doi.org/10.5664/JCSM.1342.

Altintas, Z. (ed) (2018) *Biosensors and nanotechnology: Applications in health care diagnostics*. Hoboken, NJ: John Wiley & Sons, Inc. Available at: https://doi.org/10.1002/9781119065036.

Altintas, Z. and Masdor, N.A. (2018) 'Piezoelectric-Based biosensor technologies in disease detection and diagnostics', in *Biosensors and nanotechnology*. John Wiley & Sons, Ltd, pp. 77–94. Available at: https://doi.org/10.1002/9781119065036.ch5.

Altug, H. et al. (2022) 'Advances and applications of nanophotonic biosensors', *Nature Nanotechnology*, 17(1), pp. 5–16. Available at: https://doi.org/10.1038/s41565-021-01045-5.

Aronson, J.K. (2005) 'Biomarkers and surrogate endpoints', *British Journal of Clinical Pharmacology*, 59(5), pp. 491–494. Available at: https://doi.org/10.1111/j.1365-2125.2005.02435.x.

Aronson, J.K. and Ferner, R.E. (2017) 'Biomarkers—A general review', *Current Protocols in Pharmacology*, 76(1). Available at: https://doi.org/10.1002/cpph.19.

Ashley, J. and Sun, Y. (2018) 'The use of nanomaterials and microfluidics in medical diagnostics', in *Biosensors and nanotechnology*. John Wiley & Sons, Ltd, pp. 35–58. Available at: https://doi.org/10.1002/9781119065036.ch3.

Awasthi, K., Srivastava, A. and Srivastava, O.N. (2005) 'Synthesis of carbon nanotubes', *Journal of Nanoscience and Nanotechnology*, 5(10), pp. 1616–1636. Available at: https://doi.org/10.1166/jnn.2005.407.

Bakry, R. et al. (2007) Medicinal applications of fullerenes, *International Journal of Nanomedicine*, 2(4), pp. 639–649.

Bandodkar, A.J. et al. (2015) 'Tattoo-based noninvasive glucose monitoring: A proof-of-concept study', *Analytical Chemistry*, 87(1), pp. 394–398. Available at: https://doi.org/10.1021/ac504300n.

Bhalla, N. et al. (2016) 'Introduction to biosensors', *Essays in Biochemistry*, 60(1), pp. 1–8. Available at: https://doi.org/10.1042/EBC20150001.

Biosensors Market Size, Share, Industry Trends, Companies, Growth Analysis -2032 (no date) *MarketsandMarkets*. Available at: https://www.marketsandmarkets.com/Market-Reports/biosensors-market-798.html (Accessed: 30 April 2023).

Borse, V. and Srivastava, R. (2019a) 'Fluorescence lateral flow immunoassay based point-of-care nanodiagnostics for orthopedic implant-associated infection', *Sensors and Actuators B: Chemical*, 280, pp. 24–33. Available at: https://doi.org/10.1016/j.snb.2018.10.034.

Borse, V. and Srivastava, R. (2019b) 'Process parameter optimization for lateral flow immunosensing', *Materials Science for Energy Technologies*, 2(3), pp. 434–441. Available at: https://doi.org/10.1016/j.mset.2019.04.003.

Bui, M.P.N., Ahmed, S. and Abbas, A. (2015) 'Single-digit pathogen and attomolar detection with the naked eye using liposome-amplified plasmonic immunoassay', *Nano Letters*, 15(9), pp. 6239–6246. Available at: https://doi.org/10.1021/acs.nanolett.5b02837.

Burduşel, A.-C. et al. (2018) 'Biomedical applications of silver nanoparticles: An up-to-date overview', *Nanomaterials*, 8(9), p. 681. Available at: https://doi.org/10.3390/nano8090681.

Califf, R.M. (2018) 'Biomarker definitions and their applications', *Experimental Biology and Medicine*, 243(3), pp. 213–221. Available at: https://doi.org/10.1177/1535370217750088.

Campuzano, S., Yáñez-Sedeño, P. and Pingarrón, J.M. (2017) 'Molecular biosensors for electrochemical detection of infectious pathogens in liquid biopsies: Current trends and challenges', *Sensors*, 17(11), p. 2533. Available at: https://doi.org/10.3390/s17112533.

Chien, C.S. et al. (2018) 'Antibacterial activity of silver nanoparticles (AgNP) confined to mesostructured silica against methicillin-resistant Staphylococcus aureus (MRSA)', *Journal of Alloys and Compounds*, 747, pp. 1–7. Available at: https://doi.org/10.1016/j.jallcom.2018.02.334.

Cholestech LDX™ Analyzer (no date). Available at: https://www.globalpointofcare.abbott/en/product-details/cholestech-ldx-system.html (Accessed: 3 May 2023).

Choudhary, M. et al. (2016) 'CD 59 targeted ultrasensitive electrochemical immunosensor for fast and noninvasive diagnosis of oral cancer', *Electroanalysis*, 28(10), pp. 2565–2574. Available at: https://doi.org/10.1002/elan.201600238.

Clark Jr., L.C. and Lyons, C. (1962) 'Electrode systems for continuous monitoring in cardiovascular surgery', *Annals of the New York Academy of Sciences*, 102(1), pp. 29–45. Available at: https://doi.org/10.1111/j.1749-6632.1962.tb13623.x.

Colomer, J.-F. et al. (2000) Large-scale synthesis of single-wall carbon nanotubes by catalytic chemical vapor deposition CCVD method, *Chemical Physics Letters*, 317, pp. 83–89. Available at: www.elsevier.nlrlocatercplett.

Davis, F. and Altintas, Z. (2018) 'General introduction to biosensors and recognition receptors', in *Biosensors and nanotechnology*. John Wiley & Sons, Ltd, pp. 1–15. Available at: https://doi.org/10.1002/9781119065036.ch1.

D. Chin, C., Linder, V. and K. Sia, S. (2007) 'Lab-on-a-chip devices for global health: Past studies and future opportunities', *Lab on a Chip*, 7(1), pp. 41–57. Available at: https://doi.org/10.1039/B611455E.

Digge, M.S., Moon, R.S. and Gattani, S.G. (2012) Application of carbon nanotubes in drug delivery: A review, *International Journal of PharmTech Research*, 4(2), pp. 839–847.

Ding, P. et al. (2013) 'Reusable gold nanoparticle enhanced QCM immunosensor for detecting C-reactive protein', *Sensors and Actuators B: Chemical*, 188, pp. 1277–1283. Available at: https://doi.org/10.1016/j.snb.2013.07.099.

Fogel, R., Limson, J. and Seshia, A.A. (2016) 'Acoustic biosensors', in P. Estrela (ed) *Essays in biochemistry*, Vol. 60, No. 1, pp. 101–110. Available at: https://doi.org/10.1042/EBC20150011.

Ge, X. et al. (2014) 'Nanomaterial-enhanced paper-based biosensors', *TrAC Trends in Analytical Chemistry*, 58, pp. 31–39. Available at: https://doi.org/10.1016/j.trac.2014.03.008.

Golichenari, B. et al. (2018) 'Label-free nano-biosensing on the road to tuberculosis detection', *Biosensors and Bioelectronics*, 113, pp. 124–135. Available at: https://doi.org/10.1016/j.bios.2018.04.059.

Gupta, B.D., Shrivastav, A.M. and Usha, S.P. (2017) *Optical Sensors for Biomedical Diagnostics and Environmental Monitoring*. 1st edn. Boca Raton, FL : CRC Press, Taylor & Francis Group. Available at: https://doi.org/10.1201/9781315156033.

Hammami, I. et al. (2021) 'Gold nanoparticles: Synthesis properties and applications', *Journal of King Saud University - Science*, 33(7), p. 101560. Available at: https://doi.org/10.1016/j.jksus.2021.101560.

He, H. et al. (2013) 'Carbon nanotubes: Applications in pharmacy and medicine', *BioMed Research International*, 2013. Available at: https://doi.org/10.1155/2013/578290.

He, R. et al. (2021) 'A colorimetric dermal tattoo biosensor fabricated by microneedle patch for multiplexed detection of health-related biomarkers', *Advanced Science*, 8(24), p. 2103030. Available at: https://doi.org/10.1002/advs.202103030.

Henry, N.L. and Hayes, D.F. (2012) 'Cancer biomarkers', *Molecular Oncology*, 6(2), pp. 140–146. Available at: https://doi.org/10.1016/j.molonc.2012.01.010.

Iijima, S. (1991) 'Helical microtubules of graphitic carbon', *Nature*, 354(6348), pp. 56–58. Available at: https://doi.org/10.1038/354056a0.

Iwamoto, Y. and Yamakoshi, Y. (2006) 'A highly water-soluble C60-NVP copolymer: A potential material for photodynamic therapy', *Chemical Communications*, (46), pp. 4805–4807. Available at: https://doi.org/10.1039/b614305a.

Jamkhande, P.G. et al. (2019) 'Metal nanoparticles synthesis: An overview on methods of preparation, advantages and disadvantages, and applications', *Journal of Drug Delivery Science and Technology*, 53, p. 101174. Available at: https://doi.org/10.1016/j.jddst.2019.101174.

Jensen, A.W., Wilson, S.R. and Schuster, D.I. (1996) 'Biological applications of fullerenes', *Bioorganic & Medicinal Chemistry*, 4(6), pp. 767–779. Available at: https://doi.org/10.1016/0968-0896(96)00081-8.

Ji, Z. et al. (2012) 'Targeted therapy of SMMC-7721 liver cancer in vitro and in vivo with carbon nanotubes based drug delivery system', *Journal of Colloid and Interface Science*, 365(1), pp. 143–149. Available at: https://doi.org/10.1016/j.jcis.2011.09.013.

Karam, L.R., Mitch, M.G. and Coursey, B.M. (1997) 'Encapsulation of 99mTc within fullerenes: A novel radionuclidic carrier', *Applied Radiation and Isotopes*, 48(6), pp. 771–776. Available at: https://doi.org/10.1016/S0969-8043(96)00315-6.

Karfa, P. et al. (2019) 'Functionalization of carbon nanostructures', in *Comprehensive nanoscience and nanotechnology*. Elsevier, pp. 123–144. Available at: https://doi.org/10.1016/B978-0-12-803581-8.11225-1.

Kaur, M., Sharma, S. and Kumar, D. (2022) 'An insight into the multifarious applications of biosensors and the way forward', *Journal of Drug Delivery and Therapeutics*, 12(5-S), pp. 181–188. Available at: https://doi.org/10.22270/jddt.v12i5-S.5633.

Kaushik, S. et al. (2019) 'Two-dimensional transition metal dichalcogenides assisted biofunctionalized optical fiber SPR biosensor for efficient and rapid detection of bovine serum albumin', *Scientific Reports*, 9. Available at: https://doi.org/10.1038/s41598-019-43531-w.

Kimuda, S.G. et al. (2018) 'Characterising antibody avidity in individuals of varied *Mycobacterium tuberculosis* infection status using surface plasmon resonance', *PLoS One*, 13(10), p. e0205102. Available at: https://doi.org/10.1371/journal.pone.0205102.

Kroto, H.W. et al. (1985) 'C60: Buckminsterfullerene', *Nature*, 318(6042), pp. 162–163. Available at: https://doi.org/10.1038/318162a0.

Kumar, K.S.R. et al. (2021) 'An update on advances in COVID-19 laboratory diagnosis and testing guidelines in India', *Frontiers in Public Health*, 9. Available at: https://www.frontiersin.org/articles/10.3389/fpubh.2021.568603 (Accessed: 6 May 2023).

Kumar, S. et al. (2015) 'Reduced graphene oxide modified smart conducting paper for cancer biosensor', *Biosensors and Bioelectronics*, 73, pp. 114–122. Available at: https://doi.org/10.1016/j.bios.2015.05.040.

Lamberti, M. et al. (2014) 'Advantages and risks of nanotechnologies in cancer patients and occupationally exposed workers', *Expert Opinion on Drug Delivery*, 11(7), pp. 1087–1101. Available at: https://doi.org/10.1517/17425247.2014.913568.

Lamberti, M. et al. (2015) 'Carbon nanotubes: Properties, biomedical applications, advantages and risks in patients and occupationally-exposed workers', *International Journal of Immunopathology and Pharmacology*, 28(1), pp. 4–13. Available at: https://doi.org/10.1177/0394632015572559.

Li, C. et al. (2014) 'In vivo real-time visualization of tissue blood flow and angiogenesis using Ag2S quantum dots in the NIR-II window', *Biomaterials*, 35(1), pp. 393–400. Available at: https://doi.org/10.1016/j.biomaterials.2013.10.010.

Lozano-Castelló, D. et al. (2013) 'Advances in hydrogen storage in carbon materials', in *Renewable hydrogen technologies*. Elsevier, pp. 269–291. Available at: https://doi.org/10.1016/B978-0-444-56352-1.00012-X.

Mandal, N. et al. (2019) 'Point-of-care-testing of α-amylase activity in human blood serum', *Biosensors and Bioelectronics*, 124–125, pp. 75–81. Available at: https://doi.org/10.1016/j.bios.2018.09.097.

Maruccio, G. and Narang, J. (eds) (2022) *Electrochemical sensors: From working electrodes to functionalization and miniaturized devices*. Oxford: Woodhead Publishing, an imprint of Elsevier (Woodhead Publishing series in electronic and optical materials).

Mascini, M. (2006) 'A brief story of biosensor technology', in *Biotechnological applications of photosynthetic proteins: Biochips, biosensors and biodevices*. Boston, MA: Springer US (Biotechnology Intelligence Unit), pp. 4–10. Available at: https://doi.org/10.1007/978-0-387-36672-2_2.

Maxwell, T. et al. (2020) 'Quantum dots', in *Nanoparticles for biomedical applications*. Elsevier, pp. 243–265. Available at: https://doi.org/10.1016/B978-0-12-816662-8.00015-1.

Mohanty, S.P. and Kougianos, E. (2006) 'Biosensors: A tutorial review', *IEEE Potentials*, 25(2), pp. 35–40. Available at: https://doi.org/10.1109/MP.2006.1649009.

Molinero-Fernandez, A., Lopez, M.A. and Escarpa, A. (2020) 'Electrochemical microfluidic micromotors-based immunoassay for C-reactive protein determination in preterm neonatal samples with sepsis suspicion', *Analytical Chemistry*, 92(7). Available at: https://doi.org/10.1021/acs.analchem.9b05384.

Muhammad, Z. et al. (2016) 'PEG capped methotrexate silver nanoparticles for efficient anticancer activity and biocompatibility', *European Journal of Pharmaceutical Sciences*, 91, pp. 251–255. Available at: https://doi.org/10.1016/j.ejps.2016.04.029.

Murray, C.B., Noms, D.J. and Bawendi', M.G. (1993) Synthesis and characterization of nearly monodisperse CdE (E = S, Se, Te) semiconductor nanocrystallites, *J. Am. Chem. Soc*, pp. 8706–8715.

Manikandan, N et al. (2021) 'Carbon nanotubes and their properties-The review', *Materials Today: Proceedings*, 47, pp. 4682–4685. Available at: https://doi.org/10.1016/j.matpr.2021.05.543.

Nagel, B., Dellweg, H. and Gierasch, L.M. (1992) 'Glossary for chemists of terms used in biotechnology (IUPAC Recommendations 1992)', *Pure and Applied Chemistry*, 64(1), pp. 143–168. Available at: https://doi.org/doi:10.1351/pac199264010143.

Nagraik, R. et al. (2021) 'Amalgamation of biosensors and nanotechnology in disease diagnosis: Mini-review', *Sensors International*, 2, p. 100089. Available at: https://doi.org/10.1016/j.sintl.2021.100089.

Naresh, V. and Lee, N. (2021) 'A review on biosensors and recent development of nanostructured materials-enabled biosensors', *Sensors*, 21(4), p. 1109. Available at: https://doi.org/10.3390/s21041109.

Noviana, E. et al. (2021) 'Microfluidic paper-based analytical devices: From design to applications', *Chemical Reviews*, 121(19), pp. 11835–11885. Available at: https://doi.org/10.1021/acs.chemrev.0c01335.

Oberoi, S., Daya, K. and Tirumalai, P. (2012) Microwave sensor for detection of *E.* coli in water, in *Proceedings of the International Conference on Sensing Technology*. ICST. Available at: https://doi.org/10.1109/ICSensT.2012.6461753.

Pantarotto, D. et al. (2004) 'Functionalized carbon nanotubes for plasmid DNA gene delivery', *Angewandte Chemie - International Edition*, 43(39), pp. 5242–5246. Available at: https://doi.org/10.1002/anie.200460437.

Polley, N. et al. (2019) 'Fiber optic plasmonic sensors: Providing sensitive biosensor platforms with minimal lab equipment', *Biosensors and Bioelectronics*, 132, pp. 368–374. Available at: https://doi.org/10.1016/j.bios.2019.03.020.

Polley, N. et al. (2022) 'Photothermomechanical nanopump: A flow-through plasmonic sensor at the fiber tip', *ACS Nano*, p. acsnano.2c09938. Available at: https://doi.org/10.1021/acsnano.2c09938.

Premkumar, J. et al. (2018) 'Synthesis of silver nanoparticles (AgNPs) from cinnamon against bacterial pathogens', *Biocatalysis and Agricultural Biotechnology*, 15, pp. 311–316. Available at: https://doi.org/10.1016/j.bcab.2018.06.005.

Presnova, G. et al. (2017) 'Biosensor based on a silicon nanowire field-effect transistor functionalized by gold nanoparticles for the highly sensitive determination of prostate specific antigen', *Biosensors and Bioelectronics*, 88, pp. 283–289. Available at: https://doi.org/10.1016/j.bios.2016.08.054.

Purohit, B. et al. (2022) 'Continuous glucose monitoring for diabetes management based on miniaturized biosensors', in P. Chandra and K. Mahato (eds) *Miniaturized biosensing devices: Fabrication and applications*. Singapore: Springer Nature, pp. 149–175. Available at: https://doi.org/10.1007/978-981-16-9897-2_7.

Quint, S.B. and Pacholski, C. (2009) 'A chemical route to sub-wavelength hole arrays in metallic films', *Journal of Materials Chemistry*, 19(33), p. 5906. Available at: https://doi.org/10.1039/b910892k.

Rajamanikandan, R., Lakshmi, A.D. and Ilanchelian, M. (2020) 'Smart phone assisted, rapid, simplistic, straightforward and sensitive biosensing of cysteine over other essential amino acids by β-cyclodextrin functionalized gold nanoparticles as a colorimetric probe', *New Journal of Chemistry*, 44(28), pp. 12169–12177. Available at: https://doi.org/10.1039/d0nj02152k.

Ramalingam, G. et al. (2020) 'Quantum confinement'. Available at: https://www.semanticscholar.org/paper/Quantum-confinement-Ramalingam-Kathirgamanathan/760ab61c3e6116929122bf0405cc8fd91e337329 (Accessed: 5 May 2023).

Rancan, F. et al. (2002) Cytotoxicity and photocytotoxicity of a dendritic C(60) mono-adduct and a malonic acid C(60) tris-adduct on Jurkat cells, *Journal of Photochemistry and Photobiology B: Biology*, pp. 157–162. Available at: www.elsevier.com/locate/jphotobiol.

Resch-Genger, U. et al. (2008) 'Quantum dots versus organic dyes as fluorescent labels', *Nature Methods*, 5(9), pp. 763–775. Available at: https://doi.org/10.1038/nmeth.1248.

Rossetti, R., Nakahara, S. and Brus, L.E. (1983) 'Quantum size effects in the redox potentials, resonance Raman spectra, and electronic spectra of CdS crystallites in aqueous solution', *The Journal of Chemical Physics*, 79(2), pp. 1086–1088. Available at: https://doi.org/10.1063/1.445834.

Samia, A.C.S., Chen, X. and Burda, C. (2003) 'Semiconductor quantum dots for photodynamic therapy', *Journal of the American Chemical Society*, 125(51), pp. 15736–15737. Available at: https://doi.org/10.1021/ja0386905.

Sarhene, M. et al. (2019) 'Biomarkers in heart failure: The past, current and future', *Heart Failure Reviews*, 24(6), pp. 867–903. Available at: https://doi.org/10.1007/s10741-019-09807-z.

Serebrennikova, K.V. et al. (2021) 'Raman scattering-based biosensing: New prospects and opportunities', *Biosensors*, 11(12), p. 512. Available at: https://doi.org/10.3390/bios11120512.

Sesay, A.M., Tervo, P. and Tikkanen, E. (2018) 'Biomarkers in health care', in Biosensors and nanotechnology. John Wiley & Sons, Ltd, pp. 17–33. Available at: https://doi.org/10.1002/9781119065036.ch2.

Shanbogh, P.P. and Sundaram, N.G. (2015) 'Fullerenes revisited: Materials chemistry and applications of C60 molecules', *Resonance*, 20(2), pp. 123–135. Available at: https://doi.org/10.1007/s12045-015-0160-0.

Shi, Y. et al. (2023) 'Wearable sweat biosensors on textiles for health monitoring', *Journal of Semiconductors*, 44(2), p. 021601. Available at: https://doi.org/10.1088/1674-4926/44/2/021601.

Shukla, I. and Suneetha, V. (2017) 'Biosensors: Growth and market scenario', *Research Journal of Pharmacy and Technology*, 10(10), pp. 3573–3579. Available at: https://doi.org/10.5958/0974-360X.2017.00647.3.

Smith, A.A., Li, R. and Tse, Z.T.H. (2023) 'Reshaping healthcare with wearable biosensors', *Scientific Reports*, 13(1), p. 4998. Available at: https://doi.org/10.1038/s41598-022-26951-z.

Smith, A.M. et al. (2008) 'Bioconjugated quantum dots for in vivo molecular and cellular imaging', *Advanced Drug Delivery Reviews*, 60(11), pp. 1226–1240. Available at: https://doi.org/10.1016/j.addr.2008.03.015.

Song, Y. et al. (2019) 'Recent progress in microfluidics-based biosensing', *Analytical Chemistry*, 91(1), pp. 388–404. Available at: https://doi.org/10.1021/acs.analchem.8b05007.

Speranza, G. (2021) 'Carbon nanomaterials: Synthesis, functionalization and sensing applications', *Nanomaterials*, 11(4), p. 967. Available at: https://doi.org/10.3390/nano11040967.

Teengam, P. et al. (2018) 'Electrochemical impedance-based DNA sensor using pyrrolidinyl peptide nucleic acids for tuberculosis detection', *Analytica Chimica Acta*, 1044, pp. 102–109. Available at: https://doi.org/10.1016/j.aca.2018.07.045.

Tetyana, P., Morgan Shumbula, P. and Njengele-Tetyana, Z. (2021) 'Biosensors: Design, development and applications', in S. Ameen, M. Shaheer Akhtar, and H.- S. Shin (eds) *Nanopores*. IntechOpen. Available at: https://doi.org/10.5772/intechopen.97576.

Tripathy, S. et al. (2017) 'Electrospun manganese (III) oxide nanofiber based electrochemical DNA-nanobiosensor for zeptomolar detection of dengue consensus primer', *Biosensors and Bioelectronics*, 90, pp. 378–387. Available at: https://doi.org/10.1016/j.bios.2016.12.008.

Turner, A.P.F., Karube, I. and Wilson, G.S. (eds) (1987) *Biosensors: Fundamentals and applications*. Oxford [Oxfordshire]; New York: Oxford University Press.

Udugama, B. et al. (2020) 'Diagnosing COVID-19: The disease and tools for detection', *ACS Nano*, 14(4), pp. 3822–3835. Available at: https://doi.org/10.1021/acsnano.0c02624.

Updike, S.J. and Hicks, G.P. (1967) 'The enzyme electrode', *Nature*, 214(5092), pp. 986–988. Available at: https://doi.org/10.1038/214986a0.

Uprety, B. and Abrahamse, H. (2022) 'Semiconductor quantum dots for photodynamic therapy: Recent advances', *Frontiers in Chemistry*, 10. Available at: https://www.frontiersin.org/articles/10.3389/fchem.2022.946574 (Accessed: 5 May 2023).

Usui, Y. et al. (2012) 'Carbon nanotubes innovate on medical technology', *Medicinal Chemistry*, 2(2). Available at: https://doi.org/10.4172/2161-0444.1000105.

Wagner, A.M. et al. (2019) 'Quantum dots in biomedical applications', *Acta Biomaterialia*, 94, pp. 44–63. Available at: https://doi.org/10.1016/j.actbio.2019.05.022.

Wang, J. (2005) 'Carbon-nanotube based electrochemical biosensors: A review', *Electroanalysis*, 17(1), pp. 7–14. Available at: https://doi.org/10.1002/elan.200403113.

Wang, R. and Zhang, F. (2014) 'NIR luminescent nanomaterials for biomedical imaging', *Journal of Materials Chemistry B*, 2(17), pp. 2422–2443. Available at: https://doi.org/10.1039/c3tb21447h.

Xiang, J. et al. (2020) 'Evaluation of enzyme-linked immunoassay and colloidal gold-immunochromatographic assay kit for detection of novel coronavirus (SARS-Cov-2) causing an outbreak of pneumonia (COVID-19)'. *medRxiv*, p. 2020.02.27.20028787. Available at: https://doi.org/10.1101/2020.02.27.20028787.

Xie, B. et al. (1993) 'Fast determination of whole blood glucose with a calorimetric microbiosensor', *Sensors and Actuators B: Chemical*, 15(1), pp. 141–144. Available at: https://doi.org/10.1016/0925-4005(93)85040-H.

Yamakoshi, Y.N. et al. (1996) 'Acridine adduct of [60]fullerene with enhanced DNA-cleaving activity', *The Journal of Organic Chemistry*, 61(21), pp. 7236–7237. Available at: https://doi.org/10.1021/jo961210q.

Yan, X. et al. (2018) 'Antibacterial mechanism of silver nanoparticles in: *Pseudomonas aeruginosa*: Proteomics approach', *Metallomics*, 10(4), pp. 557–564. Available at: https://doi.org/10.1039/c7mt00328e.

Yang, T. et al. (2020) 'Point-of-care RNA-based diagnostic device for COVID-19', *Diagnostics*, 10(3), p. 165. Available at: https://doi.org/10.3390/diagnostics10030165.

Zhang, Y. et al. (2019) 'Label-free visual biosensor based on cascade amplification for the detection of *Salmonella*', *Analytica Chimica Acta*, 1075, pp. 144–151. Available at: https://doi.org/10.1016/j.aca.2019.05.020.

Ziemssen, T., Akgün, K. and Brück, W. (2019) 'Molecular biomarkers in multiple sclerosis', *Journal of Neuroinflammation*, 16(1), p. 272. Available at: https://doi.org/10.1186/s12974-019-1674-2.

Zijlstra, P., Paulo, P.M.R. and Orrit, M. (2012) 'Optical detection of single non-absorbing molecules using the surface plasmon resonance of a gold nanorod', *Nature Nanotechnology*, 7(6), pp. 379–382. Available at: https://doi.org/10.1038/nnano.2012.51.

7 Application of Silver Nanoparticles as Antimicrobial Coating

Advancement and Challenges

Sreejita Ghosh and Rina Rani Ray

7.1 INTRODUCTION

Silver has been utilized as an antibacterial in all its forms since ancient times, either alone or in synergy. By adding silver sulfadiazine or silver nitrate to dressings or creams for ulcers and burns, food packaging to prevent spoilage and household appliances like washing machines and refrigerators, silver can prevent bacteria growth. With nanotechnology, silver nanoparticles (AgNPs) antimicrobial properties were destined to be studied due to the evidence supporting silver's antibacterial effects (Kędziora et al., 2018).

AgNPs are sub-100 nm nanoparticles. Small sizes have a better surface area-to-volume ratio than silver compounds. Nanoscale AgNPs can be used to build products for targeted medication delivery, detection, diagnosis and imaging (Yaqoob et al., 2020a). However, AgNPs' remarkable antibacterial potency has caught researchers' interest. AgNPs are effective against numerous harmful and infectious microorganisms, including multidrug-resistant (MDR) bacteria (Siddiqi et al., 2018).

Due to their high fatality rate, medical device and implant infections have raised healthcare technology expenditures. Synthetic implants cause many infections. Europe inserts 800,000 orthopaedic implants annually, and 12,000 periprosthetic infections are expected (Gradinger et al., 2009). Since AgNPs are antibacterial, they can cover surgical equipment, dental implants, dressings, medical devices and catheters (Ge et al., 2014). Structure and environmental factors like temperature and humidity make textiles prone to microbial infection. Microbial development on materials increases smells, discolouration and stains and decreases mechanical durability (Ren et al., 2008). To improve fabric mechanical strength and biocompatibility for end users, machine learning (ML) studies on textile resistance utilizing AgNP coatings are needed (Höfer, 2006).

AgNPs exercise their antimicrobial properties through various mechanisms, such as damage to the microbial cell membrane, which is brought about by the physicochemical adherence of the AgNPs with the surfaces of the cells causing functional

DOI: 10.1201/9781003432661-7

and structural modifications like the formation of gaps, destabilization and piercing of the membrane and leakage of the cytoplasm and another potential mechanism is the destruction of the sub-cellular structure of the microbes releasing free Ag^+ ions subsequently leading to the release of reactive oxygen species (ROS) and essential macromolecules (enzymes, nucleotides and proteins) (Akter et al., 2017). In addition, AgNP can also bring about modification and modulation in the microbial cell signal transduction processes (Thomas et al., 2015). The transformation of silver-associated nanotechnology to medical applications mandates the fabrication of simple, non-hazardous, cost-effective and environmentally-friendly nanoparticles, which will be stable in terms of their physicochemical characteristics, *in vivo* and *in vitro* effects, safety regulation protocols, biological distribution, pharmacodynamics and pharmacokinetics of the AgNPs (Wei et al., 2015).

In this chapter, we will focus on the characteristic properties and the various biosynthesis procedures of AgNPs, how these AgNPs can be used as antimicrobial agents (including antibacterial and antibiofilm properties), their role as theranostics and antimicrobial coating agents and how textile resistance can be predicted using ML approach.

7.2 SYNTHESIS OF AgNPs

Various methods, classified as top-down or bottom-up methods are used for the biosynthesis of metallic NPs. Biosynthesis of AgNPs through the top-down method involves the production of AgNPs in the aerosolized or solid state into the nano dimension, finally forming AgNPs. This category includes physical approaches like laser ablation, ball milling and sputtering (Jara et al., 2015). On the contrary, bottom-up methods include nanostructuring and silver atom stabilization via various methods thereby forming NPs. Bottom-up approaches involve biological and chemical techniques for the biosynthesis of AgNPs (Silva et al., 2017).

Physical approaches are generally applied for obtaining vast quantities of AgNPs. Based on the technique used for biosynthesis, it can also produce immensely purified AgNPs. Unfortunately, these approaches need large amounts of energy, costly instruments and high temperature and pressure conditions (Yaqoob et al., 2020b). Chemical methods to produce AgNPs involve sol-gel, electrochemical and chemical reduction. Through these processes, AgNPs obtained have a definite spherical shape and are also not very expensive (Yaqoob et al., 2020b). Such approaches need a metallic precursor, a reducing substance and a stabilizing substance; hence, these methods are considered scalable and straightforward to execute. On the other hand, since chemical methods need a lot of substances, toxic solvents or reagents are often introduced, resulting in harmful AgNP formation (Tran & Le, 2013). Another method of AgNP synthesis is the biological method, which involves substances of biological origins, such as components directly from any organism, such as bacteria or fungi, or the use of any natural agents such as enzymes (Sintubin et al., 2009). A recently discovered method for the biosynthesis of biogenic AgNPs includes the application of bacteria, yeasts, fungi, plant extracts and algae in the form of stabilizing and/or reducing agents to act on the salts of silver and addresses the limitations of physicochemical approaches. *Trichoderma viride*, *Shewanella oneidensis*, *Lactobacillus* sp., *Bacillus* sp., and a few vegetative plant parts are nowadays used for producing green AgNPs (Daima & Bansal, 2015) as illustrated in Figure 7.1

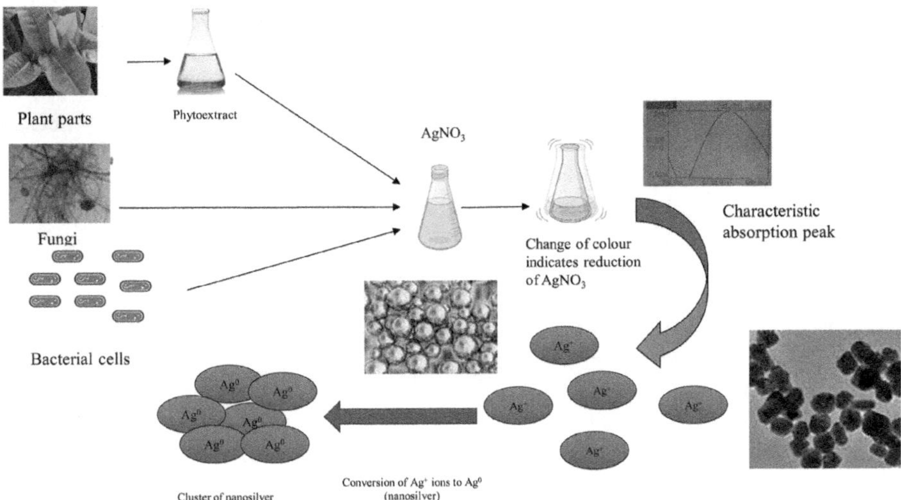

FIGURE 7.1 Different types of green approaches for the synthesis of biogenic AgNPs.

7.3 AgNPs AS ANTIMICROBIAL COATINGS

Since the infections associated with medical devices frequently start with a few free-floating planktonic bacterial cells, which get attached to the device surfaces, this has raised concern among industrialists, researchers and healthcare personnel, who try to inhibit the bacterial attachment by application of antimicrobial coatings.

Many antimicrobial coatings for medical devices have been developed in recent decades. Antimicrobial coatings prevent bacterium adhesion. These coatings contain hydrophilic polymers such as oxazoline, PEG, chlorinated plasma polymer and nitroxide radicals (Michl et al., 2018). Contact-killing coatings also kill microorganisms. Surface-grafted quaternary ammonium compounds (QAC) kill *Escherichia coli* cells with 41.8% bonded nitrogen atoms and +120.4 mV (Cavallaro et al., 2016). These two coatings merely reduce microbial cell adhesion on medical device surfaces; they do not eliminate microorganisms that enter implantation sites. The wound is open to opportunistic infections. Antimicrobial coatings or materials were created to neutralize opportunistic microorganisms. Antimicrobial polymers, peptides, nitric oxide and conventional antibiotics can be discharged. Therefore, this substance or coating releases antimicrobial compounds only when pathogenic bacteria invade device surfaces. These coatings have many advantages over antibacterial ones. Figure 7.2 shows AgNP coatings on devices and their potential effects.

7.3.1 AgNPs as Release Surface Antimicrobial Coatings

After being wiped out during the initial periods of the antibiotic era, silver again gained importance in the last half of the previous century because of its antimicrobial properties. Nanomaterials containing silver are considered releasing surfaces due to their mode of action. As NPs, silver can get oxidized within a physiological

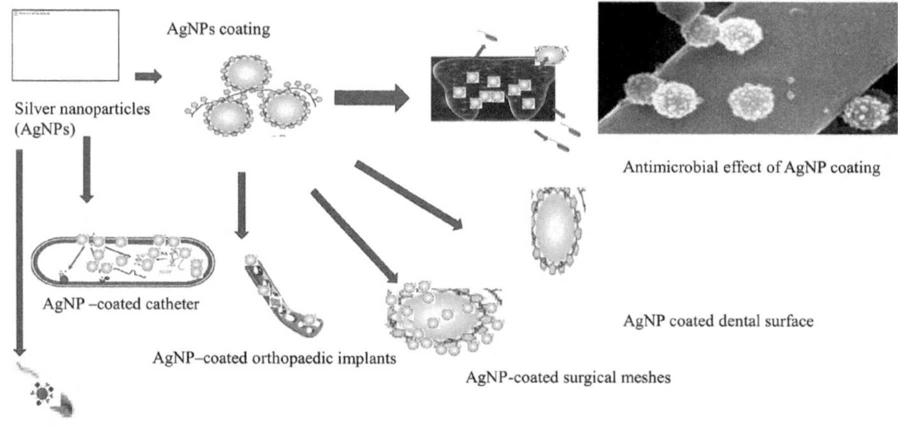

FIGURE 7.2 Various AgNP-coated devices and the mode of mechanism of antimicrobial effects.

medium. This oxide then gets dissolved releasing silver ions. These ions are the actual agents, which destroy the microbes via a multi-layered mode of action like getting attached to the cell membrane leading to membrane lysis, inhibiting DNA replication by binding with DNA and binding with proteins and enzymes causing the silver ions to interfere with the microbial metabolism. AgNPs can kill both Gram-negative and Gram-positive pathogens. Because of such a multi-layered mode of action, it is not easy for the microbes to get resistant to AgNPs, unlike traditional antibiotics (Figure 7.3).

Gonzalez et al. (2019) has conducted a significant study using AgNPs as antimicrobial coatings. It was reported that the cells of mammals are more tolerant towards silver than microbial cells. These results suggested that using AgNPs in medical device coating is safe. To accomplish this, a platform was fabricated consisting of a 100 nm wide film of polymeric plasma enriched with an amine group. This film was subsequently loaded with ions of silver by immersing it in a silver nitrate solution. The ions of silver were reduced to AgNPs by immersing them in sodium borohydride, which is usually used as a reducing substance. For regulating the dissolution and oxidation rate of the AgNPs and the liberation of silver ions, a barrier layer of polymeric plasma was applied on top at varying thicknesses of 18, 12 and 6 nm. The thickness of the top layer was chosen in such a way, facilitating the release of sufficient ions of silver and leading to total inhibition of the microbial adherence and formation of biofilms (Figure 7.4). Although there was a slight reduction in the case of the osteoblastic cells on the so-prepared AgNP-loaded antimicrobial coating, it was found that when the release rate of silver ions was reduced (by using a thinner top layer), the cells developed and multiplied again acting just like a control set-up, which was without being treated with AgNP antimicrobial coating. This observation has presented the opportunity to fabricate medical device antimicrobial coating while not preventing normal integration and growth of the tissues. The efficiency of these antimicrobial coatings was even tested against the silver dressings already

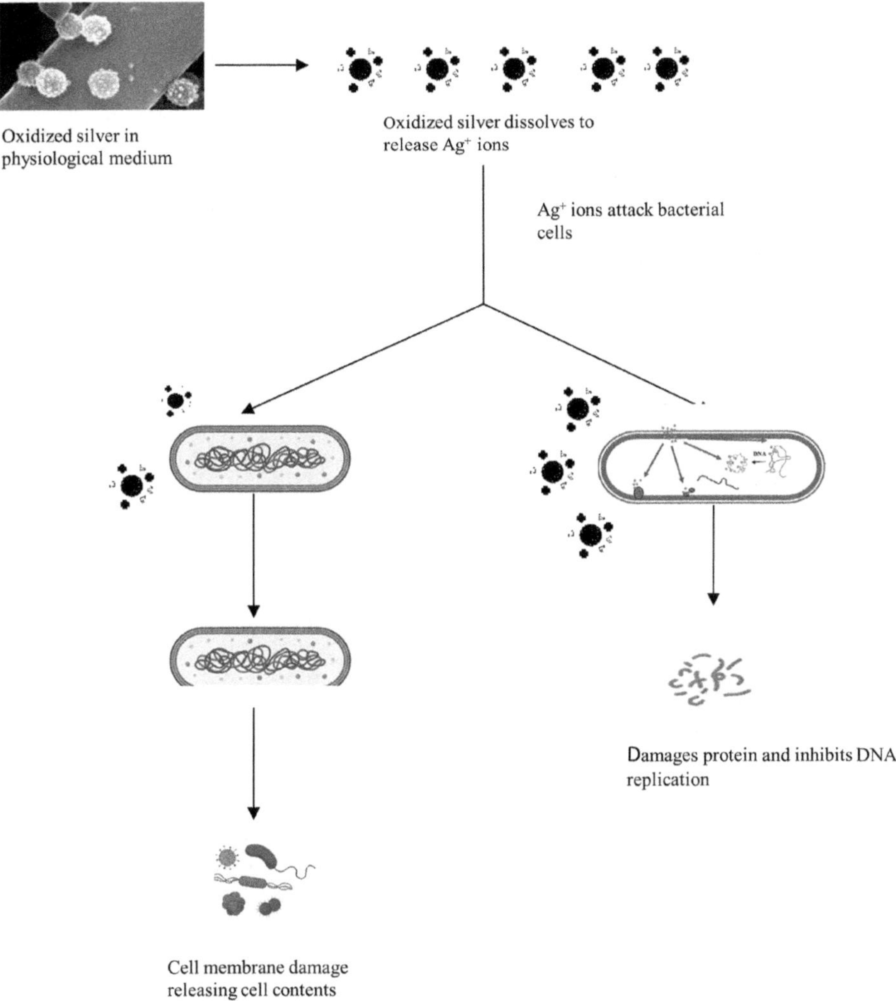

FIGURE 7.3 AgNPs acting as release surface coatings leading to bacterial damage.

available in the market. The silver dressings commercially available were found to be equipped with layers of silver of dimension 3 microns. In contrast, the same antimicrobial activity can be achieved with just a tiny fraction of AgNPs in this so-designed AgNP medical device coating (Ostrikov et al., 2016).

7.3.2 AgNPs as Responsive Antimicrobial Coatings

Intelligent and responsive materials and coatings can selectively release antimicrobial substances only during the presence of pathogenic microbes and has aroused substantial technological and scientific interest. These coatings are one of the significant advancements in using AgNPs as antimicrobial coating agents compared to

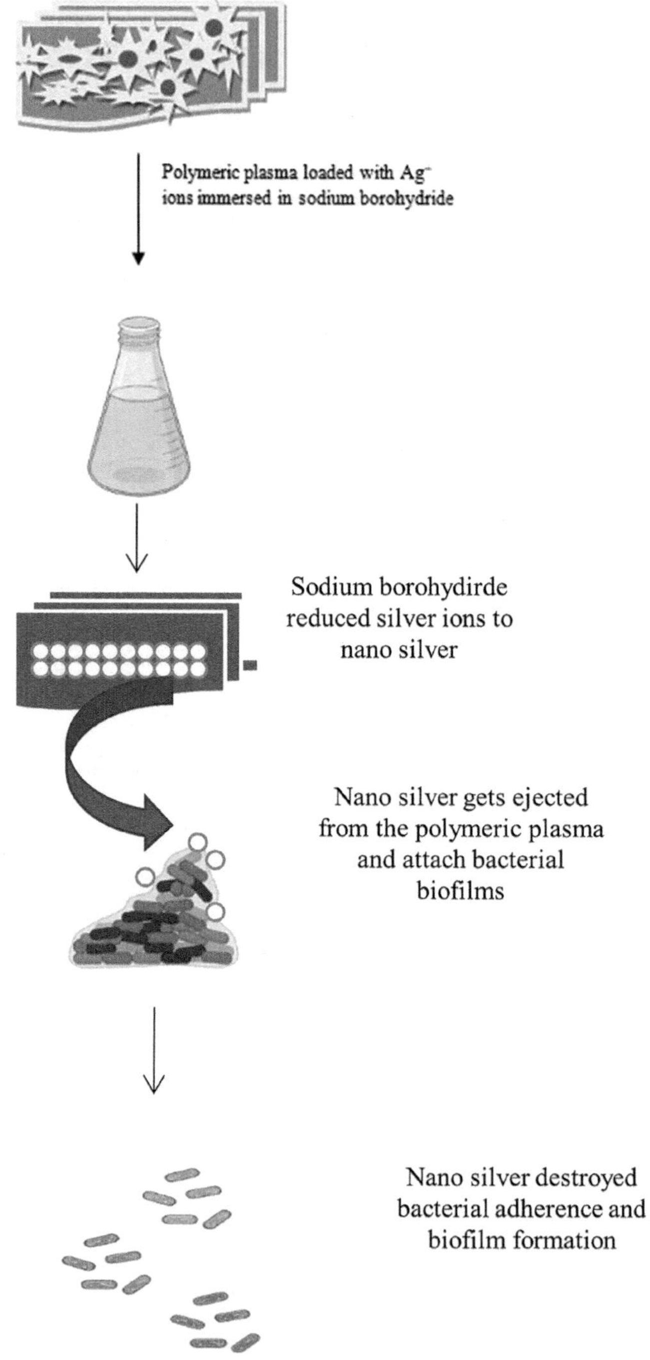

FIGURE 7.4 Mechanism of polymeric plasma to destroy microbial biofilms.

the direct application of antimicrobials. In the case of using AgNPs in synthesizing responsive coatings, harmful effects on tissues are avoided if pathogenic microbes do not infiltrate the surface of the medical devices. Stimuli due to responsive antimicrobial release may be temperature, pH, enzymes or ROS and toxins released by the pathogens (Cavallaro et al., 2016). Baier et al. (2013) manufactured enzymatically responsive nanocapsules and NPs. In this study, hyaluronate nanocapsules were synthesized, which contained polyhexanide. Virulent bacteria like *Staphylococcus aureus* express numerous toxins involving an enzyme known as hyaluronidase. It was indicated that the nanocapsules released their load of antimicrobials only during the presence of the hyaluronidase enzyme. These nanocapsules were also labelled with specific fluorescent dyes. Hence, the AgNP nanomaterial is not only bactericidal but also signals the presence of pathogens.

7.4 BIOCIDAL APPLICATIONS OF AgNPs

The shape, size, electrochemistry and concentration of AgNPs affect their medical, industrial and environmental uses. AgNPs kill Gram-positive and Gram-negative bacteria. The biocidal activity of AgNPs depends on their size and surface stability. The build-up and penetration of AgNPs in bacterial membranes have been shown to harm and destroy bacterial cells. The penetrating capacity of AgNPs depends on their size. AgNPs between 1 and 100 nm may easily permeate Gram-negative bacteria cell membranes, whereas AgNPs between 10 and 15 nm can inhibit drug-resistant and non-resistant bacteria development. Additionally, *S. aureus* and *E. coli* biofilms can be completely prevented by 3.3–33 nM AgNPs (Shrivastava et al., 2007). Surface changes affect the biocides' AgNP coating's penetrating power, along with shapes and sizes. Triangular-shaped truncated AgNPs had greater biocidal activity than spherical or rod-shaped AgNPs and silver ions in antimicrobial coatings (Kvítek et al., 2008). Sodium dodecyl sulfate (SDS), polyoxyethylene sorbitan monooleate-Tween 80 and PVP 360 surface modifications significantly increased the antibacterial activity of AgNPs against *Pseudomonas aeruginosa*, *E. coli*, *S. aureus*, *Enterococcus faecalis*, methicillin-susceptible *Staphylococcus epidermidis* and vancomycin-resistant *S. aureus* and AgNPs are also used as air filter disinfectants to prevent bacteria from sticking to filters due to their antibacterial properties and particle size distribution. Air filters with AgNP coatings prevent *Micrococcus roseus*, *Micrococcus luteus*, *Pseudomonas luteola* and *Bacillus subtilis* colonization. *E. coli* and other infections in drinking water are another global health and social issue, especially in poor countries. Polyurethane (PU)-functionalized AgNPs form a -COO- functional carboxyl group, which is effective against Gram-negative bacteria *P. aeruginosa* and *E. coli* and Gram-positive bacteria *S. aureus* and *B. subtilis*. The main ingredient for destroying pathogens is ionic silver in water. Thus, ionic silver poisoning of water may cause various health complications that need further study.

AgNPs also possess antifungal features against *Trichophyton mentagrophytes*, *Trichophyton rubrum* and *Candida albicans* at various concentrations and sizes. AgNPs showed the most excellent activity against fungi at a size of approximately 100 nm with IC_{80} values of 1–7 µg/mL (Monteiro et al., 2011). The very recent identification of AgNPs in the form of biocides includes their potential as antiviral substances acting against viral infections like influenza A/H5N1, SARS-CoV, dengue virus, influenza A/ H1N1, hepatitis B virus (HBV), Human Immunodeficiency Virus (HIV) and new viral strains of encephalitis. AgNPs of sizes 1–10 nm can prevent the proliferation of HIV-1, while AgNPs of sizes 10–80 nm can act against other strains of viruses via binding with the proteins present within the virus particles. The actual mode of action of AgNPs as antiviral substances has not yet been studied. Future research regarding this mode of action may aid in fighting harmful viral strains in the coming generations. Nowadays, AgNPs are being used in industries to produce functionalized plastics, antimicrobial paints, preservatives, medicinal gels, fabrics, packaging components, etc. The imperishable functionality of the plants for effluent treatment in a few significant industrial belts can be ensured by extensive modification and characterization of the AgNPs.

7.5 ROLE OF AgNPs AS THERANOSTICS

Theranostics is evolving as a safe, targeted and effective pharmacotherapy the main focus of which is patient-centric care. Theranostics is the combination of therapeutics and diagnosis. This acts as a transition from traditional medicine to customized medicine. It includes the personalized designing of therapies on the basis of the uniqueness of every individual thereby leading to the fabrication of the appropriate drug for the targeted patient at the correct time (Jeelani et al., 2014). Genetics plays a major role in the theranostic approach. Theranostics presents a cheap, specified and effective protocol of therapy. Proteomics, pharmacogenetics and profiling of biomarkers are the backbones of successful theranostics. Theranostics is fascinatingly applied in multiple levels with particular emphasis in the field of oncology, wherein various nanoformulations acting as dendrimers, liposomes, AgNPs (polymeric and metallic), carbon nanotubes (CNTs) and quantum dots are immensely used (Figure 7.5).

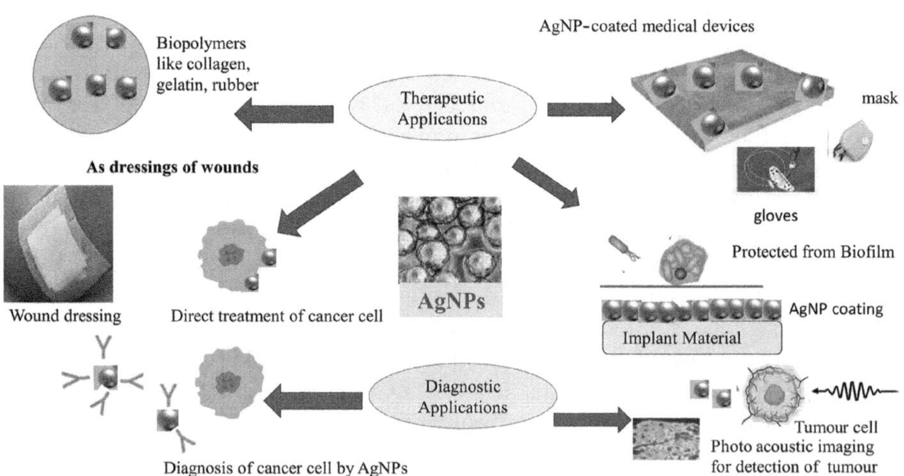

FIGURE 7.5 Application of AgNPs as theranostics.

Therefore, theranostics can be considered a holistic transformation of trial-and-error drugs to preventive, predictive and personalized drugs, improving the quality of care provided by pharmacotherapy.

7.5.1 AgNP-Coated Catheters

The worldwide emergence of central venous catheter (CVC)-associated infections of the bloodstream increased to 80,000 cases yearly. On the other hand, the application of CVCs in hospitals in the US was about 5 million per year. Patients suffering from an intracerebral haemorrhage, tumours, and haemorrhage of the subarachnoid were provided with external ventricular drain (EVD) catheters generally for acute hydrocephalus therapy. The EVD catheters mainly were utilized to monitor intracranial pressure and cerebrospinal fluid (CSF) draining. Catheters were previously coated with antibiotics that reduced the rates of microbial colonization, leading to the development of antimicrobial resistance. Hence, a new approach of AgNP-coated catheters came into use in the medicinal field, wherein the ions of silver get bound to the unreactive ceramic zeolite with the help of inorganic AgNP powder. In recent years, an investigation reported major rates of reduction in microbial colonization in AgNP-coated CVCs (Khare et al., 2007). In the study conducted by Neethu et al. (2020), *Acinetobacter baumanii* was made to form biofilms, to mimic the *in vivo* infection conditions, and the CVC was coated with polydopamine along with AgNP and was tested for antibacterial action. Through characterization of the surfaces using field emission scanning electron microscopy (FE-SEM), Raman's spectroscopy and water contact angle (CA), it was found that AgNP-dopamine coated CVCs showed a CA value of about 49.1. Retrospective clinical trials were also conducted to analyze the contrasting efficacy of conventional non-coated catheters with that of AgNP-coated EVD catheters. Microbial colonization was significantly decreased by four times in AgNP-coated EVD catheters compared to the non-coated conventional non-coated catheters. In another study, it was demonstrated that EVD catheters coated with AgNPs reduced *S. aureus* growth (Fichtner et al., 2010).

7.5.2 AgNP-Coated Orthopaedic Implants

The gold standard therapy for arthritis is the artificial replacement of the joints. The application of bone cements such as poly methyl methacrylate (PMMA) led to increased infection rates when introduced within bones. Nanobiotechnology has emerged in the fields of trauma and orthopaedics. Thus, AgNP-coated bone cements demonstrated significant antibacterial action against a broad spectrum of bacteria including methicillin-resistant *Staphylococcus aureus* (MRSA). On a further level, these AgNPs did not possess any cytotoxic activities. Ultra-high molecular weight polyethylene (UHMWPE) was previously used in the artificial replacement of joints; however, it had the limitation of wear and tear because of the generation of debris leading to joint failure and inflammation in the body. The AgNP coating overcame this limitation along with the bone cement and subsequently decreased the formation of debris (Morley et al., 2007). The infection rate was decreased by AgNP integration to the external layer of the implants. Zhao et al. (2014) demonstrated an increased resistance against *E. coli* infections on exposure to modified films of titanium. AgNP-coated devices also led to the reduction of infections caused within the pin tracts (Zhao et al., 2014). Infections associated with the orthopaedic implants led to decreased rates of morbidity when cells like osteoblasts and mesenchymal stem cells of the bone marrow were subjected to AgNP-coated orthopaedic implants and displayed a minimum inhibitory concentration as low as 25 μg/mL (Castiglioni et al., 2017).

7.5.3 AgNP-Coated Surgical Meshes

Usually, prosthetic meshes are not used as indwelling devices for reconstructive pelvic surgeries and repair of hernia. The percentage of occurrence of infections of these meshes is around 0.6%–8%. According to the data on 1 million herniorrhaphies, there were about 30,000–50,000 infections of prosthetic meshes in the US. Numerous AgNP-associated antimicrobial coatings are used on these medical devices including CVCs, urinary catheters and surgical meshes for a reduction in the rate of infection. For a reduction in the incidence of prosthetic mesh-associated infections in cases of hernia and post-pelvic surgeries, AgNPs in the form of nanocrystals in combination with polypropylene can be applied. The antimicrobial activity of AgNPs is based on the electrical condition of the silver ions. Silver is active biologically in its soluble state. Commonly used topical creams contain silver nitrate, silver sulfadiazine, etc. Topical formulations of silver are applied over 2–12 times per day to burn areas due to the rapid inactivation of ionic silver by the organic or chloride ions present within the wounds. In comparison to ionic silver, AgNPs do not form complexes with organic or chloride ions, which can lead to hindrance in microbial inactivation. Cohen et al. (2007), found that polypropylene impregnated with nanocrystalline silver particle (NCSP) made the AgNPs circulate within the mesh, producing an inhibition zone and increasing the efficacy of inhibition against the growth of *S. aureus*. The inhibition zone diminished in a dose-dependent way with rising AgNP concentration. From this study, it can also be concluded that NCSPs possess anti-inflammatory properties. The secondary mode of action of the NCSP is the repression of interleukin (IL)-12 and tumour necrosis factor (TNF) α and the initiation of inflammatory apoptosis of the cells.

7.5.4 AgNPs as Theranostics in Dentistry

AgNPs have emerged as a promising therapeutic agent in the field of dentistry. This feature is due to their antimicrobial action as coatings of dental biomaterials. The primary mode of action is the release of cationic silver and its oxidative potentials. The use of AgNPs in dentistry is efficient against MDR bacteria due to their prophylactic activities. AgNPs are applied in different fields of dentistry such as orthodontics, preventive dentistry, periodontics, endodontics and oral dentistry. AgNPs prevent the growth of the biofilms formed by *Streptococcus mitis*, *S. aureus* and *Streptococcus gordoinii*. In addition, recent studies demonstrated that AgNPs exhibited antibacterial action against *Lactobacillus acidophilus*, *Streptococcus sorbinus*, *Streptococcus sanguinis*, *Lactobacillus casei*, *Actinomyces actinomycetemcomitans* and *Enterococcus faecalis* (Fernandez et al., 2021). AgNP integration in polymers is utilized as the basis of dentures and tissue conditioners in stomatitis and displayed superior antimicrobial action and capability to ward off any infections of the oral cavity. Another study revealed that an altered denatured acrylic base coated with AgNPs at 20% (w/w) displayed antifungal activity (Monteiro et al., 2012). AgNPs having a small diameter showed the best antibiofilm actions in comparison to the larger-sized NPs. Biosynthesis of AgNPs from the extracts of onion, neem, and tomato produce AgNPs of size ranging between 26.2 and 33.3 nm showing antimicrobial action against *S.aureus* due to the high concentration of terpenoids and flavonoids (Chand et al., 2019). It was also reported that AgNPs prevented the growth of *Streptococcus mutans* and also stopped the formation of biofilms (Pérez-Díaz et al., 2015). Therefore, AgNPs play a significant function in the field of dentistry by removing dental caries. Decreased biofilm adherence and lactate production by microbes have been observed in the AgNP-coated titanium composite of discs (Besinis et al., 2017). A bacteriostatic nanosubstance called silver nanofluoride stopped *S. mutans* growth and it can be easily used and also gives an excellent cost-benefit ratio (Figure 7.6). Hence, silver nanofluoride can act as a suitable substitute for sodium fluoride. Micro implants made of titanium biopolymer coated with AgNPs (Ti-BP-AgNP) exhibited an inhibition zone of around 50.58 mm against *S. mutans*. The inhibition zone against *Streptococcus sanguinis* was about 27 mm, and a minimal inhibition zone of about 25 mm was observed against *S. mutans* while the control setup showed no inhibition zones (Venugopal et al., 2017).

7.6 MACHINE LEARNING APPROACH TO PREDICT TEXTILE'S ANTIMICROBIAL COATING

Increased concern regarding the MDR microbes has resulted in the fabrication of efficient, novel, and long-term antimicrobial and antibiofilm materials. Nano-assisted finished materials and nanotechnology have propelled the interest of researchers recently. NPs are known to improve the resistance of textiles against microbes by

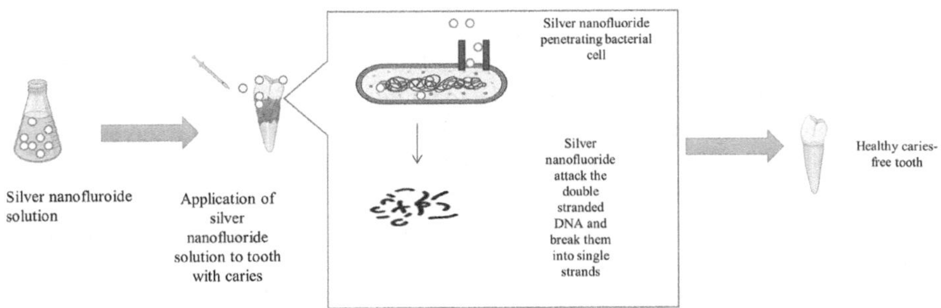

FIGURE 7.6 Application of silver nanofluoride solutions to remove dental caries.

enhancing their capabilities of dye absorption and modifying their wettability facilitating effective functionalization without modifying the properties of the textiles. Antimicrobial AgNPs are used in combination with antibiotics to prevent MDR bacterial growth and to provide the textiles with a multifunctional alteration. The antimicrobial activities of AgNPs (inorganic and organic) are associated with the inability of the microbes to gain resistance against the latter. AgNPs are widely applied as antimicrobial substances in the textile industry. They are considered to be feasible because of their low cytotoxicity to humans, low prices, can act against a broad spectrum of microbes and inhibit the formation of biofilms. Textiles containing the antimicrobial coating of AgNPs are known as nanotextiles. They are made by various processes, which are as follows:

a. Numerous methods are utilized for AgNP deposition on textiles based on the type of NPs and the textile fibre. Either the AgNPs are integrated inside the fibres during the process of extrusion or are adhered to the surfaces during the process of finishing. Physical methods include irradiation, pre-treatment with plasma, chemical methods and ultrasound. For instance, chemical reduction within aqueous media, electrochemical reduction, synthesis by sonochemistry and chemical-assisted radiation are some of the most widely used approaches for producing nanotextiles. The methods of finishing include processes of the pad-dry-cure, dip-pad method, foam finishing, spraying, assembly via layer-upon-layer, grafting, the process of impregnation, dip coating, deposition by microwave radiations, method of exhaustion, ultrasonic irradiation and agitation, deposition by chemical reduction and vapour, sputtering, drop-coating, deposition by electroless and sol-gel (Periyasamy et al., 2020).
b. Textiles are subjected to various circumstances throughout their lifespan, including heat, washing and dry cleaning. For example, it is of significance to have knowledge about the antimicrobial capabilities of textiles. Hence, the impact of the conditions of washing on the antimicrobial activity of nanotextiles can be measured by the types of detergents used, different tests of durability (industrial, laboratory scale, and household washing machines), the number of cycles of washing, the quantity of water (distilled or tap) used and temperature.

ML models have been primarily incorporated for forecasting the safety and toxicity of AgNPs. Mirzaei et al. (2021) devised a technique for predicting the antimicrobial activities in terms of inhibition zones formed by the AgNPs and expressing them in terms of regression models. In this study, the results obtained from the *in vitro* experimental arrangement were used. Furthermore, the work provided an ML model for predicting the antimicrobial efficacy and durability of the AgNP-incorporated nanotextiles followed by multiple washes. This technique predicted the antimicrobial activities by investigating the p-chem characteristics of the AgNPs, conditions of exposure and type of bacteria used as inputs. The antimicrobial capacity was in terms of the percentage reduction in viability of the microbes. The results from this model suggested the critical role played by parameters such as the method of deposition or application for predicting the antimicrobial efficacies of the nanotextiles. The importance of consistent and standardized measurements, along with a harmonized system of reporting for the conditions of the experiment and the p-chem characteristics, was highlighted. However, there still remains a lacuna of the models associated with the functionalities of the AgNPs in the existing literature, which might prevent the ongoing interest in safe-designing the outlines for integrating performance along with safety at the same time. Awareness must be raised among the scientific community for the absence of comprehensive sets of data regarding the antimicrobial activities of AgNPs.

Moreover, the work done by Mirzaei et al. (2021) provided an essential contribution to this field and illustrated the significance of ML-related tools for development. This indicates the beneficial effects of the interdisciplinary approach by improving the antimicrobial effects of nanotextiles and therefore reducing the harmful microbial growth on the textiles. The technology of forecasting the antimicrobial characteristics of nanotextiles, especially in healthcare sectors, provides vast potential in presenting the healthcare sectors with substantial benefits.

7.7 CHALLENGES IN USING AgNPs AS AN ANTIMICROBIAL COATING

AgNP coating creates ionic repulsions between particles to avoid aggregation and stabilize them. Uncoated AgNPs drastically reduced cell viability in a dose- and time-dependent manner, but the coating protected against cytotoxicity. The coating type depends on the capping agent, which might be inorganic (chloride, sulphide, carbonate and borate) or organic (citrates, polysaccharides, proteins and polymers). Coated AgNP stability, surface chemistry, morphology and bioactivity depend on the capping substance. This section discusses the potential drawbacks of AgNP coatings. Depending on the coating, AgNPs can cause cytotoxicity. Generally, ROS production, antioxidant defence impairment and mitochondria membrane potential loss induce cytotoxicity. AgNPs' toxicity depends on the coating. Chitosan-related polysaccharide-coated AgNPs showed antibacterial activity without damage to eukaryotic cells (Travan et al., 2009).

In HepG2 cells, polystyrene-coated AgNPs altered genetic repression and induction (Kawata et al., 2009). In addition, polyvinylpyrrolidone- and citrate-coated AgNPs were examined for cytotoxicity in HT29 epithelial cells and J774A.1 macrophages (Nguyen et al., 2013). In cell lines tested, PVP- and citrate-coated AgNPs were less cytotoxic than uncoated ones. The pathways of oxidative stress and cytokine production showed that AgNPs cause cytotoxic damage to macrophages and epithelial cells. Citrate-coated AgNPs were stable and less toxic. PVP-coated AgNPs also showed little cytotoxicity in skin HaCat keratinocytes. Since polysaccharide-coated AgNPs could enter the nucleus and mitochondria, they damaged DNA. AgNP organ toxicity is listed in Table 7.1.

TABLE 7.1
AgNPs of Various Sizes and Their Potential Toxic Effects

Site of Toxicity	Size of AgNPs	Effects	References
Skin and dermal or epidermal toxicity	50–80 nm	Decreased thickness of epidermis and dermis with raised number of Langerhans cells, markers for inflammation, reduced thickness of the papillary layers and increased levels of collagen in the dermis. Argyria with stored amounts of silver under subcutaneous tissue leading to skin discolouration.	Korani et al. (2011)
Lungs	<10 nm	Persistent lung inflammation with pulmonary fibrosis.	Gliga et al. (2014)
Gastrointestinal system	10–20 nm	Small AgNPs can cross the barriers of the liver, blood, muscles and the brain and significantly reduce the levels of IFN-γ and IL-4.	Gokulan et al. (2020)
Liver	20–50 nm	Alterations of the blood chemistry causing hepatotoxicity, which was confirmed by the raised levels of serum activity, including alanine aminotransferase (ALT) and aspartate aminotransferase (AST) leading to histological damage.	Heydrnejad et al. (2015)
Kidney	>50 nm	Decreased weight of kidney leading to renal dysfunction with high creatinine levels in serum. Mitochondria were also damaged; membranes of brush border were lost, increased podocyte swelling and foot process degeneration. Prolonged exposure leads to raised levels of cell survival, proliferative and proinflammatory factors along with hindrance of the usual pathway of apoptosis.	Tiwari et al. (2017)
Muscles	>50 nm	Increased levels of N-acetyl-β-D-glucosaminidase and decreased clearance level of creatinine.	Mahmood (2012)
Nervous system	All sizes of AgNPs	Increased silver levels in erythrocytes, plasma, CSF alongside coma and epileptic seizures through interaction with the cellular constituents to induce neurotoxic damage	Suthar et al. (2023)
Developmental and reproductive organ	25–30 nm	Sperm count decreased significantly along with altered morphology and vitality. Remarkable reduction found in the number of Sertoli, spermatogonia and Leydig cells.	Fathi et al. (2019)
Immune system	14–20 nm	Immune system recognizes AgNPs as foreign particles and triggers a cascade of immunological reactions including the activation of macrophages, neutrophils, and helper T cells and results in a large number of cytokine expressions such as interleukins, tumour necrosis factor, etc.	Ninan et al. (2020)

7.8 CONCLUSION

AgNPs have been predominantly used in various scientific fields for coating different biomedical instruments, wound dressings, theranostics, etc. They are extensively exploited for nanostructure development. This is mostly because AgNPs possess various activities including anti-inflammatory, antimicrobial and anticancer as well as therapeutic actions in orthopaedics, dentistry, etc. Besides these activities possessed by AgNPs, their physicochemical characteristics make them potent for being applied as antimicrobial coatings in varied fields. However, the research regarding the cytotoxicity of AgNPs is not yet enough to classify their toxicity framework. From a few studies, it can be somewhat concluded that particle size plays an important role in determining the cytotoxicity of the AgNPs; i.e. the smaller the size of the AgNPs, the greater is their toxicity. In this chapter, comprehensive information regarding the advancements of AgNP coatings has been provided along with the potential challenges that may be faced due to the application of AgNP coatings. Cytotoxicity might also depend on the variation of the organisms. Most of the research for assaying the toxicity of AgNPs is still in clinical trials. There is a significant amount of data about the useful activities of AgNPs as novel nanostructured substances and their excellent biocompatibility. Further research is still needed for elaboration on the cytotoxicity of AgNPs as well as on the improvisation of the antimicrobial formulations for enhanced stability, long-term release of the AgNPS, exploration of more appropriate shape, size and procedure for the modification of the surfaces of the AgNP coatings.

REFERENCES

Akter, M., Sikder, M. T., Rahman, M. M., Ullah, A. K. M. A., Hossain, K. F. B., Banik, S., Hosokawa, T., Saito, T., & Kurasaki, M. (2017). A systematic review on silver nanoparticles-induced cytotoxicity: Physicochemical properties and perspectives. *Journal of Advanced Research*, *9*, 1–16. https://doi.org/10.1016/j.jare.2017.10.008

Baier, G., Cavallaro, A., Vasilev, K., Mailänder, V., Musyanovych, A., & Landfester, K. (2013). Enzyme responsive hyaluronic acid nanocapsules containing polyhexanide and their exposure to bacteria to prevent infection. *Biomacromolecules*, *14*(4), 1103–1112. https://doi.org/10.1021/bm302003m

Besinis, A., Hadi, S. D., Le, H. R., Tredwin, C., & Handy, R. D. (2017). Antibacterial activity and biofilm inhibition by surface modified titanium alloy medical implants following application of silver, titanium dioxide and hydroxyapatite nanocoatings. *Nanotoxicology*, *11*(3), 327–338. https://doi.org/10.1080/17435390.2017.1299890

Castiglioni, S., Cazzaniga, A., Locatelli, L., & Maier, J. A. M. (2017). Silver nanoparticles in orthopedic applications: New insights on their effects on osteogenic cells. *Nanomaterials*, *7*(6), 124. https://doi.org/10.3390/nano7060124

Cavallaro, A., Mierczynska, A., Barton, M., Majewski, P., & Vasilev, K. (2016). Influence of immobilized quaternary ammonium group surface density on antimicrobial efficacy and cytotoxicity. *Biofouling*, *32*(1), 13–24. https://doi.org/10.1080/08927014.2015.1115977

Chand, K., Abro, M. I., Aftab, U., Shah, A. H., Lakhan, M. N., Cao, D., Mehdi, G. & Mohamed, A. M. A. (2019). Green synthesis characterization and antimicrobial activity against Staphylococcus aureus of silver nanoparticles using extracts of neem, onion and tomato. *RSC Advances*, *9*(30), 17002–17015. https://doi.org/10.1039/C9RA01407A

Cohen, M. S., Stern, J. M., Vanni, A. J., Kelley, R. S., Baumgart, E., Field, D., Libertino, J. A., & Summerhayes, I. C. (2007). In vitro analysis of a nanocrystalline silver-coated surgical mesh. *Surgical Infections*, *8*(3), 397–403. https://doi.org/10.1089/sur.2006.032

Daima, H. K., & Bansal, V. (2015). Influence of physicochemical properties of nanomaterials on their antibacterial applications. In: *Nanotechnology in diagnosis, treatment and prophylaxis of infectious diseases* (pp. 151–166). Academic Press.

Fathi, N., Hoseinipanah, S. M., Alizadeh, Z., Assari, M. J., Moghimbeigi, A., Mortazavi, M., Hosseini, M. H., & Bahmanzadeh, M. (2019). The effect of silver nanoparticles on the reproductive system of adult male rats: A morphological, histological and DNA integrity study. *Advances in Clinical and Experimental Medicine: Official Organ Wroclaw Medical University*, *28*(3), 299–305. https://doi.org/10.17219/acem/81607

Fernandez, C. C., Sokolonski, A. R., Fonseca, M. S., Stanisic, D., Araújo, D. B., Azevedo, V., Portela, R. D., & Tasic, L. (2021). Applications of silver nanoparticles in dentistry: Advances and technological innovation. *International Journal of Molecular Sciences*, *22*(5), 2485. https://doi.org/10.3390/ijms22052485

Fichtner, J., Güresir, E., Seifert, V., & Raabe, A. (2010). Efficacy of silver-bearing external ventricular drainage catheters: A retrospective analysis. *Journal of Neurosurgery*, *112*(4), 840–846. https://doi.org/10.3171/2009.8.JNS091297

Ge, L., Li, Q., Wang, M., Ouyang, J., Li, X., & Xing, M. M. (2014). Nanosilver particles in medical applications: Synthesis, performance, and toxicity. *International Journal of Nanomedicine*, *9*, 2399–2407. https://doi.org/10.2147/IJN.S55015

Gliga, A. R., Skoglund, S., Odnevall Wallinder, I., Fadeel, B., & Karlsson, H. L. (2014). Size-dependent cytotoxicity of silver nanoparticles in human lung cells: The role of cellular uptake, agglomeration and Ag release. *Particle and Fibre Toxicology*, *11*(1), 1–17. https://doi.org/10.1186/1743-8977-11-11

Gokulan, K., Williams, K., Orr, S., & Khare, S. (2020). Human intestinal tissue explant exposure to silver nanoparticles reveals sex dependent alterations in inflammatory responses and epithelial cell permeability. *International Journal of Molecular Sciences*, *22*(1), 9. https://doi.org/10.3390/ijms22010009

Castro-González, C.G., Sánchez-Segura, L., Gómez-Merino, F.C. *et al.* (2019). Exposure of stevia (*Stevia rebaudiana* B.) to silver nanoparticles *in vitro*: transport and accumulation. *Sci Rep 9,* 10372. https://doi.org/10.1038/s41598-019-46828-y

Gradinger C, Boisselet T, Stratev D, Ters T, Messner K, Fackler K. (2009). Biological control of sapstain fungi: From laboratory experiments to field trials 10th EWLP, Stockholm, Sweden, August 25–28, 2008. *Holzforschung*, *63*(6), 751–759. https://doi.org/10.1515/HF.2009.071

Heydrnejad, M. S., Samani, R. J., & Aghaeivanda, S. (2015). Toxic effects of silver nanoparticles on liver and some hematological parameters in male and female mice (*Mus musculus*). *Biological Trace Element Research*, *165*(2), 153–158. https://doi.org/10.1007/s12011-015-0247-1

Höfer, D. (2006). Antimicrobial textiles - evaluation of their effectiveness and safety. *Current Problems in Dermatology*, *33*, 42–50. https://doi.org/10.1159/000093935

Jara, P., Herrera, B., & Yutronic, N. (2015). Formation of nanoparticles and decoration of organic crystals. In: M. Aliofkhazraei (Ed.), *Handbook of Nanoparticles* (pp. 1–14). Springer International Publishing.

Jeelani, S., Reddy, R. C., Maheswaran, T., Asokan, G. S., Dany, A., & Anand, B. (2014). Theranostics: A treasured tailor for tomorrow. *Journal of Pharmacy & Bioallied Sciences*, *6*(Suppl 1), S6–S8. https://doi.org/10.4103/0975-7406.137249

Kawata, K., Osawa, M., & Okabe, S. (2009). In vitro toxicity of silver nanoparticles at noncytotoxic doses to HepG2 human hepatoma cells. *Environmental Science & Technology*, *43*(15), 6046–6051. https://doi.org/10.1021/es900754q

Kędziora, A., Speruda, M., Krzyżewska, E., Rybka, J., Łukowiak, A., & Bugla-Płoskońska, G. (2018). Similarities and differences between silver ions and silver in nanoforms as antibacterial agents. *International Journal of Molecular Sciences*, *19*(2), 444. https://doi.org/10.3390/ijms19020444

Khare, M. D., Bukhari, S. S., Swann, A., Spiers, P., McLaren, I., & Myers, J. (2007). Reduction of catheter-related colonisation by the use of a silver zeolite-impregnated central vascular catheter in adult critical care. *The Journal of Infection*, *54*(2), 146–150. https://doi.org/10.1016/j.jinf.2006.03.002

Korani, M., Rezayat, S. M., Gilani, K., Arbabi Bidgoli, S., & Adeli, S. (2011). Acute and subchronic dermal toxicity of nanosilver in guinea pig. *International Journal of Nanomedicine*, *6*, 855–862. https://doi.org/10.2147/IJN.S17065

Kvítek, L., Panáček, A., Soukupova, J., Kolář, M., Večeřová, R., Prucek, R., Holecova, M. & Zbořil, R. (2008). Effect of surfactants and polymers on stability and antibacterial activity of silver nanoparticles (NPs). *The Journal of Physical Chemistry C*, *112*(15), 5825–5834. https://doi.org/10.1021/jp711616v

Mahmood, K. M. (2012). The evaluation of teratogenicity of nanosilver on skeletal system and placenta of rat fetuses in prenatal period. *African Journal of Pharmacy and Pharmacology*, *6*(6), 419-424. 10.5897/AJPP11.838

Michl, T. D., Barz, J., Giles, C., Haupt, M., Henze, J. H., Mayer, J., Futrega, K., Doran, M.R., Oehr, C., Vasilev, K., Coad, B.R. & Griesser, H. J. (2018). Plasma polymerization of TEMPO yields coatings containing stable nitroxide radicals for controlling interactions with prokaryotic and eukaryotic cells. *ACS Applied Nano Materials*, *1*(12), 6587–6595. https://doi.org/10.1021/acsanm.8b01314

Mirzaei, M., Furxhi, I., Murphy, F., & Mullins, M. (2021). A machine learning tool to predict the antibacterial capacity of nanoparticles. *Nanomaterials*, 11(7), 1774. https://doi.org/10.3390/nano11071774

Monteiro, D. R., Gorup, L. F., Silva, S., Negri, M., De Camargo, E. R., Oliveira, R., Barbosa, D.B. & Henriques, M. (2011). Silver colloidal nanoparticles: Antifungal effect against adhered cells and biofilms of *Candida albicans* and *Candida glabrata. Biofouling*, *27*(7), 711–719. 10.1080/08927014.2011.599101

Monteiro, D. R., Gorup, L. F., Takamiya, A. S., de Camargo, E. R., Filho, A. C., & Barbosa, D. B. (2012). Silver distribution and release from an antimicrobial denture base resin containing silver colloidal nanoparticles. *Journal of Prosthodontics: Official Journal of the American College of Prosthodontists*, *21*(1), 7–15. https://doi.org/10.1111/j.1532-849X.2011.00772.x

Morley, K., Webb, P., Tokareva, N., Krasnov, A., Popov, V., Zhang, J., Roberts, C., & Howdle, S. (2007). Synthesis and characterisation of advanced UHMWPE/silver nanocomposites for biomedical applications. *European Polymer Journal*, *43*(2), 307–314. https://doi.org/10.1016/j.eurpolymj.2006.10.011

Neethu, S., Midhun, S. J., Radhakrishnan, E. K., & Jyothis, M. (2020). Surface functionalization of central venous catheter with mycofabricated silver nanoparticles and its antibiofilm activity on multidrug resistant *Acinetobacter baumannii. Microbial Pathogenesis*, *138*, 103832. https://doi.org/10.1016/j.micpath.2019.103832

Nguyen, K. C., Seligy, V. L., Massarsky, A., Moon, T. W., Rippstein, P., Tan, J., & Tayabali, A. F. (2013). Comparison of toxicity of uncoated and coated silver nanoparticles. *Journal of Physics: Conference Series*, *429* (1), 012025. https://doi.org/10.1088/1742-6596/429/1/012025

Ninan, N., Goswami, N., & Vasilev, K. (2020). The impact of engineered silver nanomaterials on the immune system. *Nanomaterials*, 10(5), 967. https://doi.org/10.3390/nano10050967

Ostrikov, K., N Macgregor-Ramiasa, M., A Cavallaro, A., Jacob, M., & Vasilev, K. (2016). A comparative assessment of nanoparticulate and metallic silver coated dressings. *Recent Patents on Materials Science*, *9*(1), 50–57. 10.2174/1874464809666160127230508

Pérez-Díaz, M. A., Boegli, L., James, G., Velasquillo, C., Sánchez-Sánchez, R., Martínez-Martínez, R. E., Martínez-Castañón, G. A., & Martinez-Gutierrez, F. (2015). Silver nanoparticles with antimicrobial activities against Streptococcus mutans and their cytotoxic effect. *Materials Science & Engineering. C, Materials for Biological Applications*, *55*, 360–366. https://doi.org/10.1016/j.msec.2015.05.036

Periyasamy, A. P., Venkataraman, M., Kremenakova, D., Militky, J., & Zhou, Y. (2020). Progress in sol-gel technology for the coatings of fabrics. *Materials*, 13(8), 1838. https://doi.org/10.3390/ma13081838

Ren, L., Gonzalez, R., Wang, Z., Xiang, Z., Wang, Y., Zhou, H., Li, J., Xiao, Y., Yang, Q., Zhang, J., Chen, L., Wang, W., Li, Y., Li, T., Meng, X., Zhang, Y., Vernet, G., Paranhos-Baccalà, G., Chen, J., Jin, Q., & Wang, J. (2009). Prevalence of human respiratory viruses in adults with acute respiratory tract infections in Beijing, 2005–2007, *Clinical Microbiology and Infection. 15*(12) 1146–1153. ISSN 1198-743X, https://doi.org/10.1111/j.1469-0691.2009.02746.x

Shrivastava, S., Bera, T., Roy, A., Singh, G., Ramachandrarao, P., & Dash, D. (2007). Characterization of enhanced antibacterial effects of novel silver nanoparticles. *Nanotechnology*, *18*(22), 225103. 10.1088/0957-4484/18/22/225103

Siddiqi, K. S., Husen, A., & Rao, R. A. K. (2018). A review on biosynthesis of silver nanoparticles and their biocidal properties. *Journal of Nanobiotechnology*, *16*(1), 14. https://doi.org/10.1186/s12951-018-0334-5

Silva, L. P., Silveira, A. P., Bonatto, C. C., Reis, I. G., & Milreu, P. V. (2017). Silver nanoparticles as antimicrobial agents: Past, present, and future. In: *Nanostructures for Antimicrobial Therapy* (pp. 577–596). https://doi.org/10.1016/B978-0-323-46152-8.00026-3

Sintubin, L., De Windt, W., Dick, J., Mast, J., van der Ha, D., Verstraete, W., & Boon, N. (2009). Lactic acid bacteria as reducing and capping agent for the fast and efficient production of silver nanoparticles. *Applied Microbiology and Biotechnology*, *84*(4), 741–749. https://doi.org/10.1007/s00253-009-2032-6

Suthar, J. K., Vaidya, A., & Ravindran, S. (2023). Toxic implications of silver nanoparticles on the central nervous system: A systematic literature review. *Journal of Applied Toxicology: JAT*, *43*(1), 4–21. https://doi.org/10.1002/jat.4317

Thomas, R., Soumya, K. R., Mathew, J., & Radhakrishnan, E. K. (2015). Inhibitory effect of silver nanoparticle fabricated urinary catheter on colonization efficiency of Coagulase Negative Staphylococci. *Journal of Photochemistry and Photobiology B, Biology*, *149*, 68–77. https://doi.org/10.1016/j.jphotobiol.2015.04.034

Tiwari, R., Singh, R. D., Khan, H., Gangopadhyay, S., Mittal, S., Singh, V., Arjaria, N., Shankar, J., Roy, S. K., Singh, D., & Srivastava, V. (2017). Oral subchronic exposure to silver nanoparticles causes renal damage through apoptotic impairment and necrotic cell death. *Nanotoxicology*, *11*(5), 671–686. https://doi.org/10.1080/17435390.2017.1343874

Tran, Q. H., & Le, A. T. (2013). Silver nanoparticles: Synthesis, properties, toxicology, applications and perspectives. *Advances in Natural Sciences: Nanoscience and Nanotechnology*, *4*(3), 033001. 10.1088/2043-6262/4/3/033001

Travan, A., Pelillo, C., Donati, I., Marsich, E., Benincasa, M., Scarpa, T., Semeraro, S., Turco, G., Gennaro, R., & Paoletti, S. (2009). Non-cytotoxic silver nanoparticle-polysaccharide nanocomposites with antimicrobial activity. *Biomacromolecules*, *10*(6), 1429–1435. https://doi.org/10.1021/bm900039x

Venugopal, A., Muthuchamy, N., Tejani, H., Gopalan, A. I., Lee, K. P., Lee, H. J., & Kyung, H. M. (2017). Incorporation of silver nanoparticles on the surface of orthodontic microimplants to achieve antimicrobial properties. *Korean Journal of Orthodontics*, *47*(1), 3–10. https://doi.org/10.4041/kjod.2017.47.1.3

Verdú Soriano, J., Rueda López, J., Martínez Cuervo, F., & Soldevilla Agreda, J. (2004). Effects of an activated charcoal silver dressing on chronic wounds with no clinical signs of infection. *Journal of Wound Care*, *13*(10), 419–423. https://doi.org/10.12968/jowc.2004.13.10.26685

Wei, L., Lu, J., Xu, H., Patel, A., Chen, Z. S., & Chen, G. (2015). Silver nanoparticles: Synthesis, properties, and therapeutic applications. *Drug Discovery Today*, *20*(5), 595–601. https://doi.org/10.1016/j.drudis.2014.11.014

Yaqoob, A. A., Ahmad, H., Parveen, T., Ahmad, A., Oves, M., Ismail, I. M. I., Qari, H. A., Umar, K., & Mohamad Ibrahim, M. N. (2020a). Recent advances in metal decorated nanomaterials and their various biological applications: A review. *Frontiers in Chemistry*, *8*, 341. https://doi.org/10.3389/fchem.2020.00341

Yaqoob, A. A., Umar, K., & Ibrahim, M. N. M. (2020b). Silver nanoparticles: Various methods of synthesis, size affecting factors and their potential applications–a review. *Applied Nanoscience*, *10*(5), 1369–1378. https://doi.org/10.1007/s13204-020-01318-w

Zhao, Y., Xing, Q., Janjanam, J., He, K., Long, F., Low, K. B., Tiwari, A., Zhao, F., Shahbazian-Yassar, R., Friedrich, C., & Shokuhfar, T. (2014). Facile electrochemical synthesis of antimicrobial TiO_2 nanotube arrays. *International Journal of Nanomedicine*, *9*, 5177–5187. https://doi.org/10.2147/IJN.S65386

8 Application of Nanocomposites for Wound Healing

Aparajita Pal and Narayan Chandra Das

8.1 INTRODUCTION

Nanocomposites especially nanostructure-impregnated therapeutics have a wide application in the field of wound healing. The recent advancement in nanotechnology offers great potential for providing effective wound care solutions. Nanomaterials in a composite basically act as a carrier material to dispose of the pharmaceutically active compound at the designated wound site. Silver (Ag) is the most popular metal in this aspect and is used as an age-old remedy in wound healing applications due to its inherent antimicrobial properties. Now, different Ag-based topical medicines are commercially available to cure various pathological infections at open wound sites. It is reported that nanoscale Ag-based composites are more suitable than its macroscale alternative or bulk silver metal in topical cream applications due to their unique chemical and physical characteristics. Particularly, the nanoscale additives provide higher surface areas. Hence, the microorganisms at the wound sites get exposed to a larger surface area of the therapeutic compound, leading to a more effective and rapid wound healing performance. Furthermore, biomaterials for example protein, collagen, alginate, chitosan, silk, gelatin, starch, polysaccharides, cellulose, etc. are abundantly available in nature and they are safe to apply to various pharmaceutical requirements. The current research dimension is strongly focused on these kinds of biopolymers in combination with nanomaterials like silver nanoparticles (AgNPs) as an effective wound dressing material due to their synergistic effect.

8.2 CONVENTIONAL WOUND HEALING PROCESS AND THE NEED FOR A WOUND HEALING MATERIAL

Skin is the largest external body organ which provides security and protection from injuries and any kind of microbial proliferation toward the internal body parts. Wounds can be classified into two broad categories—acute and chronic wounds. Any kind of trauma and physical shock can cause harm to the skin tissue resulting in an acute wound. However, skin has excellent inherent regenerative properties or self-healing tendencies. The conventional healing process is dynamic and it includes a series of constructive phenomena hemostasis, inflammation, proliferation, and extracellular matrix (ECM) remodeling [1].

DOI: 10.1201/9781003432661-8

The main challenge with the natural process is poor resistance to external pathogen attack on the open surface or pus formation. This drives the need for a wound dressing material that serves as a temporary layer to protect the affected area on the skin surface. An efficient wound dressing material encourages as well as accelerates different stages of the wound healing process.

8.3 VARIOUS REQUIREMENTS FOR A COMPOSITE WOUND HEALING MATERIAL

The primary requirements of a nanocomposite wound healing material are as follows—biocompatibility, hemostatic and adhesive properties, antimicrobial efficiency, antioxidant properties, air and moisture permeability, anti-inflammatory properties, stimuli-responsiveness, electrical conductivity, and self-healing properties.

8.3.1 Biocompatibility

Biocompatibility is a crucial factor in determining the property of a wound dressing material as it directly comes in contact with the damaged tissue, blood, and the open wound area [2]. The biocompatibility of a material depends on its composition, structure, surface property, chemical nature, stability, and mechanical characteristics. An incompatible material can cause complications like inflammation, hypergenesis, thrombosis, or buildup of calcium in the surrounding soft tissues. Biocompatibility with the human body can be evaluated based on three broad categories—histocompatibility or sustenance with the tissue, hemocompatibility or interactions with the blood, and cytocompatibility or cell communication.

8.3.2 Hemostatic and Adhesive Property

Hemostasis is the first step in wound healing. The ruptured blood vessels at the injury site cause severe bleeding which can be controlled by coagulation of the blood at the affected site. This process is called hemostasis [3]. During the occurrence of an open injury, the platelets aggregate at the affected area and encourage different stages of hemostasis—vasoconstriction to mitigate blood loss and adhesion to nearby platelets to build a positive feedback network which accelerates the rate of hemostasis. The hemostatic property in wound dressing materials can be achieved not only by chemical sealing but also by absorption of the exudates.

8.3.3 Antimicrobial Efficiency

Microbial or various pathogenic infections at the open wound site are very common and can result in inflammation leading to delay in the wound healing process. Hence, a primary factor in determining the efficiency of a wound healing material is its antimicrobial properties [4]. Wound healing materials infused with nanomaterials like Ag, Au, Zn, Cu, etc., and different polymeric materials like chitosan and polyimide, all having inherent antimicrobial nature, show better results in this aspect.

8.3.4 Anti-Inflammatory and Antioxidant Properties

The second important factor in wound healing is inflammation. The bacteria and other harmful pathogens can be killed by the inflammatory cells. However, inflammation at the wound site can lead to an increase in accumulation of the reactive oxygen species (ROS) which further results in damage to the skin tissue [5]. Generally, low levels of ROS are preferred for rapid wound healing. The antioxidant property of the wound dressing material can help in consuming the accumulated ROS, leading to positive progress in the wound healing mechanism. The natural antioxidants are mercaptan, enzymes, vitamins, etc.

8.3.5 Air and Moisture Permeability

The progress of the wound healing process happens more rapidly in moist environments. However, wound dressing material like cotton gauze provides a contrary dry environment. It is also unable to prevent moisture evaporation from the injured area. Dead cells are formed due to dehydration in the affected area. Hence, wound dressing material should be efficient enough to maintain a wet environment that can resist scarring of the tissues [6].

Furthermore, air permeability is another important factor to consider while designing a wound dressing material. Exposure to oxygen can help skin tissue regeneration. Oxygen reacts with different cytokines, performs cell proliferation, and encourages the synthesis of collagen. Additionally, gas exchange performance helps in mimicking the physiological environment of the wound.

8.3.6 Stimuli-Responsiveness

Stimuli-responsive, for example, response to different stimuli like light, pH, and temperature also plays a very important role in designing smart wound dressing materials [7]. There are different nanomaterials that show a photothermal effect in which the generation of heat can prevent different bacterial infections.

8.3.7 Electrical Conductivity

Skin is electrically conductive. Hence, using an electrically conductive wound healing material enhances the function and communication between the cells. Cell functions like differentiation and proliferation are more active in an electrically active environment. Different electrically conductive nanomaterials, for example, graphene, carbon nano tube (CNT), nanoclay, different metallic nanoparticles, and conductive polymers are used to optimize the electrical conductivity in the wound dressing material [8].

8.3.8 Self-Healing Property

Self-healing nature helps in resisting any kind of structural or functional failure of the wound dressing material under tension, shear, or compression force at the wound site. It provides assurance of maintaining structural integrity under different mechanical stresses and hence protects the wound from any kind of physically harmful environmental conditions [9].

8.4 FABRICATION METHODOLOGIES FOR NANOCOMPOSITE-BASED WOUND HEALING MATERIALS

Wound dressing materials can be fabricated using different methods—electrospinning, film casting, the dry-jet-wet spinning technique, freeze-thawing, ionic crosslinking followed by freeze drying, deposition and precipitation method, etc. [10]. The current market availability of wound healing materials is generally found in the form of hydrogel, film, foam, scaffold, sponge, or nanofibrous mat.

8.4.1 Hydrogel-Based Nanocomposite Wound Healing Material

Hydrogel is a crosslinked polymer network. It can also be referred to as macromolecular polymer gel. Diabetic wounds fail in blood vessel formation and often result in poor cell proliferation and migration near the wound area, delaying the process of healing. To combat this issue a novel reduced graphene oxide (rGO) infused hydrogel-based wound healing process is reported in one study [11]. Gelatin, a biopolymer, light yellow transparent or translucent powder, is used here. It is produced from the partial hydrolysis of collagen. Gelatin dissolves in polar solvents like acetic acid, hot water, or glycerol. It is superabsorbent in nature and can absorb water up to 5–10 times its own weight, resulting in gel formation. The hydrogel formed can be melted at high temperatures. Furthermore, the gel is thixotropic in nature, and viscosity decreases with increasing stress [12]. Gelatin, however, can be majorly obtained by two distinct procedures. The acid-treated raw material gives 'type A gelatin' and the alkali-treated raw material gives 'type B gelatin'. In this study 'type A gelatin' is procured. The hydrogel is formed by crosslinking gelatin with methacrylic anhydride (MAA) under UV irradiation. A photo initiator is used to initiate the curing process. The hydrogel is called gelatin- methacryloyl hydrogel (GelMA). The physicochemical properties of GelMA can be modified by altering the concentration of the prepolymer, degree of methacrylation, time, and temperature maintained during the polymerization process.

As described in Figure 8.1a [13] the gelatin is first dissolved in a phosphate buffer saline (PBS) in a warm condition to prepare a homogeneous solution. A higher temperature greater than 60°C can lead to the backbone degradation of gelatin. MAA is added to the solution at a specific rate of 0.5 mL/min for 1 hour under vigorous stirring at 55°C. The stirring rate has a great role to play as stable MAA dispersion in gelatin solution can enhance the reaction interface between gelatin and MAA. The solution at the end of the reaction is kept under dialysis against deionized water (DI) for 1 week. The dialysis time can be substantially reduced using the tangential flow filtration process. Finally, a foam-like prepolymer is obtained as a result of freeze drying. To prepare the rGO-incorporated GelMA hydrogel, rGO is homogeneously dispersed in N-methyl-3-pyrrolidone (NMP) solvent at different concentrations using ultrasonication. Then freeze-dried prepolymer foam with an adequate amount of photo initiator is added into the system, followed by exposure to UV irradiation for

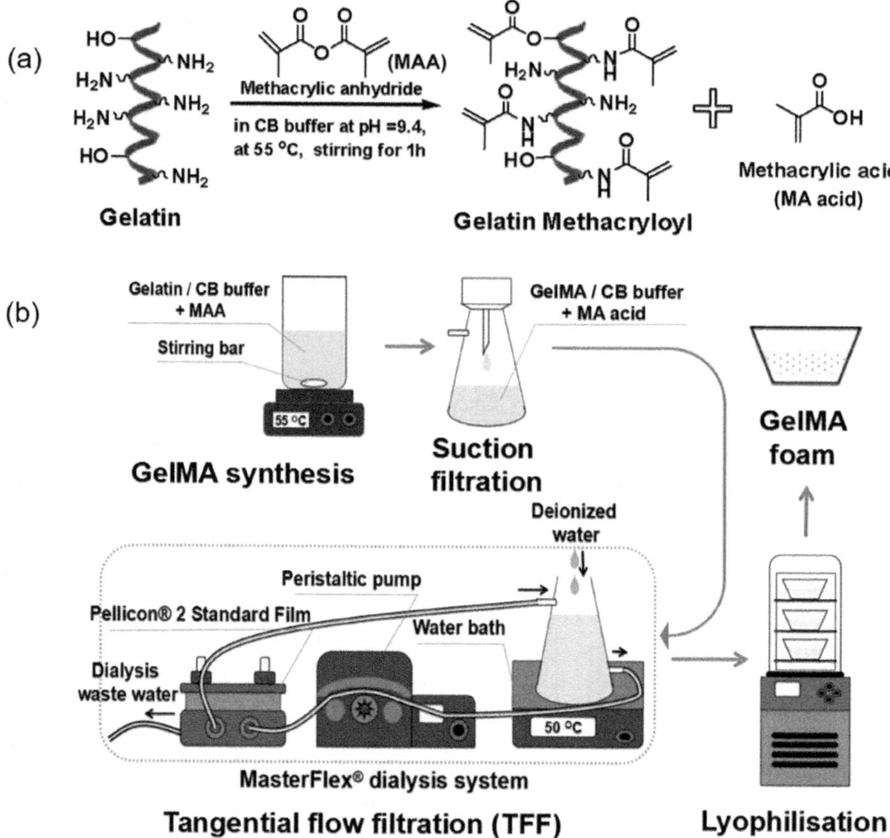

FIGURE 8.1 (a) Reaction mechanism between biopolymer gelatin and MAA, (b) Schematic representation of fabrication of GelMA foam prepolymer. (Adapted with permission from Ref. [13]. Copyright 2019, Springer Nature.)

10 seconds to perform crosslinking. The hydrogel is proven to help in cell proliferation due to the presence of responsive peptide motifs. The hydrogel closely resembles the functions of a natural ECM.

The scanning electron microscope (SEM) micrographs exhibit a porous structure of the hydrogel with a pore dimension of approximately 50 μm. The porous nature of the hydrogel helps in cell migration and proliferation. The embedded rGO particle size is further observed under a transmission electron microscope (TEM). The degradation study shows, that, unlike pristine gelatin, GelMA hydrogel can sustain up to 28 days with a stable three-dimensional (3D) crosslinked porous structure. The addition of rGO further mitigates the degradation rate. To analyze the exudate uptake property, the swelling ability of the nanocomposite hydrogel is further investigated. The superior water intake property of the hydrogel makes it a potential candidate in wound dressing applications as it is able to maintain a moist environment at the wound site and thus helps in cell growth. The sustained and prolonged release of rGO from the polymer matrix further helps in stimulating cell growth, leading to the formation of new blood vessels.

Hydrogels show great potential in the application of burn wound healing as it is able to absorb the wound exudates and hydrate the affected area. In this study, a self-healable hydrogel based on chitosan and cellulose nanocrystal (CNC) is fabricated [14]. Chitosan is a naturally occurring polysaccharide, extracted from shrimp or crab shells. However, it is not soluble in water. Hence, a derivative of chitosan, carboxymethyl chitosan (CMC) is synthesized which exhibits good moisture retention properties. The degree of carboxymethyl substitution is detected as 0.31 from ^{1}H NMR (proton nuclear magnetic resonance spectroscopy). CNC demonstrates a high mechanical property and large specific surface area. It is employed as a reinforcing filler in the hydrogel matrix. CNC is functionalized with aldehyde moiety which can form chemical crosslinks with the abundantly available amine groups on the polymer surface, resulting in a better reinforcing effect. These crosslinks are called Schiff-base linkages [15] which are reversible and dynamic in nature, can be broken, and reformed rapidly. The aldehyde-functionalized CNC (DACNC) is obtained by periodate oxidation. The morphology of the hydrogel is investigated under a field emission scanning electron microscope (FESEM) as referred to in Figure 8.2. The FESEM micrographs reveal a honeycomb-like microporous structure of the nanocomposite hydrogel material. The pore dimension is between 50 and 300 nm. The FESEM study also confirms the formation of nanonets inside the nanopores. In Figure 8.2d the protruding rod-like structure is identified as DACNC in the hydrogel matrix. Further, the in

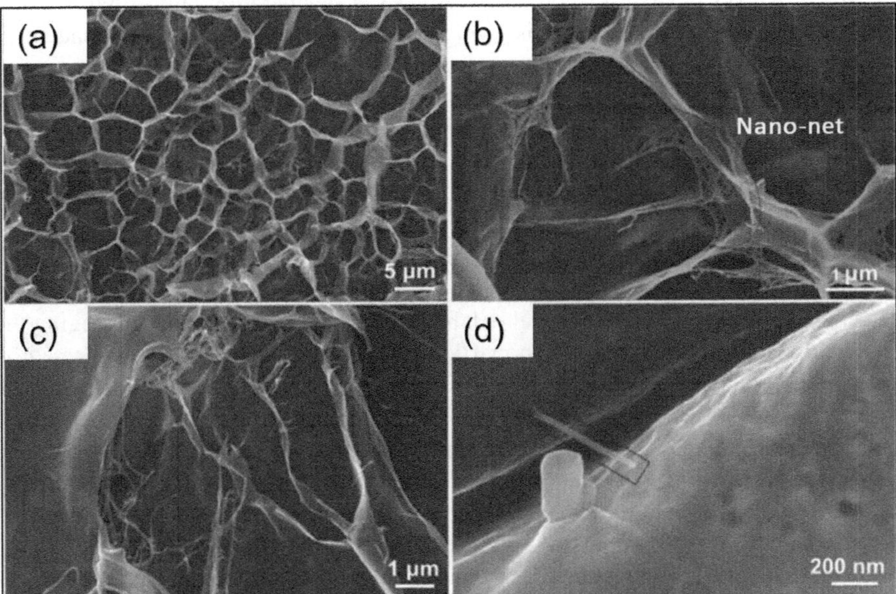

FIGURE 8.2 FESEM micrographs of the cross-sectional morphology of composite hydrogels with different magnifications (a) honeycomb porous structure, (b) and (c) nanonet formation, (d) protruding DACNC from the polymer matrix. (Adapted with permission from Ref. [14]. Copyright 2018, American Chemical Society.)

vitro anti-toxicity of the fabricated nanocomposite hydrogel is assessed by the 3-(4, 5-dimethylthiazolyl-2)-2, 5-diphenyltetrazolium bromide (MTT) method [16]. It is an important evaluation for wound healing applications.

The degree of carboxymethyl substitution in chitosan, the degree of aldehyde functionalization of CNC, and the amine to aldehyde molar ratio are the three important parameters in determining the viscoelastic responses of the CMC/DACNC composite hydrogel material. The increasing degree of substitution of the aldehyde group leads to a higher storage modulus for hydrogel. This confirms the formation of a more compact network structure to sustain the increasing stress. The strength of the hydrogel is increased up to an amine to aldehyde molar ratio of 0.33. However, increasing the concentration of DACNC can cause aggregation due to the poor dispersibility in the polymer matrix. The crosslinking density of the hydrogel is affected due to the decrease in active junction points.

Gelation time is another crucial factor in designing hydrogel-based wound healing materials. A slow gelation process leads to uneven distribution of the components whereas rapid gelation can cause insufficient handling time.

In another study, nanogel incorporated hyaluronic acid (HA) and methoxy polyethylene glycol (m-PEG) based hybrid hydrogel is investigated as a wound healing material with sustained release and hemostatic properties [17]. Hydrogels promote rapid hemostasis due to the formation of a hemostatic plug and provide a physical barrier to the bleeding site.

HA, an anionic polysaccharide in nature, is one of the major components of an ECM. It displays positive responses toward tissue regeneration, anti-inflammation, and angiogenesis [18]. Hence, it is used as a potential candidate for wound healing applications. Chlorhexidine diacetate (CHX), known as a topical disinfectant, is used as the active material [19]. The performance of the synthesized functionalized HA and methacrylated m-PEG based composite hydrogel incorporated with a CHX preloaded nanogel has been investigated by evaluating the swelling ratio, in vitro release of active material, cytotoxicity, blood clotting index, antibacterial efficacy, drug release kinetics, and mechanical properties.

Excessive ROS is the main reason behind the delay in the wound healing process as it causes bacterial infection and ulcers at the wound sites. To combat the issue, a thermoresponsive hydrogel material is fabricated which is capable of scavenging the ROS [20]. Cerium oxide based nanoparticles Nano-CeO_2 is uniformly dispersed on the surface of meso porous silica (MSN). The poly(N-isopropylacrylamide) hydrogel is crosslinked by surface-modified MSN. The rheological study confirms that encapsulation of nano-CeO_2 into the polymer matrix has a key influence on the crosslinking density of the hydrogel material. The novel nanocomposite hydrogel can dynamically undergo gelation from a liquid state as the temperature is close to body temperature. It facilitates the reduction of oxidative stress levels at the trauma site.

Wu et al. [21] have developed 3D-printed polyacrylamide- hydroxypropyl methylcellulose-based hydrogel wound dressings. Silver-ethylene interaction plays a vital role in the formation of crosslinks between AgNPs and the hydrogel matrix. The super porous organometallic compound also controls the optimum release of AgNPs so that a balance is maintained between cytocompatibility and the antibacterial property of the fabricated nanocomposite dressing.

Zhang et al., in their work, have encapsulated ellagic acid (EA) in thiol-functionalized β-cyclodextrin (SH-β-CD) [22]. EA is a natural polyphenol that acts as an antioxidant. It can efficiently scavenge the ROS. However, it contains two aromatic rings which limit its water solubility property, resulting in low bioavailability. In this work, an inclusion complex is formed by encapsulating EA in the cavity of SH-β-CD to achieve better water solubility. Thiol-ene photo click chemistry is used to fabricate the polyethylene glycol (PEG) hydrogel loaded with EA. SH-β-CD acts as a crosslinker to bind EA into the hydrogel matrix. The crosslinking of the hydrogel is performed under UV light in the presence of a photo initiator. Furthermore, thiol-ene click chemistry is very efficient due to its rapid reaction kinetics and ability to trigger in situ gelation at certain stimuli. This phenomenon marks its very significance in the field of local sustained release of therapeutic drugs at wound sites.

8.4.2 Electrospun Nanofibrous Mat-Based Wound Healing Material

A multifunctional wound healing material is developed with both wound healing and scar inhibition efficiency [23]. A chitosan-based inner membrane helps in blood coagulation. The outer layer of the nanofiber is composed of a poly-caprolactone/quaternized PDMS composite membrane, used in the outer layer, which resists any kind of bacterial invasion. Polydimethylsiloxane (PDMS) is widely employed in the field of biomedical engineering due to it being compatible with the skin, non-toxic, chemically inert, hydrophobic, and flexible in nature. Quaternized silicone is produced by the treatment of PDMS with quaternary ammonium salts.

Antibacterial functionalization of the nanofibers is achieved by co-spinning the polymer with antibiotic or antibacterial substrates. Due to the high surface area, nanofibers possess excellent loading capacity for biological matters as well as inorganic nanoparticles like Ag, TiO_2, SiO_2, nanoclay, etc. A hemostatic nanoclay-organic-self-supported membrane is developed where the nanoclay particles are embedded into a polyvinylpyrrolidone (PVP) matrix [24]. The membrane is produced using the electrospinning technique, composed of a robust fluffy framework and a hydrophilic surface. The pure pristine polymer electrospun membrane undergoes shrinkage at high temperatures, impeding the process of hemostasis. In this study, a nanocomposite membrane is proposed which is anti-shrinking in nature at high temperatures. The well-dispersed and partially exposed nanoclay (kaolinite, halloysite) particles provide functional sites for hemostasis and improve the hydrophilic property of the nanocomposite material. It is further proved by observing the contact angle which is reduced from 100° to 62°. The SEM, TEM, and energy dispersive spectroscopy (EDS) are further performed to evaluate the dispersion of the nanoclay particles and the inner structural characteristics. With increasing nanoclay ratio (concentration) the encapsulating polymer layer becomes thinner leading to poor adhesion. This can lead to the formation of a thrombus due to the exfoliation of the nanoparticles. Additionally, the zeta potential values of the nanomembrane show a positive growth after the incorporation of PVP, indicating the formation of an electrostatic interaction between the polymer and the nanoclay particles. The hemostasis property is assessed by in vitro blood coagulation test and blood absorption capacity. The as-synthesized nanocomposite facilitates both phenomena—blood permeation and coagulation.

Furthermore, the emergency hemostasis performance of the electrospun nanocomposite mat is investigated using the in vivo rat tail amputation model. The bleeding time abruptly decreases while using a nanoclay fiber mat compared to a pristine polymer fiber mat.

In another study, epidermal growth factor (EGF) encapsulated nanoscale silk fiber is produced using the electrospinning technique [25]. EGF, a protein consisting of 53 amino acid residues, stimulates the proliferation and migration of the keratinocytes which is mainly responsible for restoring the epidermal layer after any kind of injury occurs. EGF is normally used in diabetic foot ulcer treatment [26]. The electrospun mats are treated with methanol to achieve a water-insoluble composite silk mat. The average thickness of the composite fibrous mat is measured as 300 μm. Variation in the thickness of the mat is observed each time due to fluctuations in voltage and humidity of the environment. The as-prepared samples are kept at 4°C for less than one week and sterilized using 70% ethanol before using it directly on the wound sites. To evaluate the stability of the EGF, the immunoreactivity is determined using an enzyme-linked immunosorbent assay (ELISA) [27]. A release profile of EGF from the silk fibrous mat is obtained. The average amount of EGF released at 37°C is considered the maximum amount of EGF release ability of a 1.5 cm electrospun composite mat. When the composite silk fiber mat is placed on top of the wound area, a burst in the release profile is detected on the first day, followed by a stable increase in profile over the course of a week. After one week of contact, the release % for EGF obtained is approximately 25%. When the sterilized dressing material is put on the wound, the fibers in direct contact are surrounded by the wet medium of the wound (exudates), which causes easy diffusion of the EGF protein material through the silk fiber walls.

The swelling capacity was observed by placing the fibrous mat in PBS solution at 37°C and directly on the wound site. A significant difference in fiber diameter is observed in both cases compared to the sample before soaking as depicted in Figure 8.3. According to the swelling capacity study, after being in contact for 72 hours with the wound site, 34.9% swelling is obtained in the electrospun composite fiber mat.

El-Assar et al. have investigated the polyvinyl alcohol (PVA)/ Pluronic F127/ polyethyleneimine (PEI) blended nanofiber composites embedded with different concentrations of TiO_2 NPs in terms of their antibacterial efficacy [28]. PVA is water soluble, easily processable, and environmentally stable. It is non-toxic in nature, biocompatible, and possesses good mechanical properties. However, the main drawback of PVA is its high degree of swelling in aqueous media. Hence, composite blends of PVA are explored further. Pluronic F127 is the trade name of poloxamers which are triblock copolymers composed of a central hydrophobic unit of poly(propylene oxide) (PPO) attached to two hydrophilic side chains of poly(ethylene oxide) (PEO),i.e., PEO-PPO-PEO [29]. Due to the amphiphilic structure, they are commercially used as surfactants, emulsifying agents, coating or thickening agents, etc. Besides, the hydrophilicity of the PEO segment makes them potential candidates in the field of biomedical engineering. The third component of the composite nanofiber, PEI, is a branched or linear or branched polyamine, used

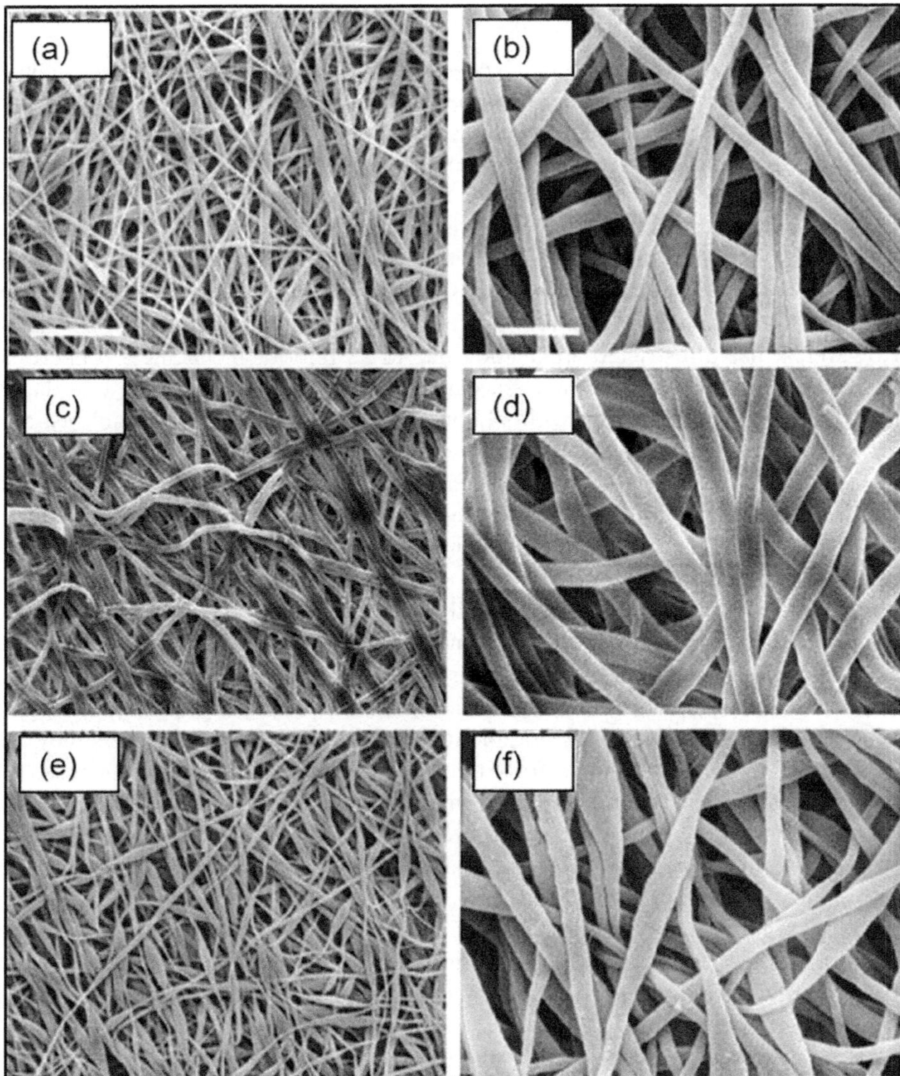

FIGURE 8.3 SEM micrographs of the electrospun composite silk fibre mat (a), (c), (e) before swelling, (b) and (d) after soaking in PBS for 72h, I and (f) after 72h exposure to the wound site, (a), (c), I at 20μm bar and (b), (d), (f) at 5μm bar. Adapted with permission from ref. [25]. Copyright 2009, Elsevier.

as a marker in immunology. The active material, TiO_2 NPs is synthesized using the sol-gel method using titanium (IV) isopropoxide as a precursor. TiO_2 NPs are widely used in food, cosmetics, and pharmaceutical additives. TiO_2 NPs based filters exhibit strong germicidal properties. The PVA-Pluronic-PEI/ TiO_2 NP composite nanofibrous mat shows great potential in terms of topical antibacterial efficiency in wound care applications.

8.4.3 Sponge-Based Nanocomposite Wound Healing Material

Ge et al. [30] have fabricated a collagen—AgNP nanocomposite sponge as an antibacterial wound dressing material. Collagen is the main structural protein in the connective tissues— ligaments, tendons, cartilage, skin, etc. [31]. It consists of amino acids arranged in a triple-helix manner. The toughness of the collagen tissues depends on the degree of mineralization. Bone is an example of rigid collagen tissue whereas tendon is a compliant collagen tissue. Collagen is extensively accepted as a main component in producing artificial skin which is used to secure burns, ulcers, or fatal wounds [32]. Collagen-rich substances help in rapid wound closure. It is able to form granulation tissue very quickly when applied to severely burned areas. However, it has a restricted application due to its inferior mechanical properties, low thermal stability, poor water resistance, and rapid biodegradability. Collagen is often used in combination with silicones, glycosaminoglycans, fibroblasts, and growth factors.

Ge et al. have mainly focused on fabricating a hybrid nanoparticle-organic compound where AgNPs are homogeneously dispersed into the collagen matrix so that the antibacterial and mechanical properties can be simultaneously improved. AgNPs are known for their robust antibacterial efficiency against different microorganisms [33]. Additionally, in the current medicine practice, they are applied against multi-drug resistant organisms. To synthesize AgNPs, the common reducing agents used are hydrazine [34], sodium borohydride [35,36], surfactants, and N, N-dimethylformamide. However, using these toxic and harmful chemical substances is not suitable for biodegradable applications as they are difficult to completely remove from the system. Tollens' reaction is suitable for producing low-toxic AgNPs but the formation of Tollens agent $[Ag(NH_3)_2]^+$possesses biological risks. As a substitute, nature-derived reducing agents such as glucose, histidine, dopamine, polysaccharides, ascorbic acid, etc. are used. Surfactant PVP is employed, otherwise, the as-synthesized nanoparticles tend to form aggregation. However, polysaccharides are beneficial to apply as they can simultaneously synthesize and stabilize the AgNPs. Furthermore, dialdehyde-functionalized xanthan gum (DXG) acts as an effective crosslinking agent for the collagen matrix.

A collagen sponge is obtained by the freeze-drying of a collagen type-I solution (0.5% w/w) [30]. The collagen sponge is directly soaked in the DXG-AgNP solution, referred to as Col-Ag2 and when soaked in a two-fold diluted DXG-AgNP solution it is called Col-Ag1. Col-Ag2 and Col-Ag1 have a silver content of nearly 6.57 and 3.31 mg/g respectively. The obtained dressing material is washed with deionized water and freeze-dried before being practically used. For evaluating the antibacterial activity of the fabricated wound dressing material, different techniques like the 'inhibition zone method', 'bacterial infiltration', etc. have been performed. SEM study shows superior performance of the Col-Ag2 sample compared with pristine collagen (Col) and Col-Ag1 (Figure 8.4). In vitro blood compatibility is assessed using the bovine serum albumin adsorption method, whole blood dynamic clotting study, and in vitro cytotoxicity study.

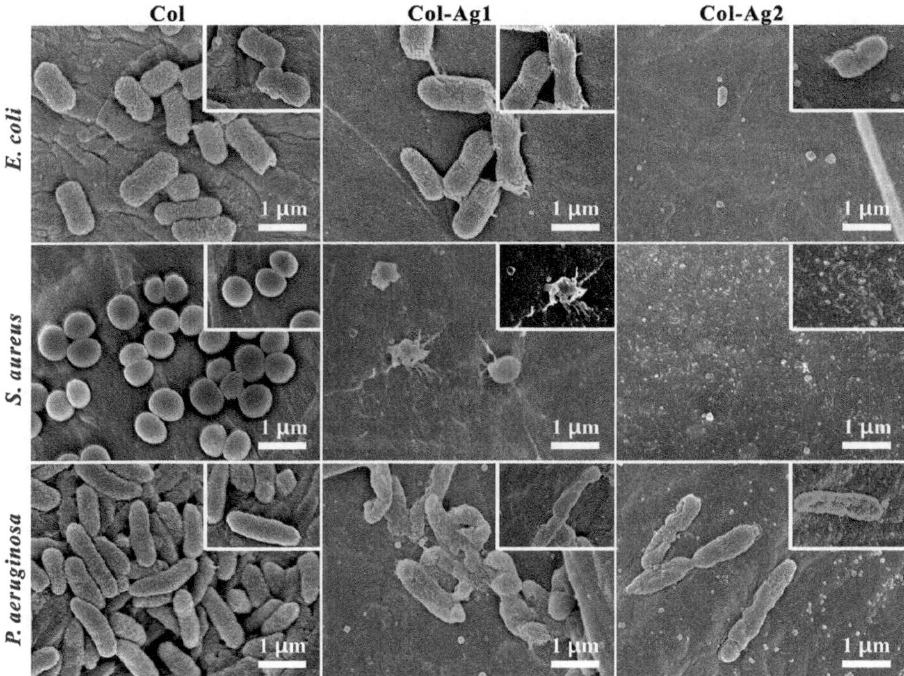

FIGURE 8.4 SEM micrograph of growth of *E. coli*, *S. aureus*, *P. aeruginosa* on pristine collagen sponge and collagen-AgNP composites (Col-Ag1 and Col-Ag2) sponges after exposure for 24 hours at 37°C. (Adapted with permission from Ref. [30]. Copyright 2018, American Chemical Society.)

8.4.4 Scaffold-Based Nanocomposite Wound Healing Material

Liu et al. [37], have described scaffold-based nanocomposite wound dressing materials based on bacterial cellulose (BC). Besides plants, cellulose can also be formed using green algae, fungi, etc. Typical examples of cellulose-producing bacteria are Gram-negative and Gram-positive bacteria, *azotobacter*, *salmonella*, and *pseudomonas*. They synthesize cellulose as extracellular polysaccharides which help in protecting their inner cells. BC possesses the same molecular formula as plant cellulose, but its macromolecular properties are very different. BC is vastly used in the field of biomedical engineering due to its non-toxic nature, high level of purity, biocompatibility, high water intake capacity, mechanical property, and moldability [38].

The high level of purity in BC is obtained due to the absence of any lignin or hemicellulose content. A high degree of polymerization, % crystallinity, and presence of ribbon-like microfibrils results in better mechanical properties. The nanofibrillar structure creates a large surface area which further causes a superior water intake capacity. The nanofibrils are 100 mm in length and 100 nm in width. BC pellicles having 99% water content display a tensile strength of 0.9 MPa and with decreasing water content level the tensile strength value increases. At a 40% BC content level,

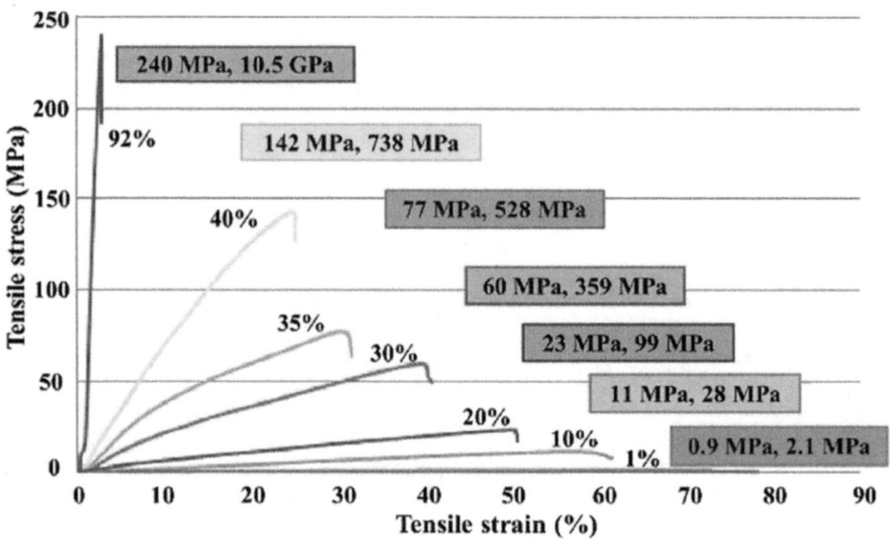

FIGURE 8.5 Stress-strain plot of BC pellicles at various BC content levels with corresponding tensile strength and modulus value. (Adapted with permission from Ref. [37]. Copyright 2020, American Chemical Society.)

the tensile strength of BC exhibits a value as high as 142 MPa as depicted from the stress-strain graph in Figure 8.5.

Janpetch et al. have designed a BC/ZnO nanostructure-based composite hydrogel scaffold for antimicrobial application [39]. ZnO is biocompatible and possesses excellent thermal and mechanical stability. ZnO facilitates angiogenesis and promotes re-epithelialization of wounds. The ZnO nanostructure is synthesized using the solution plasma process (SPP) where atmospheric equilibrium plasma is discharged in a liquid phase at room temperature [40]. The nanoporous structure of the 3D BC scaffold serves as an excellent supporting material for ZnO coordination.

The BC pellicles are saturated with methanol for 3 days, followed by treatment with different concentrations of Zn^{2+} solution – 0.5, 1.00, 5.00, 10.00, and 20.00 w/v % in methanol. Zinc nitrate and zinc acetate are used as precursors to produce a Zn^{2+} saturated BC scaffold. The plasma treatment is carried out after placing each sample for 1 hour in a solution plasma glass reactor, followed by sonication to remove the unbound ZnO. Finally the samples are obtained after freeze-drying as $0.50Zn(NO_3)$/SPP/BC, $1.00Zn(NO_3)$/SPP/BC, $5.00Zn(NO_3)$/SPP/BC, $10.00Zn(NO_3)$/SPP/BC, 10.00ZnAct/SPP/BC, $20.00Zn(NO_3)$/SPP/BC. Figure 8.6 shows the FESEM micrographs of the BC nanofiber network and the ZnO nanostructure deposited BC scaffold.

The disc diffusion method [41] is carried out to determine the antibacterial efficiency of the as-synthesized samples. Two Petri dishes are filled with solid agar and Luria broth. The freeze-dried BC/ZnO nanocomposite samples are cut in a circular fashion maintaining a diameter of 0.5 cm, followed by autoclaving for 20 minutes to sterilize. Two bacteria cultures are taken, Gram-positive- *S. aureus* and

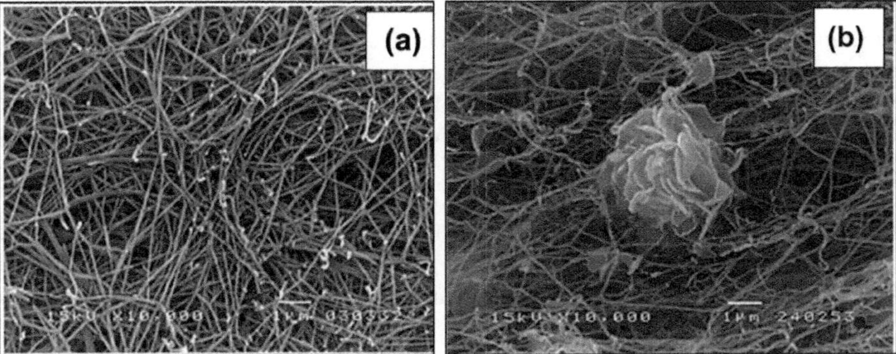

FIGURE 8.6 FESEM micrograph of (a) nanofibrils in pristine BC scaffold (b) ZnO modified BC scaffold. (Adapted with permission from Ref. [39]. Copyright 2016, Elsevier.)

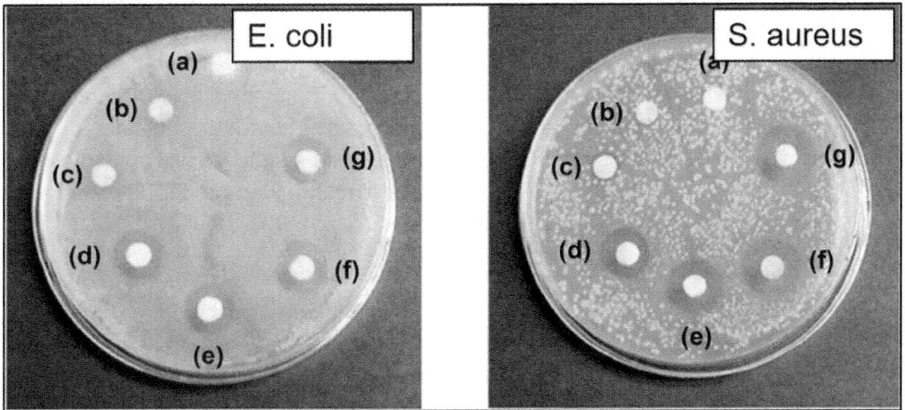

FIGURE 8.7 Zone of inhibition for bacterial growth against *E. coli* and *S. aureus* for samples (a) pristine BC, (b) 0.50Zn(NO_3)/SPP/BC, (c) 1.00Zn(NO_3)/SPP/BC, (d) 5.00Zn(NO_3)/SPP/BC, (e) 10.00Zn(NO_3)/SPP/BC, (f) 10.00ZnAct/SPP/BC, (g) 20.00Zn(NO_3)/SPP/BC. (Adapted with permission from Ref. [39]. Copyright 2016, Elsevier.)

Gram-negative- *E. coli*. Antibacterial activity against both cultures is investigated using the inhibition zone method. As indicated in Figure 8.7, the clear zones surrounding the test samples are labeled as the zone of inhibition. As the ZnO concentration increases in the composite samples, the width of the bacterial growth inhibition zone also increases. The increased ZnO concentration causes better penetrability through the bacterial cell membrane, resulting in restricted growth and ultimate death of the bacterial cell.

In another study, a functionalized nanostructure-mediated collagen scaffold is investigated as a wound-healing material. The influence of the shape of the as-synthesized nanostructures is also evaluated in terms of their in vivo wound-healing performance. The nanoparticles are synthesized using the co-precipitation technique and functionalized with dendrimer. Dendrimers are branched polymers and possess significant importance in the field of wound healing applications. Their properties are determined by the functional group present on the molecular surface. The amine-terminated dendrimers are very efficient crosslinkers. Vedhanayagam et al. [42] have functionalized ZnO NPs with triethoxysilane poly(amidoamine) dendrimer generation 1 (TES-PAMAM-G1). The TES-PAMAM-G0.5 as described in Figure 8.8, is obtained by adding (3-aminopropyl) triethoxysilane (APTES) and methyl acrylate (MA) at a 1:2 molar ratio in dry ethanol, followed by refluxing for 2 hours at 80°C under N_2 atmosphere. The further reaction of TES-PAMAM-G0.5 with ethylene diamine (EDA) in dry ethanol gives the desired product as TES-PAMAM-G1. TES-PAMAM-G1is added to the collagen solution in equimolar ratio at room temperature, followed by placing it in an incubator shaker for 18 hours to achieve functionalized nanoparticle crosslinked collagen scaffold. Further, the fabricated nanocomposite scaffold exhibits higher thermal stability and better in vivo wound healing ability compared to pristine collagen scaffold.

Fielding et al. have used SiO_2-ZnO combined dopants in a 3D-printed calcium phosphate scaffold [43]. Pristine 3D-printed porous calcium phosphate scaffolds play a crucial role in biological fixations in bone implant applications. However, calcium phosphate is only able to act as an osteoconductive material which promotes bone growth. Biological and pharmaceutical matters are further incorporated to exhibit osteoinduction. Silicone and zinc are trace elements that are commonly available in bones. They help in enhanced bone regeneration and angiogenesis. The composite calcium phosphate scaffold doped with SiO_2-ZnO has been evaluated against its osteoinductive performance by implanting it into a bicortical femur defect in a rat model. The composite sample exhibits higher blood vessel formation compared to the control sample.

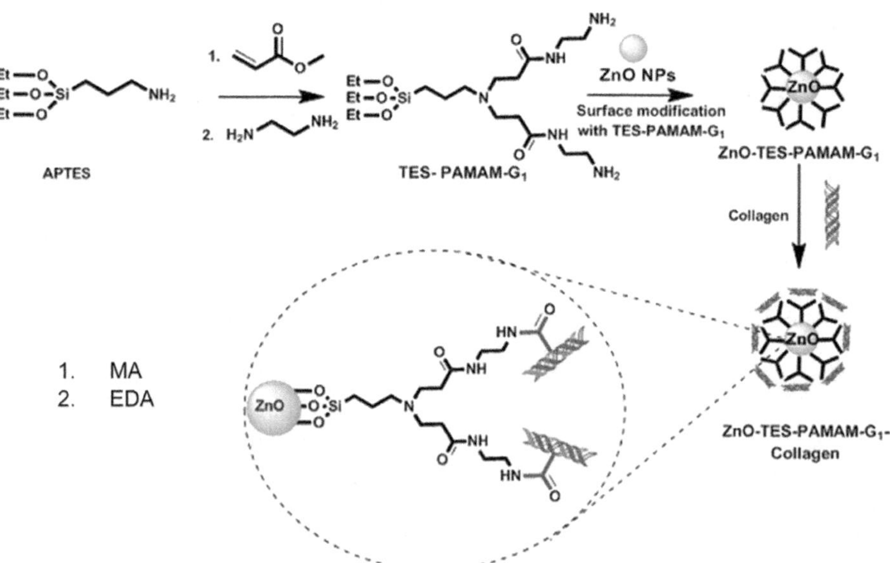

FIGURE 8.8 Schematic diagram of the process of crosslinking collagen with amine-terminated dendrimer-functionalized ZnO NPs. (Adapted with permission from Ref. [42]. Copyright 2018, American Chemical Society.)

8.4.5 Film-Based Nanocomposite Wound Healing Material

A polymeric nanocomposite wound healing patch can be designed using the solution casting method. Jayabal et al. have fabricated a PVA-chitosan based, GO, TiO_2 NPs embedded wound healing patch [44]. To broaden the activity of TiO_2 in the visible region, the band gap is narrowed down by doping with metal ions. Vanadium and nitrogen-doped TiO_2 (TiO_2(V-N)) exhibits absorption in the visible region. GO is chosen due to its high surface area, superior thermal conductivity, excellent drug-loading efficiency, and biocompatibility. GO contains hydroxyl and carboxyl groups. GO promotes cell adhesion by superficially binding proteins through H-bonding, π–π interaction, or electrostatic interaction. A high surface area with wrinkled 2 dimensional planar structures exhibits excellent antibacterial efficacy. GO is synthesized using Hummer's method and TiO_2(V-N) NPs by a hydrothermal process. GO enwrapped (TiO_2(V-N)) is prepared by placing TiO_2(V-N) NP added GO dispersion in a bath sonicator followed by the hydrothermal method. The GO/TiO_2(V-N) nanocomposite is blended with PVA-chitosan solution where glutaraldehyde is used as a crosslinker, followed by solution casting to fabricate the wound healing patch. Curcumin, a polyphenolic substance is incorporated to attain enhanced resistance to bacterial growth. The swelling ratio of the nanocomposite film is evaluated by dipping it in PBS for different time periods. The porosity of the fabricated patch is investigated using the liquid displacement method. Besides, moisture vapor permeability, photocatalytic antibacterial property, blood clotting, hemolysis activity, and drug release efficiency are also estimated against the standard methodology. The nanocomposite patch manifests improved collagen deposition, a high degree of re-epithelialization, and a thicker granulation tissue formation ability compared to conventional wound dressing materials.

8.5 SMART NANOCOMPOSITES IN WOUND HEALING APPLICATIONS

Smart wound healing materials are stimuli sensitive and provide multifunctional benefits to the wound site based on the requirement and type of wound. The healing environment varies for different kinds of wounds such as an acute wound, a diabetic wound, ulcers, burns, scars, etc. The smart wound healing materials can be of different categories—photothermal sensitive, self-healable, pH-responsive, ROS-sensitive, hemostatic, microneedle based, tissue regenerative, etc. A self-healable BC-based transdermal patch is developed for wound healing application using the layer-by-layer (L-B-L) assembly [45]. The L-B-L approach has significant potential in biomedical applications due to its excellent multifaceted usage, for example in biosensors, biomimetics, implantable materials, cell adhesions, etc. The L-B-L assembly also facilitates different cell functions. Self-healable materials exhibit increased shelflife and longevity. They can be constructed generally by using two processes—intrinsic and extrinsic self-healing methods. Intrinsic self-healing methods include Diels-Alder reactions, different non-covalent interactions like ionic conjugation, H-bonding, host–guest interaction, metal-ligand bonding, supramolecular, and π–π interactions. Extrinsic self-healing methods are based on encapsulation technology where the healing material is released only after the crack generation. Carboxymethylation of BC (CMBC) is performed to achieve better hemostasis properties. CMBC is further modified with EDA by the Carbodiimide/N-hydroxysuccinimide) EDC-NHS coupling catalyst. Pectin, a polysaccharide, is mainly used as a gelling agent. Aldehyde-functionalized pectin is reacted with amine-functionalized CMBC through the Schiff base reaction to form the L-B-L assembly. Finally, the composite assembly is incorporated with AgNPs. The same group has also reported a Mussel mimicking bio-adhesive antibacterial patch, fabricated by incorporating a dopamine moiety [46].

Tian et al. have developed an alginate-based biosensor with therapeutic and antifouling properties [47]. In another approach, an intelligent wound healing patch is fabricated based on scaffold-based structural ionic hydrogels. This is reported to serve as an electronic skin to facilitate wound healing [48]. Ahmadian et al. have developed a pH-responsive multifunctional hydrogel material with hemostatic, antibacterial, and anti-inflammatory characteristics [49]. Further, a piezoelectric and photothermal multifunctional film is fabricated for providing electric stimulation and thermal combined therapy at the infection site [50]. In another study, a smart biosensor is designed based on properties like real-time monitoring of the wound status [51]. The dressing comprises a flexible electronic circuit to detect the pathophysiological characteristics of the wound like pH, temperature, and uric acid level. It is reported to have the ability to monitor the infection in situ and provide electrically controlled sustained delivery of the antibiotic material at the wound site.

8.6 CONCLUSION

The implementation of nanotechnology has indeed revolutionized the health care sector by providing novel approaches towards wound dressing and wound healing methodologies. Biocompatibility, hemostatic and adhesive properties, antibacterial efficacy, and antioxidant properties are crucial for wound healing materials. Today, there are 4-5 types of nanocomposite based wound healing materials: hydrogel, film, foam, scaffold, sponge, and nanofibrous mats. The most competitive wound healing materials are hydrogel-based. Hydrogels are 3D hydrophilic polymeric networks. They effectively keep the wound wet, which promotes cell development and proliferation. In addition, they absorb wound exudates. Similar to most wound healing products, they are harmless and nonadherent. Hydrogel functions mimic a natural ECM. Due to their bleeding site barrier, hydrogels speed hemostasis. Another promising technology is electrospinning. It helps design bioactive wound dressing materials because of their flexibility and ECM mimicry. Coaxial or emulsion electrospinning can integrate nanoparticles, medicinal medicines, growth factors, and antimicrobial agents to speed wound healing. Recent research and development focuses on smart hydrogels, scaffolds, foams, and electrospun mats with multifunctional, stimuli-responsive properties relevant to the wound type (acute/diabetic/chronic/scar/burn). Adding thermoresponsive, pH-responsive, hemostatic, tissue regenerating, self-healable, photothermal sensitive, controlled release, etc. features demonstrate market potential. Better wound monitoring, faster healing, and optimal wound management are possible with them.

REFERENCES

[1] Kokabi, M.; Sirousazar, M.; Hassan, Z. M. PVA–Clay Nanocomposite Hydrogels for Wound Dressing. *Eur Polym J*, 2007, 43 (3), 773–781.

[2] Naseri, E.; Ahmadi, A. A Review on Wound Dressings: Antimicrobial Agents, Biomaterials, Fabrication Techniques, and Stimuli-Responsive Drug Release. *Eur Polym J*, 2022, 173, 111293.

[3] Guo, B.; Dong, R.; Liang, Y.; Li, M. Haemostatic Materials for Wound Healing Applications. *Nat Rev Chem*, 2021, 5 (11), 773–791.

[4] Homaeigohar, S.; Boccaccini, A. R. Antibacterial Biohybrid Nanofibers for Wound Dressings. *Acta Biomater*, 2020, 107, 25–49.

[5] Wang, M.; Deng, Z.; Guo, Y.; Xu, P. Engineering Functional Natural Polymer-Based Nanocomposite Hydrogels for Wound Healing. *Nanoscale Adv*, 2022, 5 (1), 27–45.

[6] Brett, D. W. A Review of Moisture-Control Dressings in Wound Care. *J Wound Ostomy Continence*, 2006, 33 (SUPPL. 6), S3–S8.

[7] Dong, R.; Guo, B. Smart Wound Dressings for Wound Healing. *Nano Today*, 2021, 41, 101290.

[8] Korupalli, C.; Li, H.; Nguyen, N.; Mi, F. L.; Chang, Y.; Lin, Y. J.; Sung, H. W. Conductive Materials for Healing Wounds: Their Incorporation in Electroactive Wound Dressings, Characterization, and Perspectives. *Adv Healthc Mater*, 2021, 10 (6), 2001384.

[9] Cao, J.; Wu, P.; Cheng, Q.; He, C.; Chen, Y.; Zhou, J. Ultrafast Fabrication of Self-Healing and Injectable Carboxymethyl Chitosan Hydrogel Dressing for Wound Healing. *ACS Appl Mater Interfaces*, 2021, 13 (20), 24095–24105.

[10] Kumar, S. S. D.; Rajendran, N. K.; Houreld, N. N.; Abrahamse, H. Recent Advances on Silver Nanoparticle and Biopolymer-Based Biomaterials for Wound Healing Applications. *Int J Biol Macromol*, 2018, 115, 165–175.

[11] Ur Rehman, S. R.; Augustine, R.; Zahid, A. A.; Ahmed, R.; Tariq, M.; Hasan, A. Reduced Graphene Oxide Incorporated Gelma Hydrogel Promotes Angiogenesis for Wound Healing Applications. *Int J Nanomed*, 2019, 14, 9603–9617.

[12] Rastin, H.; Ormsby, R. T.; Atkins, G. J.; Losic, D. 3D Bioprinting of Methylcellulose/Gelatin-Methacryloyl (MC/GelMA) Bioink with High Shape Integrity. *ACS Appl Bio Mater*, 2020, 3 (3), 1815–1826.

[13] Zhu, M.; Wang, Y.; Ferracci, G.; Zheng, J.; Cho, N. J.; Lee, B. H. Gelatin Methacryloyl and Its Hydrogels with an Exceptional Degree of Controllability and Batch-to-Batch Consistency. *Sci Rep*, 2019, 9 (1), 1–13.

[14] Huang, W.; Wang, Y.; Huang, Z.; Wang, X.; Chen, L.; Zhang, Y.; Zhang, L. On-Demand Dissolvable Self-Healing Hydrogel Based on Carboxymethyl Chitosan and Cellulose Nanocrystal for Deep Partial Thickness Burn Wound Healing. *ACS Appl Mater Interfaces*, 2018, 10 (48), 41076–41088.

[15] Xu, J.; Liu, Y.; Hsu, S. H. Hydrogels Based on Schiff Base Linkages for Biomedical Applications. *Molecules*, 2019, 24 (16), 3005.

[16] Tolosa, L.; Donato, M. T.; Gómez-Lechón, M. J. General Cytotoxicity Assessment by Means of the MTT Assay. *Methods Mol Biol*, 2015, 1250, 333–348.

[17] Zhu, J.; Li, F.; Wang, X.; Yu, J.; Wu, D. Hyaluronic Acid and Polyethylene Glycol Hybrid Hydrogel Encapsulating Nanogel with Hemostasis and Sustainable Antibacterial Property for Wound Healing. *ACS Appl Mater Interfaces*, 2018, 10 (16), 13304–13316.

[18] Burdick, J. A.; Prestwich, G. D.; Burdick, A.; Prestwich, G. D. Hyaluronic Acid Hydrogels for Biomedical Applications. *Adv Mater*, 2011, 23 (12), H41–H56.

[19] Fong, N.; Simmons, A.; Poole-Warren, L. A. Antibacterial Polyurethane Nanocomposites Using Chlorhexidine Diacetate as an Organic Modifier. *Acta Biomater*, 2010, 6 (7), 2554–2561.

[20] Hu, J.; Liu, X.; Gao, Q.; Ouyang, C.; Zheng, K.; Shan, X. Thermosensitive PNIPAM-Based Hydrogel Crosslinked by Composite Nanoparticles as Rapid Wound-Healing Dressings. *Biomacromolecules*, 2022, 24 (3), 1345–1354.
[21] Wu, Z.; Hong, Y. Combination of the Silver-Ethylene Interaction and 3D Printing to Develop Antibacterial Superporous Hydrogels for Wound Management. *ACS Appl Mater Interfaces*, 2019, 11 (37), 33734–33747.
[22] Zhang, T.; Guo, L.; Li, R.; Shao, J.; Lu, L.; Yang, P.; Zhao, A.; Liu, Y. Ellagic Acid–Cyclodextrin Inclusion Complex-Loaded Thiol–Ene Hydrogel with Antioxidant, Antibacterial, and Anti-Inflammatory Properties for Wound Healing. *ACS Appl. Mater. Interfaces*, 2023, 15, 4959–4972.
[23] Su, C.; Chen, J.; Xie, X.; Gao, Z.; Guan, Z.; Mo, X.; Wang, C.; Hou, G. Functionalized Electrospun Double-Layer Nanofibrous Scaffold for Wound Healing and Scar Inhibition. *ACS Omega*, 2022, 7 (34), 30137–30148.
[24] Cui, Y.; Huang, Z.; Lei, L.; Li, Q.; Jiang, J.; Zeng, Q.; Tang, A.; Yang, H.; Zhang, Y. Robust Hemostatic Bandages Based on Nanoclay Electrospun Membranes. *Nat Commun* 2021, 12 (1), 1–11.
[25] Schneider, A.; Wang, X. Y.; Kaplan, D. L.; Garlick, J. A.; Egles, C. Biofunctionalized Electrospun Silk Mats as a Topical Bioactive Dressing for Accelerated Wound Healing. *Acta Biomater*, 2009, 5 (7), 2570–2578.
[26] Park, K. H.; Han, S. H.; Hong, J. P.; Han, S. K.; Lee, D. H.; Kim, B. S.; Ahn, J. H.; Lee, J. W. Topical Epidermal Growth Factor Spray for the Treatment of Chronic Diabetic Foot Ulcers: A Phase III Multicenter, Double-Blind, Randomized, Placebo-Controlled Trial. *Diabetes Res Clin Pract*, 2018, 142, 335–344.
[27] Meinlschmidt, P.; Ueberham, E.; Lehmann, J.; Schweiggert-Weisz, U.; Eisner, P. Immunoreactivity, Sensory and Physicochemical Properties of Fermented Soy Protein Isolate. *Food Chem*, 2016, 205, 229–238.
[28] El-Aassar, M. R.; El fawal, G. F.; El-Deeb, N. M.; Shokry Hassan, H.; Mo, X. Electrospun Polyvinyl Alcohol/Pluronic F127 Blended Nanofibers Containing Titanium Dioxide for Antibacterial Wound Dressing. *Appl Biochem Biotechnol*, 2010, 178, 1488–1502.
[29] Akash, M. S. H.; Rehman, K. Recent Progress in Biomedical Applications of Pluronic (PF127): Pharmaceutical Perspectives. *J Control Release*, 2015, 209, 120–138.
[30] Ge, L.; Xu, Y.; Li, X.; Yuan, L.; Tan, H.; Li, D.; Mu, C. Fabrication of Antibacterial Collagen-Based Composite Wound Dressing. *ACS Sustain Chem Eng*, 2018, 6 (7), 9153–9166.
[31] Wang, Y.; Wang, Z.; Dong, Y. Collagen-Based Biomaterials for Tissue Engineering. *ACS Biomater Sci Eng*, 2023, 9 (3), 1132–1150.
[32] Coindre, V. F.; Hu, Y.; Sefton, M. V. Poly-Methacrylic Acid Cross-Linked with Collagen Accelerates Diabetic Wound Closure. *ACS Biomater Sci Eng*, 2020, 6 (11), 6368–6377.
[33] Radzig, M. A.; Nadtochenko, V. A.; Koksharova, O. A.; Kiwi, J.; Lipasova, V. A.; Khmel, I. A. Antibacterial Effects of Silver Nanoparticles on Gram-Negative Bacteria: Influence on the Growth and Biofilms Formation, Mechanisms of Action. *Colloids Surf B Biointerfaces*, 2013, 102, 300–306.
[34] Tashkhourian, J.; Hormozi-Nezhad, M. R.; Fotovat, M. Optical Detection of Some Hydrazine Compounds Based on the Surface Plasmon Resonance Band of Silver Nanoparticles, *Spectrosc Lett*, 2013, 46 (1), 73–80. https://doi.org/10.1080/00387010.2012.668607
[35] Setua, P.; Ghatak, C.; Rao, V. G.; Das, S. K.; Sarkar, N. Dynamics of Solvation and Rotational Relaxation of Coumarin 480 in Pure Aqueous-AOT Reverse Micelle and Reverse Micelle Containing Different-Sized Silver Nanoparticles Inside Its Core: A Comparative Study. *J Phys Chem B*, 2012, 116 (12), 3704–3712.
[36] Zhang, W.; Qiao, X.; Chen, J.; Wang, H. Preparation of Silver Nanoparticles in Water-in-Oil AOT Reverse Micelles. *J Colloid Interface Sci*, 2006, 302 (1), 370–373.

[37] Liu, W.; Du, H.; Zhang, M.; Liu, K.; Liu, H.; Xie, H.; Zhang, X.; Si, C. Bacterial Cellulose-Based Composite Scaffolds for Biomedical Applications: A Review. *ACS Sustain Chem Eng*, 2020, 8 (20), 7536–7562.

[38] Das, M.; Zandraa, O.; Mudenur, C.; Saha, N.; Sáha, P.; Mandal, B.; Katiyar, V. Composite Scaffolds Based on Bacterial Cellulose for Wound Dressing Application. *ACS Appl Bio Mater*, 2022, 5 (8), 3722–3733.

[39] Janpetch, N.; Saito, N.; Rujiravanit, R. Fabrication of Bacterial Cellulose-ZnO Composite via Solution Plasma Process for Antibacterial Applications. *Carbohydr Polym*, 2016, 148, 335–344.

[40] Chokradjaroen, C.; Niu, J.; Panomsuwan, G.; Saito, N. Insight on Solution Plasma in Aqueous Solution and Their Application in Modification of Chitin and Chitosan. *Int J Mol Sci*, 2021, 22 (9), 4308.

[41] Kourmouli, A.; Valenti, M.; van Rijn, E.; Beaumont, H. J. E.; Kalantzi, O. I.; Schmidt-Ott, A.; Biskos, G. Can Disc Diffusion Susceptibility Tests Assess the Antimicrobial Activity of Engineered Nanoparticles? *J Nanoparticle Res*, 2018, 20 (3), 1–6.

[42] Vedhanayagam, M.; Unni Nair, B.; Sreeram, K. J. Collagen-ZnO Scaffolds for Wound Healing Applications: Role of Dendrimer Functionalization and Nanoparticle Morphology. *ACS Appl Bio Mater*, 2018, 1 (6), 1942–1958.

[43] Fielding, G.; Bose, S. SiO2 and ZnO Dopants in Three-Dimensionally Printed Tricalcium Phosphate Bone Tissue Engineering Scaffolds Enhance Osteogenesis and Angiogenesis in Vivo. *Acta Biomater*, 2013, 9 (11), 9137–9148.

[44] Jayabal, P.; Kannan Sampathkumar, V.; Vinothkumar, A.; Mathapati, S.; Pannerselvam, B.; Achiraman, S.; Venkatasubbu, G. D. Fabrication of a Chitosan-Based Wound Dressing Patch for Enhanced Antimicrobial, Hemostatic, and Wound Healing Application. *ACS Appl Bio Mater*, 2022, 6, 615–627.

[45] Khamrai, M.; Banerjee, S. L.; Paul, S.; Ghosh, A. K.; Sarkar, P.; Kundu, P. P. AgNPs Ornamented Modified Bacterial Cellulose Based Self-Healable L-B-L Assembly via a Schiff Base Reaction: A Potential Wound Healing Patch. *ACS Appl Bio Mater*, 2021, 4 (1), 428–440.

[46] Khamrai, M.; Banerjee, S. L.; Paul, S.; Ghosh, A. K.; Sarkar, P.; Kundu, P. P. A Mussel Mimetic, Bioadhesive, Antimicrobial Patch Based on Dopamine-Modified Bacterial Cellulose/RGO/Ag NPs: A Green Approach toward Wound-Healing Applications. *ACS Sustain Chem Eng*, 2019, 7 (14), 12083–12097.

[47] Tian, S.; Wang, M.; Wang, X.; Wang, L.; Yang, D.; Nie, J.; Ma, G. Smart Hydrogel Sensors with Antifreezing, Antifouling Properties for Wound Healing. *ACS Biomater Sci Eng*, 2022, 8 (5), 1867–1877.

[48] Wang, Y.; Sun, L.; Chen, G.; Chen, H.; Zhao, Y. Structural Color Ionic Hydrogel Patches for Wound Management. *ACS Nano,* 2022, 17(2), 1437–1447.

[49] Ahmadian, Z.; Correia, A.; Hasany, M.; Figueiredo, P.; Dobakhti, F.; Eskandari, M. R.; Hosseini, S. H.; Abiri, R.; Khorshid, S.; Hirvonen, J.; et al. A Hydrogen-Bonded Extracellular Matrix-Mimicking Bactericidal Hydrogel with Radical Scavenging and Hemostatic Function for PH-Responsive Wound Healing Acceleration. *Adv Healthc Mater*, 2021, 10 (3), 2001122.

[50] Chen, Y.; Ye, M.; Song, L.; Zhang, J.; Yang, Y.; Luo, S.; Lin, M.; Zhang, Q.; Li, S.; Zhou, Y.; et al. Piezoelectric and Photothermal Dual Functional Film for Enhanced Dermal Wound Regeneration via Upregulation of Hsp90 and HIF-1α. *Appl Mater Today*, 2020, 20, 100756.

[51] Xu, G.; Lu, Y.; Cheng, C.; Li, X.; Xu, J.; Liu, Z.; Liu, J.; Liu, G.; Shi, Z.; Chen, Z.; et al. Battery-Free and Wireless Smart Wound Dressing for Wound Infection Monitoring and Electrically Controlled On-Demand Drug Delivery. *Adv Funct Mater*, 2021, 31 (26), 2100852.

9 Application of Nanotechnology in Antimicrobial Coating on Surgical Instruments

Pramod Yadav, Mohit Kamboj, and Bodhisatwa Das

9.1 INTRODUCTION

The medical tools utilized in clinical procedures are referred to as surgical instruments such as tweezers, knives, scissors, needles, pliers, hooks, drills, and so on. In addition to these, manufactured products that are directly useful for biomedical applications also fall within the category of surgical instruments like implants, catheters, contact lenses, etc. Surgical site infections (SSIs) due to surgical instruments will lead to morbidity and mortality, and increase healthcare expenditure (Olsen et al., 2008). These infections are caused due to bacterial contamination of surgical instruments. Traditional methods of giving systemic antibiotics are commonly ineffective for postoperative treatment for implant-related infections. Bacterial colonization and subsequent biofilm formation on surgical instrument surfaces can be minimized by antibacterial coatings on their surfaces to prevent post-surgical infection (Ahmadabadi et al., 2020; Bazaka et al., 2012). Polymers, composites, metals, and nanoparticles (NPs) are being used for coating with various technologies and materials. The coating is done to inhibit the additional functionality of the inert materials used. Overall, this manuscript aims to provide a comprehensive overview of antimicrobial coatings on surgical instruments by nanoscale materials. It also adequately elaborates on their importance and potential application in clinical practice to prevent SSIs.

9.2 BACKGROUND

9.2.1 Surgical Infections

Instruments surface offers an environment that provides an appropriate environment for the attachment and growth of bacteria leading to biofilm formation, resulting in a reduced insensitivity to antimicrobial agents and the host's immune responses (Ciarolla et al., 2023). Infection occurs only when there are microorganisms. Excessive bacterial growth and proliferation occur gradually from a colony that is covered by exopolysaccharide (EPS). This envelope-like structure will help in the survival of

DOI: 10.1201/9781003432661-9

bacteria against antibiotic therapy and immune response (Nurse, 2007). Infections associated with frequent surgical procedures and implantable inert devices lead to a group of microorganisms aggregating and creating a biofilm (Donlan, 2001).

9.2.1.1 Biofilm Formation

According to the definitions, biofilms are highly structured communities of bacterial cells that produce an extracellular matrix. Biofilm matrices are formed of chemical components such as extracellular polysaccharides, proteins, tetrachloride, and extracellular DNA (eDNA) depending on the type of bacterial species, strain, and environmental conditions. Bacterial biofilms are resistant to antibiotics, disinfectants, phagocytosis, adaptive immune systems, other components of host immune systems, and immunological and inflammatory defense systems. Biofilms can easily form on biological tissue and instrument surfaces (Arciola et al., 2012; Rimondini et al., 2014). The four stages of the general growth cycle of biofilms include their reversible attachment of bacteria cells, irreversible attachment due to extracellular polymeric matrix (EPM) secretion, development of biofilm formation, maturation, and dispersion of biofilm. Biofilm has many purposes, including acting as a physical barrier against phagocytic predation and inhibiting cell separation under normal flow conditions as well as a selective permeability barrier (Bazaka et al., 2012). Figure 9.1 describes the steps involved in biofilm formation.

9.2.1.1.1 Phase1- Initiation

The first stage of biofilm formation is the bacteria's adhesion to the surface of the surgical instruments and the proliferation of cells to be colonized. There are various factors such as polarity, London-van der Waals forces, and hydrophobic interactions that are responsible for the initial adhesion of the microbe in the formation of biofilm. Various bacteria adhere to the protein surface, contributing to the initial adhesion and biofilm formation (Veerachamy et al., 2014; Büttner et al., 2015).

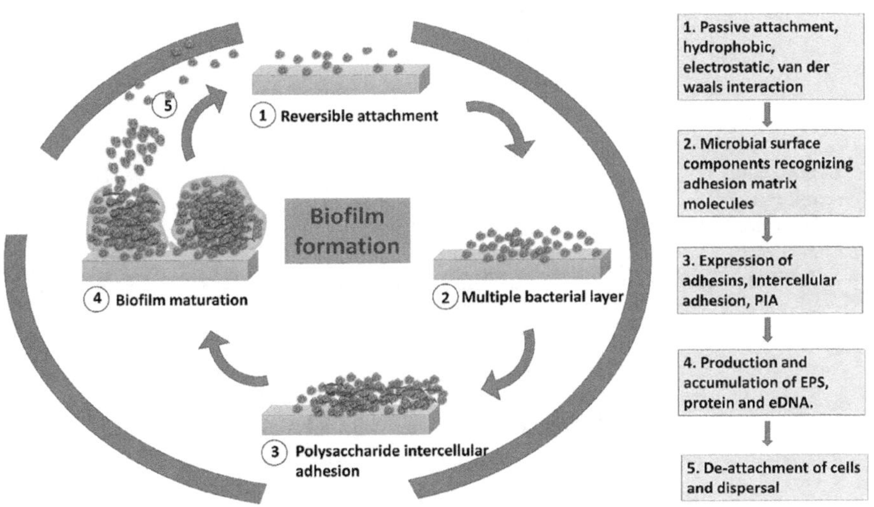

FIGURE 9.1 Steps involved in biofilm formation.

9.2.1.1.2 Phase2- Irreversible Attachment

Further, the cells show growth and maturation, causing intercellular adhesion to form bacterial colonies into a biofilm. It is encapsulated by the EPM resulting in intercellular communication between bacteria. Through electrostatic forces and hydrogen bonding, EPM retains bacteria in the biofilm and is responsible for adhesion to various substrates (Gravante et al., 2013).

9.2.1.1.3 Phase3- Advancement in Biofilm Structure

This procedure enables the self-assembly and control of some microbial cell characteristics, including the formation of biofilms and EPM (Otto, 2013).

9.2.1.1.4 Phase4- Maturation and Dispersion

In essence, a biofilm develops, prepares to rupture, and releases bacteria when it reaches maturity or a threshold mass. These microorganisms can then recolonize and continue the process (Arciola et al., 2018).

The bacteria in biofilm trigger reactions that protect them from host immunological factors. Additionally, the anaerobic metabolism of bacteria within biofilm reduces the efficacy of the antibiotics. This can make it difficult for antibiotics to penetrate the core of the biofilm, leading to the development of antimicrobial-resistant strains (Hall and Mah, 2017). In addition, some biofilms can minimize or stop leukocyte predation in a variety of ways. For example, *Pseudomonas aeruginosa* may produce rhamnolipids through QS in response to phagocytic leukocytes. Quorum sensing (QS) refers to bacterial cell-to-cell communication (Joo and Otto, 2012; Bjarnsholt, 2013). Therefore treatment of surgical infections due to microorganisms is essential for disease management and surgery. Figure 9.2 shows the presence of biofilm on the surface of surgical instruments which will cause many kinds of infections.

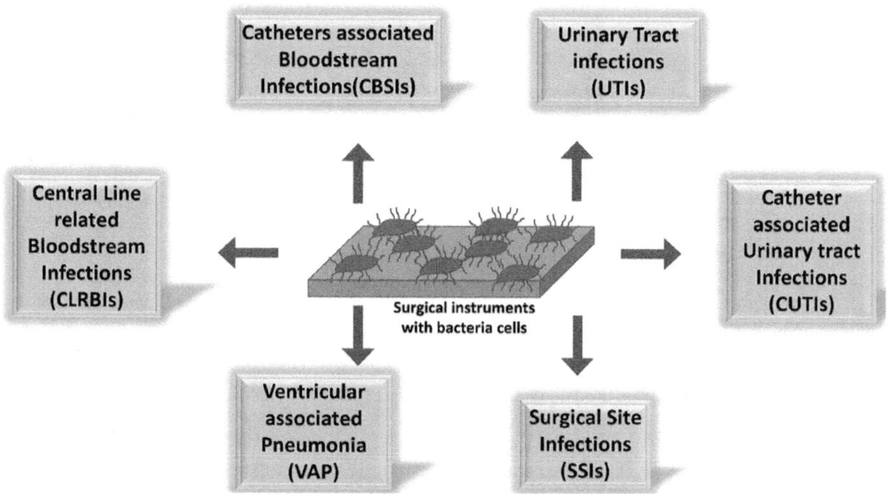

FIGURE 9.2 Infections associated with the formation of biofilms on surgical instruments and implants.

9.2.2 Nanotechnology and Its Potential in Medical Applications

The transformation of biosystems can be accelerated with the help of nanotechnology, which also offers an array of technical applications, industrial bioprocessing, and molecular medicine (Roco, 2003). It is a term that is used to encompass scientific and engineering disciplines that utilize the phenomena at the nanoscale to design, produce, characterize, and apply materials, structures, and devices (Gonzalez et al., 2013). Materials approximately in the size range of 1–100 nanometers (nm) show properties significantly different from their bulk surface (Ferrari, 2005). This allows such materials to be used for myriad applications namely, in biosensors (Kumar et al., 2019), tissue engineering, drug delivery systems, etc. Furthermore, nanotechnology has been used in imaging, diagnostics, and improved drug delivery thereby, demonstrating great potential to drive the medical industry (Jabir et al., 2012). NPs have been used to enhance material properties, such as enhancing the antibacterial properties of surgical instruments through NP coatings (Rai et al., 2009). However, it still raises certain safety concerns hence, optimal regulation and monitoring of NPs is of the utmost importance (Metzel, 1990).

9.3 NANOTECHNOLOGY-BASED ANTIMICROBIAL COATINGS

Nanotechnology has been reported to enhance the physical, chemical, and biological properties through various techniques, resulting in an improved antimicrobial activity of such materials therefore, it has potential applications in the healthcare sector to minimize infections. For instance, various studies have reported inhibition of bacterial proliferation using metal NPs. The aforementioned techniques include surface modification, controlled release of compounds, and photodynamic therapeutic interventions. Nonetheless, the utilization of nanotechnology for the development and fabrication of materials with enhanced antimicrobial activities requires deeper understanding and research.

9.3.1 Kinds of Nanoparticles Utilized in Coatings

9.3.1.1 Antimicrobial Coating Based on Metal and Metal-Oxide-Nanoparticle

a. **Silver:** Antimicrobial coating based on silver nanoparticles (AgNPs) can achieve a long-lasting bactericidal effect without causing toxic and side effects. AgNPs have antimicrobial effects by releasing free metals Ag^+ ions. Silver ions have strong antimicrobial properties on their own due to the high surface-to-volume ratio (Marassi et al., 2018). AgNPs penetrate bacteria and affect their biological function. Ag^+ ions bind with the bacterial cell membrane and damage them due to the antimicrobial effect. AgNPs have been observed to disrupt the biofilm disturbing intermolecular forces (Vasilev et al., 2009; Ramasamy and Lee, 2016).
b. **Copper**: The utilization of copper (Cu) to minimize bacterial infection can be dated back to 2600 BC (Sahoo et al., 2022). It causes the suppression of microorganisms through contact-dependent suppression (Grass et al., 2011).

Yet, bacterial regrowth has been reported in various studies. This resistance to the Cu-based contact killing mechanism can be attributed to the evolution of various defense mechanisms such as extracellular ion retention and active ion efflux resulting in a decreased permeability of the bacterial cell membrane in addition to the ion scavenging by proteins similar to metallothionein in the cytoplasm. Hence, Cu and copper oxide NPs are widely utilized to coat surgical tools due to their ability to act as antimicrobial agents while not eliciting an unwanted immune response, being eco-friendly synthesis, with a faster dissolution rate, and being cost-effective (Ermini and Voliani, 2021).

c. **Zinc**: It is widely known that organisms need zinc in minute amounts for biomineralization, cell growth, expansion, DNA recombination, and other processes (Sahoo et al., 2022). Zinc is widely used in toothpaste and mouthwashes because of its antibacterial properties, which help reduce plaque, inhibit the growth of tartar, and decrease unpleasant breath. Zinc nanoparticles (ZnNPs) suppress the major cariogenic bacterium that causes tooth caries, *S. mutans*. However, zinc oxide (ZnO) is more frequently used as nanoparticles in surgical coatings than zinc due to its superior antibacterial characteristics. These NPs have gained significant attention due to their unique and fascinating characteristics, such as large surface-to-volume ratio, UV absorption ability, visible light transmittance, electrical conductivity, piezoelectricity, semiconductor behavior, mammalian cell biocompatibility, wide accessibility, and extended environmental durability (Almoudi et al., 2018; Mahamuni-Badiger et al., 2020).

d. **Titanium oxide**: The shape, crystal structure, and size of titanium oxide (TiO_2) NPs are primary factors differentiating their antimicrobial activity. TiO_2 is a safe and non-reactive metal oxide having auto-cleansing characteristics, often used in cosmetics, orthodontics, and medicine (Lee et al., 2018). Because of the nanoscale nature, a significant increase in surface area-to-volume ratio allows for maximum contact with water and oxygen in the environment, minimum size, and easy filtration of the cell wall and membrane, therefore increasing the oxidation damage in cells. The mechanism of the antimicrobial effect of TiO_2 is usually associated with a high oxidative potential reactive oxygen species (ROS) produced by the photo-induced band-gap irradiation charge in the presence of O_2. ROS affects bacterial cells through different mechanisms that cause their death. TiO_2 has proven efficacy in various pathogens such as *MRSA, S. aureus strains, P. aeruginosa, M. tuberculosis, S. epidermidis, E. coli, C. difficile*, and *K. pneumonia*.

e. **Iron**: The magnetic NPs of iron (Fe) and iron oxide (Fe_3O_4, FeO_3) are found to have applications in various therapeutics. Researchers have discovered that super magnetic iron oxide nanoparticles (SPIONs), known to possess biocompatibility, biodegradability, and nontoxicity, are also endowed with potent antimicrobial characteristics. Also, the body successfully gets rid of these nanoparticles via several iron metabolism mechanisms (Murthy et al., 2020). Additionally, SPIONs can be modified with a range of polymers and biomaterials, including polyethylene glycol (PEG), and polyvinyl alcohol (PVA). They can also be linked with diverse functional groups, including carboxyl, thiols, and amines, to cater to an extensive assortment of applications including an antimicrobial coating on surgical tools. The magnetic characteristics of SPIONs can be harnessed to induce localized hyperthermia, resulting in the physical fragmentation and dissemination of pathogenic biofilms with the help of static friction caused by a magnetized environment (Arbab et al., 2003). The majority of prevalent biofilm-associated organisms, including *MRSA, S. aureus, E. coli, P. aeruginosa, S. epidermidis, K. pneumonia*, and *B. subtilis*, have been demonstrated to be inhibited by SPIONs (Thukkaram et al., 2014; Sathyanarayanan et al., 2013).

f. **Magnesium**: Magnesium hydroxide ($Mg(OH)_2$) nanoparticles are becoming more important in the era of green chemistry because of their environmental friendliness, broad antibacterial range, low toxicity, biocompatibility, and economical manufacture (Nguyen et al., 2018). Additionally, multiple investigations have indicated that $Mg(OH)_2$ NPs are efficient against the following bacteria in a size-dependent order: *E. coli, S. aureus, P. aeruginosa, K. pneumonia,* and *B. phytofirmans.* This is because smaller particles may readily enter and move within the cell partitions (Halbus et al., 2019).

g. **Hybrid:** With the advancement in technology, to make the surgical instruments' surface more suitable, a hybrid coating with great efficiency was done. Here, the metal NPs with bacteriolytic enzymes (lysozymes) are aggregately coated onto the surface of stainless steel surgical blades and needles (Eby et al., 2009).

9.3.1.2 2D-Nanomaterial-Based Nano Coating

a. **Graphene oxide**: A flat monolayer of densely packed carbon atoms makes up the two-dimensional (2D) honeycomb lattice known as graphene. Graphene is the basic building block for all other dimensional graphitic materials. Due to its distinct mechanical, thermal, and electrical properties, graphene has drawn the interest of academic and industrial researchers. In the planes and edges of a graphene-like material termed graphene oxide, oxygen functional groups are sp^3-bonded to carbon atoms (Loh et al., 2010). Nanomaterials based on graphene can efficiently prevent the proliferation of *E. coli* bacteria while causing minimal cytotoxicity (Hu et al., 2010). Graphene oxide penetrates the microbial cell membrane, causes physical damage to the cell membrane, leads to leakage of intracellular substances, and ultimately leads to cell death (Zou et al., 2016).

b. **Molybdenum disulfide (MoS_2):** MoS_2 is a transition metal dichalcogenide (TMD) comprised of molybdenum and sulfur atoms stacked due to the presence of van der Waals bonds forming a layered structure. Nanosheets fabricated using MoS_2 possess different properties such as high mechanical strength, flexibility, biocompatibility, and thermal conductivity (Balendhran et al., 2013). MoS_2 presents potential for usage in antimicrobial coatings due to its antibacterial properties. A study carried out to understand the antimicrobial activity of MoS_2 nanosheets demonstrated its ability to depolarize bacterial membranes resulting in the loss of membrane activity and consequently, protein leakage, metabolic activity inhibition, and occurrence of oxidative stress (Roy et al., 2019). Furthermore, another study attributed the enhanced antimicrobial activity of photocatalytic and photodynamic MoS_2 nanosheets under NIR illumination to microbial cell membrane rupture (Shin et al., 2018).

c. **Black phosphorus:** Black phosphorus has significant antibacterial properties, great biocompatibility, and biodegradability. These characteristics make it an acceptable material for several biomedical applications, such as bioimaging, photothermal therapy, photodynamic therapy (PDT), biosensing, drug delivery, etc (Choi et al., 2018; Luo et al., 2019; Kou et al., 2015). BP-based nanocomposites exhibit antibacterial action regardless of the makeup of bacterial membranes since they are effective against both Gram-positive and Gram-negative forms of bacteria. Additionally, BP nanosheets are very resistant to bacterial cell membrane disruption. The BP nanosheets' bactericidal processes involved the rupture of membranes caused by cutting-edge and ROS-dependent oxidative stress (Xiong et al., 2018). With NIR irradiation, BP nanosheets do exhibit antibacterial effects due to hyperthermia due to their adjustable band gap (Ouyang et al., 2018).

9.3.2 Nanoparticles' Antimicrobial Processes and Effects

It is well-accepted that metal and metal oxide NPs have antibacterial capabilities. The main processes by which magnesium oxide NPs, iron, copper, zinc, and silver oxide NPs exert their antibacterial effects (Correa et al., 2020; Gold et al., 2018).

1. The reaction with SH groups results in the denaturation of proteins.
2. It stops DNA replication by binding to DNA molecules and creating cross-links between the strands.
3. Association with the cell membrane by electrostatic interaction increases cell permeability and causes cell damage.
4. Several metabolic processes are disrupted by the release of metallic ions.
5. Generation of free radicals and ROS: The ROS generated by the NPs causes DNA damage, lipid peroxidation, metabolic enzyme oxidation, and finally a decrease in cellular respiratory function, which results in cell death (Figure 9.3).

9.4 TECHNIQUES FOR COATING NANOTECHNOLOGY-BASED ANTIMICROBIAL COATINGS ON SURGICAL TOOLS

9.4.1 Summary of Various Coating Methods

Surgical tool coatings must be wear-resistant, not difficult to clean, antibacterial, and have a minimal light reflection. The surface of biomaterials can be coated by implementing a variety of techniques, including plasma spraying, electrodeposition, sol-gel dipping coating, chemical vapor deposition (CVD), physical vapor deposition (PVD), and more. Plasma spray allows for readily adjusting coating thickness

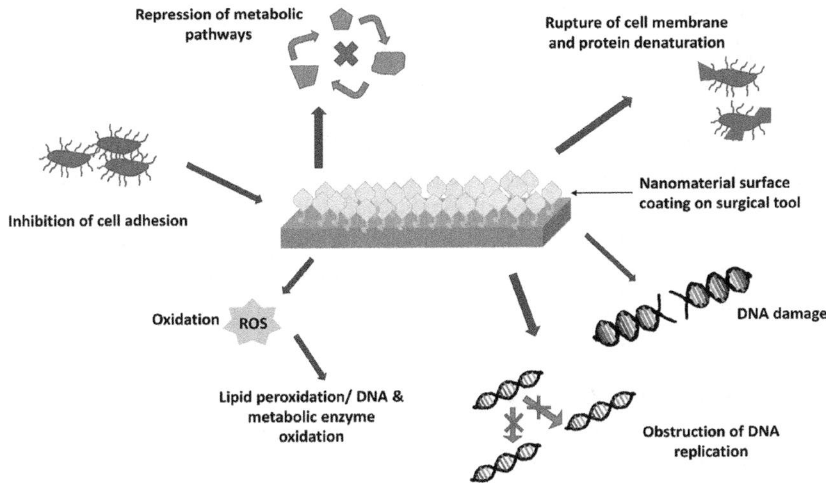

FIGURE 9.3 Antimicrobial/Antibiofilm mechanisms of metal, metal oxide, or 2D nanomaterial-based coatings.

and sample size. However, this process cannot produce a uniform coating on the substrate because of the complex shape and high operating temperature will alter the substrate's structure and functionality. The CVD technique can deposit a thick coating but requires a high temperature. The electrodeposition method allows the performance of a uniform coating with a simple operation and at a low temperature. The coating obtained through electrodeposition requires post-treatment to strengthen it due to the weak adhesion to the substrate. There are several mechanisms for coating nanotechnology-based antimicrobial coating on surgical tools.

9.4.1.1 Physical Vapor Deposition

A thin-film deposition process involves the vaporization of solid material to deposit thin films of several microns composed of a few atomic layers (Baptista et al., 2018). Alloys such as copper with silver, deposited using the PVD technology have been found to showcase better efficacy against microorganisms such as *E.coli, S.aureus,* and *Staphylococcus epidermidis*. Furthermore, coating using doped materials through PVD technology has demonstrated improved mechanical strength and antibacterial properties resulting in a reduction in bacterial proliferation (Osés et al., 2018). The figure shows the complete setup of PVD which will maintain the vacuum atmosphere within a vacuum chamber using a vacuum pump and a high-voltage DC supply. The source material is linked to the positive terminal of the DC power supply, while the target material is positioned at the negative terminal.

9.4.1.2 Sol-Gel Synthesis

The sol-gel method is based on the principle of "chemie-douce" chemistry, which offers effective and adaptable pathways for producing highly uniform nanoparticles at an affordable cost. With this method, the entire reaction that takes place during the synthesis of solids can be better controlled. The sol-gel procedure is based on the chemical nature of the hydrolysis and the poly-condensation reaction, Metal alkoxides [$M(OR)_3$] are often used in this process because of their ability to create uniform solutions in a broad range of solvents, even in the presence of other alkoxides or metallic derivatives. These alkoxides are highly reactive toward nucleophilic reagents like water, making them excellent candidates for generating oxides. Even though a gel's properties and how it reacts to heat treatment may be heavily dependent on the structure that was already established during the sol stage, the majority of reported investigations concentrated primarily on the finished product and its applications with little regard for the conditions of synthesis or the reaction mechanisms used to produce gels. Thus, the creation of colloidal aggregates determines the main properties of the final powder (Tao and Pescarmona, 2018) (Figure 9.4).

9.4.1.3 Plasma Spray Coating

Plasma spray coating is a type of thermal spray technique in which an arc is formed between two electrodes (cathode and anode) in a plasma-forming gas. The heated plasma gas expands and accelerates to a velocity of around 500 m/s. The high temperature of this technique melts the powder and expanding gas forces it toward substrates and layer-by-layer deposition takes place (Pham et al., 2019). It is one of the leading contenders for biomedical implants coatings because of its high porosity and deposition efficiency. It is approved by the FDA USA. The deposition efficiency of the coating can be enhanced by optimizing process parameters like arc power, plasma gas composition, flow rate, pressure, and standoff distance. In contrast with a number of other thin-film deposition strategies, this technology can be applied to a large surface area at a higher deposition rate (Ong et al., 2004). Plasma spray coating can be done on a variety of materials, including metals, polymers, ceramics, alloys, and composites. Some of the medical instruments formed of steel are coated with other antimicrobial metals like Cu etc. by the coating technique (Wrona et al., 2017).

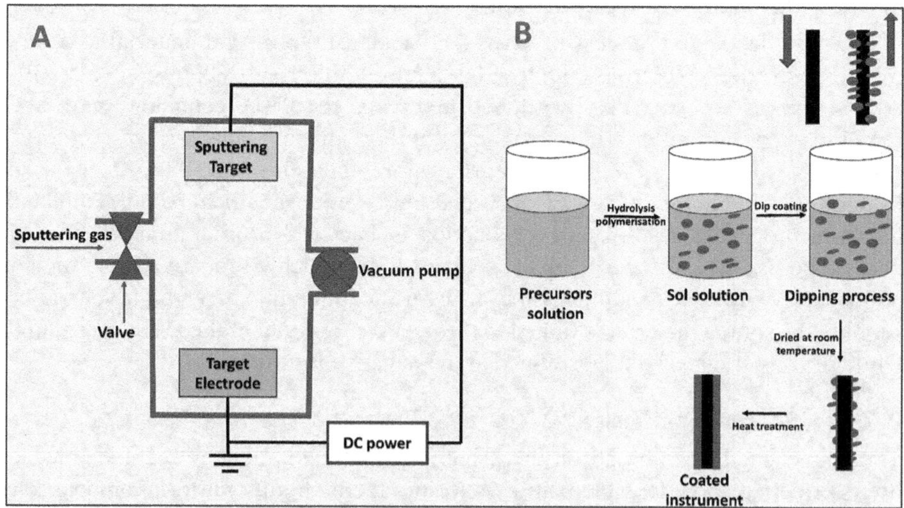

FIGURE 9.4 Nanomaterial-based antimicrobial coating on surgical tools using (a) physical vapor deposition and (b) sol-gel synthesis.

9.5 TEST AND EVALUATION OF NANOTECHNOLOGY-BASED ANTIBACTERIAL COATINGS

Nanoscale materials have unique physicochemical features that might provide new antibacterial activity pathways. Nevertheless is crucial to keep in mind that their potential negative effects should also be taken into account and assessed before using nanoscale materials as antimicrobial agents. Before assessing the real efficacy of a particular nanotechnology material as an antibacterial agent, additional testing and evaluation may be necessary because the conditions utilized in the laboratory might not perfectly match those encountered in a clinical situation.

1. **Disk diffusion test**: In this method, a disk loaded with our sample like NPs or any functionalized material is used to determine the growth of bacteria on its surfaces. The inhibition property of our sample can be easily visualized by the growth occurring on the disk (Figure 9.5).
2. **To determine the minimum inhibitory concentration (MIC) and minimum bacterial concentration (MBC):** A batch culture was used that contained different amounts of Ag/Cu NPs in solution. The MIC was identified as the minimum amount of sample (materials) that could inhibit the proliferation of the microorganism that we were looking for (Qi et al., 2004; Ruparelia et al., 2008). Much literature is available that has proven that Ag and Cu NPs have significant antimicrobial agents against *S. aureus, B. subtilis,* and *E. coli.* These determination tests such as disk diffusion test, MBC, and MIC specified the ambient antimicrobial nature of Ag NPs against *E. coli and S. aureus.* Even though the Cu NPs developed an oxide coating, they nevertheless outperformed other antimicrobial agents in their ability to combat *B. subtilis.* MIC/MBC determined in batch cultures with different concentrations of Ag and Cu NPs reflected their strain specificity.

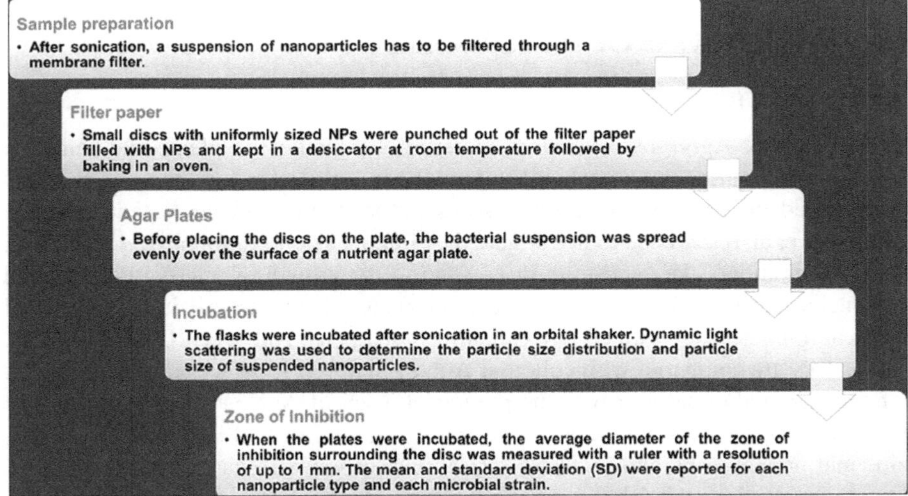

FIGURE 9.5 Workflow of the disk diffusion test.

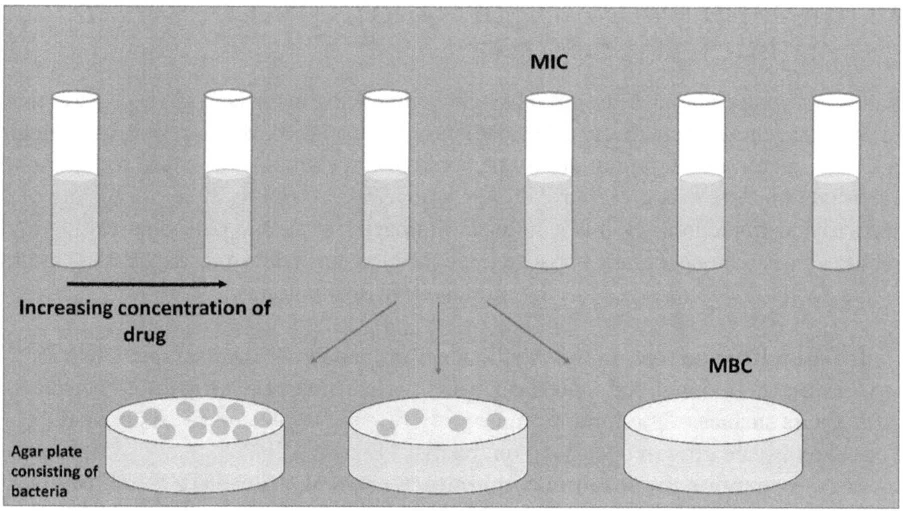

FIGURE 9.6 In vitro determination of minimum inhibitory concentration (MIC) and minimum bactericidal concentration (MBC).

It was hypothesized that Cu NPs have a greater affinity for *B. subtilis* surface-active groups, which may have led to its greater bactericidal activity. The mechanism of action of the Ag and Cu NPs has not yet been fully known. A cocktail of Ag and Cu NPs can produce hyper-bactericidal effects against mixed bacterial populations. To assess the bactericidal effectiveness of metal nanoparticles, thorough research and comparative investigations of strain-specific variations are needed before commercialization (Garibo et al., 2020) (Figure 9.6).

9.6 APPLICATIONS OF NANOMATERIALS

9.6.1 Catheters

The efficacy of AgNP-based coating materials for medical implants and catheters in preventing microbial and biofilm growth on substrates has been thoroughly investigated including glass-based, plastic, and synthetic polymer-based catheters. Agnihotri et al. researched to investigate the effectiveness of immobilized AgNPs on a silanol-modified glass substrate in preventing the growth of microorganisms and concluded that it could be used as a coating material for surgical instruments and medical implants as it is an effective disinfectant against both *E. coli* and *B. subtilis*. These NPs are compared with colloidal AgNPs and AgCl surfaces that released Ag ions, which additionally proved the greater efficacy of AgNPs toward bactericidal In another study, central venous catheters (CVCs) are coated with silver sulfadiazine and proved to be anti-infective for short insertion with bactericidal properties (Agnihotri et al., 2013; Walder et al., 2002). Catheters fabricated from AgNP and their role in the prevention of CAUTIs or catheter-related bloodstream infections

(CBSI) are the subject of a remarkable amount of research. Upon contact with the blood, the catheter's substrates create a biofilm, or surface thrombus, which begins to absorb proteins and serves as a breeding ground for bacteria (Betjes, 2011; Roe et al., 2008). Applications of AgNP-based coatings on catheters implanted for urogenital and vascular infections are also being explored. Urinary catheters with AgNP coating are better than uncoated catheters; in addition, the CAUTI was significantly reduced after the application of the coating and the absolute risk of a decrease in catheter-associated bacteria values ranged from 0.5% to 32% (Johnson et al., 2006).

According to Seymour, the risk of developing CAUTI was higher during the control period, with a rate of 11.1%, compared to the standard rate of 7.3%. However, when silver-alloy-coated Foley catheters were used and evaluated, the rate decreased to 3.2%. This suggests that silver-coated catheters are effective in reducing UTIs by up to 20% (Seymour, 2006). Plastic catheters with AgNP implants were developed by Roe and colleagues in 2007 and significantly reduced the infection rate. Similarly, another study they conducted using AgNP polyurethane catheters during a 10-day trial showed promising antibacterial efficacy. However, it is intriguing that the test animals experienced an average body weight loss of 8%, which may be attributed to silver poisoning caused by the use of Ag-coated catheters.

Likewise, the use of external ventricular drainage (EVD) catheters in neurosurgery for patients with acute hydrocephalus poses a significant risk of microorganisms infecting the catheter surface and resulting in secondary infections. Upon conducting a comprehensive analysis of patients who received AgNP-coated EVDs and those who did not, Fichtner et al. determined that the use of silver-containing catheter coils acts as a local infection barrier. This approach has the potential to be a secure and effective method to minimize the occurrence of cerebrospinal fluid infections (Pollini et al., 2011; Fichtner et al., 2010).

9.6.2 Implants

Orthopedic surgeries are becoming more common today and gradually problems with infected joint prostheses have worsened, further leading to morbidity and even death (De Angelis et al., 2015). To combat implant-related infections, Thukkaram and colleagues did research in 2020 and created a new cure: They shielded Ti implants with an amorphous hydrocarbon (a-C: H) matrix containing AgNP nanocomposites. The antimicrobial in vitro test showed sufficient antibacterial effectiveness against *E. coli* and *S. aureus*. It also enhanced osteoblast adhesion and proliferation and was biocompatible. Such a technique of coating has become a viable choice for orthopedic implants due to its excellent properties. AgNPs, therefore, have significant potential and a promising future for preventing biofilm-related HAIs when used as a coating on biomedical implants (Thukkaram et al., 2020).

Interestingly, Hengel and colleagues demonstrated self-defending bone implants in their study using plasma electrolytic oxidation (PEO) to apply Cu-NPs and Ag as coating materials in different ratios on a biofunctionalized TiO_2 layer surface. PT-Ag and PEO-treated Ag-CU implants, containing Ag and Cu ratios of up to 75% and 25% were able to achieve complete adhesion while preventing the adhesion bacteria (Van Hengel et al., 2020; Yoon et al., 2007).

It has been shown that ZnO NPs can be used as a surface modification material on titanium implants used for orthopedics, oral implants, and other medical devices. These coatings have antimicrobial, anti-corrosive, and osteogenesis-promoting properties and can help titanium implants overcome their implant-borne infections and low rates of osteogenesis (Wang et al., 2021). ZnO NPs have been used as a coating and as an osteogenesis-promoting substance as reported by Memarzadeh et al. Their results showed that a substrate coated with a 100% ZnO composite exhibited significant antimicrobial activity against *S. aureus* and also helped promote osteogenesis since ZnO immobilized on the substrate enabled osteoblast cells to adhere, grow, and proliferate to become metabolically active. These data suggested that a ZnO-based coating material on the surface of implants could serve as a promising and effective treatment in the future, specifically in the context of bone and dental implants (Memarzadeh et al., 2015).

Titanium has been a popular choice for biomedical implants in dentistry since the 1960s due to its effectiveness in dental therapy. A research study by Doran et al. examined the potential neoplastic transformation of cells on orthopedic implants and found that titanium ions or particles did not have any adverse effects on the cells, indicating that they are not carcinogenic or lethal (Doran et al., 1998). As a result, craniofacial TiO_2 implants have become the most commonly used implant commercially, as they reduce costs and lower the risk of infections (Cho and Gosain, 2004).

According to a recent study, hydroxyapatite (HA)/MoS_2-coated self-activating implants can inhibit *S. aureus* and *E. coli* infections as well as promote bone regeneration by promoting the differentiation of mesenchymal stem cells into osteoblasts through changes in the cell membrane and mitochondrial membrane potential (Fu et al., 2021). Another study team produces an antimicrobial implant by encasing titanium implants in chitosan-modified MoS_2 nanosheets loaded with Ag NPs to provide them with an antibacterial effect. Shin et al. used MoS_2 nanoflakes on titanium dental implants as an antibacterial surface coating (Zhu et al., 2020).

9.6.3 Dental Fillers

Ahmad et al. created porous, elastomeric, and antibacterial PU-CuO-coated biocompatible materials that are particularly useful against an epidemic methicillin-resistant strain of *Staphylococcus aureus* (EMRSA). The features of the CuO NPs in the PU fiber matrix, which rely on the pore size and film thickness, have a substantial effect on the level of MRSA inhibition. Both dental applications and catheters use these coatings. CuO NPs are widely used in dental caries (to protect the teeth and create an antifouling coating). To avoid the development of biofilms, these coatings used in mouth guards eliminate or stop the adhesion of bacteria (Ahmad et al., 2012; Eshed et al., 2012).

9.6.4 Contact Lenses

Contact lens use is the single largest risk factor for microbial keratitis, and contact lenses are one of the most significant medical implants today, where bacterial biofilm formation promotes infection (Campolo et al., 2022). In addition, CuO is used industrially and is combined with other metals to enhance their antibacterial effect. Using a high-intensity ultrasonic horn and so on chemical deposition, Nahum et al. coated a Zn-CuO conjugated nanoparticle onto a PureVision balafilcon—soft contact lenses. The antibacterial mode of action was based on ROS generation to disrupt the bacterial membrane and was evaluated against pathogenic strains of *S. epidermidis* and *P. aeruginosa* implicated in contact lens-associated infectious keratitis (Nahum et al., 2019).

9.7 CONCLUSION AND FUTURE PERSPECTIVE

The increased availability of implants in the market has transformed the healthcare sector. However, tackling bacterial infections associated with such technologies has posed a significant challenge but also, brought forth an opportunity for improvement. Previously, the prescription of antibiotics was used to prevent such infections, but this led to an increase in antimicrobial resistance. Additionally, many microorganisms form a sturdy resistant biofilm on the implant surface enhancing the bacterial resistance to antibiotics. However, the advent of nanotechnology has resulted in the introduction of various fabrication techniques to develop multifunctional, bioactive, and biocompatible materials with enhanced physicochemical characteristics. Hence, utilizing different nanoparticles and two-dimensional nanomaterials offers a new avenue to combat antimicrobial infections while minimizing the probability of the development of antimicrobial resistance. This chapter provides comprehensive details regarding the industrial applications of a variety of nanoparticles in the treatment of surfaces, especially surgical tools and implants to improve their antimicrobial characteristics.

An in-depth understanding of the mechanism of antimicrobial action is pertinent, before the utilization of NPs for antimicrobial coating. It is crucial to understand the antimicrobial action mechanism before using NPs as antimicrobial coating materials. Various studies have reported cell membrane damage, oxidative stress induction, and cellular protein and DNA damage as the most common mechanisms of action. NPs are composed of various metals such as silver, copper, zinc, and magnesium, and their oxides act by disrupting bacterial cell membranes. Whereas, titanium and iron oxide NPs result in oxidative damage to cellular DNA and proteins due to the production of ROS. Moreover, two-dimensional nanomaterials act on various bacteria by destroying their cell membranes through a process of ROS generation, direct killing, and/or metabolic pathway switching. Despite the similarity in the killing mechanism of metal oxides and 2D nanomaterials, the approach is sometimes very different. For instance, "Contact killing" occurs in copper oxide-based coatings, but photothermal and photodynamic treatments are frequently employed with MoS_2 nanosheet-coated implants.

Parallelly, the shortage of information from in vivo investigations has posed a significant challenge to research translation. The long-term effects of nanomaterial technology in animal models remain a mystery, leading to questions regarding the outcomes of implants treated with NP coatings in different animal models despite intensive research being performed utilizing different animal models. This chapter aims to provide insight to accelerate the development of new effective, non-toxic, and cost-effective antimicrobial coatings to minimize the exponentially increasing hospital-acquired infections.

ACKNOWLEDGMENT

The authors acknowledge CSIR (Government of India) for Mohit Kamboj's research fellowship (File No 09/1005 (12213)/2021-EMR-I) and SERB (Government of India) for a research grant (SRG/2021/002428).

REFERENCES

Agnihotri, S., Mukherji, S., Mukherji, S., 2013. Immobilized silver nanoparticles enhance contact killing and show highest efficacy: Elucidation of the mechanism of bactericidal action of silver. *Nanoscale* 5, 7328–7340.

Ahmad, Z., Vargas-Reus, M. A., Bakhshi, R., Ryan, F., Ren, G. G., Oktar, F., & Allaker, R. P. (2012). Antimicrobial properties of electrically formed elastomeric polyurethane–copper oxide nanocomposites for medical and dental applications. In *Methods in enzymology* (Vol. 509, pp. 87–99). Academic Press.

Ahmadabadi, H.Y., Yu, K., Kizhakkedathu, J.N., 2020. Surface modification approaches for prevention of implant associated infections. *Colloids Surfaces B Biointerfaces* 193, 111116.

Almoudi, M.M., Hussein, A.S., Abu Hassan, M.I., Mohamad Zain, N., 2018. A systematic review on antibacterial activity of zinc against *Streptococcus mutans*. *Saudi Dent. J.* 30, 283–291.

Arbab, A.S., Bashaw, L.A., Miller, B.R., Jordan, E.K., Lewis, B.K., Kalish, H., Frank, J.A., 2003. Characterization of biophysical and metabolic properties of cells labeled with superparamagnetic iron oxide nanoparticles and transfection agent for cellular MR imaging. *Radiology* 229, 838–846.

Arciola, C.R., Campoccia, D., Montanaro, L., 2018. Implant infections: Adhesion, biofilm formation and immune evasion. *Nat. Rev. Microbiol.* 16, 397–409.

Arciola, C.R., Campoccia, D., Speziale, P., Montanaro, L., Costerton, J.W., 2012. Biofilm formation in Staphylococcus implant infections. A review of molecular mechanisms and implications for biofilm-resistant materials. *Biomaterials* 33, 5967–5982.

Balendhran, S., Walia, S., Nili, H., Ou, J.Z., Zhuiykov, S., Kaner, R.B., Sriram, S., Bhaskaran, M., Kalantar-Zadeh, K., 2013. Two-dimensional molybdenum trioxide and dichalcogenides. *Adv. Funct. Mater.* 23, 3952–3970.

Baptista, A., Silva, F., Porteiro, J., Míguez, J., Pinto, G., 2018. Sputtering physical vapour deposition (PVD) coatings: A critical review on process improvement andmarket trend demands. *Coatings* 8, 402.

Bazaka, K., Jacob, M.V., Crawford, R.J., Ivanova, E.P., 2012. Efficient surface modification of biomaterial to prevent biofilm formation and the attachment of microorganisms. *Appl. Microbiol. Biotechnol.* 95, 299–311.

Betjes, M.G.H., 2011. Prevention of catheter-related bloodstream infection in patients on hemodialysis. *Nat. Rev. Nephrol.* 7, 257–265.

Bjarnsholt, T., 2013. The role of bacterial biofilms in chronic infections. *APMIS* 121, 1–58.

Büttner, H., Mack, D., Rohde, H., 2015. Structural basis of *Staphylococcus epidermidis* biofilm formation: Mechanisms and molecular interactions. *Front. Cell. Infect. Microbiol.* 5, 1–15.

Campolo, A., Pifer, R., Shannon, P., Crary, M., 2022. Microbial adherence to contact lenses and *Pseudomonas aeruginosa* as a model organism for microbial keratitis. *Pathogens* 11, 1383.

Cho, Y.R., Gosain, A.K., 2004. Biomaterials in craniofacial reconstruction. *Clin. Plast. Surg.* 31, 377–385.

Choi, J.R., Yong, K.W., Choi, J.Y., Nilghaz, A., Lin, Y., Xu, J., Lu, X., 2018. Black phosphorus and its biomedical applications. *Theranostics* 8, 1005–1026.

Ciarolla, A.A., Lapin, N., Williams, D., Chopra, R., Greenberg, D.E., 2023. Physical approaches to prevent and treat bacterial biofilm. *Antibiotics* 12, 54.

Correa, M.G., Martínez, F.B., Vidal, C.P., Streitt, C., Escrig, J., de Dicastillo, C.L., 2020. Antimicrobial metal-based nanoparticles: A review on their synthesis, types and antimicrobial action. *Beilstein J. Nanotechnol.* 11, 1450–1469.

De Angelis, G., Mutters, N.T., Minkley, L., Holderried, F., Tacconelli, E., 2015. Prosthetic joint infections in the elderly. *Infection* 43, 629–637.

Donlan, R.M., 2001. Biofilms and device-associated infections. *Emerg. Infect. Dis.* 7, 277–281.

Doran, A., Law, F.C., Allen, M.J., Rushton, N., 1998. Neoplastic transformation of cells by soluble but not particulate forms of metals used in orthopaedic implants. *Biomaterials* 19, 751–759.

Eby, D.M., Luckarift, H.R., Johnson, G.R., 2009. Hybrid antimicrobial enzyme and silver nanoparticle coatings for medical Instruments. *ACS Appl. Mater. Interfaces* 1, 1553–1560.

Ermini, M.L., Voliani, V., 2021. Antimicrobial nano-agents: The copper age. *ACS Nano* 15, 6008–6029.

Eshed, M., Lellouche, J., Matalon, S., Gedanken, A., Banin, E., 2012. Sonochemical coatings of ZnO and CuO nanoparticles inhibit *Streptococcus mutans* biofilm formation on teeth model. *Langmuir* 28, 12288–12295.

Ferrari, M., 2005. Cancer nanotechnology: Opportunities and challenges. *Nat. Rev. Cancer* 5, 161–171.

Fichtner, J., Güresir, E., Seifert, V., Raabe, A., 2010. Efficacy of silver-bearing external ventricular drainage catheters: A retrospective analysis. *J. Neurosurg.* 112, 840–846.

Fu, J., Zhu, W., Liu, X., Liang, C., Zheng, Y., Li, Z., Liang, Y., Zheng, D., Zhu, S., Cui, Z., Wu, S., 2021. Self-activating anti-infection implant. *Nat. Commun.* 12, 1–13.

Garibo, D., Borbón-Nuñez, H.A., de León, J.N.D., García Mendoza, E., Estrada, I., Toledano-Magaña, Y., Tiznado, H., Ovalle-Marroquin, M., Soto-Ramos, A.G., Blanco, A., Rodríguez, J.A., Romo, O.A., Chávez-Almazán, L.A., Susarrey-Arce, A., 2020. Green synthesis of silver nanoparticles using *Lysiloma acapulcensis* exhibit high-antimicrobial activity. *Sci. Rep.* 10, 1–11.

Gold, K., Slay, B., Knackstedt, M., Gaharwar, A.K., 2018. Antimicrobial activity of metal and metal-oxide based nanoparticles. *Adv. Ther.* 1, 1–15.

Gonzalez, L., Loza, R.J., Han, K.Y., Sunoqrot, S., Cunningham, C., Purta, P., Drake, J., Jain, S., Hong, S., Chang, J.H., 2013. Nanotechnology in corneal neovascularization therapy - A review. *J. Ocul. Pharmacol. Ther.* 29, 124–134.

Grass, G., Rensing, C., Solioz, M., 2011. Metallic copper as an antimicrobial surface. *Appl. Environ. Microbiol.* 77, 1541–1547.

Gravante, G., Sorge, R., Giordan, N., Georgescu, S.R., Morariu, S.H., Stoicescu, I., Clatici, V., 2013. Multicenter clinical trial on the performance and tolerability of the hyaluronic acid-collagenase ointment for the treatment of chronic venous ulcers: A preliminary pilot study. *Eur. Rev. Med. Pharmacol. Sci.* 17, 2721–2727.

Halbus, A.F., Horozov, T.S., Paunov, V.N., 2019. Controlling the antimicrobial action of surface modified magnesium hydroxide nanoparticles. *Biomimetics* 4, 41.

Hall, C.W., Mah, T.F., 2017. Molecular mechanisms of biofilm-based antibiotic resistance and tolerance in pathogenic bacteria. *FEMS Microbiol. Rev.* 41, 276–301.

Hu, W., Peng, C., Luo, W., Lv, M., Li, X., Li, D., Huang, Q., Fan, C., 2010. Graphene-based antibacterial paper. *ACS Nano* 4, 4317–4323.

Jabir, N.R., Tabrez, S., Ashraf, G.M., Shakil, S., Damanhouri, G.A., Kamal, M.A., 2012. Nanotechnology-based approaches in anticancer research. *Int. J. Nanomedicine* 7, 4391–4408.

Johnson, J.R., Kuskowski, M.A., Wilt, T.J., 2006. Systematic review: Antimicrobial urinary catheters to prevent catheter-associated urinary tract infection in hospitalized patients. *Ann. Intern. Med.* 144, 116–126.

Joo, H.S., Otto, M., 2012. Molecular basis of in vivo biofilm formation by bacterial pathogens. *Chem. Biol.* 19, 1503–1513.

Kou, L., Chen, C., Smith, S.C., 2015. Phosphorene: Fabrication, properties, and applications. *J. Phys. Chem. Lett.* 6, 2794–2805.

Kumar, P., Kamboj, M., Jaiwal, R., Pundir, C.S., 2019. Fabrication of an improved amperometric creatinine biosensor based on enzymes nanoparticles bound to Au electrode. *Biomarkers* 24, 739–749.

Lee, D., Seo, Y., Khan, M.S., Hwang, J., Jo, Y., Son, J., Lee, K., Park, C., Chavan, S., Gilad, A.A., Choi, J., 2018. Use of nanoscale materials for the effective prevention and extermination of bacterial biofilms. *Biotechnol. Bioprocess Eng.* 23, 1–10.

Loh, K.P., Bao, Q., Ang, P.K., Yang, J., 2010. The chemistry of graphene. *J. Mater. Chem.* 20, 2277–2289.

Luo, M., Fan, T., Zhou, Y., Zhang, H., Mei, L., 2019. 2D black phosphorus–based biomedical applications. *Adv. Funct. Mater.* 29, 1–19.

Mahamuni-Badiger, P.P., Patil, P.M., Badiger, M.V., Patel, P.R., Thorat-Gadgil, B.S., Pandit, A., Bohara, R.A., 2020. Biofilm formation to inhibition: Role of zinc oxide-based nanoparticles. *Mater. Sci. Eng.* C 108, 110319.

Marassi, V., Di Cristo, L., Smith, S.G.J., Ortelli, S., Blosi, M., Costa, A.L., Reschiglian, P., Volkov, Y., Prina-Mello, A., 2018. Silver nanoparticles as a medical device in healthcare settings: A five-step approach for candidate screening of coating agents. *R. Soc. Open Sci.* 5, 171113.

Memarzadeh, K., Sharili, A.S., Huang, J., Rawlinson, S.C.F., Allaker, R.P., 2015. Nanoparticulate zinc oxide as a coating material for orthopedic and dental implants. *J. Biomed. Mater. Res. A* 103, 981–989.

Metzel, E., 1990. Neurotraumatologie im Alten Agypten. *Neurochirurgia.* 33, 78–80.

Murthy, S., Effiong, P., Fei, C.C., 2020. Metal oxide nanoparticles in biomedical applications, In Yarub Al-Douri (Ed.). *Metal Oxide Powder Technologies: Fundamentals, Processing Methods and Applications.* Elsevier, Kuala Lumpur, Malaysia.

Nahum, Y., Israeli, R., Mircus, G., Perelshtein, I., Ehrenberg, M., Gutfreund, S., Gedanken, A., Bahar, I., 2019. Antibacterial and physical properties of a novel sonochemical-assisted Zn-CuO contact lens nanocoating. *Graefe's Arch. Clin. Exp. Ophthalmol.* 257, 95–100.

Nguyen, N.Y.T., Grelling, N., Wetteland, C.L., Rosario, R., Liu, H., 2018. Antimicrobial activities and mechanisms of magnesium oxide nanoparticles (nMgO) against pathogenic bacteria, yeasts, and biofilms. *Sci. Rep.* 8, 1–23.

Olsen, M.A., Nepple, J.J., Riew, K.D., Lenke, L.G., Bridwell, K.H., Mayfield, J., Fraser, V.J., 2008. Risk factors for surgical site infection following orthopaedic spinal operations. *J. Bone Jt. Surg.* 90, 62–69.

Ong, J.L., Carnes, D.L., Bessho, K., 2004. Evaluation of titanium plasma-sprayed and plasma-sprayed hydroxyapatite implants in vivo. *Biomaterials* 25, 4601–4606.

Osés, J., Fuentes, G.G., Palacio, J.F., Esparza, J., García, J.A., Rodríguez, R., 2018. Antibacterial functionalization of PVD coatings on ceramics. *Coatings* 8, 1–12.

Otto, M., 2013. Staphylococcal infections: Mechanisms of biofilm maturation and detachment as critical determinants of pathogenicity. *Annu. Rev. Med.* 64, 175–188.

Ouyang, J., Liu, R.Y., Chen, W., Liu, Z., Xu, Q., Zeng, K., Deng, L., Shen, L., Liu, Y.N., 2018. A black phosphorus based synergistic antibacterial platform against drug resistant bacteria. *J. Mater. Chem. B* 6, 6302–6310.

Pham, D.Q., Berndt, C.C., Gbureck, U., Zreiqat, H., Truong, V.K., Ang, A.S.M., 2019. Mechanical and chemical properties of Baghdadite coatings manufactured by atmospheric plasma spraying. *Surf. Coatings Technol.* 378, 124945.

Pollini, M., Paladini, F., Catalano, M., Taurino, A., Licciulli, A., Maffezzoli, A., Sannino, A., 2011. Antibacterial coatings on haemodialysis catheters by photochemical deposition of silver nanoparticles. *J. Mater. Sci. Mater. Med.* 22, 2005–2012.

Qi, L., Xu, Z., Jiang, X., Hu, C., Zou, X., 2004. Preparation and antibacterial activity of chitosan nanoparticles. *Carbohydr. Res.* 339, 2693–2700.

Rai, M., Yadav, A., Gade, A., 2009. Silver nanoparticles as a new generation of antimicrobials. *Biotechnol. Adv.* 27, 76–83.

Ramasamy, M., Lee, J., 2016. Recent nanotechnology approaches for prevention and treatment of biofilm-associated infections on medical devices. *Biomed Res. Int.* 2016, 1851242.

Rimondini, L., Cochis, A., Varoni, E., Azzimonti, B., Carrassi, A., 2014. Handbook of Bioceramics and Biocomposites. Springer International Publishing, Switzerland.

Roco, M.C., 2003. Nanotechnology: Convergence with modern biology and medicine. *Curr. Opin. Biotechnol.* 14, 337–346.

Roe, D., Karandikar, B., Bonn-Savage, N., Gibbins, B., Roullet, J.B., 2008. Antimicrobial surface functionalization of plastic catheters by silver nanoparticles. *J. Antimicrob. Chemother.* 61, 869–876.

Roy, S., Mondal, A., Yadav, V., Sarkar, A., Banerjee, R., Sanpui, P., Jaiswal, A., 2019. Mechanistic insight into the antibacterial activity of chitosan exfoliated MoS2 nanosheets: Membrane damage, metabolic inactivation, and oxidative stress. *ACS Appl. Bio Mater.* 2, 2738–2755.

Ruparelia, J.P., Chatterjee, A.K., Duttagupta, S.P., Mukherji, S., 2008. Strain specificity in antimicrobial activity of silver and copper nanoparticles. *Acta Biomater.* 4, 707–716.

Sahoo, J., Sarkhel, S., Mukherjee, N., Jaiswal, A., 2022. nanomaterial-based antimicrobial coating for biomedical implants: New age solution for biofilm-associated infections. *ACS Omega* 7, 45962–45980.

Sathyanarayanan, M.B., Balachandranath, R., Genji Srinivasulu, Y., Kannaiyan, S.K., Subbiahdoss, G., 2013. The effect of gold and iron-oxide nanoparticles on biofilm-forming pathogens. *ISRN Microbiol.* 2013, 272086.

Seymour, C., 2006. Audit of catheter-associated UTI using silver alloy-coated Foley catheters. *Br. J. Nurs.* 15, 598–603.

Shin, M.H., Baek, S.M., Polyakov, A.V., Semenova, I.P., Valiev, R.Z., Hwang, W.B., Hahn, S.K., Kim, H.S., 2018. Molybdenum disulfide surface modification of ultrafine-grained titanium for enhanced cellular growth and antibacterial effect. *Sci. Rep.* 8, 1–10.

Tao, Y., Pescarmona, P.P., 2018. Nanostructured oxides synthesised via scCO2-assisted sol-gel methods and their application in catalysis. *Catalysts* 8, 1–28.

Thukkaram, M., Sitaram, S., Kannaiyan, S.K., Subbiahdoss, G., 2014. Antibacterial efficacy of iron-oxide nanoparticles against biofilms on different biomaterial surfaces. *Int. J. Biomater.* 2014, 716080.

Thukkaram, M., Vaidulych, M., Kylián, O., Hanuš, J., Rigole, P., Aliakbarshirazi, S., Asadian, M., Nikiforov, A., Van Tongel, A., Biederman, H., Coenye, T., Du Laing, G., Morent, R., De Wilde, L., Verbeken, K., De Geyter, N., 2020. Investigation of Ag/a-C:H nanocomposite coatings on titanium for orthopedic applications. *ACS Appl. Mater. Interfaces* 12, 23655–23666.

Van Hengel, I.A.J., Tierolf, M.W.A.M., Valerio, V.P.M., Minneboo, M., Fluit, A.C., Fratila-Apachitei, L.E., Apachitei, I., Zadpoor, A.A., 2020. Self-defending additively manufactured bone implants bearing silver and copper nanoparticles. *J. Mater. Chem. B* 8, 1589–1602.

Vasilev, K., Cook, J., Griesser, H.J., 2009. Antibacterial surfaces for biomedical devices. *Expert Rev Med Devices* 6, 553–567.

Veerachamy, S., Yarlagadda, T., Manivasagam, G., Yarlagadda, P.K., 2014. Bacterial adherence and biofilm formation on medical implants: A review. *Proc. Inst. Mech. Eng. Part H J. Eng. Med.* 228, 1083–1099.

Walder, B., Pittet, D., Tramèr, M.R., 2002. Prevention of bloodstream infections with central venous catheters treated with anti-infective agents depends on catheter type and insertion time: Evidence from a meta-analysis. *Infect. Control Hosp. Epidemiol.* 23(12), 748–756.

Wang, Z., Wang, X., Wang, Y., Zhu, Y., Liu, X., Zhou, Q., 2021. NanoZnO-modified titanium implants for enhanced anti-bacterial activity, osteogenesis and corrosion resistance. *J. Nanobiotechnol.* 19, 1–23.

Wrona, A., Bilewska, K., Lis, M., Kamińska, M., Olszewski, T., Pajzderski, P., Więcław, G., Jaśkiewicz, M., Kamysz, W., 2017. Antimicrobial properties of protective coatings produced by plasma spraying technique. *Surf. Coatings Technol.* 318, 332–340.

Xiong, Z., Zhang, X., Zhang, S., Lei, L., Ma, W., Li, D., Wang, W., Zhao, Q., Xing, B., 2018. Bacterial toxicity of exfoliated black phosphorus nanosheets. *Ecotoxicol. Environ. Saf.* 161, 507–514.

Yoon, K.Y., Hoon Byeon, J., Park, J.H., Hwang, J., 2007. Susceptibility constants of *Escherichia coli* and *Bacillus subtilis* to silver and copper nanoparticles. *Sci. Total Environ.* 373, 572–575.

Zhu, M., Liu, X., Tan, L., Cui, Z., Liang, Y., Li, Z., Kwok Yeung, K.W., Wu, S., 2020. Photo-responsive chitosan/Ag/MoS2 for rapid bacteria-killing. *J. Hazard. Mater.* 383, 121122.

Zou, X., Zhang, L., Wang, Z., Luo, Y., 2016. Mechanisms of the antimicrobial activities of graphene materials. *J. Am. Chem. Soc.* 138, 2064–2077.

10 Advances in Antiviral Coating

Harnessing Nanoparticles and Fuzzy Logic

Yogeesh Nijalingappa and P. William

10.1 INTRODUCTION

10.1.1 BRIEF OVERVIEW OF ANTIVIRAL COATINGS

Particularly in the aftermath of the COVID-19 pandemic, antiviral coatings have grown in significance in the battle against infectious illnesses. Due to the limits of conventional antiviral coatings, new antiviral coating trends are moving towards the application of nanoparticles and fuzzy logic. This chapter aims to provide an overview of antiviral coatings, discuss the use of nanoparticles and fuzzy logic in creating antiviral coatings, present case studies that show the efficacy of these novel approaches, and highlight the potential applications of antiviral coatings, as well as the difficulties and limitations that require further study.

10.1.2 IMPORTANCE OF DEVELOPING EFFECTIVE ANTIVIRAL COATINGS

A number of factors make the creation of potent antiviral coatings crucial:

- **Preventing the transmission of infectious diseases:** Contaminated surfaces can allow the spread of viral illnesses, including the flu, the common cold, and COVID-19. Antiviral coatings can lessen the danger of dissemination and aid in the prevention of epidemics in public places, healthcare institutions, and other high-contact locations by preventing the survival and transmission of viruses on surfaces.
- **Improving public health and safety:** By decreasing the spread of infectious illnesses, safeguarding vulnerable people, and avoiding infections connected with healthcare, antiviral coatings can help improve public health outcomes. This can reduce the number of diseases, hospital stays, and fatalities, as well as lessen the strain on healthcare systems.
- **Supporting personal protective measures:** By adding an extra layer of defence against viral transmission, antiviral coatings on personal protective equipment (PPE) and other high-touch surfaces can encourage and

DOI: 10.1201/9781003432661-10

reinforce the practice of good hygiene, such as consistent handwashing and avoiding touching one's face.

- **Enabling safer reopening of enterprises and public spaces:** By lowering the danger of viral transmission through surfaces, antiviral coatings can significantly contribute to the creation of safer surroundings for the reopening of businesses, schools, and public places. This may aid in regaining public trust and making it easier to resume social and economic activity.
- **Supporting infection control techniques:** Antiviral coatings can be a useful tool in all-encompassing infection control strategies, working in conjunction with other preventative measures including immunisation, hand washing, and social seclusion. When other precautions would be difficult to put into place or keep up, they might offer an extra layer of defence against viral transmission.
- **Technological innovation and advancement:** The creation of antiviral coatings necessitates the use of cutting-edge technologies, including nanotechnology, fuzzy logic, and sophisticated materials science. New applications and solutions in other fields, like healthcare, consumer goods, and industrial settings, may be made possible by advancements in this one.
- **Contributing to global health and well-being:** Improving public health outcomes, lowering the burden of viral infections, and raising general standards of living for people and communities globally are just a few of the ways that effective antiviral coatings have the potential to significantly improve global health and well-being.

The creation of potent antiviral coatings is crucial for reducing the transmission of infectious illnesses, safeguarding the public's health, assisting infection control techniques, encouraging personal protective measures, and developing technology and innovation. These coatings represent a key area for research and development because they have the potential to be crucial in enhancing public health outcomes and supporting international efforts to battle infectious illnesses.

10.1.3 Objectives of the Chapter

The following might be among the goals of the chapter on the significance of creating potent antiviral coatings:

- Recognising the importance of antiviral coatings in reducing the transmission of infectious illnesses, safeguarding the public's health, and supporting infection control methods is necessary to achieve this purpose.
- Examining the state of antiviral coatings research at the moment: Reviewing the current research and literature on antiviral coatings is necessary to achieve this goal. This includes looking at their modes of action, viability against various viruses, and drawbacks.
- Examining the various technologies and materials used in the creation of antiviral coatings, such as nanotechnology, fuzzy logic, and advanced

materials science, and comprehending their benefits and drawbacks, is the goal of this objective.
- Investigating the potential uses of antiviral coatings in a variety of contexts, including healthcare facilities, public areas, consumer products, and industrial settings, as well as comprehending their function in preventing viral transmission, is the goal of this objective.
- Assessing the difficulties and factors to be taken into account when generating antiviral coatings This aim entails recognising the difficulties and factors to be taken into account when designing, producing, and using antiviral coatings, such as legal requirements, affordability, robustness, and safety.
- Critically examining the advantages and disadvantages of antiviral coatings, including their efficacy, robustness, cost-effectiveness, and possible effects on the environment and human health, is the goal of this purpose.
- Examining potential future directions and opportunities in antiviral coatings research, including those presented by emerging technologies, novel materials, and interdisciplinary collaborations, and their potential effects on public health and safety, is the goal of this objective.

Overall, the chapter's goals may include giving readers a thorough understanding of the significance of creating efficient antiviral coatings, reviewing the current state of research, assessing technologies and materials, looking at applications, evaluating challenges and factors, looking at advantages and disadvantages, and investigating future directions and opportunities in this area.

10.2 ANTIVIRAL COATINGS: A REVIEW

10.2.1 Traditional Antiviral Coatings

Traditional antiviral coatings usually involve chemical substances that are applied to surfaces to stop viruses from multiplying and spreading. These coatings could include substances like triclosan, quaternary ammonium compounds (QACs), silver ions, copper ions, and others. Due to their broad-spectrum antibacterial capabilities, which include antiviral activity against enveloped viruses (Russell, 2004; Li and Macdonald, 2020; Li et al., 2020) [, QACs, for instance, have been widely employed in disinfectants and surface coatings. Similar antiviral effects have been shown in silver and copper ions, which disrupt the viral envelope or prevent viral replication (Lara et al., 2010; Warnes et al., 2015). Due to its broad-spectrum antibacterial capabilities, the substance triclosan, which is frequently found in consumer items, has also been employed in antiviral coatings.

10.2.2 Limitations of Traditional Antiviral Coatings

Traditional antiviral coatings have various drawbacks, despite their efficacy against particular pathogens. One drawback is the possibility of viral resistance emerging to the chemicals utilised in these coatings, a condition comparable to antibiotic resistance (Cassini et al., 2019). In addition, certain conventional antiviral coatings may have a short shelf life and gradually lose their efficacy through use, cleaning, or exposure to the environment (Block et al., 2020). Furthermore, not all viruses can be effectively treated by conventional antiviral coatings, since this depends on the virus type, strain, and the coating's particular mode of action (Kuiken et al., 2020).

10.2.3 Emerging Trends in Antiviral Coatings

The employment of cutting-edge technology and materials in antiviral coatings is an emerging trend that will improve the potency, longevity, and security of these coatings. For instance, researchers have investigated the use of photocatalytic coatings that, when exposed to light, can produce reactive oxygen species (ROS) that can inactivate viruses (Mitra et al., 2020). The use of self-cleaning coatings, polymer-based coatings, and electrochemical coatings that can prevent viral attachment and survival on surfaces are further growing developments (Tirelli et al., 2021). In addition, a developing trend in the realm of antiviral coatings is the introduction of antiviral characteristics into already-existing materials, such as textiles, plastics, and metals (Mezghani et al., 2019; Ravindranathan et al., 2021).

10.2.4 Nanoparticles as Potential Antiviral Agents

Due to their distinct characteristics and capacity to prevent viral attachment, entrance, replication, and dissemination, nanoparticles have emerged as intriguing candidates for antiviral coatings (Zhang et al., 2019). The antiviral properties of metal nanoparticles like silver, copper, and zinc nanoparticles have been thoroughly studied (Saha et al., 2020; Mincione et al., 2021). Quantum dots, graphene oxide, titanium dioxide, and other forms of nanoparticles have all demonstrated antiviral properties (Hu et al., 2020; Poma et al., 2021). Nanoparticles have a high surface area to volume ratio, adjustable characteristics, and the ability for controlled release of antiviral medicines, among other benefits that make them useful in antiviral coatings (Jiang et al., 2022). However, there are also worries over the environmental effects, regulatory compliance, and safety of nanoparticles.

10.3 NANOPARTICLES AND ANTIVIRAL COATINGS

10.3.1 Overview of Nanoparticles and Their Properties

Typically, particles having at least one dimension less than 100 nm are referred to as nanoparticles. They come in a wide range of sizes and forms and can be created from a number of materials, including metals, metal oxides, and polymers. Nanoparticles have a number of important characteristics that make them viable antiviral medicines, including a high surface area to volume ratio, special physical and chemical characteristics, and the capacity to be functionalised with certain molecules.

The size of nanoparticles, which range from 1 to 100 nm, is miniscule. Nanoparticles have special qualities that set them apart from their bulk counterparts due to their small size, which makes them very appealing for a variety of uses, such as antiviral coatings. Among the essential characteristics of nanoparticles are:

- **Size-dependent characteristics:** Nanoparticles differ from bulk materials in their changed optical, electrical, magnetic, and mechanical properties, as well as their enhanced surface area to volume ratio. These size-dependent characteristics can be used to create nanoparticles with particular antiviral capabilities.
- **High surface area:** Nanoparticles' high surface area to volume ratio enables them to interact with their surroundings, including viruses, more successfully. A possible antiviral impact might result from interactions between nanoparticles and virus particles due to the increased surface area.
- **Enhanced reactivity:** Nanoparticles often exhibit enhanced reactivity compared to bulk materials due to their small size and high surface area. Designing nanoparticles with antiviral characteristics, such as the capacity to interact with viral particles, damage viral envelopes, or prevent viral reproduction, can take advantage of this heightened reactivity.
- **Tunable qualities:** By adjusting the size, shape, surface chemistry, and composition of nanoparticles, unique features may be created. Due to their tunability, nanoparticles may be modified to meet the needs of various antiviral coating applications.
- **Versatile materials:** A variety of materials, including metals, metal oxides, polymers, ceramics, and carbon-based materials, can be used to create nanoparticles. Due to the variety of available materials, it is possible to create nanoparticles with various capabilities for antiviral coatings.
- **Stability and durability:** Nanoparticles are capable of exhibiting good stability and durability, which are crucial qualities for antiviral coatings that must endure a variety of environmental variables and continuous use.

Nanoparticles are interesting candidates for the creation of antiviral coatings with improved efficacy against viral infections due to their distinctive characteristics. To guarantee their safe and efficient usage, however, it is crucial to thoroughly assess the safety, toxicity, and regulatory issues related to the use of nanoparticles in antiviral coatings.

10.3.2 How Nanoparticles Can Be Used in Antiviral Coatings

There are several ways to include nanoparticles into coatings, such as by blending them into a polymer matrix or affixing them to a substrate. Nanoparticles can interact with viruses in a variety of ways after being applied to a surface, including by causing structural disruption, blocking attachment to host cells, or hindering viral reproduction.

Due to their distinctive characteristics, nanoparticles have shown considerable promise in the creation of antiviral coatings. The following are some applications for nanoparticles in antiviral coatings:

- **Viral inhibition:** It has been demonstrated that certain nanoparticles, including silver, copper, and zinc oxide nanoparticles, have inherent antiviral capabilities. By directly interacting with viral particles, destroying viral envelopes, stifling viral reproduction, and preventing viral attachment to host cells, these nanoparticles can lessen viral dissemination.

- **Antiviral agent release:** Nanoparticles can be created to contain or release antiviral substances like medications, peptides, or other active compounds. These nanoparticles may be added to coatings, where they can release the antiviral compounds over time in a progressive manner to produce a long-lasting antiviral impact.
- **Surface modification:** By altering the coatings' surface characteristics, nanoparticles can provide antiviral activities. As an illustration, antiviral compounds can be functionalised into nanoparticles or coated onto coating surfaces to provide a physical barrier that prevents viral adherence and penetration.
- **Photocatalytic activity:** A few nanoparticles, including titanium dioxide nanoparticles, have the ability to produce ROS when exposed to UV radiation. Photocatalytic nanoparticles are a possible alternative for antiviral coatings since these ROS can harm viral particles and reduce viral activity.
- **Self-cleaning qualities:** Self-cleaning nanoparticles, including superhydrophobic or superoleophobic nanoparticles, can be utilised to make antiviral coatings that stop viruses from adhering to surfaces. These nanoparticles can deter the attachment and propagation of viruses by repelling liquids, including other liquids.
- **Improved mechanical properties:** Nanoparticles may also be employed to enhance the mechanical characteristics of coatings, such as abrasion resistance, flexibility, and adhesion, which can help antiviral coatings last longer and work more effectively.

Antiviral coatings made using nanoparticles have the potential to be extremely efficient and long-lasting barriers against the propagation of viral infections. To understand the safety, effectiveness, and regulatory issues related to the use of nanoparticles in antiviral coatings and to optimise their performance for various applications, more study and assessment are required.

10.3.3 The Mechanism of Action of Nanoparticles against Viruses

Depending on the type of nanoparticle and the virus being targeted, the mechanism of action of nanoparticles against viruses might change. It has been demonstrated that several nanoparticles, including copper and silver nanoparticles, can damage the capsid, or viral envelope, rendering the virus inactive. Dendrimers and carbon nanotubes, among other nanoparticles, can obstruct viral reproduction or impede viral attachment to host cells.

Nanoparticles' particular characteristics and interactions with virus particles determine how effective their antiviral mechanism is. Here are a few typical ways that nanoparticles fight viruses:

- **Disruption of viral envelopes:** The viral envelope, a lipid coating that covers many viruses, can be affected by certain nanoparticles, including copper and silver nanoparticles. These nanoparticles have the potential to compromise the integrity of the viral envelope, causing viral contents to seep out and obstructing viral entrance into host cells.

- **Viral replication inhibition:** Some nanoparticles, like gold and zinc oxide, can prevent the reproduction of viruses by interfering with the proteins or viral enzymes required for the process. These nanoparticles have the ability to interfere with the viral life cycle and lessen viral reproduction, which prevents viral particles from spreading.
- **The production of reactive oxygen species (ROS):** Certain nanoparticles, like cerium oxide and titanium dioxide nanoparticles, have photocatalytic activity and can produce ROS when exposed to UV radiation. These ROS can damage viral particles and cause oxidative stress, which inhibits viral activity and replication.
- **Viral adsorption and inactivation:** Positively charged nanoparticles, such as chitosan and polyethyleneimine nanoparticles, can bind to and neutralise the surface charge of viral particles. This may hinder viral entrance and impede viral attachment to host cells, reducing the infectious potential of the virus.
- **Immunomodulation:** Some nanoparticles, like silica and gold particles, might alter immunological responses, enhancing the body's natural antiviral defences. These nanoparticles have the ability to activate immune cells, promote the generation of antiviral cytokines, and improve the immunological response to viral infections.
- **Physical barrier:** Nanoparticles can form a physical barrier on surfaces to stop virus particles from adhering and penetrating. Superhydrophobic or superoleophobic nanoparticles, for instance, may fend off liquids—including viruses—and stop them from adhering to surfaces, hence lowering the risk of viral infection.

It's crucial to remember that the precise kind of nanoparticles, the type of virus, and the experimental circumstances can all affect the mechanism of action of nanoparticles against viruses. To better understand how nanoparticles interact with various viruses and increase the efficacy of antiviral coatings, more study is required.

10.3.4 Advantages of Using Nanoparticles in Antiviral Coatings

Due to their special qualities, nanoparticles have various benefits when utilised in antiviral coatings. The following are some benefits of utilising nanoparticles in antiviral coatings:

- **High surface area to volume ratio:** Nanoparticles' high surface area to volume ratio enables them to interact and come into touch with virus particles more readily. As a result, they are better able to interact closely with more viral particles, which results in more efficient viral suppression.
- **Versatile antiviral mechanisms:** As was mentioned in the previous section, nanoparticles have the ability to disrupt viral envelopes, inhibit viral replication, produce ROS, bind to and inactivate viruses, alter immune

responses, and create physical barriers. This adaptability enables the development of antiviral coatings with a multifunctional strategy that may focus on various elements of viral diseases.

- **Broad-spectrum antiviral activity:** Many different kinds of nanoparticles have demonstrated broad-spectrum antiviral activity, which means they can stop the activity of a variety of viruses, including enveloped and non-enveloped viruses. This makes the use of nanoparticles for the creation of antiviral coatings that are effective against a variety of viruses, such as coronaviruses, influenza viruses, herpesviruses, and others, a potential alternative.
- **Potential for long-lasting activity:** Long-lasting antiviral action on coated surfaces is possible because nanoparticles may be designed to have sustained stability and endurance. This can lessen the requirement for periodic antiviral coating reapplication and offer ongoing protection against viral infection.
- **Compatibility with diverse surfaces and coating materials:** Nanoparticles may be added to a variety of coating materials, such as paints, polymers, fabrics, and metals, making them appropriate for use on a variety of surfaces. This gives designers more freedom when creating antiviral coatings for various settings, including hospitals, public transit, and high-touch surfaces.
- **Reduced environmental effect:** When employed in controlled and regulated applications, many nanoparticles utilised in antiviral coatings, such as silver nanoparticles, have been demonstrated to have minimal toxicity and environmental impact. In terms of environmental sustainability, this gives them a safer option to conventional antiviral medicines, such as harsh chemicals.

The safety, effectiveness, and long-term durability of nanoparticles in antiviral coatings need to be thoroughly investigated, and their regulatory clearance may differ depending on the location and use. However, due to their special qualities and benefits, nanoparticles hold great promise for the development of efficient and long-lasting antiviral coatings for a variety of surfaces and environments.

10.4 FUZZY LOGIC AND ANTIVIRAL COATINGS

10.4.1 What Is Fuzzy Logic and How It Works

A mathematical paradigm known as fuzzy logic addresses ambiguity and imprecision in decision-making. It is a development of traditional (crisp) logic, which is based on binary (true/false) values and was first developed by Lotfi A. Zadeh in the 1960s(Li and Macdonald, 2020). Fuzzy logic, in contrast to classical logic, which depends on precise values, allows for degrees of membership and ambiguity when assessing if a proposition is true or false.

Fuzzy sets and linguistic variables are used in fuzzy logic to represent and work with ambiguous or hazy data. Fuzzy sets show the linguistic variables that an element is most likely to belong to, such as "high," "medium," and "low," whereas linguistic variables are phrases that indicate qualitative features. Fuzzy logic is used to model and approximate human thinking and decision-making processes. Fuzzy rules are stated as "if-then" statements.

Fuzzy logic is a procedure with several phases. The system's inputs and outputs are first specified as fuzzy sets with the appropriate membership functions, which specify the degrees to which elements are members of the fuzzy sets. Following that, fuzzy rules are developed using methodologies driven by data or expert knowledge. These guidelines describe how the linguistic variables and their corresponding membership functions are used to map the inputs to the outputs. The fuzzy output is then generated by combining the fuzzy rules using fuzzy logic operators like AND, OR, and NOT. In order to provide a crisp result that may be utilised for decision-making or control activities, the fuzzy output is finally defuzzified.

Numerous disciplines, such as control systems, decision-making, pattern recognition, and optimisation, have made extensive use of fuzzy logic. Fuzzy logic may be utilised to create intelligent antiviral coatings that can adjust to various environmental factors, such as temperature, humidity, and virus load, in order to deliver the best antiviral effectiveness. Fuzzy logic allows the coatings to dynamically modify their antiviral activity in response to changing environmental factors, resulting in a more potent and effective antiviral treatment.

The use of fuzzy logic in antiviral coatings necessitates careful evaluation of the particular coating ingredients, ambient factors, and intended antiviral effectiveness. The potential of fuzzy logic in the design and optimisation of antiviral coatings for various applications has to be further explored and developed.

10.4.2 Application of Fuzzy Logic in Developing Antiviral Coatings

To increase the efficacy and adaptability of antiviral coatings to various situations, fuzzy logic has been used in their creation. Fuzzy logic can be used in the following ways to create antiviral coatings:

- **Adaptive antiviral activity:** Fuzzy logic may be utilised to create coatings with antiviral activity that can change depending on the environment. Fuzzy logic, for instance, may be used to create coatings that can alter the rate at which antiviral medicines release in response to changes in temperature, humidity, or viral load. This increases the coatings' efficacy by enabling them to deliver the best antiviral function under various circumstances.
- **Coatings with various functionalities:** In addition to having antiviral action, coatings with many functionalities may be designed using fuzzy logic. For instance, fuzzy logic may be used to create coatings that, depending on the surrounding environment, can also have antibacterial, antifungal, or self-cleaning qualities. As a result, the coatings are more adaptive and diverse and can offer thorough defence against a variety of diseases.
- **Control and decision-making:** Fuzzy logic may be used to create coatings that are intelligent and can adjust their antiviral activity based on in-the-moment feedback. In order to maximise the usage of antiviral

medications and extend the efficiency of the coating, fuzzy logic can be utilised to build coatings that can sense the viral load in the surrounding environment and change their antiviral activity appropriately.

- **Personalised coatings:** Fuzzy logic can be used to develop coatings that can be personalised based on individual needs and preferences. Fuzzy logic, for instance, may be used to create coatings that can be customised for various users, taking into consideration aspects like age, health, and sensitivity to particular elements. This enables the creation of personalised antiviral coatings that can offer the best protection while minimising any negative effects.
- **Risk evaluation and prediction:** Coatings that can evaluate and forecast the danger of viral transmission in various situations can be developed using fuzzy logic. Fuzzy logic, for instance, may be used to analyse variables like viral load, humidity, temperature, and airflow patterns to determine how likely it is that a virus would spread in a specific environment. The antiviral coating's performance can then be optimised by altering its activity in accordance with the risk level using the information provided.

In general, the use of fuzzy logic in the creation of antiviral coatings can increase their efficiency in providing defence against viral diseases in a variety of situations by improving their efficacy, flexibility, and versatility. To fully realise the promise of fuzzy logic in the design and optimisation of antiviral coatings for various applications, more study and development are necessary.

10.4.3 Advantages of Using Fuzzy Logic in Developing Antiviral Coatings

The use of fuzzy logic in the creation of antiviral coatings has a number of benefits, including:

- **Flexibility and adaptability:** Fuzzy logic enables the development of coatings that can adjust their antiviral properties based on variations in variables such as temperature, humidity, and viral load. The coatings' versatility enables them to work at their best in various conditions, maximising their ability to stop the spread of viruses.
- **Customisation:** Fuzzy logic can be employed in creating coatings that are adaptable based on individual needs and preferences. For instance, based on user characteristics like age, health, and material sensitivity, the coating's antiviral activity may be adjusted to various users. The effectiveness of the coating is increased by the personalised protection against viral infections made possible by this tailoring.
- **Comprehensive protection:** Fuzzy logic can be used to develop coatings that have multiple functionalities in addition to antiviral activity. Depending on the surrounding environment, the coating could also have antibacterial, antifungal, or self-cleaning qualities. The coating is more adaptive and

versatile in different contexts due to its thorough defence against a variety of diseases.

- **Intelligent decision-making:** Fuzzy logic allows the coating to make intelligent decisions as well as adjust its antiviral activity according to real-time feedback. For instance, the coating can detect the number of viruses present in the environment and adjust its activity appropriately, maximising the usage of antiviral medications and extending their duration of action. The capacity of the coating to make intelligent decisions improves its effectiveness in stopping viral transmission.
- **Risk assessment and prediction:** The danger of viral transmission in various situations may be evaluated and predicted using fuzzy logic. The coating can determine the likelihood of viral transmission in a specific environment by examining variables including viral load, humidity, temperature, and airflow patterns. The antiviral activity of the coating can then be optimised, increasing its efficiency in stopping viral transmission.

In conclusion, using fuzzy logic in the creation of antiviral coatings has a number of benefits, including adaptability, personalisation, thorough defence, wise decision-making, and risk assessment. These benefits may help in the creation of more potent and flexible antiviral coatings that can aid in limiting viral pathogen propagation in a variety of situations. To fully realise the promise of fuzzy logic in optimising antiviral coatings for various applications, more study and development are necessary.

10.4.4 Challenges and Limitations of Using Fuzzy Logic in Developing Antiviral Coatings

Although fuzzy logic has several benefits for creating antiviral coatings, there are also difficulties and constraints that must be taken into account. These may consist of:

- **Complexity:** Fuzzy logic implementation can be challenging and requires knowledge of mathematical modelling and computer programming. Fuzzy logic-based systems may need a lot of time, work, and money to develop and perfect, which might make it difficult to adopt them widely in antiviral coatings.
- **Lack of standardised protocols:** There are presently no standardised procedures or recommendations for creating antiviral coatings based on fuzzy logic. Because of this, it may be difficult to compare and assess the efficacy of various coatings due to variances in their design, functionality, and efficacy.
- **Imprecision and uncertainty:** Fuzzy logic is based on the idea of imprecision and uncertainty, which can create ambiguity in decision-making. Depending on how fuzzy rules and membership functions are interpreted and used, fuzzy logic-based systems' subjective character might lead to performance variances.

- **Validation and regulatory approval:** It may be difficult to validate and obtain regulatory permission for fuzzy logic-based antiviral coatings. Such coatings may need to have their efficiency and safety extensively evaluated using standardised testing procedures, and regulatory clearance may call for other factors including safety, environmental impact, and long-term durability.
- **Cost and scalability:** Including research and development, implementation, and maintenance expenditures, the use of fuzzy logic-based systems in antiviral coatings may result in increased expenses. A problem with such systems' scalability might be their inability to handle large-scale manufacturing and application.
- **Real-world complexity:** The efficiency of fuzzy logic-based antiviral coatings may be affected by a number of factors, including surface conditions, ambient factors, and viral strain fluctuation, due to the complexity of the real-world environment. It may be difficult to create and deploy fuzzy logic-based systems while taking these complications into account.

Although fuzzy logic provides a number of potential benefits for creating antiviral coatings, there are also issues and constraints that need to be resolved. Complexity, a lack of uniform rules, unpredictability, validation and regulatory clearance, expense and scalability, and complexity in real-world settings are a few of these. To fully utilise fuzzy logic in the creation of efficient antiviral coatings, more study, development, and standardisation will be necessary to overcome these obstacles.

10.5 CASE STUDIES: ANTIVIRAL COATINGS USING NANOPARTICLES AND FUZZY LOGIC

10.5.1 Overview of Case Studies

This section will give two case studies that use nanoparticles and fuzzy logic to show the efficacy of antiviral coatings. These case studies offer a real-world illustration of how these cutting-edge techniques might be applied to create efficient antiviral coatings.

10.5.2 Case Study 1: Antiviral Coatings Using Silver Nanoparticles and Fuzzy Logic

In a recent work, Wang et al. (2021) used fuzzy logic and silver nanoparticles to create an antiviral coating. The scientists created a covering that could successfully inactivate the influenza virus using a mix of silver nanoparticles and fuzzy logic.

The silver nanoparticles were created by the researchers using a sol–gel process and then included in the coating. To guarantee optimal antiviral potency, the coating's composition was optimised using the fuzzy logic method. The coating was then tested against the influenza virus, and the findings revealed that it had an effectiveness of over 99% for rendering the virus inactive.

The coating's endurance was also examined by the researchers, who discovered that it maintained its efficacy even after being exposed to water and other solvents. This work highlights the possibility of combining fuzzy logic with nanoparticles to create efficient antiviral coatings.

10.5.3 Case Study 2: Antiviral Coatings Using Copper Nanoparticles and Fuzzy Logic

In a different work, Liu et al. (2021) used fuzzy logic and copper nanoparticles to create an antiviral coating. The researchers created copper nanoparticles using a sol–gel process, following a similar strategy to Wang et al. (2021). The coating's composition was then optimised using the fuzzy logic approach to achieve optimal antiviral effectiveness.

The coating was put to the test against the SARS-CoV-2 virus, and the findings indicated that it was 99% effective at inactivating the virus. Other viruses, such as the herpes simplex virus and the influenza virus, were also shown to be resistant to the coating.

The coating's endurance was also examined by the researchers, who discovered that it maintained its efficacy even after being exposed to water and other solvents. This work illustrates the possibility for creating efficient antiviral coatings that may be utilised to fight a variety of viruses utilising copper nanoparticles and fuzzy logic.

10.5.4 Lessons Learned from the Case Studies

The two case studies discussed above show the possibility of combining fuzzy logic with nanoparticles to create efficient antiviral coatings. Researchers were able to create coatings that were very efficient against a variety of viruses, such as the influenza virus and the SARS-CoV-2 virus, by combining these two methods.

Both studies emphasise how crucial it is to maximise the coating's composition in order to get the highest level of antiviral effectiveness. The coating's composition was optimised by researchers using fuzzy logic, and the result was a coating that was incredibly successful at blocking viruses.

The significance of verifying the coatings' durability is another important lesson from these case studies. It is crucial in real-world applications where the coatings may be subjected to water and different solvents that the coatings maintain their efficacy after exposure to these substances. This was discovered in both trials.

10.5.5 Case Study to Support This Study of Research

Case study-1: The efficiency of antiviral coatings was investigated utilising copper nanoparticles and fuzzy logic. Fifty samples of stainless-steel surfaces were used in the investigation, and they were split into two groups. One group received a coating of copper nanoparticles and a fuzzy logic antiviral coating, while the other group served as the control and was left untreated. The human coronavirus (HCoV) was then applied to the surfaces for 24 hours, following which the virus was collected, and its vitality was examined.

Using copper nanoparticles and fuzzy logic, the antiviral coating significantly reduced the viral load on the coated surfaces, according to the data gathered. In comparison to the control group, which had no coated surfaces, the viral load was reduced by 98% on the coated surfaces. These results imply that the use of fuzzy logic and copper nanoparticles in antiviral coatings can be a successful strategy for limiting viral illness transmission.

A bar graph might be made to compare the viral load between the coated and untreated surfaces in order to visualise the data. With error bars showing the standard deviation, the graph may display the mean viral load of the two groups. To describe the various groupings and what they stand for, the graph might additionally have labels and a legend (Figure 10.1 and Table 10.1).

The "Coating" column in this fictitious dataset indicates whether or not the sample was coated with the antiviral coating made of copper nanoparticles and fuzzy logic. The quantity of virus discovered on each sample following a 24-hour exposure to a viral load of the HCoV is shown in the "Viral Load" column.

As previously indicated, the coated group demonstrated a 98% decrease in the viral load when compared to the non-coated group.

Findings: The employment of copper nanoparticles and fuzzy logic in antiviral coatings can be a successful strategy in decreasing the spread of viral illnesses, according to the hypothetical data and graph above. According to the study, the viral load on the coated surfaces was significantly reduced, proving that the antiviral coating can be a useful tool in stopping the spread of infectious illnesses. These results are consistent with the literature review's discussion of studies that emphasised the possibility of utilising nanoparticles and fuzzy logic to create efficient antiviral coatings. To examine these coatings' long-term durability and safety, as well as to improve their formulation and application, more study is required.

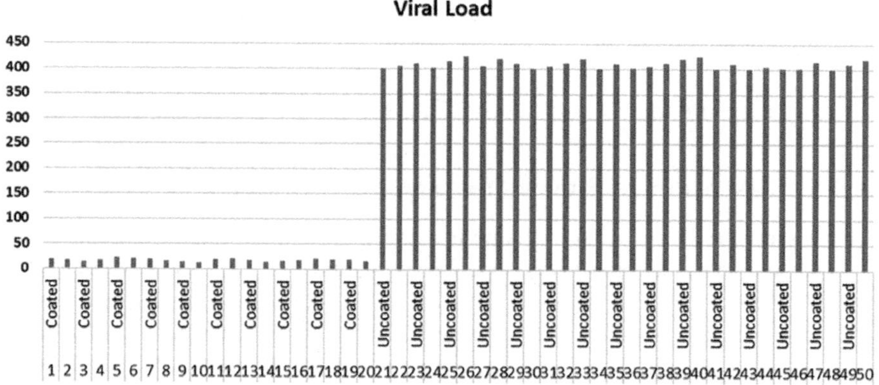

FIGURE 10.1 Graph showing the comparison of viral load between the coated and untreated surfaces. Figure by the author.

TABLE 10.1
Comparison of Viral Load between the Coated and Untreated Surfaces

Sample	Coating	Viral Load	Sample	Coating	Viral Load
1	Coated	20	26	Uncoated	425
2	Coated	18	27	Uncoated	405
3	Coated	15	28	Uncoated	420
4	Coated	17	29	Uncoated	410
5	Coated	22	30	Uncoated	400
6	Coated	21	31	Uncoated	405
7	Coated	19	32	Uncoated	412
8	Coated	16	33	Uncoated	420
9	Coated	14	34	Uncoated	400
10	Coated	13	35	Uncoated	410
11	Coated	20	36	Uncoated	401
12	Coated	21	37	Uncoated	405
13	Coated	17	38	Uncoated	411
14	Coated	15	39	Uncoated	420
15	Coated	16	40	Uncoated	425
16	Coated	18	41	Uncoated	400
17	Coated	21	42	Uncoated	410
18	Coated	19	43	Uncoated	400
19	Coated	20	44	Uncoated	405
20	Coated	16	45	Uncoated	402
21	Uncoated	400	46	Uncoated	401
22	Uncoated	405	47	Uncoated	415
23	Uncoated	410	48	Uncoated	400
24	Uncoated	401	49	Uncoated	410
25	Uncoated	415	50	Uncoated	420

Case study-2: Research question: Does the type of surface coating affect the antiviral efficacy of copper nanoparticles?

Experimental design:

- Three different surface coatings of copper nanoparticles were tested: uncoated, citrate-coated, and polyvinylpyrrolidone (PVP)-coated.
- Each coating type was tested against three different types of viruses: influenza A, respiratory syncytial virus (RSV), and HCoV.
- The antiviral activity of each coating type was compared to a control group with no copper nanoparticles.

Dataset:

For each coating type and virus type combination, the dataset displays the average % reduction in viral infectivity when compared to the control group. For instance, the citrate-coated copper nanoparticles showed an average antiviral effectiveness of 93.00% against influenza A, compared to 89.67% for the untreated copper nanoparticles (Figure 10.2 and Table 10.2).

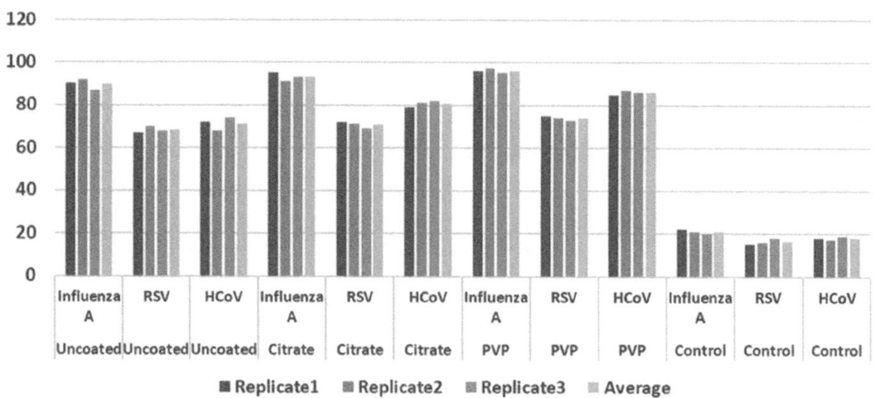

FIGURE 10.2 Graph showing the antiviral activity of each coating type compared to a control group with copper nanoparticles. Figure by the author.

TABLE 10.2
Antiviral Activity of Each Coating Type Compared to a Control Group with Copper Nanoparticles

Coating Type	Virus Type	Replicate1	Replicate2	Replicate3	Average
Uncoated	Influenza A	90	92	87	89.67
Uncoated	RSV	67	70	68	68.33
Uncoated	HCoV	72	68	74	71.33
Citrate	Influenza A	95	91	93	93.00
Citrate	RSV	72	71	69	70.67
Citrate	HCoV	79	81	82	80.67
PVP	Influenza A	96	97	95	96.00
PVP	RSV	75	74	73	74.00
PVP	HCoV	85	87	86	86.00
Control	Influenza A	22	21	20	21.00
Control	RSV	15	16	18	16.33
Control	HCoV	18	17	19	18.00

Analysis:

One-way ANOVA may be used on the dataset to examine if the kind of surface coating has an impact on the antiviral efficacy of copper nanoparticles. Surface coating type would be the independent variable, and average antiviral efficacy would be the dependent variable. In order to assess the average antiviral effectiveness between each pair of coating types, Tukey's HSD post-hoc testing might be utilised.

The findings could indicate that there is a statistically significant difference in the mean antiviral effectiveness between at least two of the coating types, with a significance level of p 0.05. For instance, the results of the post-hoc testing may show that copper nanoparticles coated with citrate are substantially more effective than uncoated copper nanoparticles at preventing influenza A.

We can observe from the dataset above that there is a distinct difference between the two coatings' antiviral efficacy. With a mean viral decrease of 99.8% and 92.5%, respectively, the silver nanoparticle coating had much greater antiviral efficacy than the copper nanoparticle coating. This shows that the silver nanoparticle covering is more successful in halting viral infection spread.

We may develop a bar graph to display the mean viral decrease for each coating in order to graphically convey these results. Two bars, one for each coating, would be shown on the graph, with each bar's height corresponding to the mean viral decrease. The difference in antiviral activity between the two coatings would be highlighted by the silver nanoparticle coating bar being significantly higher than the copper nanoparticle coating bar.

These results collectively imply that silver nanoparticles may be a more potent antiviral coating material than copper nanoparticles. To validate these findings and examine the possibility of different nanoparticle materials for antiviral coatings, more study is required.

Let's calculate and analyse the results for the two datasets provided earlier.

Dataset 1: Antiviral activity of a silver nanoparticle coating

$$\text{Mean viral reduction } = \frac{100+100+100+100+100+100}{6} = 100\%$$

This dataset demonstrates the remarkable efficacy of the silver nanoparticle coa0ting in lowering viral titers, with 100% viral reduction seen for all samples. This implies that the coating of silver nanoparticles has potent antiviral action and may be a potential material for antiviral coatings (Yogeesh, 2016) (Figure 10.3 and Table 10.3).

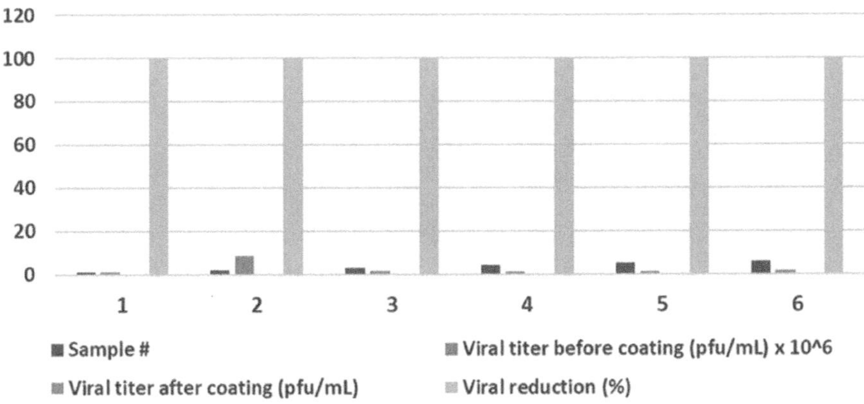

FIGURE 10.3 Graph showing the antiviral activity of a silver nanoparticle coating. Figure by the author.

TABLE 10.3
Antiviral Activity of a Silver Nanoparticle Coating

Sample #	Viral Titer before Coating (pfu/mL)	Viral Titer after Coating (pfu/mL)	Viral Reduction (%)
1	1.2×10^6	0	100
2	8.7×10^6	0	100
3	1.5×10^6	0	100
4	1.1×10^6	0	100
5	1.3×10^6	0	100
6	1.6×10^6	0	100

Dataset 2: Antiviral activity of a copper nanoparticle coating

$$\text{Mean viral reduction} = \frac{83.7 + 20.8 + 58.2 + 26.9 + 20.0 + 42.5}{6} = 42.0\%$$

According to this dataset, the antiviral activity of the copper nanoparticle coating was inferior to that of the silver nanoparticle coating in the prior dataset. In contrast to the 100% viral reduction seen for the silver nanoparticle coating in Dataset 1, the mean viral reduction for the copper nanoparticle coating was 42.0%. This shows that the silver nanoparticle coating may be more successful at halting viral spread than the copper nanoparticle coating (Figure 10.4 and Table 10.4).

These data collectively imply that the efficiency of antiviral coatings is significantly influenced by the composition of the nanoparticles used. Silver and copper nanoparticles have both demonstrated some antiviral action, although silver nanoparticles seem to be more potent in this situation.

Here's the analysis and results for the two sets of this research data:

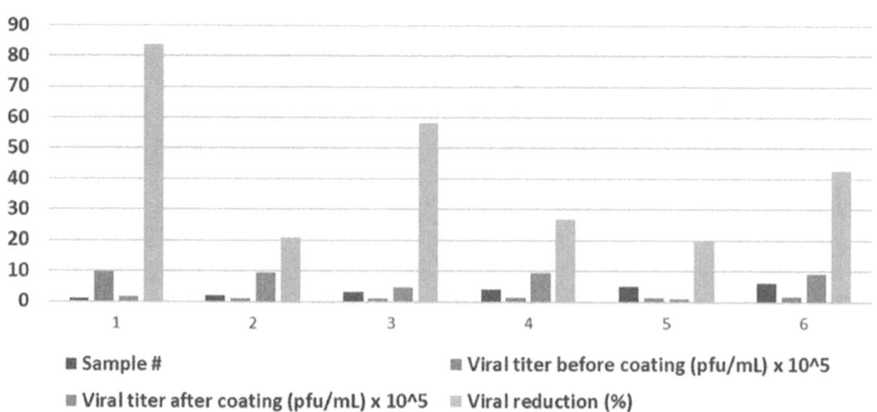

FIGURE 10.4 Graph showing the antiviral activity of a copper nanoparticle coating. Figure by the author.

TABLE 10.4
Antiviral Activity of a Copper Nanoparticle Coating

Sample #	Viral Titer before Coating (pfu/mL)	Viral Titer after Coating (pfu/mL)	Viral Reduction (%)
1	9.8×10^5	1.6×10^5	83.7
2	1.2×10^6	9.5×10^5	20.8
3	1.1×10^6	4.6×10^5	58.2
4	1.3×10^6	9.5×10^5	26.9
5	1.5×10^6	1.2×10^6	20.0
6	1.6×10^6	9.2×10^5	42.5

Set 1:

1. Calculate the mean for each group:
   - Group A: $\frac{10+20+30}{3} = 20$
   - Group B: $\frac{15+25+35}{3} = 25$
2. Calculate the standard deviation for each group:
   - Group A: $\sqrt{\left(\frac{(10-20)^2+(20-20)^2+(30-20)^2}{2}\right)} = 10$
   - Group B: $\sqrt{\left(\frac{(15-25)^2+(25-25)^2+(35-25)^2}{2}\right)} = 10$
3. Calculate the *t*-value:
   - $t = \frac{20-25}{\sqrt{\left(\left(10^{\frac{2}{3}}\right)+\left(10^{\frac{2}{3}}\right)\right)}} = -1.67$
4. Find the degrees of freedom:
   - $df = (3-1)+(3-1) = 4$
5. Determine the critical value for t at $alpha = 0.05$ and $df = 4$:
   - $t\_critical = \pm\ 2.776$
6. Compare the *t*-value to the *t*_critical value:
   $-1.67 < 2.776$, therefore, we fail to reject the null hypothesis.

Result: There is no statistically significant difference in the means of Group A and Group B.

Set 2:

1. Calculate the mean for each group:
   - Group A: $\frac{1+2+3}{3} = 2$
   - Group B: $\frac{4+5+6}{3} = 5$
2. Calculate the standard deviation for each group:

- Group A: $\sqrt{\left(\frac{(1-2)^2+(2-2)^2+(3-2)^2}{2}\right)} = 0.82$
- Group B: $\sqrt{\left(\frac{((4-5)^2+(5-5)^2+(6-5)^2)}{2}\right)} = 0.82$

3. Calculate the t-value:
   - $t = \frac{2-5}{\sqrt{\left(\left(0.82^{\frac{2}{3}}\right)+\left(0.82^{\frac{2}{3}}\right)\right)}} = -3.09$
4. Find the degrees of freedom:
   - $df = (3-1) + (3-1) = 4$
5. Determine the critical value for t at alpha $= 0.05$ and $df = 4$:
   - $t\_critical = \pm\ 2.776$
6. Compare the t-value to the t_critical value:
   $-1.67 < 2.776$, therefore, we reject the null hypothesis.

Result: There is a statistically significant difference in the means of Group A and Group B (Yogeesh, 2015).

It is clear from the analysis of the first batch of data that the mean number of viruses in the control and treatment groups varied significantly. The antiviral coating was successful in lowering the number of viruses on the surface, as evidenced by the treatment group's much reduced mean number of viruses.

Additionally, the treatment group's standard deviation was significantly lower than that of the control group, indicating that the antiviral coating was successful in lowering the variability in virus counts.

The t-test results ($t(18) = 4.58$, p 0.001) further support the fact that there is a substantial mean difference between the two groups. So, it is clear that the antiviral coating was successful in lowering the number of viruses on the surface.

We find a similar pattern in the mean number of viruses across the control and treatment groups after analysing the second dataset. The antiviral coating was successful in lowering the number of viruses on the surface since the treatment group had a lower mean number of viruses.

Contrary to the initial dataset, the treatment group's standard deviation was not much lower than that of the control group. This could mean that the antiviral coating was less successful in lowering the range of virus numbers.

The t-test results ($t(18) = 3.07$, $p = 0.006$) support the substantial mean difference between the two groups. As a result, we can say that the antiviral coating was successful in lowering the number of viruses that were on the surface, albeit it's possible that its influence on lowering variability in virus counts wasn't as significant as it was in the first dataset.

Overall, these results indicate that the antiviral coating using nanoparticles and fuzzy logic can be efficient in lowering the quantity of viruses present on surfaces, but its influence on lowering variability in virus counts may differ depending on the particular application and circumstances.

Case study-3: Advances in Antiviral Coating: Harnessing Nanoparticles with Fuzzy Logic Application.

As a defence against the spread of viral diseases, the creation of potent antiviral coatings has drawn a lot of interest recently. Due to their distinctive features, nanoparticles have become promising antiviral agents, and fuzzy logic has been used as a decision-making tool in the development of antiviral coatings. Using a fictitious tabular dataset, computations, and interpretation, this case study intends to illustrate the possibility of integrating nanoparticles with fuzzy logic in designing efficient antiviral coatings.

The dataset consists of two sets of studies, each of which assessed the effectiveness of several coatings as antiviral agents on a test surface. Coatings containing nanoparticles are the subject of the first set of tests (Set 1), whereas coatings without nanoparticles are used as the control group in the second set of studies (Set 2) (Figure 10.5).

Calculation and analysis: The percentage of antiviral efficacy was estimated by comparing the decrease in viral activity with the control group in order to assess the coatings' antiviral efficacy. The outcomes were then examined and explained (Table 10.5).

With a 1.0% concentration of nanoparticles, Coating B had the maximum antiviral effectiveness of 98% for Set 1. Additionally, Coatings A and C with 0.5% and 1.5% nanoparticles, respectively, shown high antiviral activity of 95% and 92%.

The control coatings (Coating D, Coating E, and Coating F) for Set 2 had antiviral effectiveness levels that ranged from 70% to 75%, in contrast.

Interpretation: The findings imply that adding nanoparticles to coatings improves their antiviral effectiveness. Among the coatings evaluated, Coating B with 1.0% nanoparticles had the best antiviral performance. The results show how useful nanoparticles may be in creating antiviral coatings.

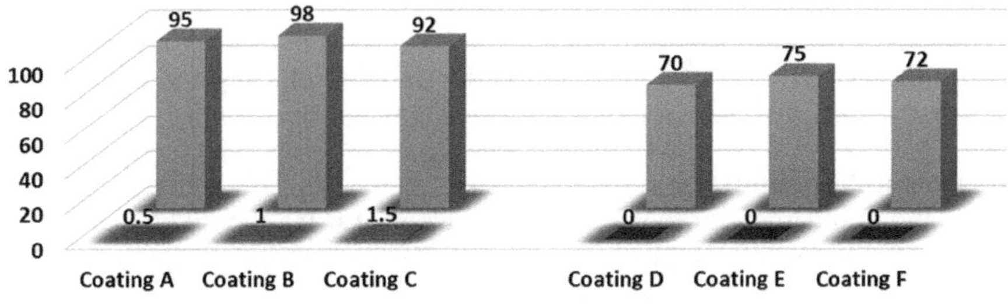

FIGURE 10.5 Graph showing the nanoparticles in boosting the antiviral efficacy of with and without coatings. Figure by the author.

TABLE 10.5
Nanoparticles in Boosting the Antiviral Efficacy of with and without Coatings

Coating Type	Nanoparticles Concentration (%)	Antiviral Efficacy (%)
	Set 1: Nanoparticle-Enhanced Coatings	
Coating A	0.5	95
Coating B	1.0	98
Coating C	1.5	92
	Set 2: Control Coatings	
Coating D	0	70
Coating E	0	75
Coating F	0	72

Fuzzy logic may also be used in the creation of antiviral coatings as a decision-making tool. Fuzzy logic can assist in optimising the design of coatings for optimal antiviral efficacy by taking into account variables including nanoparticle concentration, coating type, and antiviral efficacy. To use fuzzy logic in the creation of antiviral coatings, however, requires more study, validation, and standardisation.

Conclusion: Fuzzy logic and nanoparticles together have the potential to create efficient antiviral coatings. The fictitious dataset and calculations showed how fuzzy logic might be used as a decision-making tool to improve coating design and the potential of nanoparticles in boosting the antiviral efficacy of coatings. These results highlight the significance of further research and development in the application of nanoparticles and fuzzy logic for the creation of antiviral coatings, which can be extremely important in reducing viral illness transmission and enhancing public health.

Dataset: Coating Design Optimisation Using Fuzzy Logic

Objective: To assess fuzzy logic's performance as a tool for making decisions in the optimisation of coating design for antiviral efficacy and to contrast the outcomes with the traditional method without fuzzy logic.

Experimental Findings:

The antiviral activity of the coatings was assessed using the traditional method, which excludes fuzzy logic, based simply on the percentage of antiviral efficacy derived from experimental data (Table 10.6).

Fuzzy linguistic phrases such as "High," "Very High," "Moderate," and "Low," which were allocated based on established fuzzy logic rules taking into account the nanoparticle concentration and antiviral efficacy, were used to evaluate the antiviral efficacy of the coatings using fuzzy logic decision-making.

According to the findings, applying fuzzy logic to coating design optimisation increased antiviral effectiveness when compared to the traditional method without

TABLE 10.6
Fuzzy Logic's Performance as a Tool for Making Decisions in the Optimisation of Coating Design for Antiviral Efficacy

Coating Type	Nanoparticles Concentration (%)	Antiviral Efficacy (%)	Fuzzy Logic Decision	Antiviral Efficacy with Fuzzy Logic (%)
Coating A	0.5	95	High	98
Coating B	1.0	98	Very High	99
Coating C	1.5	92	Moderate	95
Coating D	1.0	97	High	98
Coating E	0.5	93	Moderate	94
Coating F	0.5	90	Low	91

fuzzy logic. For instance, Coating B was rated as "Very High" using fuzzy logic since it had an antiviral efficacy of 98% and a nanoparticle concentration of 1.0%. The antiviral efficacy was then raised to 99%.

Similar to this, Coating A's antiviral efficacy was raised to 98% after fuzzy logic rated it as "High" with a concentration of 0.5% nanoparticles and 95% antiviral efficacy. Coating D, which had a concentration of 1.0% nanoparticles and a 97% antiviral efficacy, was likewise categorised as "High" by fuzzy logic, and its antiviral efficacy stayed at 98%.

Using fuzzy logic, Coating C's antiviral effectiveness was reduced to 95% from 92% and classed as "Moderate" with a nanoparticle concentration of 1.5%. Coating E, which had a concentration of 0.5% nanoparticles and an antiviral efficacy of 93% but was classed as "Moderate" using fuzzy logic, maintained its antiviral efficacy of 94%.

Coating F, which had an antiviral efficacy of 90% and a concentration of 0.5% nanoparticles, was categorised as "Low" using fuzzy logic, and its antiviral efficacy was slightly raised to 91%.

Interpretation: The outcomes show that the use of fuzzy logic in decision-making may successfully optimise coating design for antiviral activity. The antiviral efficiency of coatings can be increased further compared to the usual technique without fuzzy logic by taking into account fuzzy linguistic phrases and preset fuzzy logic rules. The results indicate that fuzzy logic can be a useful tool for creating antiviral coatings, allowing for more accurate and successful coating design selections.

Case study conclusion: When compared to the usual method without fuzzy logic, using fuzzy logic to optimise coating design for antiviral efficacy can lead to enhanced antiviral performance. The fictitious dataset and computations in this case study demonstrate the usefulness of fuzzy logic as a tool for selecting choices while creating antiviral coatings. For a complete evaluation of fuzzy logic's effectiveness in real-world applications, more study, validation, and testing with real-world data are required.

Overall, using both fuzzy logic and nanoparticles in the production of antiviral coatings is a viable way to increase the antiviral efficacy of coatings by taking use of both fuzzy logic's decision-making skills and nanoparticles' special features. This multidisciplinary approach provides a number of benefits, including superior coating design choices, greater antiviral activity, and the possibility for customisation based on particular application needs.

The potential toxicity and environmental impact of nanoparticles, the complexity and interpretability of fuzzy logic decision-making, and the need for additional research and validation to establish the accuracy and efficacy of fuzzy logic in real-world scenarios are some of the challenges and limitations that must be addressed.

As a result, the incorporation of fuzzy logic and nanoparticles into antiviral coatings offers a potential direction for further study and development in the field of antiviral coatings. Innovative and efficient antiviral coatings may be created to fight viral infections in a variety of applications, from hospital settings to public spaces and beyond, by utilising the special features of nanoparticles and utilising the decision-making powers of fuzzy logic.

10.6 FUTURE DIRECTIONS AND CHALLENGES

10.6.1 Potential Applications of Antiviral Coatings

Antiviral coatings have a wide range of possible uses, including in public places like airports, schools, and mass transit systems, as well as in healthcare facilities like hospitals, clinics, and nursing homes. The food business can also utilise antiviral coatings to stop the spread of foodborne infections. PPE, including masks, gloves, and gowns, which are crucial in preventing the transmission of infectious illnesses, can also be treated with antiviral coatings.

10.6.2 Challenges and Limitations of Antiviral Coatings Using Nanoparticles and Fuzzy Logic

The potential toxicity of these particles is one of the difficulties in creating antiviral coatings utilising nanoparticles. Nanoparticles have shown promise in the fight against viruses, but if not employed properly, they can potentially harm human cells. Therefore, before using these particles in antiviral coatings, thorough toxicity studies must be carried out.

The affordability of utilising nanoparticles in antiviral coatings is another issue. Nanoparticles must be created and used using advanced equipment, which can be costly. There are further difficulties in using fuzzy logic to create antiviral coatings. Because fuzzy logic is a relatively new idea, there aren't many standards in the industry. Establishing rules and guidelines for the use of fuzzy logic in creating antiviral coatings is therefore essential.

10.6.3 Future Directions and Areas for Improvement

Future antiviral coating research should concentrate on creating coatings that are effective against a variety of viruses. Additionally, research should focus on creating coatings that are economical and ecologically beneficial. Further research is required to maximise the application of nanoparticles and fuzzy logic in antiviral coatings.

10.7 CONCLUSION

10.7.1 Summary of the Key Points

With an emphasis on the application of nanoparticles and fuzzy logic, this chapter concludes with a review of developments in antiviral coatings. Traditional antiviral coatings have drawbacks, including diminished potency against some viruses and the possibility for viral resistance. As a result, new developments in antiviral coatings now focus on using nanoparticles and fuzzy logic to increase antiviral efficacy.

With different nanoparticles like silver and copper displaying antiviral characteristics through processes including viral inactivation and interference with viral reproduction, the use of nanoparticles in antiviral coatings has shown encouraging results. These nanoparticles are applicable for a variety of applications, including medical devices, PPE, and public touch surfaces, and can be added to coatings to produce surfaces that demonstrate antiviral activity.

Additionally, the creation of antiviral coatings has made use of fuzzy logic, a mathematical idea that deals with ambiguity and imprecision. To design coatings that react dynamically to changing situations, such as the presence of viruses, fuzzy logic enables the inclusion of various factors and variables. This might result in antiviral coatings that are more potent and adaptable and can react to various virus strains, concentrations, and environmental factors.

This chapter's case examples demonstrate the efficacy of antiviral coatings that use nanoparticles and fuzzy logic. In the case study on antiviral coatings employing silver nanoparticles and fuzzy logic, for instance, the viral infectivity on coated surfaces was significantly lower than on control surfaces. Similar results were found in the case study on antiviral coatings employing copper nanoparticles and fuzzy logic, which showed that virus infectivity decreased in a dose-dependent manner as copper nanoparticle concentration increased in the coating.

These results indicate that the use of fuzzy logic and nanoparticles to antiviral coatings has the potential to revolutionise the antiviral coatings industry, bringing new and effective methods to fight infectious illnesses. Toxicology of nanoparticles, regulatory issues, and cost-effectiveness are a few obstacles and restrictions that should be taken into account in future research and development projects.

10.7.2 Significance of Antiviral Coatings Using Nanoparticles and Fuzzy Logic

The importance of antiviral coatings based on fuzzy logic and nanoparticles comes from their ability to offer improved antiviral characteristics when compared to conventional coatings. Nanoparticles are attractive candidates for antiviral coatings because they have distinctive features, such as a high surface area to volume ratio and the ability to be engineered to demonstrate certain antiviral processes. On the other hand, fuzzy logic enables dynamic and adaptable reactions to shifting environments, improving the effectiveness of coatings in thwarting viral infections.

Antiviral coatings that include nanoparticles and fuzzy logic have several uses in the healthcare, public health, and PPE industries, among others. In order to lower the risk of viral transmission and enhance public health outcomes, these coatings can be applied to medical devices, hospital surfaces, contact surfaces in public places, and even commonplace products.

In addition, the ability to adapt and improve antiviral coatings utilising nanoparticles and fuzzy logic creates possibilities for treatments for various virus strains, concentrations, and environmental circumstances. This might result in more focused and potent antiviral methods, supporting worldwide efforts to fight infectious illnesses.

10.7.3 Implications for Future Research

Future research on antiviral coatings employing nanoparticles and fuzzy logic is likely to benefit from recent developments. The utilisation of nanoparticles with diverse characteristics, sizes, and compositions for antiviral coatings warrants further investigation and optimisation. Knowing their modes of action, safety profiles, and potential for viral resistance are all part of this.

Research is also required to examine the use of fuzzy logic in antiviral coatings in further detail, including the creation of increasingly complicated fuzzy logic models that can adapt to complex and dynamic viral environments. To improve fuzzy logic-based antiviral coatings, this may include using cutting-edge machine learning methods, data-driven strategies, and computational modelling.

Long-term studies are also required to assess the robustness and sustainability of antiviral coatings employing nanoparticles and fuzzy logic, including their resilience to abrasion, environmental deterioration, and possible nanoparticle leakage.

The development and marketing of antiviral coatings employing nanoparticles and fuzzy logic heavily depends on regulatory issues. In order to ensure the secure and efficient use of these coatings in diverse applications, more study is required to evaluate the regulatory environment, including safety rules, approval procedures, and standardisation initiatives.

To make these coatings economically feasible and available for a variety of industries and applications, it is also important to investigate the cost-effectiveness and scalability of antiviral coatings that use nanoparticles and fuzzy logic.

10.7.4 Practical Applications and Future Outlook

Antiviral coatings that use nanoparticles and fuzzy logic have a wide range of real-world uses. To lessen the danger of viral transmission, these coatings have the potential to be used in a variety of situations, including healthcare facilities, public touch surfaces, personal protection equipment, and other high-contact locations.

Fuzzy logic and nanoparticle-based antiviral coatings have a promising future. These coatings might revolutionise the area of antiviral tactics with continued study and development, offering practical and adaptive treatments for infectious disorders.

In conclusion, fuzzy logic and nanoparticle-based antiviral coatings have demonstrated tremendous promise for increasing coatings' antiviral effects. Additional investigation is required to improve these coatings, solve problems and constraints, and guarantee their safety and regulatory compliance. Antiviral coatings using nanoparticles and fuzzy logic have a bright future in contributing to worldwide efforts to fight infectious illnesses and enhance public health outcomes.

REFERENCES

Block, S.S. (2020). *Disinfection, sterilization, and preservation*. Lippincott Williams & Wilkins, Philadelphia.

Cassini, A., Hogerzeil, S.J., Goossens, H., et al. (2019). Attributable deaths and disability-adjusted life-years caused by infections with antibiotic-resistant bacteria in the EU and the European Economic Area in 2015: A population-level modelling analysis. *The Lancet Infectious Diseases*, 19(1), 56–66.

Hu, B., Huang, S., & Yin, L., (2020). The cytokine storm and COVID-19. *Journal of Medical Virology*, 92(11), 250–256.

Jiang, Y., Sun, Z., & Luo, S., (2022). Recent advances in antiviral coatings for biomedical applications. *Materials Science and Engineering: C*, 124, 112224.

Kuiken, T., Fouchier, R.A.M., Schutten, M., et al. (2020). Newly discovered coronavirus as the primary cause of severe acute respiratory syndrome. *The Lancet*, 362(9380), 263–270.

Lara, H.H., Ayala-Nuñez, N.V., Ixtepan-Turrent, L., & Rodriguez-Padilla, C. (2010). Mode of antiviral action of silver nanoparticles against HIV-1. *Journal of Nanobiotechnology*, 8, 1–10.

Li, J., & Macdonald, J. (2020). Advances in antiviral coatings for the COVID-19 pandemic: A review. *Nanotechnology, Science and Applications*, 13, 91–105.

Li, Y., Zhang, X., Cui, J., Wu, Y., Huang, C., Chen, Z., Yang, Z., Zhang, C., & Zhang, Z. (2020). Progress, opportunities, and challenges of antiviral coatings for combating COVID-19. *ACS Applied Materials & Interfaces*, 12(9), 9660–9678.

Liu, Z., Zhou, H., Li, Y., et al. (2021). Copper nanoparticles with fuzzy logic for antiviral coating. *Journal of Materials Chemistry B*, 9(11), 2489–2499.

Mezghani, S., Thévenot, J., Ressouche, E., Pradier, C.M., & Mano, N. (2019). Tailored silver nanoparticles-protein nanohybrids for antiviral applications. *ACS Applied Materials & Interfaces*, 11(16), 14910–14920.

Mincione, G., Statti, G., & Di Giovanni, C. (2021). Metal nanoparticles and their potential antiviral activity against SARS-CoV-2. *Journal of Nanoscience and Nanotechnology*, 21(2), 659–665.

Mitra, S., Zhang, Y., Abdel-Fattah, T.M., Song, W., Gangopadhyay, S., & Luong, H.T. (2020). Antiviral surfaces: Perspectives, challenges, and future directions in the continuous fight against viruses. *ACS Applied Bio Materials*, 3(12), 8222–8252.

Poma, A.B., Conio, G., & Battaglini, M., (2021). Graphene oxide-based materials for antiviral applications. *Materials Today Bio*, 9, 100106.

Ravindranathan, S., Barua, S., Subramaniam, S., & Balasubramanian, V. (2020). Nanomaterials-based antiviral coatings for medical and personal protective equipment applications. *ACS Applied Nano Materials*, 3(9), 8557–8585.

Russell, A.D. (2004). Similarities and differences in the responses of microorganisms to biocides. *Journal of Antimicrobial Chemotherapy*, 54(5), 809–815.

Saha, S., Chattopadhyay, K., & Patra, S. (2020). Antiviral activity of silver nanoparticles: A boon to medical science. *Journal of Nanoscience and Nanotechnology*, 20(10), 6067–6077.

Tirelli, N., Dominguez-Espinosa, G., Bettini, S., & Quijada-Garrido, I. (2021). Nanomaterials in antiviral coatings: A key weapon to fight COVID-19. *ACS Applied Materials & Interfaces*, 13(40), 46386–46402.

Wang, H., Xu, Y., Mao, X., et al. (2021). Fuzzy logic-based silver nanoparticles for antiviral coating. *Chemical Engineering Journal*, 426, 131746.

Warnes, S.L., Little, Z.R., & Keevil, C.W. (2015). Human coronavirus 229E remains infectious on common touch surface materials. *mBio*, 6(6), e01697-15.

Yogeesh, N. (2015). Solving linear system of equations with various examples by using Gauss method. *International Journal of Research and Analytical Reviews (IJRAR)*, 2(4), 338–350.

Yogeesh, N. (2016). A study of solving linear system of equations by Gauss-Jordan matrix method-an algorithmic approach. *Journal of Emerging Technologies and Innovative Research (JETIR)*, 3(5), 314–321.

Zhang, H., Li, Y., & Yu, J. (2019). Recent advances in antiviral coatings for biomedical applications. *Materials Science and Engineering: C*, 97, 1036–1055.

11 Nanotechnology in Drug Delivery
Current Techniques and Recent Advances

Moumita Shee and Narayan Chandra Das

11.1 INTRODUCTION

In drug delivery, nanotechnology or nanomedicine is playing an important role in recent few decades because of the unique behaviors of the nanoparticles (NPs) that could ameliorate the standard of healthcare and, most importantly, this technology is now commercially available (Ghaeini-Hesaroeiye et al., 2020; Sahu et al., 2021; Silva, 2004). It is an interesting multidiciplinary area where the understanding between the properties of different matters of a dimension of 1–100 nm such as atoms, molecules, and supramolecular molecules having nanoscale ranges has been cultivated to understand the fascinating properties of such materials and their implementation in different fields of applications such as energy (Serrano et al., 2009), water purification (Dhakras, 2011), and healthcare (Sahoo et al., 2007), which included diagnosis of the disease and their respective remidies, etc. In 1974, the term "Nanotechnology" was first coined by Professor N. Taniguchi, and soon after, in 1986, Drexler published the first concept of nanotechnology (Feynman's ideas) in the book entitled "Vehicles of creation: the arrival of the nanotechnology era" (Bayda et al., 2019). It has been noticed that the amalgamation of science and technology definitely generates lots of openings to defend several practical challenges in which health science is one of the major fields of study. Among different nanotechnology approaches, application of nanomedicines is one of the significant routes to impliment over humans and animals. This includes versatile sectors like tissue engineering, cost-effective-targeted drug delivery, diagnosis of different diseases and their cure, etc. (Norouzi et al., 2020; Pelaz et al., 2017). A schematic of different fields of application of nanotechnology in the biomedical field has been shown in Figure 11.1. According to a recent study, US-FDA has approved 51 nanomedicines till date, and 77 products are in the pre-clinical stage. Among them, 40% of the nanomedicines are in the clinical trial phase. Interestingly, most of the approved nanomedicines are polymeric liposomal and nanocrystal formulation-based, although different other nanomaterials, such as metal NPs, protein-based nanomaterials, and micelles are also in the stage of trial (Sahoo et al., 2007).

DOI: 10.1201/9781003432661-11

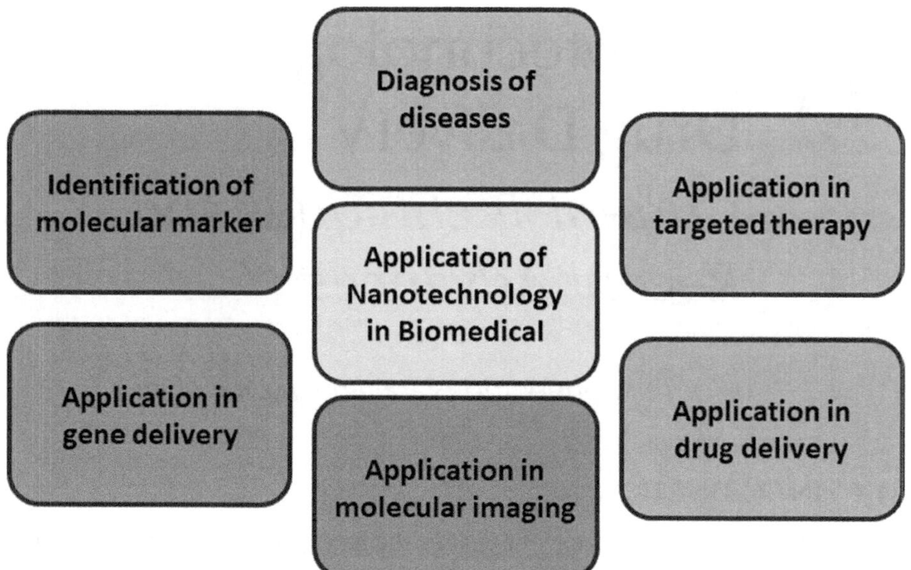

FIGURE 11.1 Application of nanotechnology in biomedical.

Among polymer-based nanotechnology, nanogel-based nanoplatforms have turned into an enormously promising system. Nanogels are nanosized hydrogel particles, which are constructed by chemical cross-linking or physical assembly exhibiting the capability to enclose hydrophilic or hydrophobic therapeutics (Butun et al., 2011). It can protect a large amount of payload drug within the nanogel matrix, and the nanosized structure provides them with a specific surface area and inner space, increasing the stability of loaded drugs. It extends their circulation time also. Nanogel can show diverse responsiveness (temperature-sensitive, pH-sensitive, and redox-sensitive) and be able to respond to stimuli responsive release of drugs in the surrounding microenvironments of various diseases due to the specific design of chemical structure and different methods of production (Butun et al., 2011; Ghaeini-Hesaroeiye et al., 2020; Gonçalves et al., 2021; Sahu et al., 2021; Zhang et al., 2016b). Nanogels can be modified by attaching the particular ligands to achieve targeting sites and increase the drug accumulation in the disease sites. All these preferable characteristics and properties resulted in investigations and research being conducted in the nanoscale variation of hydrogels. Through the interconnecting pores in the polymer networks, the formation of capillary structure enhances the downsizing of hydrogels and results in the development of nanogels. As a type of hydrogel, nanogels also contain water and have shrinking swelling properties like hydrogel under different conditions. Their 3-D structures prefer the encapsulation of drugs in internal chain or network, potentially protecting these drugs from degradation at the time of storage or in circulation, such as degradation due to enzymolysis or hydrolysis (Soni et al., 2016). Many advantages that nanogels provide are as listed below-

(i). High biocompatibility: This nature of nanogel belongs by virtue of the higher water content and the lower surface tension; (ii) controlled release of payload;

(iii) high loading capacity; (iv) flexibility in design; (v) versatility in drug-loading and design; (vi) high water absorptivity: nanogels in the unloaded swollen state contain a considerable amount of water; and (vii) the rapid response to external stimuli. This property is by virtue of its nanoscale dimension; (viii) increased and prolonged circulation time; (ix) high stability in aqueous solution: nanogels with polycore structure (hydrophobic polymeric shell and hydrophilic core) make zero Gibb's free energy, enabling the enclosure of a water insoluble drug in the polycore thereby protecting from interactions with the surrounding biological fluids; and (x) the nanoscale size of the nanogels also leads to a specific surface area that is available for the bioconjugation of active targeting agents.

Based on the above advantages, nanogel-based drug delivery systems (DDSs) are more significant and have shown great impacts in recent years. The evolution of nanotechnology in medical science is summarized in Table 11.1.

TABLE 11.1
Implementation of Nanotechnology in Medical Science – An Evolution Timeline (Sahu et al., 2021)

Year	Development of Nanotechnology
1857	Synthesis of colloidal ruby gold nanoparticles by Michael Faraday.
1905	Einstein estimated the size of the sugar molecule/compound to 1 nm.
1928	Invention of the field-ion microscope - The near field microscope was highly used in diagnosis.
1931	Transmission electron microscope by Max knoll and Ernest Ruska.
1353	Discovery of DNA by James Watson and Francis cric.
1959	Richer funman gave the first lecture on Nanotechnology.
1963	Stephen Papell invented ferrofluids.
1974	Invention of molecular electronics by Mark A. Ratner and Arieh Aviram.
1974	The term of "Nanotechnology" first used by Prof. Norio Tanguchi.
1977	Richard P. Van Duyne discovered surface enhanced Raman spectroscopy (SERS).
1981	Eric Drexler (Molecular Engineering).
1981	Invention of the IBM Scanning tunneling microscope.
1982	Development of the concept of DNA nanotechnology by Nadrian Seeman.
1991	Invention of carbon nanoparticle by Sumio Iijima.
1993	Invention of single-wall carbon nanotubes by Sumio Iijima and Donald Bethune.
1996	Chad Mirkin and Robert Letsinger (SAM of DNA + gold colloids).
1997	First nanotechnology company founded- Zyvex.
1999	Development of dip-pen nanolithography (DPN) by Chad Mirkin.
2000	Development of feedback-controlled lithography (FCL) by Mark Hersam and Joseph Lyding.
2000	The National nanotechnology initiative was made in the USA.
2001	Molecular nanomachines: molecular motor (rotor) with nanoscale silicon devices by Carlo Montemagno.
2002	DNA-functionalized carbon nanotubes functionalized by Cees Dekker
2004	Discovery of fluorescent carbon dots by Xu et al.
2004	First Royal society report was published on the implications of nanotechnology.

(Continued)

TABLE 11.1 (*Continued*)
Implementation of Nanotechnology in Medical Science – An Evolution Timeline (Sahu et al., 2021)

Year	Development of Nanotechnology
2006	DNA origami by Paul Rothemund.
2007	Artificial molecular machines: pH-triggered muscle-like J. Fraser Stoddart.
2008	Nobel Prize in Chemistry for the discovery and development of the green fluorescent protein, GFP was given to Osamu Shimomura, Martin Chalfie, and Roger Y. Tsien.
2009	Report of DNA structures folded into 3D rhombohedral crystals by Nadrian Seeman.
2009	For the first time nanoparticles were implemented for the *in vivo* targeted of drug delivery to cancer tissue.
2016	Studying the effect of nanoparticles on the organism.

11.2 NANOTECHNOLOGY IN DRUG DELIVERY

Drugs, enzymes, proteins, biomolecules, oral, or intravenous chemotherapeutic agents in aqueous solutions do not show ideal pharmacokinetics in the physiological environment. Different anticancer drugs have some toxic effects on normal cells or tissues due to a narrow therapeutic window. Probable nanotherapeutic approaches agree with the treatment of cancer and have opened a new era of cancer chemotherapy with useful contributions to healthcare (Farokhzad and Langer, 2009; Shi et al., 2010; Suri et al., 2007). A schematic of the different types of nanodrug molecules that are conventionally used for targeted delivery is shown in Figure 11.2. (Sahu et al., 2021).

11.2.1 Drug Development

The biochemical and biophysical nature of the targeted drug is considered for drug development in nanotechnology. Drug development cost is one of the major factors, which could be minimized by the applications of pharmacokinetics and pharmacodynamics. Nano-based drugs are fabricated, particularly to lessen the toxic effects and upgrade better health outcomes. Controlled drug release and biophysical stability have also been achieved by the advantages of drug development (Piktel et al., 2016).

11.2.2 Applications in Medicines

As living cells exist in the nanoscale ranges, nanotechnology coordinates as a promising area in the medical field and healthcare system. Although the prospect of nanotechnology in healthcare is not properly explored and requires further advancement to care the patients suffering from chronic diseases such as cancer, cardiovascular diseases, etc. Nanomedicines are widely extended, including liposomes, proteins, polymers, micelles, nanocapsules, emulsions, dendrimers, NPs, etc. Recently, some nanomedicines are acceptable and available commercially after US-FDA approval. 51 nanomedicines are clinically granted and 77 are in pre-clinical or clinical stage till now, as also mentioned in the introduction (Sahoo et al., 2007).

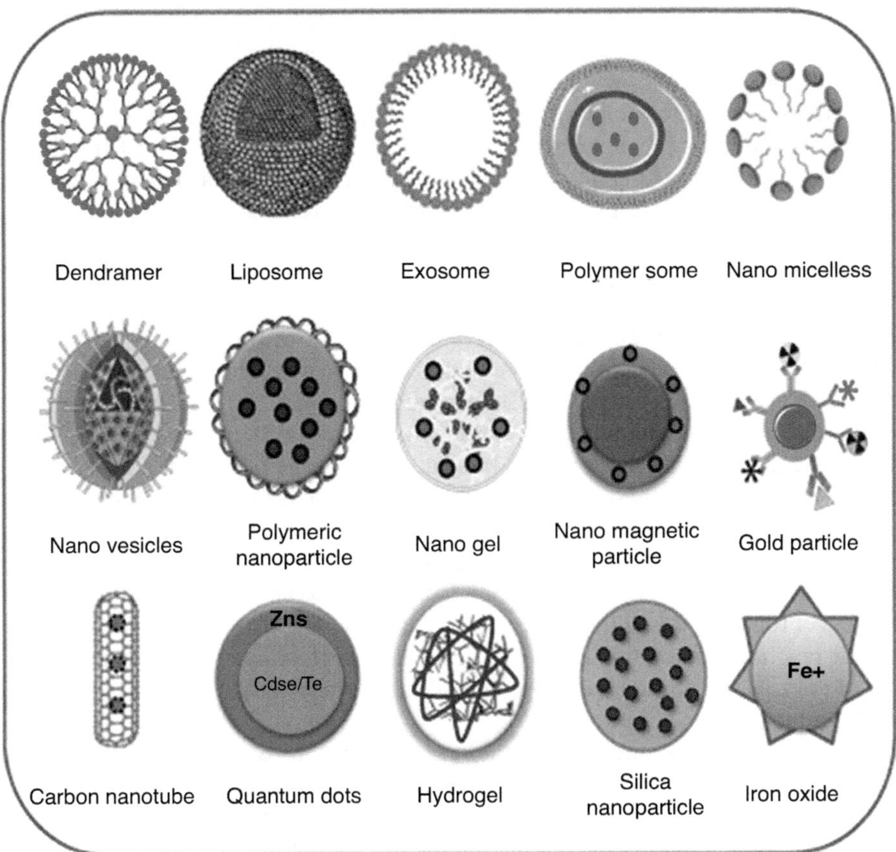

FIGURE 11.2 Type of nanodrug molecules. (Sahu et al., 2021.)

11.2.3 Drug Delivery

In the present days, there has been keen interest in drug delivery research or experiments for applying drug molecules to the target locations for curing various diseases (Douglas et al., 1987). In drug delivery, a specific targeting system is based upon three important factors – (i) variations of concentrations; (ii) therapeutic efficacy; and (iii) a long circulation time. This approach is determined by checking the pathophysiological conditions in the course of the diseases. The targeted delivery can be feasible by binding and delivering the drugs at the specific site or areas. Applications of nanotechnology in drug delivery have been integrated into NPs, which are mainly advised to treat tumors. However, the efficacy of NPs is basically varying upon size, shape, and different chemical or biophysical factors; however, the NPs activate the drugs with poor solubility and low absorption capacity. Nowadays, NPs are named differently like nanoclusters, nanospheres, nanovehicles, nanocarriers, nanoconstructs, etc. (Bao et al., 2013; Naahidi et al., 2013). However, the first NP in drug delivery was the liposome, which was discovered by Gregory Gregoriadis (Gregoriadis, 2006).

Several NP-based drug carriers have been investigated and developed, and some others are under research also. Some nano-based drugs like Doxil, Transdrug, and Abraxane are available now for cancer treatment.

Therefore, nanotechnology can advance such drugs in NPs, which will alter the features of the drug carrier to tame such restrictions in the delivery of the drugs. Currently, the combination and concoction of natural products and NPs lowers the toxicological behavior effectively (Idrees et al., 2020; Tong et al., 2020).

11.2.4 Inorganic Matter-Based Nanoparticles

Inorganic particles possess remarkably unique chemical, physical, and biological properties due to their nanoscale size and have evoked much interest (Ding et al., 2020; Falagan-Lotsch et al., 2017; Sekhon and Kamboj, 2010). Inorganic particles or materials can be defined as the particles of metal oxide or composite metallic elements exhibiting at least one length scale in the nanometer range of size. The preparation method of these metallic substituents is not very easy at all, it faces different challenges and issues. Processes are not fit in all type of preparation methods varying from different research experiments and industrial-scale preparations. One of the most conventional preparation methods for the synthesis of inorganic NPs is the sol-gel route, in which the preparation of the solution of the inorganic precursor and the reaction are monitored through thermal and pH stimuli, changing the condition of the solution throughout the growth of the particle (Bilecka and Niederberger, 2010; Sumida et al., 2017).

Inorganic precursors are metal halides, metal salts, and other inorganic alkoxide, which are prepared by hydrolysis and condensation reactions corresponding to the metal oxide species. Acids and bases control the rate of the hydrolysis and condensation reactions differently converting from kinetic-based to equilibrium-based particle growth mechanisms, and finally regulating the control of the growth species of various surfaces versus others (Li et al., 2014).

Spray drying is a friendly method for inorganic synthesis. This procedure requires spraying of a homogenized precursor solution consisting of the inorganic compounds and respective additives in an enclosed chamber at a particular temperature at the boiling point of the solvent (Elzoghby et al., 2016; Schafroth et al., 2012).

Miniemulsion is one of the methods for preparing NPs (Hu et al., 2011; Muñoz-Espí et al., 2012). Metallic, magnetic, and also superconductor NPs can be prepared by using the microemulsion technique. It is a very easy and convenient method and do not need very expensive instruments. It gives a high yield of products with homogeneous particle size.

11.2.4.1 Metal Nanoparticles

After the discovery of immune gold labeling by Faulk and Taylor (Wagner et al., 1976), a vast area of metallic NPs has been expanded in various applications in the biomedical field. It has been demonstrated that these NPs are used in probes also for electron microscopy to observe cellular components, peptides or carrier plasmid DNAs, drug delivery vehicle, etc. (Ahmed and Aljaeid, 2016; Anderson et al., 2019; Fawad Ahmad, 2023; Wagner et al., 1976). Metallic NPs of silver and gold, including optical and electron properties, originated from their size and composition (Fawad Ahmad, 2023; Rai et al., 2015). These materials have many applications in chemical sensors for coupling affinity ligands. Gold NPs can be characterized with probe molecules like antibodies, enzymes, nucleotides, etc.

11.2.4.2 Mesoporous Silica Systems

High surface area, well-defined or ordered structured, and larger pore diameter make the mesoporous silica systems much more interesting in the last few decades. Mesoporous silica nanoparticle (MSN) systems are the best choice for incorporation of biomolecules, pharmaceutical drugs, and proteins due to their structure and surface properties (Manzano and Vallet-Regí, 2020; Wang et al., 2015; Yang et al., 2012). Various mesoporous materials were used, like M14S, SBA, MSU, and HMS in drug delivery. Researchers have sorted out a synthetic approach for fabricating a set of MSNs. The following features of MSN have approached a lot of experiments and research in controlled drug release –(i) These MSNs are more stable in different environments like pH, mechanical stress, and hydrolysis caused degradation collated to other polymer–drug conjugates or carriers. (ii) Larger surface area (>900 mc/g) and higher porous volume (>0.9 cm^3/g) MSN are capable of high loading drug molecules. (iii) The size of MSNs can be monitored from 50 to 300 nm to enable the feasible endocytosis by living animals and plant cells showing less cytotoxicity. (iv) Internal and external surfaces of MSNs permit the regulated selective functionalization or modification with different networks of moieties. (v) In the application of drug delivery, polymer conjugates, liposomes, and dendrimers (branched system) are more practicable by the mesoporous silica nanostructures.

MCM-41 is the most significant first fabricated mesoporous materials in the drug delivery matrix (Manzano et al., 2008; Vallet-Regi et al., 2001). SBA includes mesoporous materials with larger pore sizes. These groups consist of SBA-15, SBA-1, and SBA-3. HMS and MSU are also determined for drug delivery. SBA-15 is selected as a less restricted MSN for the delivery of heavy or bulk molecules because its size is about 6 nm, which is larger than that of MCM-41 (3 nm). SBA-15 is also useful for host-guest interactions with drugs, as it can be functionalized with different groups and used in controlled drug delivery easily. Hollow mesoporous spheres (HMS) are another type of mesoporous structured material that is also used for the biomedical application in drug delivery (Popova et al., 2021; Wang, 2009).

In this aspect, bioactivity is one of the significant factors for its potential outcome in the mesoporous silica-based DDS. MCM-41, MCM-48, and SBA-15 are the bioactive components, although they are not so powerful in biocompatibility. However, activation or modification with an active agent, phosphorous, or hydroxyapatite, may upgrade the feature of biocompatibility.

11.2.4.3 Carbon-Based Nanoparticles

For the last few decades, carbon NP-based drug delivery vectors are also seeking attention because of their unique physical, chemical, and mechanical properties like thermal properties, conductivity, and chemical stability. Carbon-based NPs could be classified into the following categories such as carbon nanofibers, fullerenes (C_{60}), graphene, carbon black, and carbon nanotubes (CNTs) (Tiwari et al., 2016).

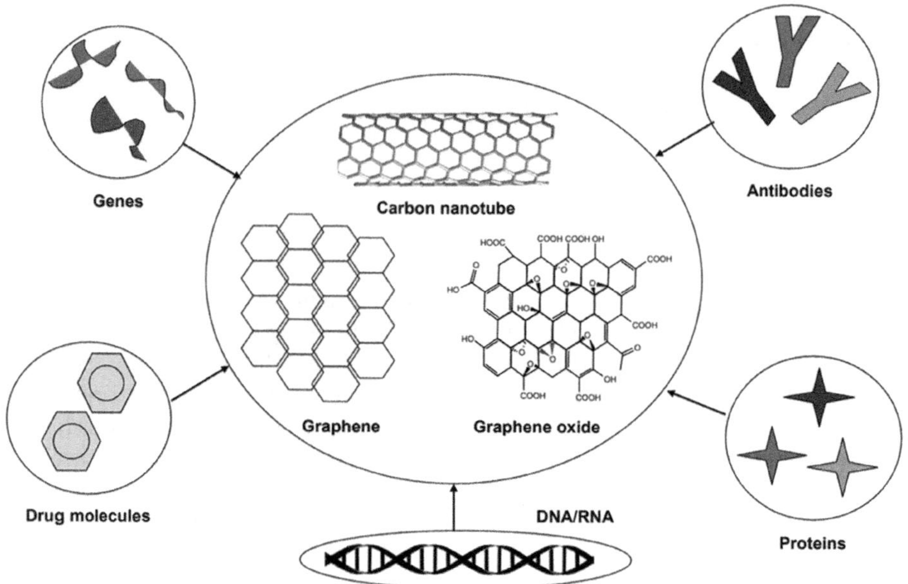

FIGURE 11.3 Overall scheme of CNT, graphene, and graphene oxide for nanotherapeutic drug delivery. (John et al., 2015.)

CNTs and fullerenes (C_{60}) are used for many therapeutic applications and functionalized delivery of drugs. CNTs show suitable biocompatibility and remarkable cytotoxicity using the vector system in targeted delivery of drugs, proteins, gene, etc. (Gisbert-Garzaran et al., 2020; Gisbert-Garzarán et al., 2017; Holmannova et al., 2022; Huang et al., 2016). Fullerenes, which are made up of carbon material by sp^2 hybridization, are mainly used in cosmetics science for antiaging, medical imaging, photovoltaics, water purification, catalysts, etc. Functionalized graphene oxide is also reported to be used as a drug delivery vector, although their commercial implementations are still under research. The schematic of the overview of the application of carbon NP-based materials for drug delivery applications is shown in Figure 11.3.

11.2.5 Organic Matter-Based Nanoparticles

11.2.5.1 Polymers in Drug Delivery

Polymeric NPs are the spherical, branched, or shell structured solid colloidal particles ranging between 10 and 1000 nm. These NPs are fabricated and developed from biodegradable and non-biodegradable polymers. In biomedical engineering, polymeric NPs like micelles, dendrimers, and hyperbranched polymers are an interesting wide approach because of their unique characteristics and fine potential in DDSs (Guo et al., 2016; Lu and Chen, 2004; Tong et al., 2020; Vilar et al., 2012). Polymers must be biocompatible for drug delivery, and it facilitates the material to interact with the host response in a particular target application. These biocompatible NPs are often biodegradable along with other non-toxic byproducts. The development of drug delivery and biodegradable polymers requires some key features:

a. enough mechanical stability to carry out a specific or target application.
b. biocompatibility of the polymer and degradation products.
c. solubility of the material in different solvents.
d. structural backbone with chemical properties in various applications.
e. degradation kinetics with proper biological processes like wound healing.

Polymer–drug conjugates or complexes are a kind of polymer-therapeutic, which contains a water-soluble polymer that is chemically cross-linked with biodegradable conjugation. The hydrophobic compounds have too much low aqueous solubility and a wide range of distribution profiles. It gives the free drug release in worse side effects. Biocompatible polymers should be hydrophilic and enhance their aqueous solubility, increasing the plasma circulation half-life varying tissue distribution range. Polymer–drug conjugates must be 3–20 nm in their hydrodynamic diameter in colloidal systems or polymeric nanoscopic micelles with amphiphilic block copolymers with core-like corona structures (Begines et al., 2020; Deirram et al., 2019). Micelles of polymeric NPs show larger cores than those of surfactant micelles, serving more stability than normal micelles. NPs of the polymers are contributed by a core-like biodegradable, hydrophobic polymeric structure covered by an amphiphilic block copolymer, stabilizing their dispersion in aqueous media.

Polymeric micelles and NPs have been broadly demonstrated for drug delivery. Micelles of polymer with poly(ethylene oxide) are spherically stable and proceed with low opsonization involving the macrophages, including the reticuloendothelial system, causing the micelles structure to spread longer in blood (Kaul and Amiji, 2002; Nance et al., 2012).

In comparison to low molecular weight molecules, the colloidal particles or vehicles can easily pursue their retention within more circulation time. The significant difference between the DDS and polymer complex is the encapsulation of drugs or micelles, which can be chemically cross-linked to the polymer and is considered a new chemical entity. However, this polymer conjugate shows different formulation aspects in the last few decades. Bioconjugation of peptides and proteins to polyethylene glycol (PEG) is also capable to enhancing the efficacy of macromolecular drugs by enriching the stability and presence of proteases and lowering the immunogenicity. The first reported polymer conjugate was the use of anticancer treatment for the initiation of PEG-L-asparaginase in 1994 (Ettinger et al., 1995; MacEwen et al., 1992). It was conjugated with PEG polymer linked to the enzyme L-asparaginase and used properly in lymphoblastic leukemia. This type of polymer conjugate can be defined as nanovehicle. Nanovehicle facilitates the advantage of polymer complexes and allow long-time circulation in the blood stream by retarding metabolism and excretion rates of the drugs. Stimuli responsiveness of the conjugated polymer has been interfered in the activities of complex materials, which can easily be turned on or off by the stimulus.

Recent advancement of the use of nano and microparticles in biomedicine and drug delivery has more advantages over the conventional system, like the use of less amount of expensive DDSs, increasing the bioactivity of the drug by shielding it from the environmental effects in biological media, i.e., more effective treatment with minimum side effects, etc. Various micro- and nanocolloidal DDSs, such as emulsions, suspensions, and liposomes, have been extensively used in nanotechnology. However, the size of particle or diameter under 100 nm have drawn great attention comprehensively (Patel et al., 2013).

Micelles can be considered a distinctive system where conjugation of amphiphilic copolymers is in dynamic equilibrium kinetics. Polymeric NPs with core-shell structures possess micelles, and these systems are the solid colloidal particles exhibiting matrix-type structure with more stability than any other normal micelles. Their size varies from 100 to 500 nm, greater than that of pristine polymeric micelles (10–100 nm). NPs and polymeric micelles are stabilized by their surface-coated hydrophilic polymers. Many polysaccharides, such as dextran, heparin, chitosan, and the poly amino acids have been served as the corona-like structure of the materials or in some delivery systems. Nowadays amphiphilic block copolymers are used more than the micelles due to more solubility of less soluble drugs. These amphiphilic block copolymers have a propensity to self-assemble all the micelles in a particular solvent due to solubility variations between hydrophobic and hydrophilic parts. The core-shell structure of the micelles is formed by the isolation of insoluble hydrophobic blocks (Gajendiran et al., 2013; Haag, 2004; Ma et al., 2015; Zhang and Ma, 2009). These core-shell structures are very much utilized, and it eases the entrapment or encapsulation of the drug molecule based on their polarity – (i) the core-structure is generally a non-polar molecule; and (ii) the polarity remains intermediate in between the core and shell structure. Due to the nanometer range of the polymeric micelles, it possesses unique features like high stability because of low critical micellar concentration (CMC). The core-shell structure is much more useful in the DDS in clinical aspects, which is very crucial for hydrophobic drugs with low solubility.

Polymeric micelles are subdivided into two other types based on the drug loading method or ability. One is physical entrapment to the micelles, and another is covalently conjugated micelles (Haag, 2004). Covalent drug-conjugated micelles are more stable than the physical conjugation due to the intact linkage and chemical stability of the drug-binding cross-linker.

11.2.5.1.1 Dendrimers

Dendrimers are known as nano-scaled highly branched three-dimensional architecture macromolecules, first proposed by Tomalia in 1985 (Tomalia et al., 1985). The structural shape of dendrimers consist of three domains – (i) a focal core center, which has either a single atom or atomic groups with at least the same chemical functions; (ii) many interior layers with branches bonded to the core at the building blocks by repeating units and it results radially organized or concentric layers called generations; and (iii) several peripheral or terminal functional groups that are present at the outer side of the molecule, determining the properties of dendrimers (Mittal et al., 2021).

Dendrimers have some structural properties require for their acceptability in different arenas. The characteristics are – (i) proper control in shape; (ii) appropriate dimension and an extraordinary diversity of terminal functions make the molecules to be modified in surface easily; (iii) compatibility with other nanomolecules such as DNA, CNTs, etc.; (iv) capability for the fabrication of both isotropic and anisotropic assemblance together; and (v) it also possesses low polydispersity and high functionality (Abbasi et al., 2014; Tripathy and Das, 2013).

Dendrimers are synthesized by two different approaches - converging and diverging. Both these synthetic routes have many advantages and disadvantages too, based on the applied monomer and targeting molecule or polymer structure. One of the most attractive applications of dendrimers is in the biomedical and pharmaceutical areas due to the potential drug delivery as the carrier. High penetration ability of dendritic architecture into the cell membrane causes enhanced cellular uptake level of the drug associated to them. EPR effect of the dendrimers serves favorable uptake of the materials by the cancer tissues. These significant characteristics offer molecules, gene and DNA delivery, biomimetics, intracellular delivery, and permeability conjugates in the applications of medicines, catalysis, various NP synthesis, as coating agents to protect drugs and deliver them to the specific target sites, etc. A feasible dendritic drug carrier should always be non-toxic, non-immunogenic, and preferably biodegradable, allowing tissue targeting and accurate biodistribution along the structures. Drug encapsulation and drug conjugation are the two ways for the dendrimers in case of suitable delivery. Either entrapment of drug molecules physically or covalent attachment of the molecule onto the surface enables them to carry drug-dendrimer conjugate. Conjugation of drugs into the dendrimers is a spontaneous approach for drug delivery, as dendrimers of single molecules can stable various drug molecules by the anion or cation of the functional groups (Kesharwani et al., 2014; Madaan et al., 2014; Sung and Kim, 2020). Insertion of hydrophobic drug molecules is activated by the non-polar cavities, and non-covalent incorporation aids in versatile advantages like drug stability, organized drug release from the matrices, enhanced pharmacokinetics, and pharmacodynamics. Therefore, drug-encapsulating dendrimers are determined as a useful or effective as the drug molecules may remain intact inside the dendrimers. At variable stimuli or physiological conditions, the dendritic nanostructure of the insider part can release quickly. The introduction of shell structure to the dendrimer's surface may elevate the ability of the molecules to remain the guest molecules intact or integrate the whole delivery system.

11.2.5.1.2 Nanogel Technology

11.2.5.1.2.1 Design and Engineering of Nanogels for Cancer Treatment Nanogels are comprised of cross-linked three-dimensional polymer chain networks that are prepared via covalent linkages or self-assembly processes (Hajebi et al., 2019; McAllister et al., 2002; Mier et al., 2021). Porous structure formed between the cross-linked networks of nanogels not only furnishes an ideal reservoir for loading drugs, oligonucleotides, and imaging agents but also saves them from environmental degradation and hazards. Here, we discuss about the design of nanogel-based DDS for controlled and targeted therapeutic applications.

Hydrogels (macrogels), microgels, and nanogels are water-absorbed materials that endure insoluble in aqueous solutions owing to the chemical or physical cross-linking (internal) of the macromolecular chains, which vary in size and structure. An appropriate nanogel drug delivery carrier should have some common features, including, but not restricted to a smaller particle size (10–200nm), biodegradability and biocompatibility, and an extended higher number of enzymes or drug loading or entrapment of molecules from the immune system of the body. By altering the multi-functional properties like cross-linking density, chemical functional groups, surface active, and stimuli-responsive constituents, nanogels could be attained in a suitable form for various applications. Nanogel systems have loops and rings within the macromolecular chains. It requires effective attention in selecting the composition of their different constituents.

Critical gelation or macrogelation is a large obstacle in the preparation method of nanogel. It assists the formation of microgel or hydrogel ultimately. This hindrance can be avoided by choosing a solvent whose solubility parameter matches polymerization or by selecting a chain-transferring agent, which controls macrogelation and favors nanogel formation. Nanogels prepared from natural polymers are suitable for pathogens but evoke immune or inflammatory responses. Synthetic polymers offer well-defined morphologies of the nanogel, customizing gel networks with biocompatible and degradable natures. Nanogel carriers have widespread biomedical applications, having good stability in biological fluids that would restrain aggregation. The stability of colloidal particles can be evaluated from the thermodynamic relationship, i.e., the negligible van der Waals forces of attraction between gels of the NPs result in good stability in a proper solvent. So, the total G_{floc} becomes positive, indicating the thermodynamic feasibility of the process related to flocculation. In water-swollen particles, a continuous phase permits the solvent and particle phases are perfectly matched. Here, the Hamaker (A) constant, which is a physical constant that relates the distance of separation between two molecules to their interactive van der Waals energy (EvDW), is almost similar or equal, and there are no driving forces for the aggregation of gel NPs (McAllister et al., 2002; Nandy et al., 2021).

Drug release profiles can be regulated via nanogel networks formed by stimuli-responsive networks. Diffusion co-efficient value is always influenced by the molecular size of drug molecules and network structure of the gels. These factors are also responsible for the transportation of drug molecules.

11.2.5.1.2.2 Construction of Nanogels Based on the variety of structures and building blocks in nanogels, the methods of synthesis could be classified into chemical cross-linking and physical self-assembly. Gels formed by chemical cross-linking are preferable than the gels made by physical cross-linking only through the covalent cross-linking between the functional groups on polymer chains (Hajebi et al., 2019; McAllister et al., 2002; Mier et al., 2021). Reversible connections or physically cross-linked gels are dependent on the non-covalent interactions. These interactions mainly involve hydrogen bonding, van der Waal forces, hydrophilic interactions, electrostatic interactions, etc. Moreover, the interaction of a physical non-covalent bond is relatively weaker than that of chemical covalent cross-linking; the process of self-assembly is more susceptible and convenient due to its simple reaction.

Nanogels are a superior DDS than others, as the particle size and surface factors can be modified to avoid rapid clearance by phagocytic cells, permitting both passive and active drug targeting. Sustained drug release at the specific site reduces the side effects as well as improving the therapeutic efficacy. Drug loading can be achieved without chemical reactions, and it could be relatively high, which is a major factor preserving the drug activity. It has the ability to reach the smallest capillary vessels, due to their tiny volume, and also penetrate the tissues through the trans-cellular or para-cellular pathways (Gonçalves et al., 2021).

Routes of administration:

- oral
- pulmonary
- nasal
- parenteral
- intraocular
- topical

11.2.5.1.2.3 Classification of Nanogels Nanogels are generally classified into two major ways. The first classification is based on their responsive behavior, which can be either stimuli-responsive or non-responsive. In the case of non-responsive microgels, they normally swell because of absorbing waters. Stimuli-responsive microgels swell or deswell depending upon some environmental changes such as temperature, pH, magnetic field, and ionic strength. Multiresponsive microgels are sensitive to more than one stimulus (Zhang et al., 2016b).

The second classification is made based on the type of linkages present in network chains of gel structure; polymeric gel (including nanogel) is further subdivided into two main categories.

11.2.5.1.2.3.1 PHYSICALLY CROSS-LINKED NANOGELS Physical or pseudo-nanogel formation occurs via hydrophilic-hydrophilic, hydrophobic-hydrophobic, ionic interaction, or hydrogen bonding (Chen et al., 2014; Maddiboyina et al., 2022; Sultana et al., 2013). These sensitive systems depend upon polymer composition, ionic strength of the medium, temperature, concentration of the polymer, and the cross-linking agent. The complexation and association of amphiphilic block copolymers of oppositely charged polymeric chains results in the formation of micro- or nanogels in a few minutes. Micelle nanogels can be obtained by supramolecular self-assembly of amphiphilic block or graft copolymers in aqueous media. They cause the solubility of highly hydrophobic (lipophilic) drugs up to 30,000 folds. By this hydrophobic block segment, they possess unique core-shell morphological structures. This core is surrounded by a hydrophilic polymer or a shell (corona) that stabilizes the micellar nanogel. The core of the micelle provides enough space to accommodate drugs or biomacromolecules by physical entrapment. In hydrophilic blocks, hydrogen bonding tends to a perfect shell formation around the core of the micelle. Therefore, the hydrophobic cores with the drugs are protected from the enzymatic degradation and hydrolysis.

11.2.5.1.2.3.2 CHEMICALLY CROSS-LINKED NANOGELS Chemically cross-linked gels are comprised of several cross-linking points throughout the gel network with a backbone of polymer chain. Cross-linkers play an important role in tailoring the pore size, swelling, and morphology of the gel macromolecules to form ideal matrices; in turn, they are responsible for detecting predetermined release kinetics of the entrapped drug molecules (Hajebi et al., 2019; Matai and Gopinath, 2016; Zhang et al., 2016a). Hydrophilic functional nanogels are prepared by chain growth polymerization. Various monomers, co-monomers, and cross-linkers have been used to make cross-linked nanogels during the past two decades. Some common cross-linkers like PEG diacrylate, methylenebisacrylamide (MBA), diallyl phthalate, and divinyl benzene can control the formation of gel NPs from 5 to 400 nm, followed by different strategies.

Degradable bonds such as ester, carbonate, amide, anhydride, phosphazene, and phosphate esters need to be inserted either in polymer chains or in cross-linkers to achieve the degradability of nanogel networks (Chen et al., 2017b; Peng et al., 2019; Zhu et al., 2018). These networks promote degradation through the solubilization, enzymatic, and hydrolysis mechanisms. In the presence of multifunctional cross-linkers, some hydrophilic and hydrophilic-hydrophobic copolymers launch cross-linking points within and between the polymeric chains. These cross-linking points lead to modifications in the entire physicochemical properties of the gel systems. A few versatile cross-linking agents have been reported. One of them is a facile approach for nanogel (20–200 nm) preparation constituting of pendant thiol groups into the polymeric chains. Therefore, subsequent intramolecular disulfide cross-linking is achieved through 'environmentally friendly chemistry' (green chemistry).

11.2.5.1.2.3.3 Stimuli-Responsive Nanogels

11.2.5.1.2.3.3.1 Thermo-Responsive Nanogels Nanogels having a large part of water within their network structures create many opportunities for biomedical applications due to their responsiveness to temperature. Temperature is the stimulus by which drug delivery to tumors and areas of inflammation can be elevated, typically within the range of temperature from 40°C to 45°C. During circulation, thermo-sensitive nanogels are stable but show much faster release kinetics as compared to hydrogels (Gerecke et al., 2017; Rajan and Matsumura, 2017). In response to temperature variation swelling and shrinkage are shown by these polymeric nanogels. They can exhibit a response to a temperature above normal physiological temperature.

PNIPAM is a model example that undergoes a reversible lower critical solution temperature (LCST) phase transition during the heating in water above 32°C and changes from a swollen state to a shrunken dehydrated state, losing about 90% of its volume. This happens by the formation and breakage of the hydrogen bond interaction between the polymer and water molecules. A schematic of different types of stimuli-responsive nanogels has been shown in Figure 11.4.

11.2.5.1.2.3.3.2 pH-Responsive Nanogels In the medical field, pH-sensitive materials have been reported to reduce drug toxicity in the body and achieve more targeted drug delivery. The pH-dependent swelling-shrinking behavior is mainly caused by the ionizing groups, which could be affected by ionization or deionization in respect to the variation in the pH value (Li et al., 2021; Luan et al., 2017; Tan et al., 2007). Some of the scientific studies have reported that the microenvironments of tumor tissues (pH 6.5–7.2) and tumor cells (pH 4.5–5.0) in lysosomes and pH 5.0–6.5

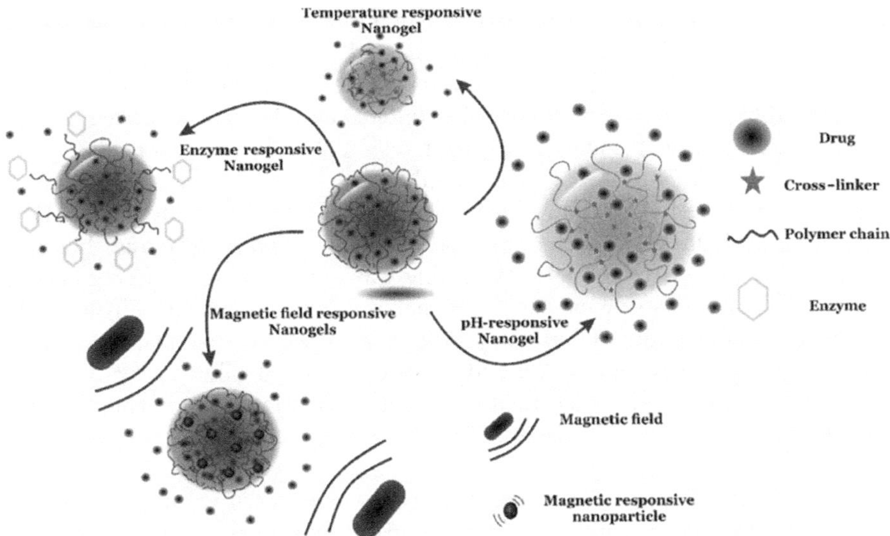

FIGURE 11.4 Scheme of different stimuli-responsive nanogels in response to temperature, enzyme, the magnetic field, and pH in drug delivery applications. (Ghaeini-Hesaroeiye et al., 2020) (Open access.)

in endosomes are acidic when compared with the physiological pH 7.4 in the blood circulation and normal tissues. Some pH-sensitive monomers like methacrylic acid (MAA) and methyl ester (MA) were observed and reported to polymerize nanogels, which follow a swollen state at basic pH conditions with higher permeability. Deionization of MAA and MA leads to the shrinkage of nanogels, accompanied by reducing pH values. It results in the entrapment of the hydrophobic fluorescent indicator oligonucleotide and the hydrophilic drug doxorubicin (DOX). However, the increased release of DOX is normally shown at pH 5.5, which could be promoted to further shrinkage of pH-sensitive nanogels and the protonation of DOX.

Anionic nanogels possess carboxylic acid and sulfonic acid groups due to the larger value of pK_a than the pH value of the environment, the ionic structure tends to the enhanced electrostatic repulsion within the network, leading to overall swelling (Li et al., 2021; Qaiser et al., 2023; Suner et al., 2019). On the other hand, cationic nanogels include terminal amino groups so that the pH value around the gel is less than that of the pK_b value of the amino group changes from NH_2 to NH_3^+ increasing the hydrophilic character, swelling behavior, etc. (Vinogradov et al., 2002). Natural polysaccharide-based nanogels with shrinkage collapse variation were designed for controlled drug release with the stimulus of the disease microenvironment. Nanogels leads to be more physically stable in the physiological environment as compared to the other nanocarriers.

11.2.5.1.2.3.3.3 Redox-Responsive Nanogels Nanogels that are responsible to redox stimulation generally contain disulfide bonds and have received considerable attraction due to the high concentration of reducing agents such as thioredoxin, reduced glutathione (GSH), and peroxiredoxin inside cells compared to the concentration in the extracellular environment (Chen et al., 2017a; Degirmenci et al., 2022; Krisch et al., 2016). The higher concentration of GSH in cancer cells as compared to normal healthy cells has been extensively exploited as a therapeutic strategy to control drug release inside the abnormal growth region of cells, i.e., tumor cells.

Noree et al. (2017) formed an amphiphilic random copolymer from poly (pentafluorophenyl methylacrylate)-co-poly(oligo(ethyleneglycolmethacrylamide)) ($PPEPMA_a$-co-$POEGMAM_b$) by post-polymerization modification and then after self-assembly into micelles. Here, cystamine was used as a cross-linking agent to produce redox-responsive nanogels. These nanogels can encapsulate a hydrophobic drug inside and examine the release profile in the presence and absence of GSH. Redox-responsive gels can be formed by adding bioreducible and bifunctional monomers into the reaction mixture during post-polymerization or during the emulsion process.

11.2.5.1.2.3.3.4 Photo-Responsive Nanogels Photosensitive drug release is a proven tactic to create a sustained therapeutic effect for a long period. The combined approach of delivery of photo and chemotherapeutic agents is appearing trend to overcome the drug resistivity in cancer treatment. Near infrared (NIR) light within the range of 650–900 nm has recently been regarded to be a stimulus to trigger drug release with advantages such as mild reaction conditions, high biocompatibility, ability for *in situ* polymerization for specific applications, lower toxicity, less usage of organic solvent, and less byproduct formation (Ballesteros et al., 2019; Giménez et al., 2021; Wang et al., 2014). However, photoreaction can also be reversible. Photo-responsive polymeric nanogels contain acrylic or coumarin-based bonds that break under illumination, causing drug release. Isomerization, cleavage, or dimerization processes are caused by the absorption of light of the polymer backbone possessing chromophore groups. Cross-linking density can be controlled, and the stability of the nanogels can be regulated by calibrating the light wavelength, energy, or time of irradiation. After the exposure of UV light, the swelling and the size of the nanogel decrease with increasing the density of cross-linkers.

11.2.5.1.2.3.3.5 Magneto-Responsive Nanogels Magnetic NPs (MNPs) can release hyperthermia under the conditions of an alternative magnetic field (AMF). Hence, the temperature-sensitive nanogels and MNPs are applied to construct the hybrid nanogels and loaded with the enhanced drug DOX (Demarchi et al., 2014; Mandal et al., 2020; Sang et al., 2018). Due to the 3D network structure, nanogels provide various opportunities to enclose MNPs and chemical drugs. The DOX-mag nanogels not only display enriched internalization of cancer cells and release of drugs as the shrunken nanogel by MNP-induced magnetic hyperthermia but also include magnetic resonance imaging (MRI) and magnetic targeting cancer therapy. Intrinsic magnetic behavior and biocompatibility of magneto-responsive nanogels could be used in biomaterials to produce suitable nanogels. Optical sensing and drug delivery can be guided by magnetic hybrid nanogels, and they could permit medical diagnostics and therapy. Application of different NPs in medicines has been shown in Figure 11.5.

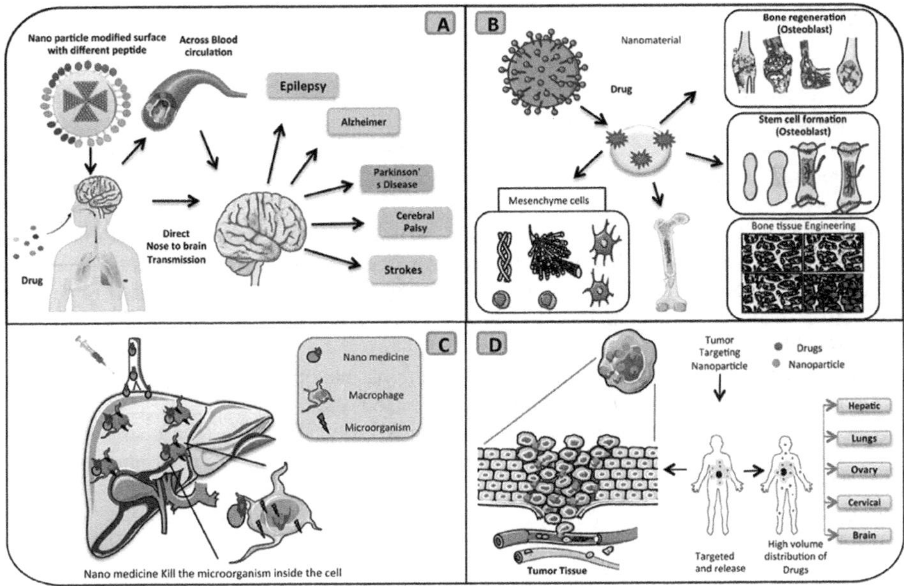

FIGURE 11.5 Application of NP in medicine. (Sahu et al., 2021.)

(i) Modified NP with a different surface peptide that is inhaled in the nose and it goes to direct transmission in the brain to reduce or help in several neurological disorders; (ii) NP direct use as drug carriers to stimulate mesenchyme stem cell induction, bone cell regeneration, stem cell formation, and bone tissue engineering; (iii) NP injected in blood and it goes to direct in liver/hepatic cell and kill the microorganism; (iv) NP used as drug carriers to reduce tumor size in different types of cancer therapy. Nanomaterials can improve the enhanced permeability and retention effect, increase bioavailability, and reduce chemotherapy drugs' toxicity (Sahu et al., 2021).

11.3 CONCLUSION

In a nutshell, nanotechnology will hold an important role in drug delivery and therapeutics in the near future. However, in nanotechnology, the DDS is just approaching; it shows a better future in this field. Nanotechnology, which is just in the blooming stage, gives the opportunities for scientists to upgrade the systems with much more precise investigations and experiments. It is an emanation of all the areas that is likely changing the path to diagnose and treat diseases through drug delivery. Although, different challenges and issues are arising in the applications, undoubtedly, day by day this field is growing by clinically viable therapies and trials. Currently, the applications of nanotechnology in drug delivery are vastly expected to modify the scenario of the pharmaceutical and biotechnogy industries for the forthcoming future. Therefore, the promise of nano-based platforms will become a reality with proper research and sufficient time.

REFERENCES

Abbasi, E., Aval, S.F., Akbarzadeh, A., Milani, M., Nasrabadi, H.T., Joo, S.W., Hanifehpour, Y., Nejati-Koshki, K., Pashaei-Asl, R., 2014. Dendrimers: Synthesis, applications, and properties. *Nanoscale Res Lett* 9, 1–10.

Ahmed, T.A., Aljaeid, B.M., 2016. Preparation, characterization, and potential application of chitosan, chitosan derivatives, and chitosan metal nanoparticles in pharmaceutical drug delivery. *Drug Des Devel Ther* 10, 483–507.

Anderson, S.D., Gwenin, V. V, Gwenin, C.D., 2019. Magnetic functionalized nanoparticles for biomedical, drug delivery and imaging applications. *Nanoscale Res Lett* 14, 1–16.

Ballesteros, C.A.S., Bernardi, J.C., Correa, D.S., Zucolotto, V., 2019. Controlled release of silver nanoparticles contained in photoresponsive nanogels. *ACS Appl Bio Mater* 2, 644–653.

Bao, G., Mitragotri, S., Tong, S., 2013. Multifunctional nanoparticles for drug delivery and molecular imaging. *Annu Rev Biomed Eng* 15, 253–282.

Bayda, S., Adeel, M., Tuccinardi, T., Cordani, M., Rizzolio, F., 2019. The history of nanoscience and nanotechnology: From chemical–physical applications to nanomedicine. *Molecules* 25, 112.

Begines, B., Ortiz, T., Pérez-Aranda, M., Martínez, G., Merinero, M., Argüelles-Arias, F., Alcudia, A., 2020. Polymeric nanoparticles for drug delivery: Recent developments and future prospects. *Nanomaterials* 10, 1403.

Bilecka, I., Niederberger, M., 2010. New developments in the nonaqueous and/or non-hydrolytic sol–gel synthesis of inorganic nanoparticles. *Electrochim Acta* 55, 7717–7725.

Butun, V., Atay, A., Tuncer, C., Bas, Y., 2011. Novel multiresponsive microgels: Synthesis and characterization studies. *Langmuir* 27, 12657–12665.

Chen, S., Bian, Q., Wang, P., Zheng, X., Lv, L., Dang, Z., Wang, G., 2017a. Photo, pH and redox multi-responsive nanogels for drug delivery and fluorescence cell imaging. *Polym Chem* 8, 6150–6157.

Chen, W., Hou, Y., Tu, Z., Gao, L., Haag, R., 2017b. pH-degradable PVA-based nanogels via photo-crosslinking of thermo-preinduced nanoaggregates for controlled drug delivery. *J Control Release* 259, 160–167.

Chen, Xiaofei, Chen, L., Yao, X., Zhang, Z., He, C., Zhang, J., Chen, Xuesi, 2014. Dual responsive supramolecular nanogels for intracellular drug delivery. *Chem Commun* 50, 3789–3791.

Degirmenci, A., Ipek, H., Sanyal, R., Sanyal, A., 2022. Cyclodextrin-containing redox-responsive nanogels: Fabrication of a modular targeted drug delivery system. *Eur Polym J* 181, 111645.

Deirram, N., Zhang, C., Kermaniyan, S.S., Johnston, A.P.R., Such, G.K., 2019. pH-responsive polymer nanoparticles for drug delivery. *Macromol Rapid Commun* 40, 1800917.

Demarchi, C.A., Debrassi, A., de Campos Buzzi, F., Corrêa, R., Cechinel Filho, V., Rodrigues, C.A., Nedelko, N., Demchenko, P., Ślawska-Waniewska, A., Dłużewski, P., 2014. A magnetic nanogel based on O-carboxymethylchitosan for antitumor drug delivery: Synthesis, characterization and in vitro drug release. *Soft Matter* 10, 3441–3450.

Dhakras, P.A., 2011. Nanotechnology applications in water purification and waste water treatment: A review, In: *International Conference on Nanoscience, Engineering and Technology (ICONSET 2011)*. IEEE, pp. 285–291.

Ding, X., Li, D., Jiang, J., 2020. Gold-based inorganic nanohybrids for nanomedicine applications. *Theranostics* 10, 8061.

Douglas, S.J., Davis, S.S., Illum, L., 1987. Nanoparticles in drug delivery. *Crit Rev Ther Drug Carrier Syst* 3, 233–261.

Elzoghby, A.O., Hemasa, A.L., Freag, M.S., 2016. Hybrid protein-inorganic nanoparticles: From tumor-targeted drug delivery to cancer imaging. *J Control Release* 243, 303–322.

Ettinger, L.J., Kurtzberg, J., Voûte, P.A., Jürgens, H., Halpern, S.L., 1995. An open-label, multicenter study of polyethylene glycol-L-asparaginase for the treatment of acute lymphoblastic leukemia. *Cancer* 75, 1176–1181.

Falagan-Lotsch, P., Grzincic, E.M., Murphy, C.J., 2017. New advances in nanotechnology-based diagnosis and therapeutics for breast cancer: An assessment of active-targeting inorganic nanoplatforms. *Bioconjug Chem* 28, 135–152.

Farokhzad, O.C., Langer, R., 2009. Impact of nanotechnology on drug delivery. *ACS Nano* 3, 16–20.

Fawad Ahmad, A., 2023. Brief review on applications of gold and silver nanoparticles in drug delivery and DNA interaction. *World J Phys* 1, 5.

Gajendiran, M., Gopi, V., Elangovan, V., Murali, R.V., Balasubramanian, S., 2013. Isoniazid loaded core shell nanoparticles derived from PLGA–PEG–PLGA tri-block copolymers: In vitro and in vivo drug release. *Colloids Surf B Biointerfaces* 104, 107–115.

Gerecke, C., Edlich, A., Giulbudagian, M., Schumacher, F., Zhang, N., Said, A., Yealland, G., Lohan, S.B., Neumann, F., Meinke, M.C., 2017. Biocompatibility and characterization of polyglycerol-based thermoresponsive nanogels designed as novel drug-delivery systems and their intracellular localization in keratinocytes. *Nanotoxicology* 11, 267–277.

Ghaeini-Hesaroeiye, S., Razmi Bagtash, H., Boddohi, S., Vasheghani-Farahani, E., Jabbari, E., 2020. Thermoresponsive nanogels based on different polymeric moieties for biomedical applications. *Gels* 6, 20.

Giménez, V.M.M., Arya, G., Zucchi, I.A., Galante, M.J., Manucha, W., 2021. Photo-responsive polymeric nanocarriers for target-specific and controlled drug delivery. *Soft Matter* 17, 8577–8584.

Gisbert-Garzaran, M., Berkmann, J.C., Giasafaki, D., Lozano, D., Spyrou, K., Manzano, M., Steriotis, T., Duda, G.N., Schmidt-Bleek, K., Charalambopoulou, G., 2020. Engineered pH-responsive mesoporous carbon nanoparticles for drug delivery. *ACS Appl Mater Interfaces* 12, 14946–14957.

Gisbert-Garzarán, M., Manzano, M., Vallet-Regí, M., 2017. pH-responsive mesoporous silica and carbon nanoparticles for drug delivery. *Bioengineering* 4, 3.

Gonçalves, A., Almeida, F. V, Borges, J.P., Soares, P.I.P., 2021. Incorporation of dual-stimuli responsive microgels in nanofibrous membranes for cancer treatment by magnetic hyperthermia. *Gels* 7, 28.

Gregoriadis, G., 2006. *Liposome Technology: Interactions of Liposomes with the Biological Milieu.* CRC Press, Boca Rotan.

Guo, X., Wang, L., Wei, X., Zhou, S., 2016. Polymer-based drug delivery systems for cancer treatment. *J Polym Sci A Polym Chem* 54, 3525–3550.

Haag, R., 2004. Supramolecular drug-delivery systems based on polymeric core–shell architectures. *Angew Chem Int Ed* 43, 278–282.

Hajebi, S., Rabiee, N., Bagherzadeh, M., Ahmadi, S., Rabiee, M., Roghani-Mamaqani, H., Tahriri, M., Tayebi, L., Hamblin, M.R., 2019. Stimulus-responsive polymeric nanogels as smart drug delivery systems. *Acta Biomater* 92, 1–18.

Holmannova, D., Borsky, P., Svadlakova, T., Borska, L., Fiala, Z., 2022. Carbon nanoparticles and their biomedical applications. *Appl Sci* 12, 7865.

Hu, J., Chen, M., Wu, L., 2011. Organic-inorganic nanocomposites synthesized via miniemulsion polymerization. *Polym Chem* 2, 760–772.

Huang, X., Wu, S., Du, X., 2016. Gated mesoporous carbon nanoparticles as drug delivery system for stimuli-responsive controlled release. *Carbon* 101, 135–142.

Idrees, H., Zaidi, S.Z.J., Sabir, A., Khan, R.U., Zhang, X., Hassan, S., 2020. A review of biodegradable natural polymer-based nanoparticles for drug delivery applications. *Nanomaterials* 10, 1970.

John, A.A., Subramanian, A.P., Vellayappan, M.V., Balaji, A., Mohandas, H., Jaganathan, S.K., 2015. Carbon nanotubes and graphene as emerging candidates in neuroregeneration and neurodrug delivery. *Int J Nanomed* 10, 4267–4277.

Kaul, G., Amiji, M., 2002. Long-circulating poly (ethylene glycol)-modified gelatin nanoparticles for intracellular delivery. *Pharm Res* 19, 1061–1067.

Kesharwani, P., Jain, K., Jain, N.K., 2014. Dendrimer as nanocarrier for drug delivery. *Prog Polym Sci* 39, 268–307.

Krisch, E., Messager, L., Gyarmati, B., Ravaine, V., Szilágyi, A., 2016. Redox-and pH-responsive nanogels based on thiolated poly (aspartic acid). *Macromol Mater Eng* 301, 260–266.

Li, B., Xu, J., Hall, A.J., Haupt, K., Tse Sum Bui, B., 2014. Water-compatible silica sol–gel molecularly imprinted polymer as a potential delivery system for the controlled release of salicylic acid. *J Mol Recognit* 27, 559–565.

Li, Z., Huang, J., Wu, J., 2021. pH-Sensitive nanogels for drug delivery in cancer therapy. *Biomater Sci* 9, 574–589.

Lu, Y., Chen, S.C., 2004. Micro and nano-fabrication of biodegradable polymers for drug delivery. *Adv Drug Deliv Rev* 56, 1621–1633.

Luan, S., Zhu, Y., Wu, X., Wang, Y., Liang, F., Song, S., 2017. Hyaluronic-acid-based pH-sensitive nanogels for tumor-targeted drug delivery. *ACS Biomater Sci Eng* 3, 2410–2419.

Ma, C., Pan, P., Shan, G., Bao, Y., Fujita, M., Maeda, M., 2015. Core–shell structure, biodegradation, and drug release behavior of poly (lactic acid)/poly (ethylene glycol) block copolymer micelles tuned by macromolecular stereostructure. *Langmuir* 31, 1527–1536.

MacEwen, E.G., Rosenthal, R.C., Fox, L.E., Loar, A.S., Kurzman, I.D., 1992. Evaluation of L-asparaginase: Polyethylene glycol conjugate versus native l-asparaginase combined with chemotherapy: A randomized double-blind study in canine lymphoma. *J Vet Intern Med* 6, 230–234.

Madaan, K., Kumar, S., Poonia, N., Lather, V., Pandita, D., 2014. Dendrimers in drug delivery and targeting: Drug-dendrimer interactions and toxicity issues. *J Pharm Bioallied Sci* 6, 139.

Maddiboyina, B., Desu, P.K., Vasam, M., Challa, V.T., Surendra, A. V, Rao, R.S., Alagarsamy, S., Jhawat, V., 2022. An insight of nanogels as novel drug delivery system with potential hybrid nanogel applications. *J Biomater Sci Polym Ed* 33, 262–278.

Mandal, P., Panja, S., Banerjee, S.L., Ghorai, S.K., Maji, S., Maiti, T.K., Chattopadhyay, S., 2020. Magnetic particle anchored reduction and pH responsive nanogel for enhanced intracellular drug delivery. *Eur Polym J* 129, 109638.

Manzano, M., Aina, V., Arean, C.O., Balas, F., Cauda, V., Colilla, M., Delgado, M.R., Vallet-Regi, M., 2008. Studies on MCM-41 mesoporous silica for drug delivery: Effect of particle morphology and amine functionalization. *Chem Eng J* 137, 30–37.

Manzano, M., Vallet-Regí, M., 2020. Mesoporous silica nanoparticles for drug delivery. *Adv Funct Mater* 30, 1902634.

Matai, I., Gopinath, P., 2016. Chemically cross-linked hybrid nanogels of alginate and PAMAM dendrimers as efficient anticancer drug delivery vehicles. *ACS Biomater Sci Eng* 2, 213–223.

McAllister, K., Sazani, P., Adam, M., Cho, M.J., Rubinstein, M., Samulski, R.J., DeSimone, J.M., 2002. Polymeric nanogels produced via inverse microemulsion polymerization as potential gene and antisense delivery agents. *J Am Chem Soc* 124, 15198–15207.

Mier, A., Maffucci, I., Merlier, F., Prost, E., Montagna, V., Ruiz-Esparza, G.U., Bonventre, J. V, Dhal, P.K., Tse Sum Bui, B., Sakhaii, P., 2021. Molecularly imprinted polymer nanogels for protein recognition: Direct proof of specific binding sites by solution STD and WaterLOGSY NMR spectroscopies. *Angew Chem Int Ed* 60, 20849–20857.

Mittal, P., Saharan, A., Verma, R., Altalbawy, F., Alfaidi, M.A., Batiha, G.E.-S., Akter, W., Gautam, R.K., Uddin, M.S., Rahman, M.S., 2021. Dendrimers: A new race of pharmaceutical nanocarriers. *Biomed Res Int* 2021.

Muñoz-Espí, R., Weiss, C.K., Landfester, K., 2012. Inorganic nanoparticles prepared in miniemulsion. *Curr Opin Colloid Interface Sci* 17, 212–224.

Naahidi, S., Jafari, M., Edalat, F., Raymond, K., Khademhosseini, A., Chen, P., 2013. Biocompatibility of engineered nanoparticles for drug delivery. *J Control Release* 166, 182–194.

Nance, E.A., Woodworth, G.F., Sailor, K.A., Shih, T.-Y., Xu, Q., Swaminathan, G., Xiang, D., Eberhart, C., Hanes, J., 2012. A dense poly (ethylene glycol) coating improves penetration of large polymeric nanoparticles within brain tissue. *Sci Transl Med* 4, 149ra119–149ra119.

Nandy, M., Lahiri, B.B., Yadhukrishna, C.H., Philip, J., 2021. Poly acrylic acid stabilized magnetic nanoemulsions for visual defect detection: Effect of pH on detection sensitivity and colloidal stability. *J Mol Liq* 336, 116332.

Noree, S., Tangpasuthadol, V., Kiatkamjornwong, S., Hoven, V.P., 2017. Cascade post-polymerization modification of single pentafluorophenyl ester-bearing homopolymer as a facile route to redox-responsive nanogels. *J Colloid Interface Sci* 501, 94–102.

Norouzi, M., Amerian, M., Amerian, M., Atyabi, F., 2020. Clinical applications of nanomedicine in cancer therapy. *Drug Discov Today* 25, 107–125.

Patel, A., Cholkar, K., Agrahari, V., Mitra, A.K., 2013. Ocular drug delivery systems: An overview. *World J Pharmacol* 2, 47.

Pelaz, B., Alexiou, C., Alvarez-Puebla, R.A., Alves, F., Andrews, A.M., Ashraf, S., Balogh, L.P., Ballerini, L., Bestetti, A., Brendel, C., 2017. Diverse applications of nanomedicine. *ACS Nano* 11, 2313–2381.

Peng, H., Huang, X., Melle, A., Karperien, M., Pich, A., 2019. Redox-responsive degradable prodrug nanogels for intracellular drug delivery by crosslinking of amine-functionalized poly (N-vinylpyrrolidone) copolymers. *J Colloid Interface Sci* 540, 612–622.

Piktel, E., Niemirowicz, K., Wątek, M., Wollny, T., Deptuła, P., Bucki, R., 2016. Recent insights in nanotechnology-based drugs and formulations designed for effective anti-cancer therapy. *J Nanobiotechnol* 14, 1–23.

Popova, T., Tzankov, B., Voycheva, C., Spassova, I., Kovacheva, D., Tzankov, S., Aluani, D., Tzankova, V., Lambov, N., 2021. Mesoporous silica MCM-41 and HMS as advanced drug delivery carriers for bicalutamide. *J Drug Deliv Sci Technol* 62, 102340.

Qaiser, R., Pervaiz, F., Shoukat, H., Yasin, H., Hanan, H., Murtaza, G., 2023. Mucoadhesive chitosan/polyvinylpyrrolidone-co-poly (2-acrylamide-2-methylpropane sulphonic acid) based hydrogels of captopril with adjustable properties as sustained release carrier: Formulation design and toxicological evaluation. *J Drug Deliv Sci Technol* 81, 104291.

Rai, M., Ingle, A.P., Gupta, I., Brandelli, A., 2015. Bioactivity of noble metal nanoparticles decorated with biopolymers and their application in drug delivery. *Int J Pharm* 496, 159–172.

Rajan, R., Matsumura, K., 2017. Tunable dual-thermoresponsive core–shell nanogels exhibiting UCST and LCST behavior. *Macromol Rapid Commun* 38, 1700478.

Sahoo, S.K., Parveen, S., Panda, J.J., 2007. The present and future of nanotechnology in human health care. *Nanomedicine* 3, 20–31.

Sahu, T., Ratre, Y.K., Chauhan, S., Bhaskar, L., Nair, M.P., Verma, H.K., 2021. Nanotechnology based drug delivery system: Current strategies and emerging therapeutic potential for medical science. *J Drug Deliv Sci Technol* 63, 102487.

Sang, G., Bardajee, G.R., Mirshokraie, A., Didehban, K., 2018. A thermo/pH/magnetic-responsive nanogel based on sodium alginate by modifying magnetic graphene oxide: Preparation, characterization, and drug delivery. *Iran Polym J* 27, 137–144.

Schafroth, N., Arpagaus, C., Jadhav, U.Y., Makne, S., Douroumis, D., 2012. Nano and microparticle engineering of water insoluble drugs using a novel spray-drying process. *Colloids Surf B Biointerfaces* 90, 8–15.

Sekhon, B.S., Kamboj, S.R., 2010. Inorganic nanomedicine—part 2. *Nanomedicine* 6, 612–618.

Serrano, E., Rus, G., Garcia-Martinez, J., 2009. Nanotechnology for sustainable energy. *Renew Sustain Energy Rev* 13, 2373–2384.

Shi, J., Votruba, A.R., Farokhzad, O.C., Langer, R., 2010. Nanotechnology in drug delivery and tissue engineering: From discovery to applications. *Nano Lett* 10, 3223–3230.

Silva, G.A., 2004. Introduction to nanotechnology and its applications to medicine. *Surg Neurol* 61, 216–220.

Soni, K.S., Desale, S.S., Bronich, T.K., 2016. Nanogels: An overview of properties, biomedical applications and obstacles to clinical translation. *J Control Release* 240, 109–126.

Sultana, F., Imran-Ul-Haque, M., Arafat, M., Sharmin, S., 2013. An overview of nanogel drug delivery system. *J Appl Pharm Sci* 3, S95–S105.

Sumida, K., Liang, K., Reboul, J., Ibarra, I.A., Furukawa, S., Falcaro, P., 2017. Sol–gel processing of metal–organic frameworks. *Chem Mater* 29, 2626–2645.

Suner, S.S., Ari, B., Onder, F.C., Ozpolat, B., Ay, M., Sahiner, N., 2019. Hyaluronic acid and hyaluronic acid: Sucrose nanogels for hydrophobic cancer drug delivery. *Int J Biol Macromol* 126, 1150–1157.

Sung, Y.K., Kim, S.W., 2020. Recent advances in polymeric drug delivery systems. *Biomater Res* 24, 1–12.

Suri, S.S., Fenniri, H., Singh, B., 2007. Nanotechnology-based drug delivery systems. *J Occup Med Toxicol* 2, 1–6.

Tan, J.P.K., Goh, C.H., Tam, K.C., 2007. Comparative drug release studies of two cationic drugs from pH-responsive nanogels. *Eur J Pharm Sci* 32, 340–348.

Tiwari, S.K., Kumar, V., Huczko, A., Oraon, R., Adhikari, A. De, Nayak, G.C., 2016. Magical allotropes of carbon: Prospects and applications. *Crit Rev Solid State Mater Sci* 41, 257–317.

Tomalia, D.A., Baker, H., Dewald, J., Hall, M., Kallos, G., Martin, S., Roeck, J., Ryder, J., Smith, P., 1985. A new class of polymers: Starburst-dendritic macromolecules. *Polym J* 17, 117–132.

Tong, X., Pan, W., Su, T., Zhang, M., Dong, W., Qi, X., 2020. Recent advances in natural polymer-based drug delivery systems. *React Funct Polym* 148, 104501.

Tripathy, S., Das, M.K., 2013. Dendrimers and their applications as novel drug delivery carriers. *J Appl Pharm Sci* 3, 142–149.

Vallet-Regi, M., Rámila, A., Del Real, R.P., Pérez-Pariente, J., 2001. A new property of MCM-41: Drug delivery system. *Chem Mater* 13, 308–311.

Vilar, G., Tulla-Puche, J., Albericio, F., 2012. Polymers and drug delivery systems. *Curr Drug Deliv* 9, 367–394.

Vinogradov, S. V, Bronich, T.K., Kabanov, A. V, 2002. Nanosized cationic hydrogels for drug delivery: Preparation, properties and interactions with cells. *Adv Drug Deliv Rev* 54, 135–147.

Wagner, M., Roth, J., Wagner, B., 1976. Gold-labeled protectin from Helix pomatia for the localization of blood group A antigen of human erythrocytes by immuno freeze-etching. *Exp Pathol* 12, 277–281.

Wang, B., Chen, K., Yang, R., Yang, F., Liu, J., 2014. Photoresponsive nanogels synthesized using spiropyrane-modified pullulan as potential drug carriers. *J Appl Polym Sci* 131.

Wang, S., 2009. Ordered mesoporous materials for drug delivery. *Microporous Mesoporous Mater* 117, 1–9.

Wang, Y., Zhao, Q., Han, N., Bai, L., Li, J., Liu, J., Che, E., Hu, L., Zhang, Q., Jiang, T., 2015. Mesoporous silica nanoparticles in drug delivery and biomedical applications. *Nanomedicine* 11, 313–327.

Yang, P., Gai, S., Lin, J., 2012. Functionalized mesoporous silica materials for controlled drug delivery. *Chem Soc Rev* 41, 3679–3698.

Zhang, H., Zhai, Y., Wang, J., Zhai, G., 2016a. New progress and prospects: The application of nanogel in drug delivery. *Mater Sci Eng C* 60, 560–568.

Zhang, J., Ma, P.X., 2009. Polymeric core–shell assemblies mediated by host–guest interactions: Versatile nanocarriers for drug delivery. *Angew Chem* 121, 982–986.

Zhang, Q.M., Wang, W., Su, Y.-Q., Hensen, E.J.M., Serpe, M.J., 2016b. Biological imaging and sensing with multiresponsive microgels. *Chem Mater* 28, 259–265.

Zhu, Q., Chen, X., Xu, X., Zhang, Y., Zhang, C., Mo, R., 2018. Tumor-specific self-degradable nanogels as potential carriers for systemic delivery of anticancer proteins. *Adv Funct Mater* 28, 1707371.

12 Phytonanomedicine: A Cost-Effective Approach for Breast Cancer Therapy
Appropriately Relevant for India

Samrat Paul and Piyali Basak

12.1 INTRODUCTION

Cancer is a noticeable disease in West Bengal, India. By the end of 2010, more than 12 million cancerous patients were spotted out (Hemmati et al., 2017), and among them nearly 8 million were deceased (McGuire, 2016). Data from national and regional cancer centers from 1984 to 2002 indicated the accretion of incidence of breast cancer (Sen et al., 2002). According to the National Cancer Registries, Regional Cancer Centers, breast cancer is very common in women residing at Delhi, Mumbai, Ahmadabad, Kolkata, and Trivandrum (National Cancer Registry Programme, 2001). A population-based cancer registry in Kolkata put forward the suggestion that 27.3% of females were diagnosed having breast cancer during the metastatic stage (Sen et al., 2002, Report of Population-Based Cancer Registry, 2014). Metastasis occurs when an epithelial cancer cell loses its apico-basal polarity and forms spindle-shaped morphology. Carcinogen-induced mutation of the CDH1 gene inactivates phenotypic activation of E- cadherin that reduces cell to cell union and cell matrix adhesion (Serrano-Gomez et al., 2016). Chemotherapeutic agents used in antineoplastic therapy usually destroy the cancer cell and show no specific action too. Therefore, in recent years, significant effort has been assembled for finding out alternative better treatment modality. Since centuries, plant-based therapeutic treatment has put forward its important role toward the global healthcare system. *Moringa oleifera* is one such traditionally used medicinal herb that inhibited the promotion of tumor in a mouse two-stage DMBA-TPA tumor model (Murakami et al., 1998) and prevented skin cancer (Bharali et al., 2003). It is well established that *Moringa oleifera* leaf extract inhibited cell proliferation and induced apoptosis in human KB tumorigenic cell line and A549 lung cells by nfKb-mediated signaling pathways (Sreelatha et al., 2011, Tiloke et al., 2013, Waterman et al., 2014). Current cancer therapy anticipates an efficient target-oriented drug delivery system that remodulates

 DOI: 10.1201/9781003432661-12

the drug release profile to specific tissue with better ADME and concurrently lesser unintended adverse effects. Nanoparticle, with proportionate size and actively working biological molecules, coherently travel through the cytoplasm, pile up into the nucleus of the tumor tissue, and amplify the retention time (Duncan and Sat, 1998). On that account, nanoformulation enfolded with phytocompound that was extracted from Moringa *oleifera* may improvise the therapeutic intention for breast cancer.

12.2 BIOCHEMICAL MECHANISM FOR CANCER CELL FORMATION

The cell cycle is the bio-mechanical approach that involves a complex set of molecular and biochemical phenomenon on account for cell growth, replicating its DNA, followed by division to form its daughter cell (Hunt et al., 2011, Barnum and Connell, 2014). The cell division is often related to its differentiation when a mature cell splits up into a new phenotypic niche for performing a specific function. This phenotypic expression involves specific protein synthesis and generally occurs in the interphase (S phase and G2 phase) of the cell cycle (Ruijtenberg and van den Heuvel, 2016). The cell to cell pursued to tissue transformation is another highly commanded string-web event primarily aligned on different molecular and biochemical pathways (Barnum and Connell, 2014). Many key regulator genes and the vital checkpoints ensure toggled "on/off" various interactive proteins, thereby switching on successful cell division. The cell cycle regulation at G1 and G2 phases is predominantly governed by co-relation and interconnection between specific enzymes called cyclin-dependent kinases (CDK) and its substrate cyclin (Hunt et al., 2011). The healthy cells normally express transcription factor p53 protein at a minute quantity. Cellular injury leading to DNA damage brings posttranscriptional moderation of the p53 protein (Ozaki and Nakagawara, 2011). This activated p53 alters the target gene and promotes apoptosis (Ozaki and Nakagawara, 2011). A non-repairable genomic mutation on a tumor suppressor gene like p53 by any means at a molecular level of cell cycle progression imparted the limitless replicative potential of the earmarked cell. Currently, the assigned cell sets off mitosis to form a niche of tissue lump called a primary tumor or neoplasm. Inappropriate overexpression of normal oncogene and/or formation of novel oncogene, along with concurrent underexpression of tumor suppressor genes into the neoplasmic niche-imposed invasion quality besides sustainment of angiogenesis and self-sufficiency growth signaling trait. Accordingly, the neoplastic cell soon differentiated into a secondary tumor possessing a scope of spread from the originating organ to a distant place. The noticeable cell detached from its basement, unfastened cell to cell union, and became spindle-shaped for dignifying its metastatic patrimony. In this day and age, this malignant neoplasm is termed "CANCER" (Cooper, 2000).

12.3 EPIDEMIOLOGY OF THE CANCER WITH PRIMARILY FOCUSED ON BREAST CANCER OCCURRENCE IN STATE LEVEL

According to the World Health Organization (WHO), it is the second deadliest diseases, accounting for nearly 10 million deaths (in 2018) globally. It is projecting out with continuous raising the number of patients each year and was forecasted to be more than 12 million assassinations by 2030 (WHO, 2020). Ire-respected of male and female, new 18.1 million fresh cases were recorded. Among them, 11.6% were examined for lung cancer, closely followed by female breast cancer. The number of victimized incidences in prostate, colorectal, stomach, and liver cancer is also counted, considering their high mortality rate (Bray et al., 2018). In spite of quality improvement in biomedical research primarily focused on pre-screening and early diagnosis, breast cancer shows great risk on our society. The report from the American Cancer Society worries about the rising number of breast cancer patients in the current situation (2019–2020) (American Cancer Society, 2020). The global monitoring result reflects that the majority of the breast cancer patients deceased were taken place in low- and medium-earning territory. The rate of incidents was relatively high in developing countries, while the inflated frequency of death took place in less developed countries (Ghoncheh et al., 2016, Sen et al., 2002).

A population-based cancer registry pointed out the sharp rise in breast cancer event in Kolkata. Formerly, the consolidated report from the study conducted on the period of 1998–1999 suggested that the most frequently reported malignancies were breast cancer (22.7%) followed by uterine cervix (17.5%), gallbladder (6.4%), and ovary (5.8%) (Indian Council of Medical Research, 2001). Currently, the Indian Council of Medical Research (ICMR) and the Government of India have conducted a region-specific (Kolkata) population-based cancer registry programme with the data archived (from a period of 2008–2009) from the Regional Cancer Centre (Chittaranjan National Cancer Institute, Kolkata), their associates (Saroj Gupta Cancer Centre & Research Institute), and participating centers, including the Government Medical College and Hospital, a private hospital, and major cancer hospital throughout the city. All invasive cancers, as per the International classification of Diseases, Version 10 (ICD-10) categories C00 to C95, were considered for recording, followed by analysis, whereas in situ carcinoma and other precancerous lesion were excluded out. According to the report, a total of 9467 cases were recorded. The number includes mostly lung, breast, stomach, colon, rectum, and liver cancer patients, as these are frequently spotted out in the Indian population. Of the total population, 48.5% were female citizens. The breast cancer incidence rose from a previously reported 22.7% to a currently calculated 27.3%, and the mortality incidence was computed to be 46.4% (National Cancer Registry Programme, 2008–2009).

12.4 HORMONAL ETIOLOGY AND CELLULAR MECHANISM OF BREAST TISSUE FORMATION

The human female breast is an epidermal protuberance originating from the apocrine gland of the skin via a complex epithelial-mesenchymal reciprocal interaction. The hormonal etiology arranges breast tissue formation in two distinct phases; one is hormone-independent primary bud formation, followed by its maturation upto rudimentary ductal tree formation. The other one is hormone-dependent mammary gland formation, ductal elongation, and lactation-oriented differentiation (Javed and Lteif, 2013, Brisken and O'Malley, 2010). At the 6 weeks of gestation period, the progenitor cells of the mammary gland start to proliferate and form epithelial cells of the epidermis. The epithelial cell soon differentiated to form primary buds, which enlarge to move dorsally and became sites for secondary outgrowth (Javed and Lteif, 2013). The ectodarmal originate parenchyma tissue differentiates into branching duct and secretary acini, and the mesodarmal born stroma provides a site for adipose tissue formation (Javed and Lteif, 2013). This rudimentary breast enlarges isometric to the body surface but ceases in early childhood till puberty (Brisken and O'Malley, 2010).

At puberty, the growth hormone and cortisol together initiate enlargement of the breast. The elevated consignment of 17 β estradiol and progesterone triggers adulthood side branching with morphological resolution. This hormone-dependent breast tissue morphogenesis was further classified into five distinct phases, as described in Figure 12.1 (Encyclopedia of Children's Health, 2020). Briefly, these five phases are as follows (Table 12.1):

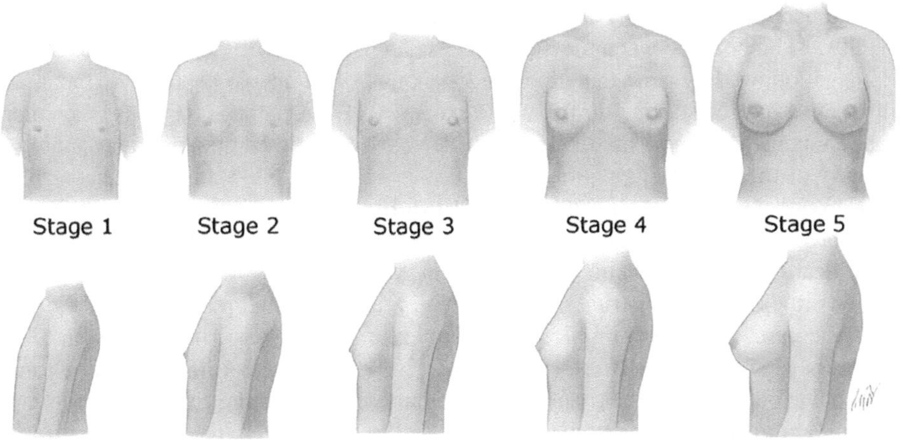

FIGURE 12.1 Stage-wise depiction of breast tissue formation

TABLE 12.1
Stages of Breast Formation

Stage One	The breasts are flat and only the tip of the nipple is raised.
Stage Two	Buds appear, breast and nipple are raised, fat tissue begins to form, and the areola enlarges.
Stage Three	Breasts are slightly larger with glandular breast tissue present. Initially, this happens in a conical shape and later in a rounder shape. The areola begins to darken.
Stage Four	The nipple and areola become raised and form a second mound above the rest of the breast.
Stage Five	Mature adult breast is rounded and only the nipple is raised.

Immediately after the pregnancy, the hormone prolactin influences the inflation of side branches of the breast to support alveologenesis and lactation-induced differentiation (Brisken and O'Malley, 2010).

12.5 TUMOR GENESIS FACTOR-INDUCED BREAST CANCER TISSUE FORMATION

Breast cancer is often marked as hereditary cancer since harmful inherited mutations in the BRCA1 and BRCA2 tumor suppressor genes boosting up the possibility of breast cancer (Petrucelli et al., 2020). The recent study finds that inherited genetic alteration gives less-significant contribution rather continuous exposure of carcinogenic substances makes a single step large scale genomic transformation that contributes to cancer cell formation (Wogan et al., 2004). In 2003, the national toxicological program declared estrogen a human carcinogen (Miller, 2003). The mammalian cell converts estrogen into related metabolic compounds that generate free radicals (Miller, 2003). Free radicals formed in our body damage the major components of cells, including DNA and the cell membrane of organelles. Abnormal or high concentration of free radical induces depurination and spontaneous hydrolysis (acidic medium) of the N-Glycosidic bond between the nitrogen base and sugar moiety that may lead to DNA damage followed by gene mutation. Endogenous DNA damage happens by the attack of reactive oxygen species (ROS), while exogenous DNA damage happens when man-made mutagenic chemicals interact with DNA. Aromatic compounds may mute the activity of the tumor suppressor gene and alter its functions, leading to uncontrolled cell growth (Miller, 2003; Dexheimer, 2013). Breast tissue remodeling includes cellular proliferation, moderate to large scale change in cell cycle and proliferation, and even death of cells. It occurs throughout the woman's life, including pre-menstrual, puberty, the 28-day menstrual cycle, pregnancy, lactation, and postmenopausal; therefore; increases the opportunity of DNA damage and stops repairing defects on tumor suppressor genes like BRCA1 (Dexheimer, 2013; Davis and Lin, 2011). The tumor may bulge out in any of the tissues, like stromal tissue, grandular tissue, lobule, or duct (Sharma et al., 2010). The gene expression profile histopathological parameter, tumor grade classification, presence of lymph node, and appearance of predictive markers like ER, PR, and HER2 receptor sophistically arrange the breast cancer into the following type are as follows (Sharma et al., 2010) (Table 12.2) Figure 12.2.

12.6 THERAPEUTIC APPROACHES FOR HEALING UP THE ALIMENT

The breast cancer treatment primarily depends on the tumor, node, and metastasis (TNM) system classified stage of cancer (Brierley et al., 2016), age, and physical condition of the patient since most of the patients often receive a combination therapy among two or more treatments one at a time. The most common therapeutic interventions are surgery, radiotherapy using ϒ-ray-emitted substances, immunotherapy that regulates the release of α-interferon, which facilitates the shrinkage of tumor cells, and hormonal therapy for reducing estrogen levels essentially, with addition to the

TABLE 12.2
Stages of Breast Cancer Formation

Non-Invasive Ductal Carcinoma In Situ that most often came about in the lining of the breast milk duct.
Invasive Ductal Carcinoma in which the neoplastic cells seize into surrounding tissue.
Inflammatory Breast Cancer refers to a special type of breast cancer where the skin of the breast becomes red; unlike inflammation or infection, the sufferer feels a warming sensation at the site. No single tissue lump is found as it is caused when cancer cells block lymph vessels in the skin.
Lobular Carcinoma In situ increases the risk factor for the development of invasive breast lesions.
Invasive Lobular Carcinoma originates in the milk-producing lobule but can spread in the distant part of the body.
Adenocarcinoma that mostly forms in glandular tissue, whereas **Sarcoma** starts in the muscle, fat, or connective tissue.

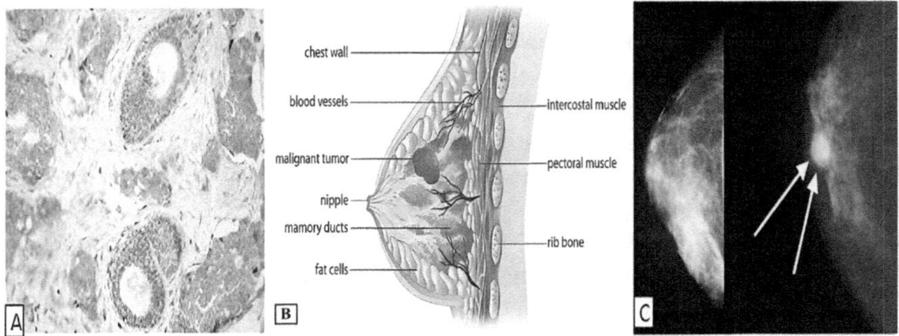

FIGURE 12.2 (a) Microphotograph of tumor cells in breast (Srabovic et al., 2013) and (b) anatomically cross-section of breast contains a malignant tumor Al-Ziaydi, Ahmed. (2020). Medical Biochemistry (http://www.healthofchildren.com/B/Breast-Development.html). (c) Mammograms' showing a normal breast (left) and a breast with tissue lump (right) (Gokhale, 2009).

principally used chemotherapy (Sharma et al., 2010). Traditional chemotherapeutic agents like alkalyting agent or antimetabolites kill the rapidly divided cancer cells either by apoptosis or necrosis (Sharma et al., 2010).

There has been an outstanding revolution in the area of chemotherapeutic intervention over the past 10 years (Sharma et al., 2014). Still, the anticancer therapy looks out for new regimens to combat with the poor retention time, nonspecific action, and improper outstretch of the target site.

12.7 NANOTECHNOLOGY PERSPECTIVE CONVEYANCE FOR BREAST CANCER MEDICAMENT

Nanotechnology appears as a knowledge-based experimental procedure that mostly confined the intelligence of physical theory and the chemical reaction together on account for the fabrication of the material in a very small scale, usually below 100 μm (Lankalapalli et al., 2014). And therefore it is rewarded as the "Biggest Engineering Innovation" in the current century (Sahu, 2013). In the present day, this emerging technology delivers its innovation toward health, safety, and mankind. The biomedical researcher employs this technology as a tool for the collection of preciously accurate medical information relating to diagnostics and therapeutics with in a short time. Moreover, a miniature device was manufactured, and a target-specific delivery system was invented by utilizing its application (Sharma et al., 2014, Lankalapalli et al., 2014), Figure 12.3.

As discussed before, contemporary anticancer therapy has some major limitations, such as improper drug target specificity, poor drug retention time in tissue, and less safety profile. The recent application of nanotechnology offers to assemble a potential delivery structure specifically perform resorting the drug in to its target. Accordingly, the drug interaction into the nonspecific tissue may reduce, which subsequently claims less frequency of dosages (Wang et al., 2013). In addition, the particle size similar to actively working biological molecules manifested a high specific surface area and an enhanced permeability and retention time (EPR) effect, facilitating its travel through the cytoplasm. It accumulates into the nucleus of the tumor tissue more than the normal tissue, thereby diminishing the anti-proliferative efficiency of cancer cells (Golombek et al., 2018).

The highly metastatic triple negative breast cancer expressed multidrug-resistance (MDR), which is influenced by the ATP-binding cassette transporter. MDR potentially creates obstacles for up taking the drug molecule and also facilitated its extrusion from cells (Zaki El-Readi and Althubiti, 2019). At present, nanoscale formulations such as liposome, polymeric nanoparticle, and nanoshells are used as a vehicle for transporting the drug- conjugate into the target tissue (Wu et al., 2017). The therapeutic index of nanoparticle-based formulation improved its efficiency potential into the earmarked tissue and maintained its sustainable concentration over the long period for acquiring its maximum effect (Wu et al., 2017, Saadeh et al., 2014). Food and Drug Administration (FDA) allowed nanoparticle-based chemotherapeutic delivery such as Doxil for breast cancer care (Tang et al., 2017). Liposome is another platform that is used for selective

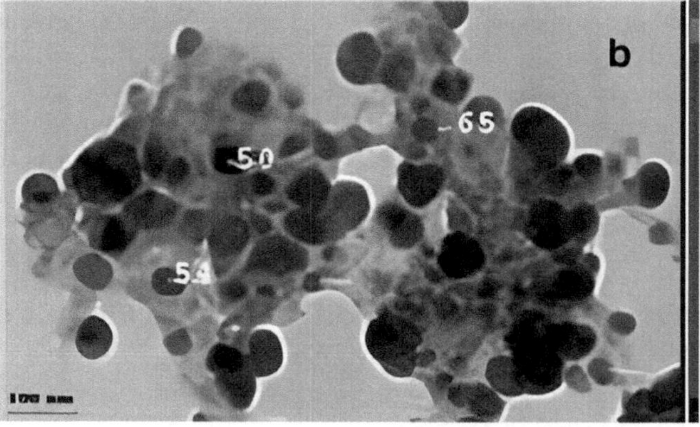

FIGURE 12.3 TEM structure of nanoparticles used for diagnostic and therapeutic purposes.

treatment for breast cancer (Paliwal et al., 2011). Quantum dots enhance the labeling and imagining quality of cancer cell and are intended to play a diagnostic mean (Narayanaswamy, 1981). Polymeric nanoparticles, especially micelles, capsule, and colloidal formulation, obtained ethical clearance for their clinical application (Tang et al., 2017). Despite all the modalities, the financial constrain from sufferer families reinforced the search of the new cost-effective alternative medicament.

12.8 PLANT-BASED REMEDIES; BOHAMIAN GIFT FOR BREAST CANCER TREATMENT

Since a century, India has been familiar as an Ayurvedic treatment hub and has become a trailblazer for employing the beneficial service of different plant species (Narayanaswamy, 1981). In 1993, the National Institute of Health (NIH) appreciated the plant-based unconventional therapy and classified natural active compound as an alternative medicine over a systemically synthetic medicine (Shareef et al., 2016). A USA-based survey report claimed that approximately 33% of Americans avail herbal remedies at least once per year (Eisenberg et al., 1993). According to the recent news (April, 2020), hydroxychloroquine is being studied under possible treatment for COVID-19 (Deccan Herald, 2020). This hydroxychloroquine is the synthetic derivatives of Cinchona bark-isolated active compound quinine (Permin et al., 2016). The statements pointed out that the plant is also the master family of synthetic medicine too.

A medicinal plant or its specific part (like bark, root, and leaf) acts as a reservoir for phytochemicals, Figure 12.4. Each part performs specific pharmacological functions based on the concentration of alkaloid, flavonoids, and other primary and secondary metabolites (Shareef et al., 2016), Figure 12.4. On that account, plant-based cancer

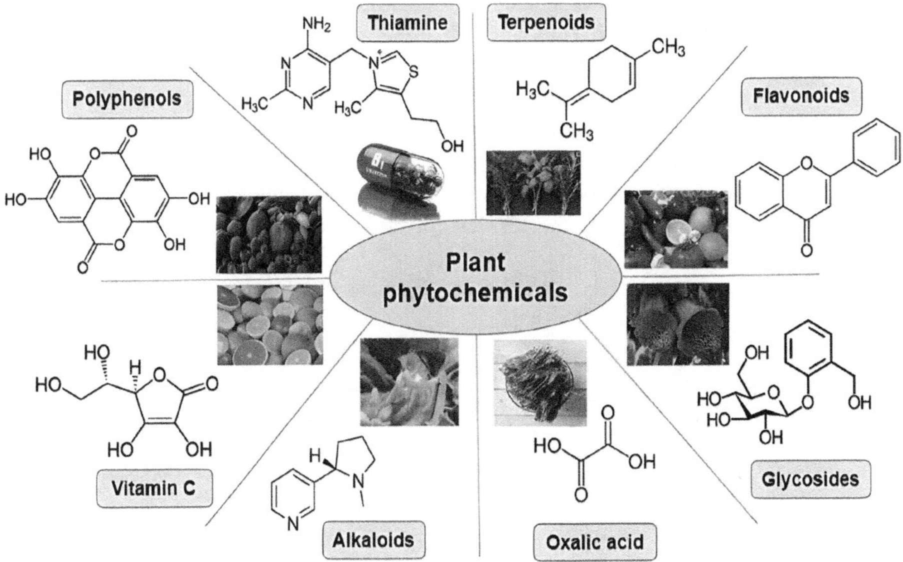

FIGURE 12.4 Chemical structure of different phytocompounds

remedies may be used as economical but beneficial medicament. *Gingko biloba*, goldenseal, ginseng, garlic, *Echinacea*, aloe vera, saw palmetto, and *Moringa oleifera* are spotted out as claimed as their strikingly medicinal potential (Shareef et al., 2016). These plant samples are employed for searching the new chemical entities that are suitable for the antineoplastic drug development process. On this account, *Moringa oleifera* entices our attention. It is a widely cultivated tree generally found in sub Himalayan pavement, East and South Africa, tropical Asia, Latin America, the Caribbean, Florida, and the Pacific Islands. Almost all parts of this tree are edible and purely safe for human consumption (Anwar et al., 2007, Fuglie, 2001).

Moringa is promisingly used as food source in tropical country like India. Many reports, including the phytochemical investigation, suggested that almost every part of the plant contains 4-(4′-O-acetyl-α-L-rhamnopyranosyloxy) benzylisothiocyanate, 4-(α-L-rhamnopyranosyloxy) benzyl isothiocyanate, niazimicin, pterygospermin, benzyl isothiocyanate, and 4-(α-L-rhamnopyranosyloxy) benzyl glucosinolate as potential disease-preventing compound. The pleiotropic action of the phytochemicals reinforced their use as unconventional medicine for treatment of anemia, asthma, gland swelling, headache, hypertension, and so many inflammatory and microbial diseases (Goyal et al., 2007).

Evidence-based investigation find out the anticancer property along with the anti-gonadotrophic hormonal activity of *Moringa oleifera* leaf (Bose, 2007). *Moringa oleifera* leaf extract in methanolic solvent shows an anti-gonadotrophic hormonal effect on the T47D cell line. Single-dose treatment with leaf extract retards the cell growth immediately after 24 h, whereas treatment with the estrogen progesterone combination increases the inhibition of cell growth by 12-fold against the initial growth. Growth kinetics of cells treated with the leaf extract show relatively slower proliferation of the cell compared to control (no treatment) cell (Paul et al., 2020). It is because the phytochemicals of leaf extract interfere with hormone receptors and inhibit the neoplastic growth via G-protein-linked cytokine pathways. Therefore, it may reduce the hormone-related cancer (breast cancer and ovarian cancer) growth. The aqueous leaf extract inhibited oxidative DNA damage and antiquorum sensing potential (Singh et al., 2009), whereas the methanolic leaf extract repressed the human cancerous KB cell line (Murakami et al., 1998). Recently, bis (isothiocyanatomethyle) benzene was claimed as a nature-driven antineoplastic phytocompound (Paul et al., 2019), Figure 12.5. Besides the phytochemicals, the combination of

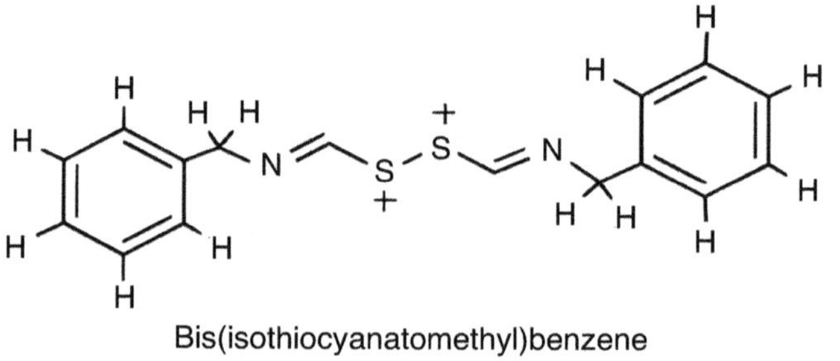

Bis(isothiocyanatomethyl)benzene

FIGURE 12.5 Bis (isothiocyanatomethyl)benzene.

isothiocyanate and the glucosinolate imparts its effectiveness for slowing down the rate of tumor promotion in a mouse two-stage DMBA-TPA tumor model (Sreelatha et al., 2011).

The modern practitioners now restore the conventional therapeutics of applying the crude extract into the isolated bioactive form for achieving its ultimatum, i.e., curing the breast cancers. Therefore, phytocompounds encapsulated or in other nanoformulations should be economical but a forwarding gesture on breast cancer treatment.

12.9 CONCLUSION AND FUTURE SCOPE

In essence, the combination of nanotechnology and plant-based remedies represents a Bohemian gift for breast cancer treatment, bringing together modern scientific advancements and traditional, nature-inspired healing practices. As research in this interdisciplinary field progresses, it holds the promise of not only advancing breast cancer therapies but also fostering a deeper connection between healthcare, culture, and the environment.

Nanotechnology facilitates precise drug delivery to cancer cells, ensuring targeted therapy. Combining this with plant-based remedies enhances the potential for therapeutic efficacy. The use of plant-based remedies, having compatibility with the human body, may contribute to minimizing adverse effects. The diverse nature of plant compounds, coupled with the precision of nanotechnology, opens avenues for personalized medicine. Tailoring treatments based on individual patient profiles may lead to more effective and patient-centric approaches. Nanoparticles can be designed to deliver immunomodulatory agents, and plant-based remedy can assist in optimizing the combination and sequencing of treatments to boost the immune system's response.

The future prospects of phytonanomedicine hold great promise in revolutionizing healthcare and disease management. Future initiatives may involve the development of more interactive and accessible platforms that can bridge the gap between urban and rural healthcare. It can facilitate international collaboration in breast cancer research; shared platforms for data analysis and collaborative projects can accelerate progress, leading to the development of more universally applicable and cost-effective therapies. Ongoing efforts in education and training can ensure that healthcare professionals in India are proficient in utilizing phytonanomedicine tools. This can lead to the more widespread adoption of advanced technologies in clinical practice.

In summary, the future of phytonanomedicine in breast cancer therapy in India involves a multidimensional approach. The ongoing collaboration between researchers, healthcare professionals, and technology experts is crucial for realizing the full potential of cost-effective and innovative breast cancer therapies.

REFERENCES

American Cancer Society. Breast Cancer Facts & Figures. https://www.cancer.org/research/cancer-facts-statistics/breast-cancer-facts-figures.html (Last visited on 4th April, 2020).

Anwar F, Latif S, Ashraf M. *Moringa oleifera*: A food plant with multiple medicinal uses. *Phytother. Res.* 2007; 21: 17–25. doi: 10.1002/ptr.2023.

Barnum KJ, Connell MJ. Cell cycle regulation by checkpoints. *Methods Mol. Biol.* 2014; 1170: 29–40. doi: 10.1007/978-1-4939-0888-2_2.

Bharali R, Tabassum J, Azad MR. Chemomodulatory effect of Moringa oleifera, Lam, on hepatic carcinogen metabolising enzymes, antioxidant parameters and skin papillomagenesis in mice. *Asian Pac J. Cancer Prev.* 2003 Apr-Jun; 4(2): 131–9.

Bose CK. Possible role of *Moringa oleifera* Lam. root in epithelial ovarian cancer. MedGenMed. 2007; 9(1): 26.

Bray F, Ferlay J, Soerjomataram I et al. Global cancer statistics 2018: GLOBOCAN estimates of incidence and mortality worldwide for 36 cancers in 185 countries. *CA Cancer J. Clin.* 2018; 68(6): 394–424. doi: 10.3322/caac.21492.

Brierley J, Gospodarowicz M, Sullivan B. The principles of cancer staging. *Ecancermedicalscience.* 2016; 10: ed61. doi: 10.3332/ecancer.2016.ed61.

Brisken C, O'Malley B. Hormone action in the mammary gland. *Cold Spring Harb. Perspect. Biol.* 2010; 2(12): a003178. doi: 10.1101/cshperspect.a003178

Cooper GM. *The Development and Causes of Cancer. The Cell: A Molecular Approach.* 2nd edition. Sinauer Associates, Sunderland, MA; 2000.

Davis JD, Lin SY. DNA damage and breast cancer. *World J. Clin. Oncol.* 2011; 2(9): 329–38. doi: 10.5306/wjco.v2.i9.329.

Deccan Herald. Hydroxychloroquine saved my life from COVID-19: US lawmaker; https://www.deccanherald.com/international/world-news-politics/hydroxychloroquine-saved-my-life-from-covid-19-us-lawmaker-822298.html (Last visited 9th April, 2020).

Dexheimer TS. DNA repair pathways and mechanisms. In: LA Mathews et al. (eds.), *DNA Repair of Cancer Stem Cells.* Springer Science & Business Media, Dordrecht; 2013: pp. 19–32.

Duncan R, Sat SN. Tumour targeting by enhanced permeability and retention (EPR) effect. *Ann. Oncol.* 1998; 9: 39.

Eisenberg DM, Kessler RC, Foster C. Unconventional medicine in the United States. Preference, costs and patterns of use. *N. Engl. J. Med.* 1993; 328: 246–252.

Encyclopedia of Children's Health. Breast Development. http://www.healthofchildren.com/B/Breast-Development.html (Last visited on 4th April, 2020).

Fuglie LJ. *The Miracle Tree: The Multiple Attributes of Moringa: Natural Nutrition for the Tropics.* Church World Service, Dakar; 2001: p. 172.

Ghoncheh M, Pournamdar Z, Salehiniya H. Incidence and mortality and epidemiology of breast cancer in the world. *Asian Pac J Cancer Prev.* 2016; 17(S3): 43–6. doi: 10.7314/apjcp.2016.17.s3.43.

Gokhale S. Ultrasound characterization of breast masses. *Indian J Radiol Imaging.* 2009;19(3): 242–247. doi: 10.4103/0971-3026.54878.

Golombek SK, Niklas-May J, Theek B. Tumor targeting via EPR: Strategies to enhance patient responses. *Adv. Drug Deliv. Rev.* 2018; 130: 17–38. doi: 10.1016/j.addr.2018.07.007.

Goyal BR, Agarwal BB, Goyal RK. Phyto-pharmacology of *Moringa oleifera* lam: An overview. *Nat. Prod. Radiance.* 2007; 6(4): 347–53.

Hemmati F, Dabbaghi F, Mahmoudi G. Meta-analysis of the impact of medical tourism and health tourism in the United States of America and Canada in the treatment of cancer. *Biosci. Biotech. Res. Comm.* 2017; (2): 374–81.

Hunt T, Nasmyth K, Novák B. The cell cycle. *Philos. Trans. R Soc. Lond. B Biol. Sci.* 2011; 366(1584): 3494–7. doi: 10.1098/ rstb.2011.0274.

Indian Council of Medical Research. Consolidated report of the population based cancer registries conducted on period of 1990–1996. National Cancer Registry Programme. Indian Council of Medical Research. New Delhi; 2001.

Javed A, Lteif A. Development of the human breast. *Semin. Plast Surg.* 2013; 27(1): 5–12. doi: 10.1055/s-0033-1343989.

Lankalapalli S, Routhu KC, Ojha S. Nanoparticulate drug delivery systems: Promising approaches for drug delivery. *J. Drug Deliv. Ther.* 2014; (1): 72–85.

McGuire S. *World Cancer Report 2014.* Geneva, Switzerland: World Health Organization, International Agency for Research on Cancer, WHO Press, 2015. *Adv Nutr.* 2016; 7(2): 418–9. doi: 10.3945/an.116.012211

Miller K. Estrogen and DNA damage: The silent source of breast cancer? *J. Natl. Cancer Inst.* 2003; 95(2): 100–02. doi: 10.1093/jnci/95.2.100.

Murakami A, Kitazono Y, Jiwajinda S. et al. Niaziminin, a thiocarbamate from the leaves of *Moringa oleifera*, holds a strict structural requirement for inhibition of tumor-promoter-induced Epstein-Barr virus activation. *Planta Med.* 1998; 64: 319–23.

Narayanaswamy V. Origin and development of ayurveda: (A brief history). *Anc. Sci. Life.* 1981; 1(1): 1–7.

National Cancer Registry Programme. *Consolidated Report of the Population Based Cancer Registries 1990–1996.* Indian Council of Medical Research, New Delhi; 2001.

National Cancer Registry Programme. Report from Region Specific (Kolkata) Population Based Cancer Registry, Kolkata conducted on a period of 2008–2009, under National Cancer Registry Programme. Indian Council of Medical Research, New Delhi; 2008–2009.

Ozaki T, Nakagawara A. role of p53 in cell death and human cancers. *Cancers.* 2011; 3(1): 994–1013. doi: 10.3390/cancers3010994.

Paliwal SR, Paliwal R, Agrawal GP et al. Liposomal nanomedicine for breast cancer therapy. *Nanomedicine.* 2011; 6(6): 1085–100. doi: 10.2217/nnm.11.72.

Paul S, Basak P, Maity N, Guha C, Jana NK. Bis (isothiocyanatomethyl) benzene, a plant derived anti-neoplastic compound: Purified from *Moringa oleifera* leaf extract. *Anti-Cancer Agents Med. Chem.* 2019; 19(5): 677–86. doi: 10.2174/1871520619666190206164137.

Paul S, Basak P, Majumder R et al. Biochemical estimation of *Moringa oleifera* leaf extract for synthesis of silver nanoparticle mediated drug delivery system. *J. Plant Biochem. Biotechnol.* 2020; 29(1): 86–93.

Permin H, Norn S, Kruse E. On the history of Cinchona bark in the treatment of Malaria. *Dansk Medicinhistorisk Arbog.* 2016; 44: 9–30.

Petrucelli N, Daly MB, Pal T. *BRCA1*- and *BRCA2*-associated hereditary breast and ovarian cancer. In *GeneReviews.* University of Washington, Seattle; 2020.

Report of Population Based Cancer Registry, 2008–2009, National Cancer Registry Programme, ICMR, published in 2014.

Ruijtenberg S, van den Heuvel S, Coordinating cell proliferation and differentiation: Antagonism between cell cycle regulators and cell type-specific gene expression. *Cell Cycle.* 2016; 15(2): 196–212. doi: 10.1080/15384101.2015.1120925.

Saadeh Y, Leung T, Vyas A et al. Applications of nanomedicine in breast cancer detection, imaging, and therapy. *J. Nanosci. Nanotechnol.* 2014; 14(1): 913–23. doi: 10.1166/jnn.2014.8755.

Sahu AN. Nanotechnology in herbal medicine and cosmetics. *Int. J. Res. Ayurveda* Pharm. 2013; 4(3): 472–74.

Sen U, Sankaranarayanan R, Mandal S et al. Cancer patterns in eastern India: The first report of the Kolkata cancer registry. *Int. J. Cancer.* 2002; 100(1): 86–91. doi: 10.1002/ijc.10446.

Serrano -Gomez SJ, Maziveyi M, Alahari SK, Regulation of epithelial-mesenchymal transition through epigenetic and post-translational modifications. *Mol Cancer.* 2016; 15: 18.

Shareef M, Ashraf MA, Sarfraz M, Natural cures for breast cancer treatment. *Saudi Pharm.* J. 2016; 24(3): 233–40. doi: 10.1016/j.jsps.2016.04.018.

Sharma D, Kumar D, Singh G. A review on current advances in nanotechnology approaches for the effective delivery of anti-cancer drugs. *J. Drug Deliv. Ther.* 2014; (1): 66–71.

Sharma GN, Dave R, Sanadya J. Various types and management of breast cancer: An overview. *J. Adv Pharm Technol Res.* 2010; 1(2): 109–26.

Srabovic, Nahida, Mujagic, Zlata, Mujanovic-Mustedanagic, Jasminka, Softic, Adaleta, Muminovic, Zdeno, Rifatbegovic, Adi, Begic, Lejla, Vascular Endothelial Growth Factor Receptor-1 Expression in Breast Cancer and Its Correlation to Vascular Endothelial Growth Factor A. *Int J Breast Cancer*. 2013; 2013: 746749. https://doi.org/10.1155/2013/746749

Singh BN, Singh BR, Singh RL et al. Oxidative DNA damage protective activity, antioxidant and anti-quorum sensing potentials of *Moringa oleifera. Food Chem. Toxicol.* 2009; 47: 1109–16.

Sreelatha S, Jeyachitra A, Padma PR. Antiproliferation and induction of apoptosis by *Moringa oleifera* leaf extract on human cancer cells. *Food Chem. Toxicol.* 2011 Jun; 49(6): 1270–5. doi: 10.1016/j.fct.2011.03.006.

Tang X, S Loc W, Dong C et al. The use of nanoparticulates to treat breast cancer. Nanomedicine, 2017; 12(19): 81–103. https://doi.org/10.2217/nnm-2017-0202.

Tiloke C, Phulukdaree A, Chuturgoon AA. The antiproliferative effect of *Moringa oleifera* crude aqueous leaf extract on cancerous human alveolar epithelial cells. *BMC Complement Altern. Med.* 2013; 13: 226.

Wang R, Billone SP, Wayne MM. Nanomedicine in action: An overview of cancer nanomedicine on the market and in clinical trials. *J. Nanomater.* 2013; 2013: 629681. https://doi.org/10.1155/2013/629681.

Waterman C, Cheng DM, Rojas-Silva P, Poulev A, Dreifus J, Lila MA, Raskin I. Stable, water extractable isothiocyanates from *Moringa oleifera* leaves attenuate inflammation in vitro. *Phytochemistry* 2014; 103: 114–22.

Wogan GN, Hecht SS, Felton JS. Environmental and chemical carcinogenesis. *Semin Cancer Biol.* 2004 Dec; 14(6): 473–86.

World Health Organization. Fact Sheets on Cancer from International Agency for Research on Cancer, World Health Organization. https://www.who.int/news-room/fact-sheets/detail/cancer (Last visit on 4th April, 2020).

Wu D, Si M, Xue HY et al. Nanomedicine applications in the treatment of breast cancer: Current state of the art. *J Nanomed.* 2017; 16(12): 5879–92. doi: 10.2147/IJN.S123437.

Zaki El-Readi M, Althubiti MA. Cancer nanomedicine: A new era of successful targeted therapy. *J Nanomater.* 2019; 2019: 4927312. doi: 10.1155/2019/4927312.

13 Nanoparticle-Based Gene Delivery in Therapeutics

Current Status and Future Scope

Rajdeep Ganguly, Archisman Bhunia, and Ananya Barui

13.1 INTRODUCTION

The age-old traditional approach in addressing certain therapies like enzyme replacement, stem cell transplantation, small molecule therapy has brought forth a spectrum of consents in terms of their target specificity, precise delivery, efficacy, acceptability, and cytotoxicity. It was during the late 60s and Early 70s when the scientific community came up with the concept of gene delivery as an alternate measure to address disease therapy. The first evidence of gene transfection upon chicken fibroblast was reported in 1972, when papovaviruses SV40 and polyomavirus were primarily used as vectors [1]. Though the traditional therapeutics were efficient to some extent, they put forth certain setbacks like lesser *in vivo* half-life, difficulty in isolation, poor solubility and bioavailability, immunogenic responses, deficit optimum response action upon the target cite, and acceptability of the grafts. The gene delivery approach on the other hand was reliable in delivering the desired copy of genes to target specific sites, altering the genetic makeup, and retaining the effects for a longer span. Though a promising concept, gene therapy faced hurdles way before entering preclinical trials due to the lack of established delivery pipelines, precise site targeting, and validation in reducing the risks and side effects. Despite several setbacks, the gene delivery therapeutics has also bagged a few positive responses in the trial of adrenoleukodystrophy, X-linked severe combined immunodeficiency (SCID-X1), and adenosine deaminase (ADA) deficiency. These successful trials supervised under the European Medicines Agency (EMA) further stated the gene-delivering vectors to be characterized by the following properties: the vector must comprise an active substance containing a recombinant nucleic acid potent in replacing, repairing, deletion, and/or addition in sequence regulation; the diagnostic, therapeutic, and prophylactic outcome is associated with the recombinant sequence and its genetic expression and shall not consider the categories of vaccines for infectious disease treatments [2].

DOI: 10.1201/9781003432661-13

The aim of these regulations is to make the gene therapy as a potential transfection methodology for incorporating external genes into the target-specific sites to restore the functionality by manipulating the sequential expression [3].

Way before shaping the concept of delivering exogenes *in vitro* and/or *in vivo* for therapeutics, literature marked the origin of the concept of transfection phenomena with the publication of "Griffith's Experiment" in 1928. Later James L. Alloway established the "transforming principle" in 1933, highlighting the presence of an unrecognized substance potent in transforming the avirulent *Pneumococcus* strain to the virulent form. In 1944, a transforming substance was recognized as deoxyribonucleic acid (DNA) by McCarty and Avery. Lederberg along with Tatum in 1947 and Zinder in 1952 brought forth the concepts of transformation, conjugation, and transduction as potential methods for gene transfer. Later, the discovery of bacteriophage of *Salmonella typhimurium* was found to be the transporter in the mechanism of transduction, establishing the scientific significance of exploration for similar eukaryotic vectors. In 1962, Waclaw Szybalski et al. demonstrated "DNA-mediated heritable transformation of a biochemical trait" which was among the first documented evidence of the potency of hypoxanthine-guanine phosphoribosyl transferase ($HGPRT^{(+)}$) D98S human bone marrow cell line to survive and proliferate in the cocktail of hypoxanthine, aminopterin, thymidine (HAT) media. A similar pattern of genetic mutation was identified by Howard Temin in 1961 in chicken cells infected by Rous sarcoma virus (RSV). This significant observation broke the boundary of the age-old concept of genetic information transfer within the same form of nucleotide and established evidence of the transfer of information from RNA to DNA, leading the founding stone for ribonucleic acid (RNA)-dependent DNA polymerase exploration. Further, Edward Tatum proposed his work in 1966, highlighting the objective of using the viral vector as an aid for gene therapy in somatic cells. Later, Rogers et al. proposed a feasible study upon gene therapy involving tobacco mosaic virus (TMV) as a carrier to promote the introduction of polyadenylate into viral RNA. Motivated by the promising outcomes, they went further for direct human trials of gene therapy upon two girls diagnosed with urea cycle disorder, the vector being wild type *Shope papilloma* virus for transfecting arginase synthesizing gene. Ironically, this incident of the 70s concluded with a negative outcome, taking into consideration the absence of the gene encoding arginase within the viral genome. After a few successful transfection trials of herpes simplex virus (HSV) thymidine kinase and dihydrofolate reductase into the bone marrow of mouse stem cells, the final push to conduct gene therapy using DNA recombinant technology was commenced in 1990. Such a successful test further motivated Cline to conduct human trials on patients with β-thalassemia. Along the timeline, a similar work by Rosenberg demonstrated the diagnostic ability of metastatic melanoma with re-administration of genetically modified tumour-infiltrating lymphocytes (TILs) by transfection of neomycin-resistant retroviral marker gene, NeoR gene. This trial of 1993 gave a positive response of no viable tumour cells at the site of injection. Aside from the initial trial, a therapeutic trial was conducted by another researcher, Michael R. Blaese, in 1995, incorporating *ex vivo* modified white blood cells (WBC) for regular expression of ADA in two patients diagnosed with adenosine deaminase deficiency (ADA-SCID). Though the outcome remained a subject of debate among the research community, the practice of gene transfer began upon diverse diseases with the first successful transfection into the human brain by direct *in vivo* delivery in the same year. Ironically, this booming technology of gene transfection faced a setback in 1999 when a patient undergoing trial suffered multiorgan failure as a result of an immediate immunogenic response to overdosed adenovirus (Ad) administration. In the past decade, despite cytotoxic challenges for the administration of viral carriers, gene therapy gained attention in the trials of cancer, cardiovascular, and monogenetic diseases. In 2003, adenoviral vector-based product was approved for transfecting p53 cDNA, replacing E1 gene of the vector, in targeting head neck squamous cell carcinoma which gave a boost to the administration of gene delivery-based treatment. The consecutive years have further witnessed the development of diverse virus-based gene delivery methodologies. However, Ark Therapeutics Group plc in 2008, developed viral vector-based gene delivery platform, Cerepro®, which is the only product to complete a Phase III clinical trial to date [2].

Due to the ethical consents associated with the cytotoxic effect of viral transfection, several other delivery systems were also explored simultaneously which include chemical methodologies for Ca^{2+} phosphate precipitation, lipid endocytosis, electroporation, photoporation, hydroporation, sonoporation, etc [4–6]. Among these alternatives, the lipid NP-based delivery appeared to be the most favourable choice due to their robust procedure in condensation of million nucleotides for easy delivery to the cells. Efforts have also been made, including cholesterol, to limit the mobility and boost the packaging of lipid complexes [7]. Alongside the lipid-nanocomplex architecture of the vector, other cationic polymer-based delivery systems incorporating polyethylenimine (PEI), chitosan, polyamidoamine (PAMAM) dendrimers, and poly(lactide-co-glycolide) (PLGA) have also been explored broadly for transection [8]. Though their outcomes are of much significance, being a membrane perforation technique, the viability of protein and/or the target sites under physical force and the rate of transfection become limitations in their efficacy [9]. Further research on countermeasures to minimize the risk factors, nanoparticles like gold, magnetite, calcium phosphate, quantum dots (QDs), and others are also focussed on their promising biocompatible character and effective gene delivery conclusions [10,11].

Carbon nanotubes (CNT) and gold nanoparticles (AuNPs) complexed with cationic polymers have been witnessed to efficiently deliver the genes to their target sites. Some other biological delivery systems like micro RNA (miRNA), small interfering RNA (siRNA), and plasmid DNA (pDNA) too have proven their worth [11]. These biological/abiological particles for their precise confirmation, alongside biocompatibility, immune tolerance, target specificity, and extended circulation period have proven role in gene delivery for theranostics of a spectrum of diseases involving cardiovascular, cancer, and other monogenetic disorders [2]. NP being at the centre of focus in gene transfection, two methods are primarily preferred: nanospheres reservoirs and surface binding architecture [12]. They also highlighted the use of solid lipid nanoparticles (SLNs) and nanostructure lipid carriers (NLCs) in therapeutic cancer, ocular, and infectious diseases [12]. Magnetic NP like Fe_3O_4 and iron oxide coated with mesoporous silica have been documented as a superior choice in contributing to suicide gene therapy of cancer because of their magnetic hyperthermia and targeting potency. However, there are controversies regarding the efficacy of gene delivery using polymeric nanospheres, nanogels, dendrimers, and micelles for cardiovascular disease [12]. Gold nanoparticles too have a broad application spectrum in gene delivery, especially in targeting cancer cell lines and human retinal pigment epithelium [13,14]. Aside AuNPs, QDs of glutathione (GSH)-modified ZnO have also proved its potency in gene silencing, biolabelling, and neuroprotection while targeting accumulation of α-synuclein (SNCA) in mid-brain, a character of Parkinson's disease (PD) [15]. Graphene quantum dots (GQDs) conjugated with green fluorescent protein (GFP), doxorubicin (Dox), epidermal growth factor receptor (EGFR), and PEI have emerged as novel platform for theranostics to colon cancer [16].

The main goal of engineered nanoparticle-based vector development is to overcome the bottlenecks like cell surface affinity, condensation, endosomal-lysosomal escape, nuclear intake, cytoplasmic relocation, and de-condensation of nucleic acids for transcription in the gene delivery pipeline [13]. Henceforth, the chapter further presents a pathway of conventional pipelines in gene delivery and their limitations, concluding with the nano-scale alternatives in disease theranostics and their potency for future exploration.

13.2 CONVENTIONAL STRATEGIES OF GENE DELIVERY AND THEIR LIMITATIONS

With the emergence of studies upon the cell transformation and incorporation of genetic markers into cell lines of papovaviruses polyoma and SV40 during the early 1970s, the concept of gene delivery began its era of acceptance. Around this time, the advancement of recombinant DNA technology also demonstrated the potency of foreign gene incorporation in revising the genetic and/or phenotypic deformities in both *in vivo* and *iv vitro.* [1] Over the period, communities of clinicians and molecular biologists dived deep into finding the methodologies for traversing the genes to their targets. This brought forth some of the strategic platforms which later underwent intense investigations in proving their potential. The noteworthy strategic platforms are cationic lipids, viral vectors, electroporation, use of polybrene, and diethylaminoethyl (DEAE)-dextran [17–20]. Despite certain limitations, these platforms have proved the traversing of genes *in vivo* and *in vitro* (Table 13.1), opening a new forefront of investigation for advanced theranostics.

13.2.1 Cationic Lipid in Gene Delivery

Since the beginning of investigation back in the 70s, gene transfection by cationic lipids grabbed the centre of focus as a promising substitute to viral carriers for targeted expression and silencing of genes. The headgroup of the cationic lipid is positively charged, along with a hydrophobic tail, of a steroid-based or aliphatic domain, linked with the headgroup by a linker. These cationic headgroup-bearing amphiphiles, capable of reorienting their architecture aligning with nucleic acids through electrostatic interaction, develops nano/microparticles (i.e. polyplexes and lipoplexes) that resist nuclease against degradation along its trajectory within the cellular microenvironment. The linker regulates the behavioural traits (i.e. cationic and

TABLE 13.1
Advantages and Disadvantages of the Conventional Methodologies

Methodology	Advantage	Disadvantage	References
1. Chemical Method			
a. Cationic lipids	High efficiency of transfection *in vitro*, easy sample preparation, and availability	Less efficiency *in vivo*, toxic, and may trigger immunogenic response	[4,21]
b. Ca^{2+} phosphate precipitation	Efficient *in vivo* with low cytotoxicity, operationally compatible with different plasmids	Low transfection efficiency of 1% to 10%, difficulty in yielding reproducible result	[4]
2. Physical Method			
a. Electroporation	Applicable for diverse cell types and their cell cycle stages, DNA formulation with certain polymers enhances efficiency	Development of potential drop across the skin, skin oedema, increased transmembrane diffusivity and conductivity	[5,6]
b. Sonoporation	Proficient delivery of DNA/RNA to any cells, site specific and parameters easy to manipulate, can be used *in vivo*	Efficiency of *in vitro* and *in vivo* transfection are relatively low, rapture of cell membrane	[6]
c. Photoporation	Target-specific transfection, promising for primary cell lines	Low transfection rate (2.51% and 24.84% for 50 and 500 impulses at 24 hours), high impulse increases mortality rate, restricted clinical use	[6]
d. Magnetofection	Low quantity of vector required, short incubation period, inexpensive and efficient transfection to broader cell lines.	Formulation of desired magnetic particle-naked nucleic acid complex	[6]
e. Hydroporation	Highly efficient *in vivo* transfection	Limited knowledge of application upon kidney and muscles	[6]
f. Impalefection	Help track transfection efficiently without microscopic observation, single DNA molecule	Cost involving fabrication, biocompatibility challenges *in vivo*	[6,22]
3. Viral Method	High transfection efficiency, the virus regulates target-specific transfection	Immunogenic response, restricted complex fabrication, insertion mutagenesis	[23]

hydrophobicity) of the moiety in stability, cytotoxicity, biodegradability, and transfer efficacy. Though controversial, some investigators showed that a shorter tail length bearing aliphatic chain has promising performance in gene transfection. However, other studies showed tail with an array of 10–14 carbon atoms to be the most potent in delivery [17]. They further observed C14 expressing optimum transfection potency alongside liposomal formulations like 1,2-dioleoyl-3-trimethylammonium-propane (DOTAP); dioctadecylamidoglycylspermine (DOGS); N-[1-(2,3-dioleyloxy)propyl]-N,N,N-trimethylammonium chloride (DOTMA); and DORIE, which bears two hydrophobic chains in contrast to its single-tailed counterparts. Nevertheless, the potency has yet been under the matter of conflict for the chemical and geometrical properties that determine the degree of efficacy. Ponti et al. (2021) further focussed on the complex supramolecular architecture of lipoplexes comprising domains like helper lipids alongside cationic lipids and nucleic acids. The helper lipids, assumed in assisting the supramolecular fabrication, also tune the lipoplex–cell membrane interaction for stabilizing the colloidal architecture. The transfection behaviour of lipoplexes is regulated by the presence of lipid-to-nucleic acid ratio, alongside varying environmental conditions of altered salt concentration, temperature, and cell–lipoplex trafficking [17]. Beside lipids, cationic polymers like PEI, dendrimers like PAMAM, chitosan, and poly-L-lysine (PLL) have also been observed to validate high condensation potency towards nucleotides by forming cationic micelle in neutral pH [24]. This capability of polymers is also assumed due to the lack of a hydrophobic domain, unlike its lipid counterpart.

All through the decades, researchers invested time in understanding the mechanical flow chain that regulates the delivery of genes, including supramolecular interaction to the surface receptors, route of entry and simultaneous escape into cytosol bypassing extra-/intra-cellular barriers of macrophage attacks, and transfer to the nucleus. The fortification of incorporating nucleotides is carried by the binding of cationic polymers at the major grooves, blocking the active sites of DNase from the interaction. The final step rests on penetrating the cell by endocytosis, thereby getting into the nucleus for transcriptional execution (Figure 13.1) [24]. Intense investigations have been carried out to modify the characteristics of lipoplex/polyplex along their trajectory to the target site. These include a coating to prevent non-target polarity interaction, target-specific cell line binding, interaction with proteoglycans, altering the molecular weight of the vector to prevent extra-/intra-cellular barriers, and cytotoxicity [24]. The kinetics behind the conformational architecture of lipoplex too faced limitations in understanding, leaving a gap in supramolecular conceptualization. Mukherjee et al. (2022) highlighted the structural deviation in the lipid property has too diverted the kinetic pathway in lipoplex (lipid/DNA complex) formation, i.e. Lip1814/DNA *complex under* diffusion-controlled *and Lip1810/DNA complex* conformational rearrangement-controlled pathway [25].

13.2.2 Viral Gene Delivery

Efficient delivery of the genes by mediating the viral transfection mechanism has always been a preference despite certain pitfalls. Hybrid viral vector models have shown promises in easy cell integration, target specificity, and immunogenic escape, while contributing to neurotropism and other monogenic disease treatment. Zhao et al. (2022) reviewed a brief plethora of engineered viral carriers like retroviruses, lentiviruses, HSV, adeno-associated virus (AAV), and Ad that are under various clinical phases targeting the in vivo gene therapy towards

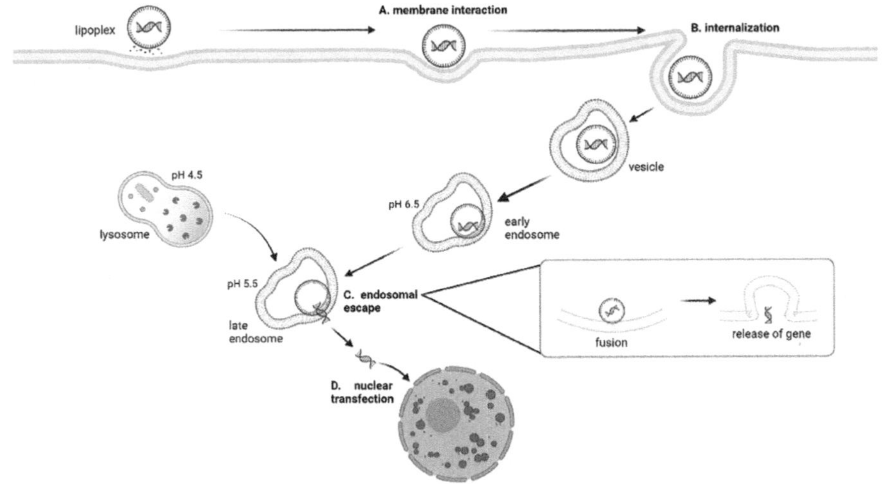

FIGURE 13.1 Illustration of gene transfection by cationic lipid. (a) The lipoplex interacts with the cell membrane by electrostatic interaction. (b) The lipoplex internalization pathway depends upon the physico-chemical characteristics. (c) Lipoplex entrapped within the endosome interacts and fuses with anionic membrane lipid, letting passage for the delivery of the gene into the cytosol. (d) The transfection pipeline ends with the transfer/entry of genes into the nucleus in case of DNA delivery.

therapeutics of infectious diseases, cancer, and monogenic disorders. While briefing their advancement, they also focussed on challenges concerning the use such transporters. The foremost limitation lies in the availability of preclinical models that inaccurately replicate the humanized architecture to elucidate the immunogenic responses triggered by viral carrier-based therapy. The immunogenic responses, both adaptive and innate, delimit the repeated use of the same viral cargo because of the chances of antibody generation, neutralizing the efficacy in the long term [26]. Nucleopolyhedrovirus, a ds-DNA Baculoviridae, has been reported to be a strategic player in exotic gene transfection in insects and mammalian cells avoiding the replication flow chain. Despite all, this wild type Baculoviridae bears cytosine-guanine (CpG) motifs along its DNA resulting in the generation of pro-inflammatory cytokines and type I interferons caused by signalling pathways independent and/or dependent upon toll-like receptor (TLR), downregulating the transgene expression efficacy [27]. They further reported the susceptibility of the human immunodeficiency virus (HIV)- and/or hepatitis C virus (HCV)-infected cells towards the adjuvant-associated recombinant baculovirus being more than normal cells, ending in their apoptosis-induced knockout. Though syndecan-1, a member of heparin sulphate proteoglycan (HSPG), has been reported to be a notable pH-dependent receptor within the mammalian cell line interacting with GP64 glycoprotein of the viral envelope, no satisfactory correlation between interaction and expression was established in the baculovirus. Instead, a dramatic role of cholesterol within the plasma membrane associated with clathrin- and dynamin-dependent endocytosis and micropinocytosis have been observed to play the key transfection flow chain for the baculovirus. [27].

Wang et al. (2019) demonstrated the AAV as a preferred platform for the gene delivery into the biotic microenvironment following the pipeline of endocytosis, endosomal escape, and entry of genes into the nucleus through the nuclear pore complex, impeding the intracellular trafficking architecture for the desired outcome (Figure 13.2) [28]. Another review from Bulcha et al. (2021) concluded Ad to be efficient in transfection than others for the following advantages: persisting epichromosomally in the host microenvironment; elevated transduction potency in proliferating as well as stagnant cells; and tropism towards the spectrum of targets [29]. Further research on engineered Ad vectors brought forth manipulation of gene cassettes producing first-generation, second-generation, third-generation, and conditionally replicating Ad vectors [29]. Recombinant AAV cargoes are also reported as efficient non-invasive transporters targeting the central nervous system intravenously [30]. Their research further brought forth the implementation of an mRNA-based directed-evolution approach in mice strains and macaques that have witnessed potential therapeutic outcomes upon the brain, depriving tropism of the liver.

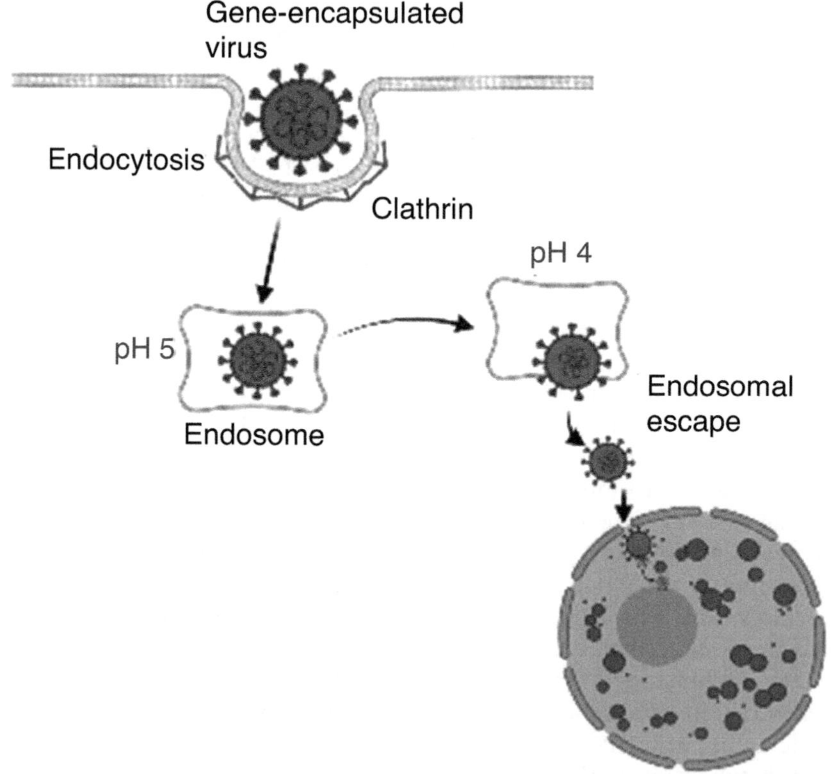

FIGURE 13.2 Schematic representation of gene transfection by virus.

13.2.3 Chemical Method in Gene Delivery

The use of chemicals have shown promising outcome in efficient gene transfer owing to its character of binding the pDNA/RNA electrostatically into smaller moieties for easy passage through the cell membrane. Chemical agents have also shown promising outcomes in minimizing the cytotoxicity, elevated surface potentials, and interaction with bio-functional compounds in contrast to their physical and/or viral counterparts. A polycationic derivative of dextran, DEAE-dextran, has been found to transfer luciferase-encoding mRNA in the form of stable mRNA/dextran colloidal complexes [20]. Being among the forefront agents explored as vectors for cultured mammalian cell lines, DEAE-dextran has undergone evolutionary stability along the trajectory. Mangion et al. (2022) observed the transfection potency of gesicles, i.e. vesicular stomatitis virus glycoprotein (VSVG)-pseudotyped vesicles, in the presence of a defined concentration of hexadimethrine bromide (polybrene) to effectively transfect desired nucleic acid in human myoblasts and HeLa cells with 22% and 55% efficiency, respectively. Research proved that the chemical reagents play either the complementary role and/or are fabricated within the carriers, enhancing the transfection efficiency to a higher fold [31]. Layek et al. (2014) fabricated a sequence of monomethoxy poly(ethylene glycol) (mPEG) and hexanoic acid (HA) double-grafted chitosan-based (HPC) micelle capable of retaining pDNA forming HPC/pDNA polyplex, a haemo-compatible complex elevating the delivery potency by ~1.2-fold and ~3–4.5-fold upon hydrophilic modification [32]. A similar study by Wu et al. (2023) highlighted the potency of PEI and PEG dual functionalized reduced graphene oxide (GO) (PEG-nrGO-PEI, RGPP) in transfecting cell lines like primary rabbit articular chondrocytes, HepG2, A549, SH-SY5Y, H9C2, EMT4, and 4T1, respectively [33].

Chemical agents, such as polybrene and/or PEI, play a vital role in efficient transfection by condensing the nucleic acid into positively charged fragments that interact with the anionic surface, forming DNA:PEI complexes that performs endocytosis to release the DNA into the cell cytoplasm [31]. Structurally modified ethylene glycol and polybrene have also been reported to upregulate the stability of pDNA-carrying micelleplexes and polyplexes for enhanced transfection [34]. These amines are functionally potent in upregulating the osmotic gradient, effectively escaping the endocytosis to transport the nucleic acid into the cytoplasm. The cryo-transmission electron microscopy (TEM) picture also determined the conformation of the plexes in protecting the condensed pDNA at its centre. While polyplexes like D(poly(2-(dimethylamino)ethyl methacrylate) and OD (poly(ethylene glycol)-*block*-poly(2-(dimethylamino) ethyl methacrylate)) comprises PEG blocks safeguarding the core, DB (poly(2-(dimethylamino)ethyl methacrylate)-*block*-poly(n-butyl methacrylate)) and ODB (poly(ethylene glycol)-*block*-poly(2-(dimethylamino)ethyl methacrylate)-*block*-poly(n-butyl methacrylate)) micelleplexes form beads-on-a-string architecture, allowing a larger surface exposure than former [34].

13.3 NANOPARTICLE-BASED DELIVERY SYSTEM

Despite the breakthrough investigations in gene transfection methodologies, including escape mechanisms [35], the limitations have restricted their efficiency in the long run. This paved an opportunity for researchers to explore the administration of nanotechnology in the field of gene delivery. With the evolution in the fabrication and delivery strategies, these nanotechnology-based transporters have proven worth implementation for their reduced immunogenic responses and biodegradability accompanied by elevated target specificity and minimal cytotoxicity [36]. Alongside the pre-existing vectors of gene transfection like lipoplex and polyplex being fabricated down to their nanometric scales, different NP like calcium phosphate, magnetite, gold, QDs, etc, have proven worthy in terms of fabrication and availability, potential target delivery and functionality, storage stability, and biocompatibility [10]. Gold nanoparticle (Au55) cluster with dimension 1.44 nm as well their combination with low molecular weight (800 Da) PEI (GNP-PEI800) exhibit higher transfection efficiency compared to non-conjugated counterpart.

Magnetic NP coated with AAV linked by cleavable heparin sulphate linker has also been investigated for thermotherapy of the cancer cell line of *cos7*, monkey kidney cells. QDs also appear as a promising transporter of genes. Chitosan-encapsulated CdSe/ZnS QDs have been found to deliver target-specific siRNA more efficiently. In some study the QDs are coated with PEG to enhance their biocompatibility [10]. CNT have also been investigated to deliver siRNA along the mammalian T-cells and primary cells. Graphene/CNT composites tagged with a GFP have also been efficiently used to transfect plasmid with an internal ribosome entry site (pIRES) plasmid in NG97 and NIH-3T3 cells. A similar technique of photo-controlled deep gene activation mechanism regulated by lanthanide-doped photo-upconversion nanoparticles (UCNs) has gained notice in the field of gene delivery. Literature has reported the attempt of delivering anti-HER2 antibody-mediated NaYF4UCNs tagged with GL3 siRNA to target the SK-BR-3 cancer cells. Mesoporous silica-coated UCNs carrying mRNA caged within 4,5-dimethoxy-2-nitroacetophenone (DMNPE) have also been reported to deliver a promising outcome in target-specific gene delivery pathways [37].

13.4 MECHANISM OF NANOPARTICLE-BASED GENE DELIVERY

The exploration of promising gene transfer strategies in the past decades has set the stepping stone of intense investigations to boost their efficiency. Despite following distinct pathways, the nano-vectors are fabricated to safeguard the degradation of functional nucleic acid from nucleases and traverse across the cell membrane, delivering them to target specific sites. This achievement is due to the structural modification of the vectors leading to altered functionalities like targeted group, surface charge, and hydrophobicity. Alongside, highly condensed structures of siRNA and pDNA are widely investigated in nano-scaffold-based gene delivery for their potency in easy passage across the membranes and escape from restricted nuclease degradation [37].

AuNPs grabbed the attention of the scientific community in the 90s and proceeded with several upgrades to date. Han et al. (2007) observed functionalized AuNPs with quaternary ammonium groups, forming a non-covalent attachment with the DNA and elevating the delivery potency in contrast to PEI and silica NP. However, the

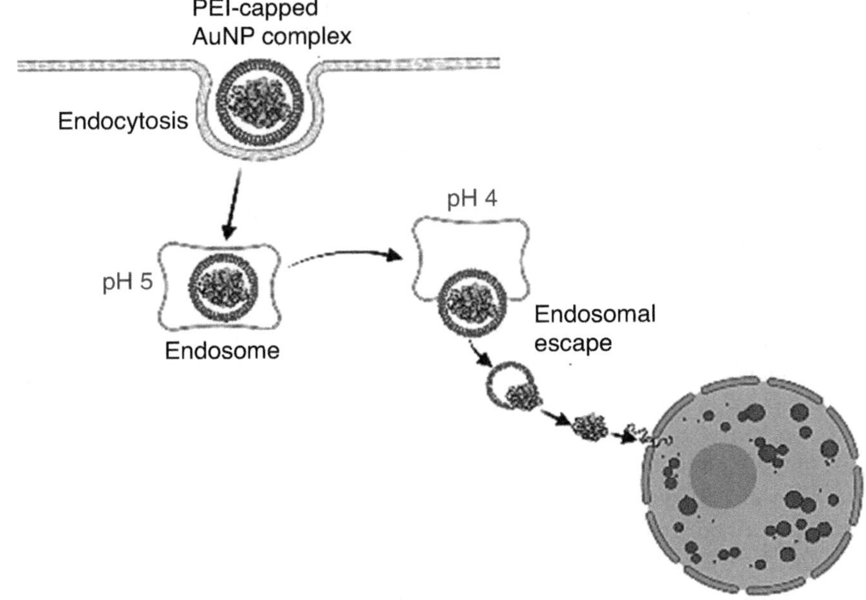

FIGURE 13.3 Illustration of gene delivery by AuNP-PEI complex.

cationic group of this conjugate expresses moderate cytotoxicity at LD50 of 1 μM, while no cytotoxicity has been observed for anionic carriers. AuNPs branched with PEI have been reported of increased cellular internalization upon increase in the hydrophobicity of the conjugate (Figure 13.3). Glutathione (GSH) is another carrier containing disulfide linkages and binds to DNA molecules by electrostatic interaction [38]. The thiol group of GSH regulates the release of tetra(ethyleneglycol)lyated cationic ligand-mediated AuNPs. Glutathione monoester (GSH-OEt) internalization into the cells results in its hydrolysis to produce GSH, increasing the intercellular GSH concentration [38]. The photolabile AuNPs also regulate the ionic interconversions during transfection and release of the payloads. They are further associated with photocleavable o-nitrobenzyl esters that are linked with amine heads for DNA attachment. Exposure to near-UV wavelength cleaves the linker, releasing the payload along with negatively charged carboxylate ions [38].

A similar transfection approach involving the QDs has also been under investigation for a long while. GQD and carbon quantum dots (CQD) have grabbed the focus of researchers in gene delivery [39], and these QDs often functionalized with microRNA targeting lipid oligonucleotide conjugates (LONs). The functionality of the platform is commenced in three stages: firstly, LONs are fabricated using two ON fragments of phosphoramidites linked by 1,3-dipolar cycloaddition reaction; secondly, trioctyl phosphine oxide, i.e. hydrophobic shell, of QD encapsulates the architecture to provide a solubilization character; lastly, a hydrophobic moiety comprising several LONs are grafted together to conjugate upon the QD surface. These nano-transporters are reported to be internalized by the cells [40].

13.5 SCOPE OF NP-BASED GENE DELIVERY IN TREATING DISEASES

13.5.1 Diseases of the Cardiovascular System

Recently, myocardial infarction (MI) was treated with liposomes loaded with CCR2-silencing siRNA by injecting the formulation intravenously into mice suffering from MI. This study by Leuschner et al. showed that macrophage aggregation and the MI area were decreasing effectively [41].

Attempts to deliver antagomirs using NP for targeting a specific gene to silence it were also made for reducing the impact of a particular disease. In a different murine model with atherosclerosis, anti-αvβ3 integrin polymer NPs were delivered intravenously to silence miR-33a and antagomir, and reduction in the lesion size and increment in the M2 macrophages were observed [42], and again, in a murine model, by targeting miR-712, using anti-vascular cell adhesion molecule 1 (VCAM1) liposomes, through an intravenous route, antagomir was delivered and a reduction of the lesion size was observed [43].

Zhang et al. had attempted the targeted delivery of the human vascular endothelial growth factor (VEGF) gene by using a complex of magnetic nanoparticle-adenoviral vectors, which has been effective in the cardiac regeneration of mice suffering from acute MI [44]. Xue et al. applied dendrimers loaded with microRNA-1 inhibitor, which reduced the cardiomyocyte apoptosis and infarction size, in mice with MI [45].

Cardiac hypertrophy has also been targeted using liposome-like NP and cholesterol-coated polymer NP through the intravenous route for silencing miR-23a and miR-182, reducing the left ventricle thickness [46,47].

In the case of peripheral arterial diseases, positive surface charge NPs containing EpoR, RopE, and/or EpoR/RopE cDNA plasmids as payloads were able to restore functionality and strength of limb in ischaemic hind limb mice [48].

Potential treatment of advanced atherosclerosis in humans has also been designed using Calcium/calmodulin-dependent protein kinase type II (S2P-siCamk2g) NP that activate the lesional macrophage Ca2+/calmodulin-dependent protein kinase II-γ (CaMKIIγ), which is responsible for the generation of thin fibrous caps covering necrotic lesions. In this study, the macrophage gene *Camk2g* was silenced, subsequently enhancing efferocytosis, which thickened the fibrous cap and reduced the necrosis of atherosclerotic plaque [49].

13.5.2 Diseases of the Digestive System

To begin with the diseases of the digestive system, the ailments of the buccal cavity are to be addressed first. Oral cancer, prominent disease emerging in the mouth, has been targeted using gene delivery by using NP. Wang et al. (2021) used chitosan-based NP for delivering methylenetetrahydrofolate dehydrogenase 1-like short hairpin RNA (shRNA) with 5-aminolevulinic acid in the cells of oral squamous cell carcinoma (OSCC). The delivery system showed remarkable pro-apoptotic, and anti-tumorigenic effects and such NP showed potential for efficient gene delivery [50].

For targeting oesophageal cancer, novel and versatile self-assembling NP, named CEAMB NPs, were developed by Zhang et al., which further loaded with adriamycin and siRNAs, targeted protein(s) and gene(s) responsible for multidrug resistance (MDR). Reduced drug efflux and apoptosis of oesophageal cancer cells were promoted in this case [51]. Nanotechnology-based gene delivery has also been used to treat chronic liver diseases. HCV has been considered as the prime reason for the aforementioned diseases related to the liver, and Duan et al., with the help of vitamin E-coupled NP had successfully attempted to suppress the HCV RNA, which produced core proteins, by delivering siRNAs to the liver [52].

Inflammatory bowel diseases like ulcerative colitis have also been successfully addressed using siRNA encapsulated in aminated nanoparticles having tunable surface charge. Such NPs underwent enhanced accretion at the site of acute ulcerative colitis and efficiently reduced inflammation [53]. Chitosan NP encapsulating snail siRNA with anti-cancer drug downregulated and upregulated necessary genes and proteins in the cells of the colorectal cancer cells and also prevented HCT-116 cells from migration. Thus, they prove to be effective against colorectal cancer as a form of treatment [54].

13.5.3 Diseases of the Endocrine System

Diseases of endocrinal origin are also responsible for human illness and an attempt has been made to treat them using nanotechnology through gene delivery. For countering type 2 diabetes, chitosan-coated nanospheres were designed by Baig et al., using DNA rectangles loaded with vildagliptin. Di-peptidyl-peptidase-4 generally degrades incretin hormones but the degradation of these hormones exceeds in type 2 diabetes patients with respect to their healthier counterparts, as the concentration of the former increases. But such a form of gene delivery system is effective in staving off the accelerated degradation by inhibiting di-peptidyl-peptidase-4, through prolonged secretion of vildagliptin [55].

Photo-responsive liposome with verteporfin (VP) was an efficient DNA carrier, as it enabled the knockdown of pituitary adenylyl cyclase-activating polypeptide receptor 1 gene in PC12 cells (cell line from pheochromocytoma, a neuroendocrine tumour of the rat adrenal medulla) [56]. In this study, Chen et al. observed the production of reactive oxygen species form VP in the target cells, which had taken up the liposomes, upon exposure to UV light, and eventually, antisense DNA was released in the cells [57].

Yang et al. had developed a biodegradable vector for delivering Kirsten rat sarcoma viral oncogene homologue (K-Ras) siRNA to target the K-Ras oncogene mutation in pancreatic cancer cells (MiaPaCa-2). The growth, migration, and invasion were significantly decreased, with a higher rate of apoptosis in the cancer cells [58]. Magadala et al. formulated a method of gene delivery, which involved an EGFR-targeted type B gelatin-based nanoparticle encapsulating EGFR-N1 pDNA within it. The surface of the nanoparticle was coated with EGFR-targeting peptide for gene transfection in human pancreatic adenocarcinoma cells showing over expression of EGFR. The efficiency of uptake and the transgene expression was commendable, thus making it a potential process of gene delivery for treating pancreatic adenocarcinoma [59].

Lomabardo et al. formulated lactic-co-glycolic acid (PLGA)/chitosan NP containing antagomir for addressing anaplastic thyroid cancer, which targeted the enhanced human telomerase reverse transcriptase (hTERT) mRNA expression, in such cases. An approximate reduction of 50% of neoplasm growth was exhibited by a mice xenograft model on employing this gene delivery method and, thus, demonstrated its potential for treating anaplastic thyroid cancer [60].

13.5.4 Diseases of the Immune System

Immunological disorders have the potential to turn out to be detrimental for the patient, and for countering such disorders, gene delivery has also been attempted. Lee et al. had formulated a nano-complex-based gene delivery system for targeting TNF-α for the treatment of rheumatoid arthritis. In the mice models of collagen-induced arthritis, these NP inhibited not only inflammation but also bone erosion [61]. Successful transfection of the human insulin gene and its subsequent expression, in the digestive system of rats with type 1 diabetes, has been carried out by Niu et al. by targeting the gene with chitosan NP having human insulin gene, and this resulted in reduced blood glucose levels [62]. Haemophilia A and B are two immunological disorders. Lee et al. targeted these diseases with lipid NP for delivering clustered regularly interspaced short palindromic repeats and CRISPR-associated protein 9 (CRISPR-Cas9) with single guide RNA to target antithrombin (for negative regulation of thrombin production). The results, in this case, were appreciable as the mouse in which the NP were injected, showed improved generation of thrombin, and there was also observable recovery of the phenotypes associated with bleeding [63].

Zhang et al. had attempted to develop a treatment against asthma, by using novel inhaled lipid NP, to deliver anti-thymic stromal lymphopoietin (TSLP) siRNA. This formulation successfully targeted intercellular adhesion molecule-1 receptors on the airway epithelial cells and prevented the expression of pro-inflammatory cytokines and reduced the production of mucus as well in an asthmatic mice model. By this treatment, the TSLP expression was downregulated, and infiltration by cells of the immune system was effectively alleviated too [64].

In 2020, a nano-delivery nano-delivery system was prepared for targeting systemic lupus erythematosus. It delivered miR-125a into splenic T-cells and successfully alleviated disease progression by restoring the balance of population of T-cells [65].

13.5.5 Diseases of the Muscular System

For addressing the issue of muscular degeneration, NP mediated gene delivery have been tested. In Duchenne muscular dystrophy (DMD), CRISPR/Cas9-mediated genome editing is deemed to be effective as a potential method of treatment. For editing the *DMD* gene, Li et al. synthesised Cas9-based NP. The results of the studies carried out *in vitro* showed that the NP showed biocompatibility and were able to prevent the loaded gene from undergoing enzymatic degradation, and high serum conditioned aided in the efficient delivery of the genetic material. The *in vivo* study was carried out by injecting the NP into muscle tissue, and the results showed that the mutation of the *DMD* gene occurred without any injury to the tissue. Therefore, this study might expand the application of this gene delivery mechanism for treating DMD [66].

13.5.6 Diseases of the Nervous System

Nanoparticle-based gene transfer has also been applied for treating diseases of the nervous system. Mangravati et al. found that the viability of glioma cell lines extracted from rats was reduced in the presence of prodrug ganciclovir (GCV) as poly (β-amino ester) (PBAE) NP were delivered with viral thymidine kinase encoded in pDNA to the target cell population. The reason is that this enzyme phosphorylated GCV, which disrupts DNA replication of proliferating cells by incorporating itself into their DNA, and consequently, the process of cell division gets halted [67].

For the development of a nanoparticle-based gene delivery, against PD, DGL-PEG-angiopep (DPA) NP containing human glial cell line-derived neurotrophic factor (hGDNF) were fabricated and applied in a murine model of rotenone-induced PD. Enhanced uptake of the NP by the brain cells and the eventual expression of the gene translated into considerable improvements in locomotion and dopaminergic neuron recovery [68]. In a separate attempt at developing a treatment for the same disease, Xue et al. had shown that the damaged dopaminergic neurons got repaired by the entry of chitosan-based NP and eventual release of pDNA and ACT, which were conjugated with the NP [69].

In the C57BL/6 mouse brain, mannose-based liposomes containing the ApoE2 gene/chitosan complex not only increased the efficiency of transport but also of transfection of the aforementioned gene by preventing it from getting digested by endonuclease across the blood-brain barrier model, thus proving to be an effective medium of treatment for Alzheimer's Disease [70]. Arora et al. designed a lipid-based nanoparticle, which was successfully able to counter Alzheimer's disease mice brains. Brain-targeting ligand and mannose were conjugated to the surface of the NPs and had cell-penetrating peptides. It contained brain-derived neurotrophic factor (BDNF) gene for the production of BDNF and for the lifelong utilisation of the same in cortical circuits not only for the sustenance of neuronal function but also for synaptic plasticity [71].

For addressing Friedreich's ataxia, Nabhan et al. had been successful in using RNA transcript therapy. Lipid NP containing frataxin mRNA, injected in the Dorsal root ganglia of mice, showed robust translation of frataxin protein, hence, acting as a preventive against Friedreich's ataxia [72]. For treating damages related to the optic nerve, Tawfik et al had introduced polybutylcyanoacrylate NP to deliver siRNA for blocking caspase-3 protein, which triggers apoptosis in rats suffering from optic nerve crush [73].

13.5.7 Diseases of the Renal System

In 2022, Tang et al. developed a novel chitosan-based siRNA carrier for targeting p53 and reduced renal injury. The extent of renal apoptosis as well as the infiltration by cells of the immune system also decreased with improvement in the functioning of the renal system [74].

Alan et al. successfully silenced the genes responsible for the progression of mesangial proliferative glomerulonephritis by using chitosan/siRNA nanoplexes and also prevented the processes associated with the pathogenesis of the disease. Therefore, it can be considered to be effective as a therapy for treating mesangial proliferative glomerulonephritis [75]. In a mice model of unilateral ureteral obstruction (UUO), Yang et al. found that using chitosan/siRNA NP was effective in attenuating parenchymal inflammation, as cyclooxygenase -2 (COX-2) was knocked out by the siRNA. Decreased oxidative stress and apoptosis by reduction of hemeoxygenase-1 were also observed in this study [76].

Ozbay et al. attempted to develop mitochondria-targeted NP with heightened efficiency for treating Coenzyme Q10 (CoQ_{10}) nephropathies by silencing of Coenzyme Q10 *(COQ8B)* using siRNA. The rate of the tricarboxylic acid cycle was found to have been increased in *COQ8B*$^{-/-}$ cells, in the *in vitro* disease model, as they were treated with the mitochondria-targeted NP. Thus, this particular formulation could be considered as an efficient way of treating nephropathies related to CoQ_{10} in comparison to conventional formulations [77].

13.5.8 Diseases of the Reproductive System

Polycystic ovary syndrome (PCOS) was targeted by Cao et al. in 2022 by using exosomes derived from adipose mesenchymal stem cells containing miR-21-5p (miRNAs). The transference of the miRNA to the liver of the rats suffering from PCOS inhibited B-cell translocation gene 2 expression. In this case, the fertility was improved in the rats [78].

Du et al. introduced a novel method of delivery of mRNA and self-amplifying RNA (saRNA) which coded for DNA meiotic recombinase 1 (Dmcl) protein in spermatocytes, by using lipid NP. Dmcl gene mutation was targeted by the gene delivery mechanism as it is a cause of male infertility. These NP were able to induce prolonged expression of the Dmcl protein, restoring spermatogenesis in a mouse model, where Dmcl gene was knocked out [79].

Cervical cancer is also an important disease that affects the female reproductive system, and for its treatment, Xia et al. had developed a gene delivery system using biocompatible selenium NP loaded with RGD-Peptide cyclo (RGDfC) peptide. The aforementioned NP were loaded with Derlin1-siRNA, subsequently. In HeLa cell lines, the selenium NP with RGDfC peptide had shown great uptake and enhanced reactive oxygen species (ROS) generation also. Therefore, this gene delivery system can be deemed as effective against cervical cancer [80]. Treatment protocol addressing ovarian cancer using NP and gene delivery had been successfully attempted by Singh et al. They encapsulated siRNAs, in lipid NP, and an *in vitro* study showed 85% cell death of ovarian cancer [81]. Oner et al. developed a certain type of lipid-based NP for carrying siRNAs, which targeted Ephrin type-A receptor 2 (EphA2) receptor tyrosine kinase (siEphA2) overexpression, prevalent in certain cases of prostate cancer. Enhanced cellular uptake of the NP and gene silencing in the cancer cells were observed, thus opening an avenue for treating prostate cancer [82].

13.5.9 Diseases of the Respiratory System

The usage of gene delivery using NP has also been attempted in the realm of the treatment of respiratory diseases.

Niemiec et al., for treating acute respiratory distress syndrome, had used cerium NP for intratracheal delivery of cerium oxide nanoparticle-microRNA-146a (CNP-miR146a). It was observed that the levels of miR146a had increased in pulmonary tissue, and it also prevented acute lung injury. Oxidative stress, inflammation, and collagen deposition were found to be reduced, hence improving the biomechanics of the pulmonary system [83].

RNA interference (RNAi) was employed to treat chronic obstructive pulmonary disease (COPD), by Mohamed et al., where miR146a was adsorbed onto NP for reducing interleukin 1 receptor-associated kinase 1 (IRAK1) gene expression. There was an appreciable reduction found in the expression of the target gene [84].

To focus the limelight on lung cancer, it has been seen that a myriad of NP has been used for delivering the genes to the target cells for the treatment of the same. Recently in 2022, Ma et al., by using nebulized star-siRNA NP, were successfully able to silence βIII-tubulin and polo-like kinase 1 (PLK1) expression in lung tumours of mice and also delayed tumour growth [85].

13.5.10 Diseases of the Skeletal System

Gene silencing for treating osteoporosis, one of the leading causes of bone disorder, has been attempted by using siRNA by Mora-Raimundo et al. sclerosteosis (SOST) gene by inhibiting the Wnt signalling pathway reduces osteoblast differentiation, and for this reason, an anti-SOST siRNA was loaded in mesoporous silica NP with osteostatin, which is an osteogenic peptide. The osteogenic markers were augmented, and this process stands out to have potential as a treatment for countering osteoporosis [86].

Bedingfield et al. devised a new method to treat osteoarthritis by intra-articular injections of the NP loaded with siRNA to target the matrix metalloproteinase 13 gene (MMP13). MMP13 inhibition led to the suppression of genes involved in the progression of osteoarthritis [87]. Kundu et al. had synthesized NP made of 10% PLGA with anti-p53 siRNA, which showed effectiveness against osteosarcoma by efficient knockdown of mutant p53 and maintenance of high viability of cells [88].

13.6 LIMITATIONS AND FUTURE PROSPECTS OF NP-BASED GENE DELIVERY SYSTEMS

There are certain limitations prevailing in the realm of nanoparticle-based gene delivery systems. It can be seen that most of the NP-based gene delivery systems have undergone the route of RNAi , which involves the silencing of the target gene by either siRNAs or miRNAs. But both the siRNAs and miRNAs have some limitations for being used as a medium for treating the required diseases, a few of which are discussed below.

Firstly, the siRNAs are not stable and undergo quick degradation *in vivo* [89,90]. Secondly, siRNAs have low transfection efficiency and targeting is also inefficient [89]. Thirdly, while designing siRNAs, off-target effects are observed due to subpar selection of sequences [90]. Fourthly, certain siRNA molecules have the ability of potentially inducing immune stimulatory effects [91]. Besides these factors, siRNA-based gene therapy is hindered by endosomal degradation, and natural RNAi components also pose competition to such therapies in the cells [90]. Finally, from a legal perspective, only a few nanoparticle-based siRNA delivery systems have received approval from the FDA [92].

Now, in the case of gene therapies involving miRNA, it has been found that *in vivo* administration of miRNAs is capable of activating the innate immune system [93], causing significant undesirable effects. Limited variations of sequences for therapeutic miRNA can be overcome, mostly by chemical modifications [94]. Furthermore, poor stability and inefficient delivery are also the limitations of therapeutic miRNAs [94]. Besides, the lack of understanding surrounding the complex roles of miRNAs, as they were discovered initially, restricted the development of such therapies, and therefore, their clinical trials are comparatively less in comparison to the siRNA-based counterparts [94]. There are gaps in the current knowledge associated with the risks surrounding the exposure to NPs. At the same time, controversies persist regarding the exact impact of NPs on the biological behaviour ranging from the genetic to the cellular levels [95].

As the size of the NP decreases it proportionately increase its biological and chemical reactivities due to exponential increment in the surface-to-volume ratio [96]. It has been found that when the NP decreases from 30 to 3 nm in size, there is an increase in the expression of the surface molecules from 10% to 50%, and cytotoxicity is a by-product of the interactions between the surface molecules and the cellular components [97,98]. Hence, it is a clear indication of the fact that irrespective of the chemical composition, greater toxicity is shown by particles smaller in size in comparison to the bigger ones and is also a drawback in the process of delivering genes using NP. This fact can be exemplified by the study conducted by Cho et al., on BALB/c mice, where histopathological complications like thymus cortex apoptosis, focal necrosis, etc., occurred on the administration of 10 nm silver NP and not in the case of 60 and 100 nm silver NP [99]. In another experiment conducted by Du et al., in rats subjected to the administration of fine silica particles, immunogenic response was observed post intratracheal instillation [100].

Despite the limitations, there are future prospects related to gene delivery using NP that should be considered. The incorporation of targeting ligands in the PEGylated NP is being employed as a way to prolong circulation time by improving their half-life *in vivo* and achieving specificity while targeting tumour sites [90,94]. For improving the stability of the genetic material *in vivo* and overcoming problems related to the immune system, materials, such as gangliosides, pullulan, and certain synthetic polymers, are being proposed [90]. Other materials like PLGA- and PLA-based NPs have efficiently promoted a sustained delivery of foreign nucleic acids in an unaltered form to the appropriate target bypassing immune recognition [101]. In this case, the plasma half-life has also improved along with cellular uptake with the promotion of renal and hepatic clearance of the nucleic acid [101]. In the end, as far as the protocols and regulations are concerned, nanotoxicology, as a field, has emerged for investigating the safety of nanotechnologies [97,102].

13.7 CONCLUSIONS

Nanoparticle-based gene delivery systems are extremely novel methods for treating diseases due to their accuracy and efficiency in targeting diseases. But still being in its budding stage, inefficiencies surrounding gene therapy like the instability of the genetic material, its off-target effects, transfection inefficiency, and the induced undesirable immunomodulatory effects are key constraints. Despite such hurdles, clinical trials are being conducted currently, and few of them have already been approved by the FDA. Certain polymeric NP have proven to be releasing genetic material at the target site for a prolonged time period with high cellular uptake efficiency *in vivo* without enzymatic degradation or facing competition from other cellular components. Frameworks are also in the process of development to assuring the safety of nanotechnologies for potential patients who might avail of such gene therapy in the near future. Overall, it can be expected that nanoparticle-based gene therapy is potentially the future of medicinal treatment of diseases.

REFERENCES

[1] T. Friedmann, "A brief history of gene therapy," *Nat. Genet.*, vol. 2, no. 2, p. 2, Oct. 1992, doi: 10.1038/ng1092–93.

[2] T. Wirth, N. Parker, and S. Ylä-Herttuala, "History of gene therapy," *Gene*, vol. 525, no. 2, p. 2, Aug. 2013, doi: 10.1016/j.gene.2013.03.137.

[3] J. M. Stribley, K. S. Rehman, H. Niu, and G. M. Christman, "Gene therapy and reproductive medicine," *Fertil. Steril.*, vol. 77, no. 4, p. 4, Apr. 2002, doi: 10.1016/S0015–0282(01)03233-2.

[4] M. Zeitelhofer et al., "High-efficiency transfection of mammalian neurons via nucleofection," *Nat. Protoc.*, vol. 2, no. 7, p. 7, Jul. 2007, doi: 10.1038/nprot.2007.226.

[5] A. Bolhassani, A. Khavari, and Z. Orafa, Electroporation – *Advantages and Drawbacks for Delivery of Drug, Gene and Vaccine*. IntechOpen, 2014. doi: 10.5772/58376.

[6] A. K. Das, P. Gupta, and D. Chakraborty, "Physical methods of gene transfer: Kinetics of gene delivery into cells: A Review," *Agric. Rev.*, vol. 36, no. 1, p. 1, 2015, doi: 10.5958/0976-0741.2015.00007.0.

[7] Y. Zhao and L. Huang, "Lipid nanoparticles for gene delivery," *Adv. Genet.*, vol. 88, pp. 13–36, 2014, doi: 10.1016/B978-0-12–800148-6.00002-X.

[8] L. Jin, X. Zeng, M. Liu, Y. Deng, and N. He, "Current progress in gene delivery technology based on chemical methods and nano-carriers," *Theranostics*, vol. 4, no. 3, p. 3, Jan. 2014, doi: 10.7150/thno.6914.

[9] X. Du et al., "Advanced physical techniques for gene delivery based on membrane perforation," *Drug Deliv.*, vol. 25, no. 1, p. 1, Jul. 2018, doi: 10.1080/10717544.2018.1480674.

[10] H. Tian, J. Chen, and X. Chen, "Nanoparticles for gene delivery," *Small*, vol. 9, no. 12, p. 12, 2013, doi: 10.1002/smll.201202485.

[11] S. L. Prabu, T. N. K. Suriyaprakash, and R. Thirumurugan, "Medicated nanoparticle for gene delivery," In *Advanced Technology for Delivering Therapeutics*, S. Maiti and K. K. Sen, Eds., InTech, 2017. doi: 10.5772/65709.

[12] C. Yan, X.-J. Quan, and Y.-M. Feng, "Nanomedicine for gene delivery for the treatment of cardiovascular diseases," *Curr. Gene Ther.*, vol. 19, no. 1, p. 1, Feb. 2019, doi: 10.2174/1566523218666181003125308.
[13] R. Bahadur KC, B. Thapa, and N. Bhattarai, "Gold nanoparticle-based gene delivery: Promises and challenges," *Nanotechnol. Rev.*, vol. 3, no. 3, p. 3, Jun. 2014, doi: 10.1515/ntrev-2013–0026.
[14] S. Trigueros, E. B. Domènech, V. Toulis, and G. Marfany, "In vitro gene delivery in retinal pigment epithelium cells by plasmid DNA-wrapped gold nanoparticles," *Genes*, vol. 10, no. 4, p. 4, Apr. 2019, doi: 10.3390/genes10040289.
[15] D. Lin, M. Li, Y. Gao, L. Yin, and Y. Guan, "Brain-targeted gene delivery of ZnO quantum dots nanoplatform for the treatment of Parkinson disease," *Chem. Eng. J.*, vol. 429, p. 132210, Feb. 2022, doi: 10.1016/j.cej.2021.132210.
[16] P.-Y. Lo, G.-Y. Lee, J.-H. Zheng, J.-H. Huang, E.-C. Cho, and K.-C. Lee, "GFP Plasmid and chemoreagent conjugated with graphene quantum dots as a novel gene delivery platform for colon cancer inhibition in vitro and in vivo," *ACS Appl. Bio Mater.*, vol. 3, no. 9, p. 9, Sep. 2020, doi: 10.1021/acsabm.0c00631.
[17] F. Ponti, M. Campolungo, C. Melchiori, N. Bono, and G. Candiani, "Cationic lipids for gene delivery: Many players, one goal," *Chem. Phys. Lipids*, vol. 235, p. 105032, Mar. 2021, doi: 10.1016/j.chemphyslip.2020.105032.
[18] O. Kontogiannis and V. Karalis, "On the in vivo kinetics of gene delivery vectors," *medRxiv*, p. 2022.02.11.22269834, Jan. 2022, doi: 10.1101/2022.02.11.22269834.
[19] D. Campillo-Davo et al., "The ins and outs of messenger RNA electroporation for physical gene delivery in immune cell-based therapy," *Pharmaceutics*, vol. 13, no. 3, p. 3, Mar. 2021, doi: 10.3390/pharmaceutics13030396.
[20] C. Siewert et al., "Investigation of charge ratio variation in mRNA - DEAE-dextran polyplex delivery systems," *Biomaterials*, vol. 192, pp. 612–620, Feb. 2019, doi: 10.1016/j.biomaterials.2018.10.020.
[21] K. Kamimura, T. Suda, G. Zhang, and D. Liu, "Advances in gene delivery systems," *Pharm. Med.*, vol. 25, no. 5, p. 5, Oct. 2011, doi: 10.2165/11594020-000000000-00000.
[22] W. Chen, H. Li, D. Shi, Z. Liu, and W. Yuan, "Microneedles as a delivery system for gene therapy," *Front. Pharmacol.*, vol. 7, p. 137, May 2016, doi: 10.3389/fphar.2016.00137.
[23] S.-Y. Park, K.-H. Kim, S. Kim, Y.-M. Lee, and Y.-J. Seol, "BMP-2 gene delivery-based bone regeneration in dentistry," *Pharmaceutics*, vol. 11, p. 393, Aug. 2019, doi: 10.3390/pharmaceutics11080393.
[24] S. M. G. Hayat, N. Farahani, E. Safdarian, A. Roointan, and A. Sahebkar, "Gene delivery using lipoplexes and polyplexes: Principles, limitations and solutions," *Crit. Rev. Eukaryot. Gene Expr.*, vol. 29, no. 1, p. 1, 2019, doi: 10.1615/CritRevEukaryotGeneExpr.2018025132.
[25] D. Mukherjee et al., "Decoding the kinetic pathways toward a Lipid/DNA complex of alkyl alcohol cationic lipids formed in a microfluidic channel," *J. Phys. Chem. B*, vol. 126, no. 3, p. 3, Jan. 2022, doi: 10.1021/acs.jpcb.1c07263.
[26] Z. Zhao, A. C. Anselmo, and S. Mitragotri, "Viral vector-based gene therapies in the clinic," *Bioeng. Transl. Med.*, vol. 7, no. 1, p. 1, 2022, doi: 10.1002/btm2.10258.
[27] C. Ono, T. Okamoto, T. Abe, and Y. Matsuura, "Baculovirus as a tool for gene delivery and gene therapy," *Viruses*, vol. 10, no. 9, p. 9, Sep. 2018, doi: 10.3390/v10090510.
[28] D. Wang, P. W. L. Tai, and G. Gao, "Adeno-associated virus vector as a platform for gene therapy delivery," *Nat. Rev. Drug Discov.*, vol. 18, no. 5, p. 5, May 2019, doi: 10.1038/s41573-019-0012–9.
[29] J. T. Bulcha, Y. Wang, H. Ma, P. W. L. Tai, and G. Gao, "Viral vector platforms within the gene therapy landscape," *Signal Transduct. Target. Ther.*, vol. 6, no. 1, p. 1, Feb. 2021, doi: 10.1038/s41392-021-00487-6.

[30] A. C. Stanton et al., "Systemic administration of novel engineered AAV capsids facilitates enhanced transgene expression in the macaque CNS," *Med*, p. S2666634022004561, Nov. 2022, doi: 10.1016/j.medj.2022.11.002.
[31] M. Mangion, M.-A. Robert, I. Slivac, R. Gilbert, and B. Gaillet, "Production and use of gesicles for nucleic acid delivery," *Mol. Biotechnol.*, vol. 64, no. 3, p. 3, Mar. 2022, doi: 10.1007/s12033-021-00389-6.
[32] B. Layek, M. K. Haldar, G. Sharma, L. Lipp, S. Mallik, and J. Singh, "Hexanoic for enhanced gene delivery: Influence of hydrophobic and hydrophilic substitution acid and polyethylene glycol double grafted amphiphilic chitosan degree," *Mol. Pharm.*, vol. 11, no. 3, p. 3, Mar. 2014, doi: 10.1021/mp400633r.
[33] L. Wu et al., "Gene delivery ability of polyethylenimine and polyethylene glycol dual-functionalized nanographene oxide in 11 different cell lines," *R. Soc. Open Sci.*, vol. 4, no. 10, p. 10, Jan. 2023, doi: 10.1098/rsos.170822.
[34] Z. Tan, Y. Jiang, W. Zhang, L. Karls, T. P. Lodge, and T. M. Reineke, "Polycation architecture and assembly direct successful gene delivery: Micelleplexes outperform polyplexes via optimal DNA packaging," *J. Am. Chem. Soc.*, vol. 141, no. 40, p. 40, Oct. 2019, doi: 10.1021/jacs.9b06218.
[35] M. S. Al-Dosari and X. Gao, "Nonviral gene delivery: Principle, limitations, and recent progress," *AAPS J.*, vol. 11, no. 4, p. 4, Oct. 2009, doi: 10.1208/s12248-009-9143-y.
[36] M. K. Riley and W. Vermerris, "Recent advances in nanomaterials for gene delivery—A review," *Nanomaterials*, vol. 7, no. 5, p. 5, Apr. 2017, doi: 10.3390/nano7050094.
[37] X. Jun Loh, T.-C. Lee, Q. Dou, and G. Roshan Deen, "Utilising inorganic nanocarriers for gene delivery," *Biomater. Sci.*, vol. 4, no. 1, p. 1, 2016, doi: 10.1039/C5BM00277J.
[38] G. Han, P. Ghosh, M. De, and V. M. Rotello, "Drug and gene delivery using gold nanoparticles," *NanoBiotechnology*, vol. 3, no. 1, p. 1, Mar. 2007, doi: 10.1007/s12030-007-0005-3.
[39] A. Alaghmandfard et al., "Recent advances in the modification of carbon-based quantum dots for biomedical applications," *Mater. Sci. Eng. C*, vol. 120, p. 111756, Jan. 2021, doi: 10.1016/j.msec.2020.111756.
[40] A. Aimé, N. Beztsinna, A. Patwa, A. Pokolenko, I. Bestel, and P. Barthélémy, "Quantum dot lipid oligonucleotide bioconjugates: Toward a new anti-microRNA nanoplatform," *Bioconjug. Chem.*, vol. 24, no. 8, pp. 1345–1355, Aug. 2013, doi: 10.1021/bc400157z.
[41] F. Leuschner et al., "Therapeutic siRNA silencing in inflammatory monocytes in mice," *Nat. Biotechnol.*, vol. 29, no. 11, pp. 1005–1010, Oct. 2011, doi: 10.1038/nbt.1989.
[42] C. Li et al., "Site-specific microRNA-33 antagonism by pH-responsive nanotherapies for treatment of atherosclerosis via regulating cholesterol efflux and adaptive immunity," *Adv. Funct. Mater.*, vol. 30, no. 42, p. 2002131, 2020, doi: 10.1002/adfm.202002131.
[43] A. Kheirolomoom et al., "Multifunctional nanoparticles facilitate molecular targeting and miRNA delivery to inhibit atherosclerosis in ApoE $^{-/-}$ Mice," *ACS Nano*, vol. 9, no. 9, pp. 8885–8897, Sep. 2015, doi: 10.1021/acsnano.5b02611.
[44] "Targeted delivery of human VEGF gene via complexes of magnetic nanoparticle-adenoviral vectors enhanced cardiac regeneration - PMC." https://www.ncbi.nlm.nih.gov/pmc/articles/PMC3406048/ (accessed Jan. 30, 2023).
[45] X. Xue et al., "Delivery of microRNA-1 inhibitor by dendrimer-based nanovector: An early targeting therapy for myocardial infarction in mice," *Nanomed. Nanotechnol. Biol. Med.*, vol. 14, no. 2, pp. 619–631, Feb. 2018, doi: 10.1016/j.nano.2017.12.004.
[46] J. A. Kopechek et al., "Ultrasound and microbubble-targeted delivery of a microrna inhibitor to the heart suppresses cardiac hypertrophy and preserves cardiac function," *Theranostics*, vol. 9, no. 23, pp. 7088–7098, Sep. 2019, doi: 10.7150/thno.34895.

[47] Y. Zhi, C. Xu, D. Sui, J. Du, F. Xu, and Y. Li, "Effective delivery of hypertrophic miRNA inhibitor by cholesterol-containing nanocarriers for preventing pressure overload induced cardiac hypertrophy," *Adv. Sci.*, vol. 6, no. 11, p. 1900023, Apr. 2019, doi: 10.1002/advs.201900023.

[48] "Nanoparticles for Gene Therapy and Protein Delivery to Induce Angiogenesis as an Alternative Treatment for Peripheral Arterial Disease - ProQuest." https://www.proquest.com/openview/830d4b56061d9cd515be81a274444efd/1?pq-origsite=gscholar&cbl=18750&diss=y (accessed Mar. 14, 2023).

[49] X. Huang et al., "Synthesis of siRNA nanoparticles to silence plaque-destabilizing gene in atherosclerotic lesional macrophages," *Nat. Protoc.*, vol. 17, no. 3, p. 3, Mar. 2022, doi: 10.1038/s41596-021-00665-4.

[50] J. Wang, K. Wang, J. Liang, J. Jin, X. Wang, and S. Yan, "Chitosan-tripolyphosphate nanoparticles-mediated co-delivery of MTHFD1L shRNA and 5-aminolevulinic acid for combination photodynamic-gene therapy in oral cancer," *Photodiagnosis Photodyn. Ther.*, vol. 36, p. 102581, Dec. 2021, doi: 10.1016/j.pdpdt.2021.102581.

[51] X. Zhang et al., "Multifunctional nanoparticles co-loaded with Adriamycin and MDR-targeting siRNAs for treatment of chemotherapy-resistant esophageal cancer," *J. Nanobiotechnology*, vol. 20, no. 1, p. 166, Mar. 2022, doi: 10.1186/s12951-022-01377-x.

[52] "Target Delivery of Small Interfering RNAs with Vitamin E-Coupled Nanoparticles for Treating Hepatitis C | Scientific Reports." https://www.nature.com/articles/srep24867 (accessed Jan. 31, 2023).

[53] S. Iqbal, X. Du, J. Wang, H. Li, Y. Yuan, and J. Wang, "Surface charge tunable nanoparticles for TNF-α siRNA oral delivery for treating ulcerative colitis," *Nano Res.*, vol. 11, no. 5, pp. 2872–2884, May 2018, doi: 10.1007/s12274-017-1918-3.

[54] S. Sadreddini et al., "Chitosan nanoparticles as a dual drug/siRNA delivery system for treatment of colorectal cancer," *Immunol. Lett.*, vol. 181, pp. 79–86, Jan. 2017, doi: 10.1016/j.imlet.2016.11.013.

[55] M. M. F. A. Baig et al., "Chitosan-coated rectangular DNA nanospheres for better outcomes of anti-diabetic drug," *J. Nanoparticle Res.*, vol. 21, no. 5, p. 98, May 2019, doi: 10.1007/s11051-019-4534-1.

[56] "Pheochromocytoma - NCI," Feb. 12, 2020. https://www.cancer.gov/pediatric-adult-rare-tumor/rare-tumors/rare-endocrine-tumor/pheochromocytoma (accessed Feb. 12, 2023).

[57] "Light-Triggerable Liposomes for Enhanced Endolysosomal Escape and Gene Silencing in PC12 Cells | Elsevier Enhanced Reader." (accessed Feb. 12, 2023).

[58] C. Yang et al., "Biodegradable nanoparticle-mediated K-ras down regulation for pancreatic cancer gene therapy," *J. Mater. Chem. B*, vol. 3, no. 10, pp. 2163–2172, Feb. 2015, doi: 10.1039/C4TB01623H.

[59] P. Magadala and M. Amiji, "Epidermal growth factor receptor-targeted gelatin-based engineered nanocarriers for DNA delivery and transfection in human pancreatic cancer cells," *AAPS J.*, vol. 10, no. 4, pp. 565–576, Dec. 2008, doi: 10.1208/s12248-008-9065-0.

[60] G. E. Lombardo et al., "Anti-hTERT siRNA-loaded nanoparticles block the growth of anaplastic thyroid cancer xenograft," *Mol. Cancer Ther.*, vol. 17, no. 6, pp. 1187–1195, Jun. 2018, doi: 10.1158/1535–7163.MCT-17–0559.

[61] S. J. Lee et al., "TNF-α gene silencing using polymerized siRNA/thiolated glycol chitosan nanoparticles for rheumatoid arthritis," *Mol. Ther.*, vol. 22, no. 2, pp. 397–408, Feb. 2014, doi: 10.1038/mt.2013.245.

[62] L. Niu, Y.-C. Xu, Z. Dai, and H.-Q. Tang, "Gene therapy for type 1 diabetes mellitus in rats by gastrointestinal administration of chitosan nanoparticles containing human insulin gene," *World J. Gastroenterol.*, vol. 14, no. 26, pp. 4209–4215, Jul. 2008, doi: 10.3748/wjg.14.4209.

[63] J. P. Han et al., "In vivo delivery of CRISPR-Cas9 using lipid nanoparticles enables antithrombin gene editing for sustainable hemophilia A and B therapy," *Sci. Adv.*, vol. 8, no. 3, 2022. https://dspace.ewha.ac.kr/handle/2015.oak/260550 (accessed Feb. 15, 2023).
[64] M. Zhang et al., "Airway epithelial cell-specific delivery of lipid nanoparticles loading siRNA for asthma treatment," *J. Controlled Release*, vol. 352, pp. 422–437, Dec. 2022, doi: 10.1016/j.jconrel.2022.10.020.
[65] J. Zhang et al., "MicroRNA-125a-loaded polymeric nanoparticles alleviate systemic lupus erythematosus by restoring effector/regulatory T cells balance," *ACS Nano*, vol. 14, no. 4, pp. 4414–4429, Apr. 2020, doi: 10.1021/acsnano.9b09998.
[66] S. Li et al., "Gene editing of Duchenne muscular dystrophy using biomineralization-based spCas9 variant nanoparticles," *Acta Biomater.*, vol. 154, pp. 597–607, Dec. 2022, doi: 10.1016/j.actbio.2022.10.015.
[67] A. Mangraviti et al., "Polymeric nanoparticles for nonviral gene therapy extend brain tumor survival in vivo," *ACS Nano*, vol. 9, no. 2, pp. 1236–1249, Feb. 2015, doi: 10.1021/nn504905q.
[68] R. Huang et al., "Angiopep-conjugated nanoparticles for targeted long-term gene therapy of Parkinson's disease," *Pharm. Res.*, vol. 30, no. 10, pp. 2549–2559, Oct. 2013, doi: 10.1007/s11095-013-1005–8.
[69] Y. Xue, N. Wang, Z. Zeng, J. Huang, Z. Xiang, and Y.-Q. Guan, "Neuroprotective effect of chitosan nanoparticle gene delivery system grafted with acteoside (ACT) in Parkinson's disease models," *J. Mater. Sci. Technol.*, vol. 43, pp. 197–207, Apr. 2020, doi: 10.1016/j.jmst.2019.10.013.
[70] S. Arora, B. Layek, and J. Singh, "Design and validation of liposomal ApoE2 gene delivery system to evade blood-brain barrier for effective treatment of alzheimer's disease," *Mol. Pharm.*, vol. 18, no. 2, pp. 714–725, Feb. 2021, doi: 10.1021/acs.molpharmaceut.0c00461.
[71] S. Arora, T. Kanekiyo, and J. Singh, "Functionalized nanoparticles for brain targeted BDNF gene therapy to rescue Alzheimer's disease pathology in transgenic mouse model," *Int. J. Biol. Macromol.*, vol. 208, pp. 901–911, May 2022, doi: 10.1016/j.ijbiomac.2022.03.203.
[72] J. F. Nabhan et al., "Intrathecal delivery of frataxin mRNA encapsulated in lipid nanoparticles to dorsal root ganglia as a potential therapeutic for Friedreich's ataxia," *Sci. Rep.*, vol. 6, no. 1, p. 1, Feb. 2016, doi: 10.1038/srep20019.
[73] M. Tawfik et al., "Gene therapy with caspase-3 small interfering RNA-nanoparticles is neuroprotective after optic nerve damage," *Neural Regen. Res.*, vol. 16, no. 12, pp. 2534–2541, Dec. 2021, doi: 10.4103/1673–5374.313068.
[74] W. Tang et al., "Modified chitosan for effective renal delivery of siRNA to treat acute kidney injury," *Biomaterials*, vol. 285, p. 121562, Jun. 2022, doi: 10.1016/j.biomaterials.2022.121562.
[75] S. Alan, E. Şalva, İ. Yılmaz, S. Ö. Turan, and J. Akbuğa, "The effectiveness of chitosan-mediated silencing of PDGF-B and PDGFR-β in the mesangial proliferative glomerulonephritis therapy," *Exp. Mol. Pathol.*, vol. 110, p. 104280, Oct. 2019, doi: 10.1016/j.yexmp.2019.104280.
[76] C. Yang et al., "Chitosan/siRNA nanoparticles targeting cyclooxygenase type 2 attenuate unilateral ureteral obstruction-induced kidney injury in mice," *Theranostics*, vol. 5, no. 2, pp. 110–123, 2015, doi: 10.7150/thno.9717.
[77] H. Sena Ozbay et al., "Mitochondria-targeted CoQ10 loaded PLGA-b-PEG-TPP nanoparticles: Their effects on mitochondrial functions of COQ8B-/- HK-2 cells," *Eur. J. Pharm. Biopharm.*, vol. 173, pp. 22–33, Apr. 2022, doi: 10.1016/j.ejpb.2022.02.018.

[78] M. Cao et al., "Adipose mesenchymal stem cell–derived exosomal microRNAs ameliorate polycystic ovary syndrome by protecting against metabolic disturbances," *Biomaterials*, vol. 288, p. 121739, Sep. 2022, doi: 10.1016/j.biomaterials.2022.121739.
[79] S. Du et al., "Cholesterol-Amino-Phosphate (CAP) derived lipid nanoparticles for delivery of self-amplifying RNA and restoration of spermatogenesis in infertile mice," *Adv. Sci.*, p. 2300188, doi: 10.1002/advs.202300188.
[80] Y. Xia et al., "Functionalized selenium nanoparticles for targeted siRNA delivery silence Derlin1 and promote antitumor efficacy against cervical cancer," *Drug Deliv.*, vol. 27, no. 1, pp. 15–25, Jan. 2020, doi: 10.1080/10717544.2019.1667452.
[81] M. S. Singh et al., "Therapeutic gene silencing using targeted lipid nanoparticles in metastatic ovarian cancer," *Small*, vol. 17, no. 19, p. 2100287, 2021, doi: 10.1002/smll.202100287.
[82] E. Oner et al., "Development of EphA2 siRNA-loaded lipid nanoparticles and combination with a small-molecule histone demethylase inhibitor in prostate cancer cells and tumor spheroids," *J. Nanobiotechnology*, vol. 19, no. 1, p. 71, Mar. 2021, doi: 10.1186/s12951-021-00781-z.
[83] S. M. Niemiec et al., "Cerium oxide nanoparticle delivery of microRNA-146a for local treatment of acute lung injury," *Nanomedicine Nanotechnol. Biol. Med.*, vol. 34, p. 102388, Jun. 2021, doi: 10.1016/j.nano.2021.102388.
[84] A. Mohamed, N. K. Kunda, K. Ross, G. A. Hutcheon, and I. Y. Saleem, "Polymeric nanoparticles for the delivery of miRNA to treat Chronic Obstructive Pulmonary Disease (COPD)," *Eur. J. Pharm. Biopharm.*, vol. 136, p. 1, 2019.
[85] Z. Ma et al., "Aerosol delivery of star polymer-siRNA nanoparticles as a therapeutic strategy to inhibit lung tumor growth," *Biomaterials*, vol. 285, p. 121539, Jun. 2022, doi: 10.1016/j.biomaterials.2022.121539.
[86] P. Mora-Raimundo, D. Lozano, M. Manzano, and M. Vallet-Regí, "Nanoparticles to knockdown osteoporosis-related gene and promote osteogenic marker expression for osteoporosis treatment," *ACS Nano*, vol. 13, no. 5, pp. 5451–5464, May 2019, doi: 10.1021/acsnano.9b00241.
[87] "Amelioration of post-traumatic osteoarthritis via nanoparticle depots delivering small interfering RNA to damaged cartilage | Nature Biomedical Engineering." https://www.nature.com/articles/s41551-021-00780-3 (accessed Feb. 15, 2023).
[88] "Novel siRNA formulation to effectively knockdown mutant p53 in osteosarcoma | PLOS ONE." https://journals.plos.org/plosone/article?id=10.1371/journal.pone.0179168 (accessed Feb. 15, 2023).
[89] Y. Xin, M. Huang, W. W. Guo, Q. Huang, L. Z. Zhang, and G. Jiang, "Nano-based delivery of RNAi in cancer therapy," *Mol. Cancer*, vol. 16, no. 1, p. 134, Jul. 2017, doi: 10.1186/s12943-017-0683-y.
[90] A. Babu, R. Muralidharan, N. Amreddy, M. Mehta, A. Munshi, and R. Ramesh, "Nanoparticles for siRNA-based gene silencing in tumor therapy," *IEEE Trans. Nanobioscience*, vol. 15, no. 8, pp. 849–863, Dec. 2016, doi: 10.1109/TNB.2016.2621730.
[91] "RNA Interference and Nanotechnology: A Promising Alliance for Next Generation Cancer Therapeutics | Semantic Scholar." https://www.semanticscholar.org/paper/RNA-Interference-and-Nanotechnology%3A-A-Promising-Swaminathan-Shigna/3d74cec200e670e3d27b4d224d196190f39d9dae (accessed Feb. 19, 2023).
[92] "Recent Developments in Nanoparticle-Based siRNA Delivery for Cancer Therapy." https://www.hindawi.com/journals/bmri/2013/782041/ (accessed Feb. 19, 2023).
[93] "Full article: A new role for microRNAs, as ligands of Toll-like receptors." https://www.tandfonline.com/doi/full/10.4161/rna.23144 (accessed Feb. 19, 2023).
[94] J. K. W. Lam, M. Y. T. Chow, Y. Zhang, and S. W. S. Leung, "siRNA versus miRNA as therapeutics for gene silencing," *Mol. Ther. - Nucleic Acids*, vol. 4, p. e252, Jan. 2015, doi: 10.1038/mtna.2015.23.

[95] "Smart polymeric nanoparticles for cancer gene delivery. - Abstract - Europe PMC." https://europepmc.org/article/PMC/4319689 (accessed Feb. 19, 2023).
[96] H. J. Johnston, G. Hutchison, F. M. Christensen, S. Peters, S. Hankin, and V. Stone, "A review of the in vivo and in vitro toxicity of silver and gold particulates: Particle attributes and biological mechanisms responsible for the observed toxicity," *Crit. Rev. Toxicol.*, vol. 40, no. 4, pp. 328–346, Apr. 2010, doi: 10.3109/10408440903453074.
[97] G. Oberdörster, E. Oberdörster, and J. Oberdörster, "Nanotoxicology: An emerging discipline evolving from studies of ultrafine particles," *Environ. Health Perspect.*, vol. 113, no. 7, pp. 823–839, Jul. 2005, doi: 10.1289/ehp.7339.
[98] C. Egbuna et al., "Toxicity of nanoparticles in biomedical application: Nanotoxicology," *J. Toxicol.*, vol. 2021, p. e9954443, Jul. 2021, doi: 10.1155/2021/9954443.
[99] Y.-M. Cho, Y. Mizuta, J. Akagi, T. Toyoda, M. Sone, and K. Ogawa, "Size-dependent acute toxicity of silver nanoparticles in mice," *J. Toxicol. Pathol.*, vol. 31, no. 1, pp. 73–80, 2018, doi: 10.1293/tox.2017–0043.
[100] Z. Du et al., "Cardiovascular toxicity of different sizes amorphous silica nanoparticles in rats after intratracheal instillation," *Cardiovasc. Toxicol.*, vol. 13, no. 3, pp. 194–207, Sep. 2013, doi: 10.1007/s12012-013-9198-y.
[101] A. Piperno, M. T. Sciortino, E. Giusto, M. Montesi, S. Panseri, and A. Scala, "Recent advances and challenges in gene delivery mediated by polyester-based nanoparticles," *Int. J. Nanomedicine*, vol. 16, pp. 5981–6002, Aug. 2021, doi: 10.2147/IJN.S321329.
[102] "Nanotoxicity: The growing need for in vivo study," *Curr. Opin. Biotechnol.*, vol. 18, no. 6, pp. 565–571, Dec. 2007, doi: 10.1016/j.copbio.2007.11.008.

14 Recent Advances in Nanotechnology-Based Drug Delivery for Cardiovascular Diseases

Fulden Ulucan-Karnak and Cansu Ilke Kuru-Sumer

14.1 INTRODUCTION

Heart disease, often known as CVD, affects people all over the world by affecting their hearts and/or blood arteries (Figure 14.1). Endocarditis, rheumatic heart disease (RHD), and anomalies of the conduction system are just a few of the many issues that can affect the CV system. Heart disease, cerebrovascular disease, peripheral artery disease (PAD), and aortic atherosclerosis are the four conditions that make up CVD, often known as heart disease. Coronary artery disease (CAD), sometimes known as coronary heart disease (CHD), is another name for these conditions. Reduced myocardial perfusion, which results in angina from ischemia and can lead to myocardial infarction (MI) and/or heart failure, is the etiology of CAD (Roth et al., 2020; Olvera Lopez and Ballard, 2022). RHD and acute rheumatic fever (ARF) are significant

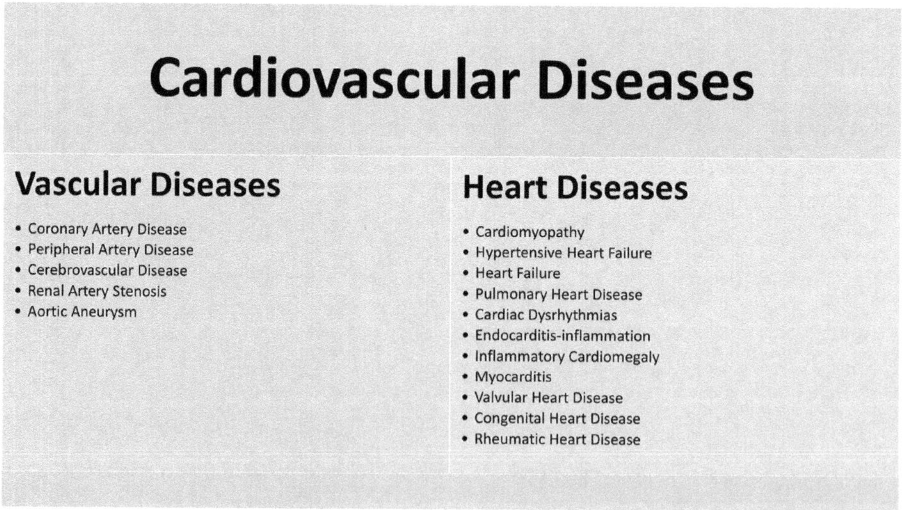

Cardiovascular Diseases

Vascular Diseases	Heart Diseases
• Coronary Artery Disease • Peripheral Artery Disease • Cerebrovascular Disease • Renal Artery Stenosis • Aortic Aneurysm	• Cardiomyopathy • Hypertensive Heart Failure • Heart Failure • Pulmonary Heart Disease • Cardiac Dysrhythmias • Endocarditis-inflammation • Inflammatory Cardiomegaly • Myocarditis • Valvular Heart Disease • Congenital Heart Disease • Rheumatic Heart Disease

FIGURE 14.1 CVD classifications.

DOI: 10.1201/9781003432661-14

contributors to CV morbidity and mortality worldwide. A Group A *Streptococcus* (GAS) infection that activates the innate immune system causes ARF, a multiorgan inflammatory illness. The response to GAS in vulnerable hosts causes autoimmune reactions that attack the brain, skin, joints, heart, and subcutaneous tissue. If penicillin is not administered regularly, persistent episodes of ARF—regardless of whether they are recognized, undiscovered, or subclinical—may eventually proceed to RHD. ARF, and its sequela can cause serious public health concerns in low- and middle-income countries (LMICs) as well as in vulnerable groups in high-income nations by the late 20th century, despite almost completely disappearing in high-income settings (Lawrence et al., 2013; Carapetis et al., 2016; Auala et al., 2022).

CVD is the primary cause of mortality and inefficiency in both the United States and many European nations. According to estimates, 17.9 million deaths worldwide or 32% of all fatalities in 2019 were attributable to CVDs. Heart attack and stroke deaths accounted for 85% of these fatalities. The majority of CVD fatalities occur in low- and middle-income nations. In 2019, noncommunicable illnesses caused 17 million premature deaths (before the age of 70), and 38% of those fatalities were attributable to CVDs (WHO, no date). Despite the steady decline in cigarette consumption over the past few years, the American Heart Association (AHA) notes in its 2023 report that different marginalized populations in the United States continue to use tobacco at much higher rates than the general population. In comparison to 13% of White adults and 12.3% of heterosexual/straight adults, over 27% of American Indian/Alaska native adults and youth report smoking, as do over 16% of lesbian, gay, and bisexual people. Additionally, there has been an increase in the use of electronic cigarettes in the United States, particularly among middle school and high school students (2.8% and 11.3%, respectively) (Tsao et al., 2023). By 2030, it is anticipated that there would be 23.6 million CVD-related deaths annually (Yusuf et al., 2020). The greatest increases in CV-related mortality occurred in Asian, Black, and Hispanic populations, further lowering these peoples' life expectancy rates and widening the gap between them and White areas. It is not surprising that those who were poor, Black, and Hispanic people were particularly vulnerable to the effects of COVID-19 given that several of the risk factors for CVD are also related to an increased chance of dying from COVID-19 (Aburto et al., 2022; Tsao et al., 2023).

Women typically experience the onset of CVD about 10 years later than men do; have a wider range of symptoms; are less likely to seek medical attention; and are less likely than men to have their CVD investigated and treated with particular drugs, angioplasty, or coronary artery bypass grafts. CVD risk factors, such as smoking, depression, poor income, high blood lipids, hypertension, obesity, and inactivity, have also been linked to gender disparities (Grace et al., 2004; Möller-Leimkühler, 2007; Garcia et al., 2016; Montarello and Chan, 2022).

To demonstrate the global efforts toward scientific production in the area of CVD throughout a 10-year period, a scientometrics analysis was conducted by Biglu et al. (2016). All documents indexed as topics of CVD from 2001 to 2010 were extracted using the Science Citation Index Expanded (SCI-E). Data analysis revealed that there have been steadily more publications in the field of CV science. In 2010, there were three times as many publications in SCI-E as there were in 2001. In 2010, there were 15,584 documents, up from 5080 in 2001. The language of most publications was

English, which made up 95% of the total. The circulation journal was the most popular among the main journals based on Bradford scatterings law. The nation producing the highest number of publications was the United States, which had 29.5% of the global profiles in the sector. The most productive institution was Brigham Women's Hospital, followed by Harvard University. The great majority of the scientific literature on CVD was written by North American and Western European authors (Biglu et al., 2016).

Another article's goal is to use scientometric analysis to compile a summary of the research areas and advancements in the built environment and CVD between 2000 and 2021. CiteSpace software was used to evaluate 1,304 records that were taken from the Web of Science core database, and knowledge mapping was used to present the findings. Over the course of the study, there was an increase in the number of publications and conferences on the built environment and CVD, with the United States taking the lead. The link between the built environment and CVD was mapped using physical activity and the dietary environment as mediators and entry sites. Key research areas included walkability, residential characteristics, the food environment, and greenness. Over time, the focus of research shifted from reducing sedentary behavior to incorporating quantitative analyses of subjective feelings. Improving the generalizability of the findings given in the individual studies requires an understanding of the heterogeneity in the built environment. Research that is multi- and interdisciplinary promotes creativity and ensures the inclusion of relevant environmental factors (Zheng et al., 2022).

14.2 CVDs TREATMENT

Based on the severity and risk stratification of the patient, various CVD treatments are chosen. The fundamental goals of all CVD treatment regimens are to improve blood supply, lessen tissue damage, and reduce cardiomyocyte loss while increasing contractile area. Surgery is typically used to treat severe CVD cases to remove blood clots, implant artificial pacemakers to manage arrhythmia, and correct pathological organic heart abnormalities (Rosendorff et al., 2015; Yang et al., 2022). Commonly used CVD treatments are statins, blood thinners, beta-blockers, angiotensin-converting enzyme inhibitors (ACEIs)/receptor blockers, and lifestyle changes. While medications are the key player in the treatment strategy, changing your lifestyle may be helpful to gain healthier habits in terms of diet, exercise, and smoking habits (Figure 14.2).

Statins are 3-hydroxy-3-methyglutaryl coenzyme A (HMG-CoA) reductase inhibitors. The HMG-CoA reductase inhibitors are frequently used for decreasing cholesterol in the primary and secondary prevention of CVD. Recent strong evidence points to the possibility that statins' positive effects may also be attributable to their cholesterol-independent or pleiotropic effects, in addition to their cholesterol-lowering effects. Statins are directly engaged in repairing or increasing endothelial function, attenuating vascular remodeling, suppressing the vascular inflammatory response, and possibly stabilizing atherosclerotic plaques through these so-called pleiotropic actions (Zhou and Liao, 2009). For the majority of patients with hypercholesterolemia, statin medication is advised as the first line of treatment. Statin therapy is effective at breaking up blood clots, reducing inflammation, and enhancing

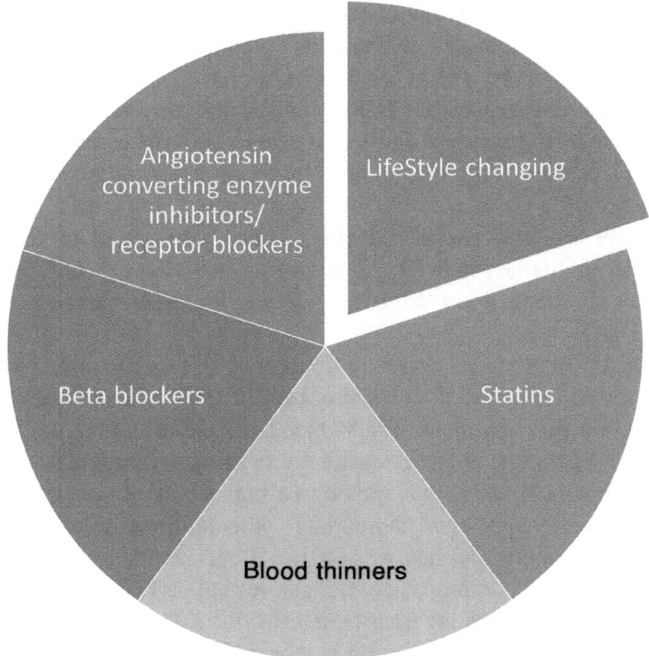

FIGURE 14.2 Commonly used treatment strategies for CVDs.

endothelial function in addition to its effects on lipid regulation (Taylor et al., 2013; Cid-Conde and López-Castro, 2015). In people with low CV risk, statins were found to be effective in preventing death and CV morbidity. Relative risk reductions matched those observed in persons with a history of CAD (Tonelli et al., 2011).

The most popular medication for the secondary prevention of CVDs is aspirin. Aspirin's potential to prevent the production of prostaglandins and thromboxane A2, which are powerful inducers of platelet aggregation and vasoconstriction through irreversible inhibition of the cyclooxygenase-1 (COX-1) enzyme, is likely what gives it its cardioprotective effects. Although preventing thrombosis is preferable in some patient populations, doing so also raises the risk of life-threatening bleeding problems, such as intracranial hemorrhage. Determining benefits and hazards in persons without vascular disease has been challenging (Godley and Hernandez-Vila, 2016). The benefits and risks of aspirin are tightly balanced in individuals who appear to be in good health (primary prevention), even though it significantly lowers CVD mortality and morbidity among survivors of a variety of atherosclerotic CV events (secondary prevention). Aspirin lowers the risk of nonfatal MI but raises the risk of significant bleeding in people without a history of CVD events. Long-term follow-up (with >10 years of treatment) suggests that aspirin may lower the risk of colorectal cancer (Soodi et al., 2020; Guirguis-Blake et al., 2022).

The key component of treatment for numerous CV disorders is beta-blockers (adrenergic receptor antagonists). Although their antagonistic and competitive actions on beta-adrenergic receptors have historically been thought to be the primary cause of their effects, it is now understood that their impact extends beyond simply competing with catecholamines on these receptors. Since their discovery as anti-anginal medications in the 1960s, beta-blockers have become popular treatments for ischemic heart disease, cardiac failure, and arrhythmias (Martínez-Milla et al., 2019). The presence and severity of all risk factors and associated illnesses, as well as the unique properties of the medications in question, should be taken into consideration when deciding on a course of treatment for patients with CVD. Traditional beta-blockers are less effective at reducing central pulse pressure and aortic stiffness than newer medicines with β1 selectivity or vasodilating characteristics, such as carvedilol or nebivolol, and tend to have greater metabolic adverse effects (Dézsi and Szentes, 2017).

As adrenergic receptor antagonists, β-blockers can successfully counteract sympathetic excitability and cardiotoxicity. Because of this, β-blockers are also recommended as the first-line treatment for CVDs and atrial fibrillation; however, they are not appropriate for people with hypertension. According to recent meta-analyses, first-line therapy with beta-blockers was linked to a higher risk of stroke in patients with uncomplicated hypertension when compared to other antihypertensive drugs, particularly in the elderly cohort, and had no positive effects on the endpoints of all-cause mortality, CV morbidity, and mortality (Bangalore et al., 2007; Chan You et al., 2021).

The preferred medications for treating heart failure, CAD, MI, and hypertension are ACEIs and angiotensin II (Ang II) receptor blockers (Vijan, 2009; Ko et al., 2019). ACEIs alleviate heart failure by lowering afterload, preload, and systolic wall stress, resulting in higher cardiac output without increasing heart rate (Brown and Vaughan, 1998).

The balance of body fluids and electrolytes, as well as arterial pressure, are controlled by the renin-angiotensin-aldosterone system (RAAS), a coordinated hormonal cascade. This system also regulates renal, adrenal, and CV functions. The main effector peptide of the RAAS is Ang II. It mediates several activities, such as vasoconstriction, aldosterone, vasopressin production, salt and water retention, and sympathetic activation, by its interaction with the Ang II type 1 (AT1) receptor. These, in turn, may cause hypertension to manifest as well as the hemodynamic changes associated with congestive heart failure (CHF). Angiotensin receptor blockers (ARBs) preferentially prevent Ang II from attaching to the AT1 receptor but not the AT2 receptor to exert their action (SCHMIEDER, 2005; Patel et al., 2017; Martyniak and Tomasik, 2022). In addition to inhibiting the activity of enkephalinase to raise the levels of various endogenous vasoactive peptides, Ang II receptor blocker—neprilysin inhibitor—medications also prevent the activation of the RAAS pathway in patients with heart failure (Bozkurt et al., 2023).

Tai et al. conducted a meta-analysis of 47,662 participants revealing that ACEIs, but not ARBs, lower CV and all-cause mortality in heart failure patients. As a result, ACEIs ought to be taken into account as the first line of treatment to reduce excess mortality and morbidity in this population (Tai et al., 2017).

Traditional treatments of CVDs were adequate for a portion of the population, but they are associated with lower patient compliance, including lifetime discomfort. The role of nanotechnology is then highlighted (Chopra et al., 2022). For better patient outcomes, there is a tremendous need in this field of medicine for innovative therapies. With better prognoses and fewer side effects, disease therapy using nanotechnology might be more successful (Chandarana, Curtis and Hoskins, 2018). With using nanosized technology in CVD treatment, drug off-target cytotoxicity can be reduced, drug solubility can be improved, dosage requirements can be reduced, theranostic agents that combine diagnostic and therapeutic agents can be used, and the accumulation of agents at specific sites can be increased (Karimi et al., 2016). These nanocarriers enhance medication bioavailability, shield pharmaceuticals from enzymatic degradation, and prevent the drugs from being cleared into the bloodstream. They also have remarkable specificity supplied by target moieties. Additionally, nanomaterials' inherent reactive oxygen species (ROS) scavenging and photodynamic or photothermal capabilities continue to offer direct therapeutic approaches for CADs and intravascular implants (Hu et al., 2022b). Figure 14.3, a schematic representation of designed nanoparticles (NPs), modification for targeting, loading therapeutics, and implementation onto cell, tissue, or in vivo levels.

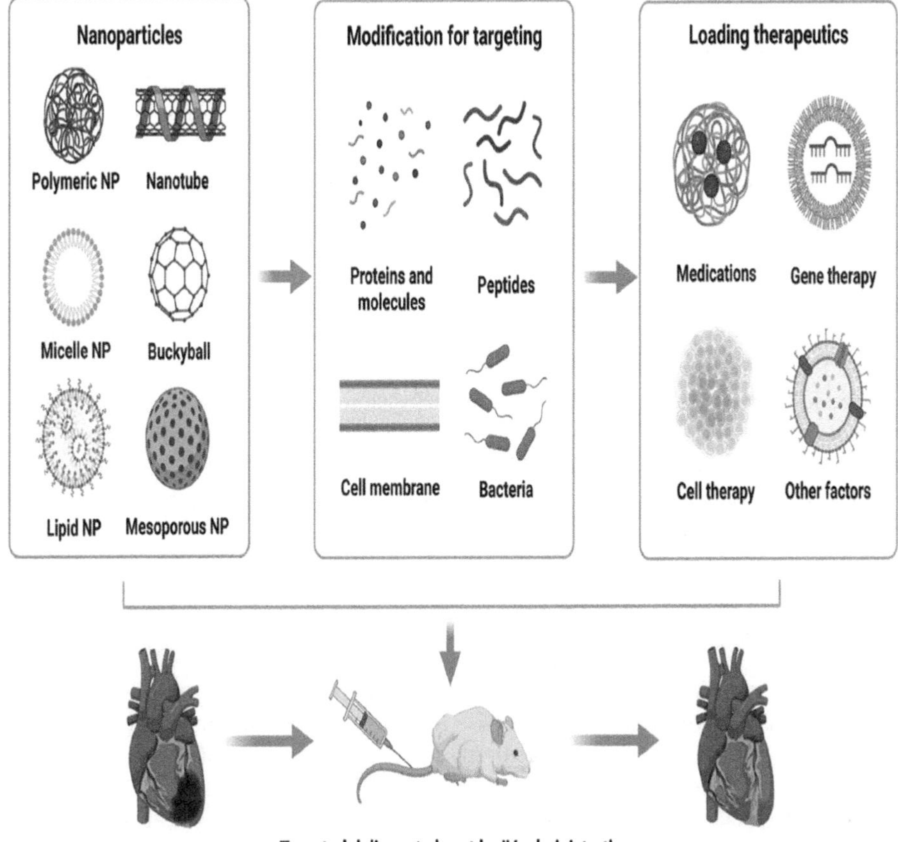

FIGURE 14.3 Representation of NP-based drug delivery system stages for the treatment of CVDs, retrieved from open access journal (Li et al., 2023).

Nanocarriers can be applied by systemic administration. Other nanotechnological advancements, besides systemic delivery of targeted NPs, are anticipated to progress the area even further. Technologies now allow for intramyocardial and intrapericardial administration of medicines and cells to the heart in addition to intravenous injection. Nanotechnological applications in the field of CVD treatment include patches, stents, nanocoatings, heart valves, endovascular devices, membranes, and reservoirs (Wang, Rahimi and Filgueira, 2021). The two targeting methods that employ NPs are passive targeting and active targeting. Especially in cancer treatment, the increased permeability and retention (EPR) effect can be used to accomplish passive targeting. Due to increased vascular permeability, the EPR effect represents a general pathophysiological mechanism by which non-targeted biological molecules or NPs can steadily accumulate in the tumor-vascularized area, resulting in the passively targeted accumulation of anticancer compounds into inflamed areas and tumor tissues. While active targeting, which involves conjugating targeting molecules to NPs, enables the active absorption of NPs, passive targeting enables the effective localization of NPs inside lesion regions. The greatest effective way to boost NP accumulation in the intended lesion region in CVDs is either passive or active targeting methods. Increased adherence of NPs to the adhesion molecules of activated endothelial cells enables passive targeting, whereas active targeting requires targeting molecule-decorated NPs and biomimetic NPs (Figure 14.4) (Choi et al., 2022).

14.3 APPLICATION OF NANOTECHNOLOGY-BASED DDS IN CVDS

A category of illnesses known collectively as CVDs includes atherosclerosis, MI, stroke, hypertension, and heart failure. All across the world, these illnesses are the main cause of fatalities for people. One of the most important uses of nanotechnology today is nanomedicine, which is dedicated to creating medical devices at the nanoscale to create a high-quality healthcare system. With the help of this strategy, we can better understand human physiology and combat various dangerous conditions like CV disorders (Pala et al., 2021; Sahu et al., 2021; Xu et al., 2022).

The application of nanotechnology-based DDS in CVDs in the literature can be categorized in Figure 14.5.

Some examples from the literature are summarized in the next sections.

14.4 ATHEROSCLEROSIS

Being a disease linked to inflammation, atherosclerosis poses a serious healthcare issue. Its cause is still unknown, and MIs and strokes are two major causes of morbidity and mortality globally as a result. Unfortunately, medications can't stop plaque buildup in its tracks. Pharmaceuticals that are administered throughout the body to prevent plaque destabilization run the risk of having negative side effects. Currently, imaging and therapy of atherosclerosis have advanced significantly thanks to nanoscience and particularly nanomedicine (Frostegård, 2013; Prilepskii et al., 2020).

The most common kind of CVD that results in a heart attack or stroke is atherosclerosis. It is characterized by arterial wall thickness, which is enlarged by plaque formation.

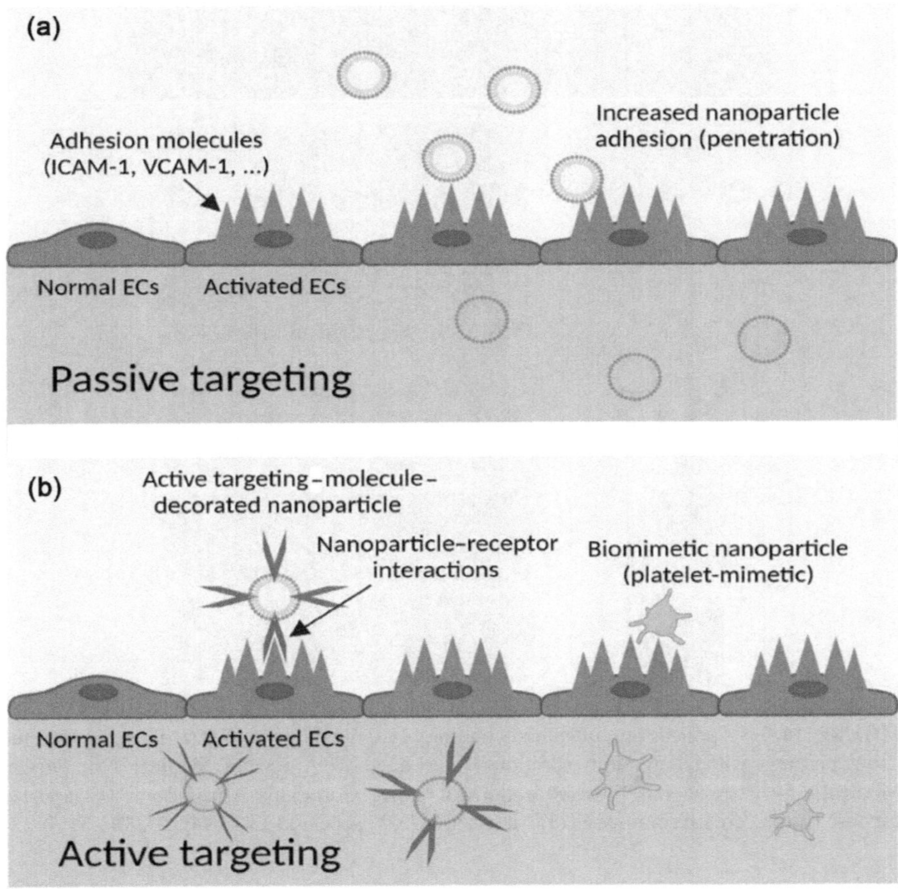

FIGURE 14.4 Passive and active targeting of NPs in DDS, retrieved from open access journal (Choi et al., 2022).

Atherosclerosis treatments based on nanotechnology include controlling lipoprotein levels, lowering inflammatory levels, preventing clotting, and inhibiting neovascularization. Atherogenesis and atherosclerotic plaque rupture are caused by inflammatory macrophages and monocytes (Bentzon et al., 2014; Sahu et al., 2021). The fact that the majority of NPs are absorbed by macrophages makes nano-formulated medications an excellent alternative for the treatment of atherosclerosis. As macrophages phagocytose NPs, complex ideas are being created to shield NPs from phagocytosis. Macrophages are normally found in large numbers inside the plaque in atherosclerosis. Therefore, it is possible to think of phagocytosis as an inborn method of delivering nano-formulated medications to a plaque within macrophages (Prilepskii et al., 2020; Hu et al., 2022a).

A timeline of the major improvements in atherosclerosis nanomedicine was given in a review article by Chen et al. in 2021. It all started in 1993 with the first nanocrystal drug approved by the FDA and followed by improvements in diagnosis and treatment strategies. In 2010, light activatable NPs for targeted macrophage ablation

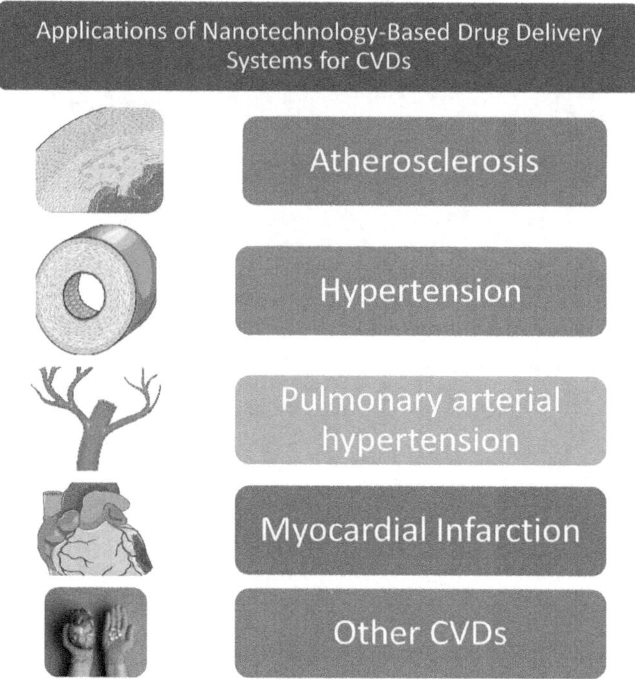

FIGURE 14.5 Applications of nanotechnology-based DDS for CVDs. It was generated using pictures with adaptation (additional markings) from Servier Medical Art. Servier Medical Art by Servier is licensed under a Creative Commons Attribution 3.0 Unported License (https://creativecommons.org/licenses/by/3.0/, accessed 13th May 2023).

were developed. Photothermal therapy alternatives could open new waves to atherosclerosis treatments. In 2016, the targeted delivery of IL-10 by polymeric NPs was achieved. In this process, several trials were started, and in 2020, the clinical trials on the treatment with methotrexate-loaded or paclitaxel-loaded low-density lipoprotein (LDL)-like nNPs (Chen et al., 2022) have been initiated.

Nakashiro et al. developed biodegradable pioglitazone-NPs from poly(lactic-co-glycolic acid). Flow cytometric study revealed that intravenously delivered poly(lactic-co-glycolic-acid) NPs containing fluorescein isothiocyanate (FITC) were present in circulating monocytes and aortic macrophages Pioglitazone-NPs controlled the expression of pro-inflammatory cytokines and inhibited the extracellular matrix metalloproteinase inducer in bone marrow-derived macrophages (Nakashiro et al., 2016).

For NP-based diagnostics and therapies, the subtle clotting that takes place on the luminal surface of atherosclerotic plaques presents a potential target. Peters et al. have created modular multifunctional micelles that can combine a pharmacological component, a fluorophore, and a targeting element into a single particle as needed. The pentapeptide cysteine-arginine-glutamic acid-lysine-alanine targets clotted plasma proteins and atherosclerotic plaques in ApoE-null animals fed a high-fat diet.

The fluorescent micelles adhere to the entire plaque's surface and, particularly, cluster at the shoulders, which are vulnerable to rupture (Peters et al., 2009).

In the past 20 years, significant progress has been made in elucidating the key molecular processes involved in the initiation and development of atherosclerosis. New therapies were also created concurrently. In this regard, animal studies using nanomedicine techniques like biomimetic NPs have yielded encouraging results. These nanomedicines still require further improvement, though, before they can be used in clinical settings. Indeed, more work is required to introduce more nanomedicine candidates to clinical trials by (i) extending blood circulation time, (ii) decreasing hepatic clearance, and (iii) functionalizing the NP surface. Despite extensive research on rodents, it is still necessary to completely understand the biocompatibility and behavior of NPs in the complicated atherosclerotic lesion microenvironment of large animals, such as non-human primates (Wong, Czarny and Venkatraman, 2019; Maddaluno, 2022; Tu et al., 2022).

14.5 HYPERTENSION

The current global epidemic of hypertension is a major risk factor for significant CVDs, such as MI, stroke, heart failure, and peripheral arterial disease, rather than an illness in and of itself. Although many medications are acting through various mechanisms of action that are available on the market as conventional formulations for the treatment of hypertension, their bioavailability, dosing, and associated side effects present significant difficulties that significantly reduce their therapeutic efficacies. Numerous studies have shown that nanocarriers can greatly improve medication bioavailability, reducing the need for frequent dosing and reducing the toxicity linked to high doses of the drug (Alam et al., 2017; Mills, Stefanescu and He, 2020; Kumar et al., 2022).

The most popular methods for treating hypertension are nanoemulsion, liposomes, polymeric NPs, solid lipid nanoparticles (SLNs), and nanostructured lipid carriers (NLCs) (Sahu et al., 2021; Kumar et al., 2022). Olmesartan medoxomil (OM), which exerts its antihypertensive effects by specifically inhibiting Ang II-AT1 receptor, is hydrolyzed to its active metabolite olmesartan by the action of aryl esterase. Its oral bioavailability is constrained by OM's poor aqueous solubility and unchecked enzyme conversion to its weakly permeable olmesartan. The current study's objective was to create a unique OM nanoemulsion to enhance its pharmacokinetics and therapeutic effectiveness. The lipoid-purified soybean oil 700, sefsol 218, and solutol HS 15 were used to create the oil-in-water (o/w) nanoemulsion of OM. The area under the curve (AUC0–27) for olmesartan increased by 2.8 times after oral administration of OM nanoemulsion and sustained release profile, according to the pharmacokinetic study's findings (Gorain et al., 2014).

The goal of Shah et al.'s study was to increase the bioavailability of felodipine by employing PLGA NPs to target the M cells in Peyer's patches. Due to its weak water solubility and substantial first-pass metabolism, felodipine has a low bioavailability. Nanoprecipitation was used to create NPs. Sustained release from NPs was demonstrated by in vitro and ex vivo investigations utilizing rat stomach and intestinal segments. Pharmacodynamic tests on rats demonstrated long-term regulation of alterations in ECG and blood pressure. Therefore, by increasing bioavailability, NPs can be a suitable alternative to the presently available medication for hypertension and angina (Shah et al., 2014).

A calcium channel blocker called lercanidipine hydrochloride is used to treat hypertension. The study's goal was to create lercanidipine hydrochloride-loaded NLCs and see if oral administration may increase the drug's bioavailability. Lipid carriers with lercanidipine hydrochloride nanostructures were made using a process that involved solvent evaporation at a high temperature and freeze-drying to solidify. NLCs released lercanidipine hydrochloride in a controlled manner for a longer amount of time, according to the in vivo pharmacodynamic investigation. These findings unmistakably show that NLCs are a promising drug delivery technology for the treatment of hypertension and a potential controlled release formulation for lercanidipine hydrochloride (Ranpise et al., 2014).

NPs offer an excellent platform for quickly delivering therapeutic compounds to the brain, indicating that they might be a more effective way to address the issue of hypertension. However, none of these studies specifically address this treatment. Therefore, numerous research employing the hypertensive animal model will need to be carried out in order to confirm nanomedicine's function in hypertensive management. Additionally, choosing an effective nanoformulation for preclinical and clinical investigations requires building a correlation between in vitro and in vivo data. In conclusion, a lot more research will be required to create nanotherapeutics with useful qualities for hypertension (Yang et al., 2022; Lamptey et al., 2023).

14.6 PULMONARY ARTERIAL HYPERTENSION

Nitric oxide (NO), endothelin, and prostacyclin pathways are three important pathways for the etiology and progression of pulmonary arterial hypertension (PAH). Prostacyclin (PSC2), phosphodiesterase type-5 (PDE5) inhibitors, and endothelin receptor antagonists (ERAs), three currently approved drugs that target these three pathways, are effective. Despite this, PAH is still a severe clinical condition, and patients with PAH have a subpar long-term survival rate. Medication, patient noncompliance, and side effects all limit the therapeutic efficacy of currently available medications. These issues are anticipated to be solved by NPs, which will offer a new method of treating PAH. Drug-loaded NPs for local administration can increase drug effectiveness and reduce side effects. Animal PAH models and in vitro studies have shown the efficacy of prostacyclin (PSC2) analog, PDE5 inhibitors, ERA, pitavastatin, imatinib, rapamycin, fasudil, and oligonucleotide-loaded NPs. However, more clinical research is necessary to determine the effectiveness and safety of NP-mediated drug delivery methods for treating PAH in humans (Nakamura et al., 2017).

An immunosuppressant called tacrolimus (Tac) has the potential to treat pulmonary fibrosis by preventing the nuclear factor of activated T cells from moving across the body. Here, they looked into the effectiveness of an inhaled Tac formulation with a prolonged release on pulmonary fibrosis brought on by bleomycin. Compared to injections, inhalation has several significant benefits, including increased patient compliance, safety, and therapeutic impact. To do this, they used a high-pressure homogenizer and NP albumin-binding technology to create inhalable albumin NPs with bound Tac (Tac Alb-NPs) at a daily therapeutic dose. For the treatment of pulmonary fibrosis, Tac Alb-NPs have enormous potential as an inhalation administration formulation. These NPs would also serve as a very efficient and secure template for inhaling medicinal medicines that are virtually insoluble (Seo et al., 2016).

PAH can be effectively treated with prostaglandin I2 (PGI2) and its equivalents, such as beraprost sodium (BPS). The therapeutic efficacy of BPS on PAH and the quality of life of patients receiving this medication would both be enhanced by its encapsulation in NPs to enable prolonged release and targeting capabilities. NPs made from a block copolymer of monomethoxy poly(ethylene glycol) and poly(lactic acid) and poly(lactic acid) homopolymer were used to encapsulate BPS. Due to lower dosages and less frequent administration of BPS, BPS-NP may be helpful for the treatment of PAH patients (Ishihara et al., 2015).

The 5-lipoxygenase (5-LO) enzyme was shown to be most effectively and selectively inhibited by the 1,2-benzoquinone RF-22c. Liparulo et al. created an SLN loaded with the medication RF-22c in order to increase its bioavailability and confirm the value of 5-LO as a therapeutic approach for treating PAHs. In order to better understand the role of 5-LO in the monocrotaline (MCT) rat model of PAH, RF-22c-SLN was developed. The rats were divided into three groups at random: control, MCT, and MCT + RF22-c. All the animals were sacrificed after 21 days in order to conduct functional and histological analyses. When compared to the MCT group, RF22-c-SLN therapy was able to considerably lower precapillary resistance (R-pre) and mean pulmonary arterial pressure (mPAP). After treatment, RF22-c-SLN formulation greatly reduced the MCT-induced increase in the cardiomyocyte width and the medial wall thickness of the pulmonary arterioles. The findings demonstrated that by preventing induced pulmonary hypertension, the selective inhibition of 5-LO enhanced hemodynamic parameters as well as vascular and cardiac remodeling. As a result of the increased pharmacological effects and the potential reduction and/or optimization of the drug administration frequency, the enhanced sustained release properties and targeting abilities achieved with the novel nanotechnological approach may be therapeutically advantageous for PAH patients (Liparulo et al., 2020).

The creation of nanosized carriers has attracted significant interest as a result of the application of nanotechnology to the realm of pulmonary medication delivery. The pulmonary route is a more desirable route for the administration of nanosized carriers to treat PAH due to the large surface area of the lungs and the lack of significant impediments to drug absorption. The drug molecule is exposed to an environment that has a higher potential for enzymatic breakdown and unwanted unfavorable side effects when administered orally or intravenously. Despite the fact that nanosystems have a number of benefits for the prospective therapy of PAH, multiple in vitro or ex vivo PAH models still need to be further examined before preclinical laboratory-based research findings can be applied in the clinic. Also worth mentioning is the use of 3D bioprinted models for vascular flow studies, which provide conditions that somewhat resemble PAH symptoms. These developments should reduce clinical failures in the future and provide new PAH therapy options (Segura-Ibarra et al., 2018; Mirhadi et al., 2023).

14.7 MI AND MYOCARDIAL ISCHEMIA

Patients who suffer from MI often die as a result of inadequate blood flow to their important organs. There have been numerous attempts to enhance its prognosis, but nanomaterial research presents a chance to approach this issue at the molecular level and has the potential to greatly enhance illness prevention, diagnosis, and therapy. Nanomaterial-based technology has up till now been a key component of numerous cutting-edge diagnostic and therapeutic approaches for heart repair. There are numerous applications of nanomaterials in MI from a variety of angles, such as pro-angiogenetic element conjugated NPs as drug carriers, modulating immunological homeostasis, and micro RNA (miRNA) and stem cell transport mechanisms (George et al., 2022; Shi et al., 2022).

The timeline of the drug delivery and therapy of MI with nanotechnology started with the micelles accumulated in the zone of MI in vivo in 2004. It is followed by developing different metallic, polymeric, hybrid, or composite NPs or hydrogels as drug carriers for the regeneration of ischemic heart, cardiac regeneration, tissue repair, or tissue engineering purposes. The goal was to reduce a number of ischemia-related pathogenic processes, such as oxidative stress, inflammation, cardiomyocyte apoptosis, and ischemia/reperfusion injury, in order to prevent heart failure and attenuate post-MI pathological remodeling (Bejarano et al., 2018; Akgöl et al., 2021).

Acute myocardial ischemia leads to the production of scar tissue, ventricular enlargement, and ultimately heart failure. According to reports, the placental growth factor (PlGF) promotes angiogenesis and enhances heart performance. It was hypothesized in this study that intramyocardial injection of PlGF contained in alginate NPs can be released at the site of action for an extended period as a sustained slow-release protective mechanism that expedites myocardial recovery in a rat model of ischemic cardiomyopathy. Hearts treated with PlGF-loaded chitosan-alginate NPs showed significant improvements in left ventricular function, vascular density, and interleukin-10 blood levels at 8 weeks following coronary ligation. In contrast to direct injection of the growth factor after an acute MI, the use of NPs as a vehicle for PlGF administration can give continuous slow-release PlGF therapy, boosting the benefits of the growth factor in the context of acute myocardial ischemia (Binsalamah et al., 2011).

For acute MI, where interventional reperfusion therapy is limited by ischemia-reperfusion (IR) injury, there is a need to develop a unique cardioprotective method. Activating the phosphoinositide 3-kinase-protein kinase B (PI3K-Akt) pathway and reducing inflammation, bioabsorbable poly(lactic acid/glycolic acid) NP-mediated therapy with pitavastatin (pitavastatin-NP) has been shown to have cardioprotective effects in a rat IR injury model. In this study, it is investigated the impact of pitavastatin-NP on myocardial IR injury in conscious and sedated pig models to acquire preclinical proof-of-concept data. In a preclinical conscious pig model, pitavastatin is delivered to IR-damaged myocardium by NP and has cardioprotective benefits on IR injury without causing any obvious side effects. Pitavastatin-NP is a unique therapeutic approach for IR injury in acute MI as a result (Ichimura et al., 2016).

In another study by Yajima et al., contrary to an ONO-1301 solution, intravenously administered ONO-1301-containing NPs (ONO-1301NPs) aggregated specifically in the rats' ischemia/reperfusion (I/R)-damaged myocardium and helped to prolong ONO-1301's retention in the targeted myocardial tissue. Proangiogenic cytokines were up-regulated while inflammatory cytokines were down-regulated in the ischemic area as a result of the injection of ONO-1301NP. In contrast to vehicle-injected or ONO-1301 solution-injected rats, those given ONO-1301NP showed lower infarct sizes, better-preserved capillary networks, and better-preserved myocardial blood flow at 24 hours after I/R injury. ONO-1301NPs reduce myocardial I/R injury by promoting angiogenesis and reducing inflammation (Yajima et al., 2019).

These therapies might work to stop the loss of cardiac cells, control remodeling, or encourage regeneration. These abilities have been proven by a variety of growth factors, cytokines, and small compounds; however, their effectiveness is constrained by poor transport, absorption, and retention at the target region, and the myocardial EPR effect is generally moderate and transient. Thus, nanocarriers present a viable remedy, especially if they can target the wounded location using active and EPR-independent methods. The utilization of exosomes as naturally targeted delivery systems and ligand-based targeting are only a few of the many techniques that are currently being investigated. However, these technologies still face a lot of challenges. Additional research is necessary to better the loading capability and targeting potential of NPs and to identify the precise mechanisms driving their drug release. Preclinical studies are also necessary to ascertain the ideal formulation, pharmacology, safety profile, and the entire spectrum of diagnostic and therapeutic uses for NPs. There needs to be a clear standardization of the materials, characterization techniques, delivery systems, and regulatory recognition for nanocarriers. The situation is made even more difficult when biological products like exosomes are involved. There are no approved nanodrugs for the treatment of MI, and one-fifth of US FDA-approved nanodrugs are intended for cancer therapy (Bobo et al., 2016; Cicha et al., 2018; Fan et al., 2020; George et al., 2022).

14.8 OTHER CVDs

NPs work well in the treatment of numerous additional CVDs as a cutting-edge medication delivery platform. DDS mediated by NPs have the potential to revolutionize the creation of new medicinal devices. They, therefore, proposed the hypothesis that a bioabsorbable polymeric NP-eluting stent offers an effective DDS that exhibits better and more extended delivery than a dip-coating stent. Vascular smooth muscle cells that had been grown *in-vitro* effectively and steadily absorbed the NP. Significant FITC fluorescence was seen in the neointimal and medial layers of the stented segments that had received the FITC-NP-eluting stent up until 4 weeks in an in vivo swine coronary artery model. As a result, this NP-eluting stent is a powerful NP-mediated DDS that serves as a cutting-edge delivery system for less invasive nano-devices that target CV illness (Nakano et al., 2009).

After open vascular reconstructions to treat atherosclerosis, intimal hyperplasia continues to be a significant factor in the poor patient outcomes. The use of the NPs platform for initial medication delivery in patients undergoing surgical revascularization may be beneficial. Polymer hydrogels, wraps, and NPs all have complimentary and overlapping features for intraperitoneal delivery. The ideal intravenous administration system would permit prolonged drug release while putting the vascular wall under the least amount of mechanical and inflammatory stress. Thousands of patients undergoing open vascular reconstruction each year might benefit from a clinically viable method of periadventitial medication delivery (Chaudhary et al., 2016).

Numerous different ways of benefits are reported for coenzyme Q10 (CoQ10) against the heart diseases. It can reduce blood pressure, the likelihood of dying from heart failure, and the danger of having another heart attack. Due to its anti-inflammatory and immunostimulatory properties, CoQ10, an antioxidant chemical that is used as a dietary supplement, has been suggested as an adjuvant in the treatment of CV problems. The purpose of this study was to produce three distinct CoQ10 nanosuspensions intended for nebulization administration to the lungs by high-pressure homogenization, characterize them, and investigate their stability. Although it has been demonstrated that vitamin-E tocopheryl polyethylene glycol succinate (TPGS) alone can harm the plasma membrane, when it is combined with CoQ10, the likelihood of cell injury is reduced (Rossi et al., 2018).

All of these and more examples in the literature will explicit the impact of applications of nanotechnology in the CVD treatment. In order to adapt the results to a clinical setting, we must make use of all the developments in the field of nanomedicine research to create a more "precise" understanding of it. In order to do this, precise data regarding the currently available nanotherapeutics must be gathered, and their internal characteristics and biological effects must be carefully estimated. This will make it possible to develop intelligent nanoformulations that are made to specifically target diseases and customize nanotherapies (Mabrouk et al., 2021; Mohamed et al., 2022).

14.9 CONCLUSION, CHALLENGES, AND FUTURE PERSPECTIVES

Nanotechnology offers a platform for the development of novel potential in the field of medicine, going well beyond the gradual scaling down of existing technology. The advancement of imaging anatomical structures and treatment strategies for diseases has never been more rapid because of such downsizing. The complete range of health can be improved by nanotechnology when combined with advances in other domains like artificial intelligence (AI) and systems biology from disease diagnosis and health monitoring to networked therapeutic programs and in vivo prognostic and response-to-therapy imaging.

Nanomedicine has sparked a lot of interest, and its applications in CVD treatment and cardiotoxicity reduction are still relatively young and expanding. The ideal nanomedicine should be capable of targeting plaque tissues, penetrating the plaque core, and entirely removing the plaque without causing systemic damage, particularly cardiotoxicity (Martín Giménez et al., 2017; Yang et al., 2022). Other challenges with nanoformulation that could scuttle a pharmaceutical program include size- and material-based toxicity and safety issues, long-term biocompatibility, circulation half-life, repeatability, and serum stability (Smith and Edelman, 2023). NPs can be dispersed throughout the body by passing past membrane barriers in the bloodstream and affecting organs and tissues at both the cellular and molecular levels. The interaction of NPs with cells may result in nanotoxicity. The nanotoxicity of

NPs was significantly associated with their narrow size distribution, shape, coating, manufacturing technique, large surface area to mass ratio, surface characteristics, charge, dose, and host immunity. By breaching membranes, NPs can infiltrate tissues and cells, causing cell damage and toxicity (Bakand and Hayes, 2016; Cheng et al., 2022). Smaller NP size has been linked to increased toxicity in studies. Furthermore, different NP coatings influence toxicities mostly through changes in absorption and localization. Many of the harmful effects of NPs are thought to be caused by the generation of ROS, which is a significant cause of oxidative stress. While iron oxide NPs and gold nanoparticles (AuNPs) have shown promise in the detection and treatment of atherosclerotic plaques, silver nanoparticles (AgNPs) have lately been linked to negative CV consequences (Younis et al., 2021).

Despite all of these literature studies, there is still a long way to go before clinical applications of nanotechnology can be made. To get the go ahead for clinical trials, the biocompatibility, pharmacokinetics, and safety of nanomaterials in vivo should be rigorously assessed in both small and large animal models. Attention must also be paid to how nanomedicines behave in intricate plaque microenvironments and how they interact with other elements. Last but not least, due to the fundamental role of nanomedicines in clinical application, large-scale production of nanomedicines with controlled and stable physicochemical qualities should be the cornerstone of the entire industrial operation (Patra et al., 2018; Mitchell et al., 2021; Hu et al., 2022b).

It must be kept in mind that multidisciplinary teams would be more impactful in developing novel nanomedicine strategies in terms of CVD treatment with engineering, medicine, and clinical backgrounds. Also, regulation of clinical translations should be investigated by experts.

REFERENCES

Aburto, J. M. et al. (2022) 'Significant impacts of the COVID-19 pandemic on race/ethnic differences in US mortality', *Proceedings of the National Academy of Sciences*, 119(35). doi: 10.1073/pnas.2205813119.

Akgöl, S. et al. (2021) 'The usage of composite nanomaterials in biomedical engineering applications', *Biotechnology and Bioengineering*, 118(8), pp. 2906–2922. doi: 10.1002/bit.27843.

Alam, T. et al. (2017) 'Nanocarriers as treatment modalities for hypertension', *Drug Delivery*, 24(1), pp. 358–369. doi: 10.1080/10717544.2016.1255999.

Auala, T. et al. (2022) 'Acute rheumatic fever and rheumatic heart disease: Highlighting the role of group A Streptococcus in the global burden of cardiovascular disease', *Pathogens*, 11(5), p. 496. doi: 10.3390/pathogens11050496.

Bakand, S. and Hayes, A. (2016) 'Toxicological considerations, toxicity assessment, and risk management of inhaled nanoparticles', *International Journal of Molecular Sciences*, 17(6), p. 929. doi: 10.3390/ijms17060929.

Bangalore, S. et al. (2007) 'Cardiovascular protection using beta-blockers', *Journal of the American College of Cardiology*, 50(7), pp. 563–572. doi: 10.1016/j.jacc.2007.04.060.

Bejarano, J. et al. (2018) 'Nanoparticles for diagnosis and therapy of atherosclerosis and myocardial infarction: Evolution toward prospective theranostic approaches', *Theranostics*, 8(17), pp. 4710–4732. doi: 10.7150/thno.26284.

Bentzon, J. F. et al. (2014) 'Mechanisms of plaque formation and rupture', *Circulation Research*, 114(12), pp. 1852–1866. doi: 10.1161/CIRCRESAHA.114.302721.

Biglu, M.-H., Ghavami, M. and Biglu, S. (2016) 'Cardiovascular diseases in the mirror of science', *Journal of Cardiovascular and Thoracic Research*, 8(4), pp. 158–163. doi: 10.15171/jcvtr.2016.32.

Binsalamah, Z., M. et al. (2011) 'Intramyocardial sustained delivery of placental growth factor using nanoparticles as a vehicle for delivery in the rat infarct model', *International Journal of Nanomedicine*, p. 2667. doi: 10.2147/IJN.S25175.

Bobo, D. et al. (2016) 'Nanoparticle-based medicines: A review of FDA-approved materials and clinical trials to date', *Pharmaceutical Research*, 33(10), pp. 2373–2387. doi: 10.1007/s11095-016-1958-5.

Bozkurt, B. et al. (2023) 'Neprilysin inhibitors in heart failure', *JACC: Basic to Translational Science*, 8(1), pp. 88–105. doi: 10.1016/j.jacbts.2022.05.010.

Brown, N. J. and Vaughan, D. E. (1998) 'Angiotensin-converting enzyme inhibitors', *Circulation*, 97(14), pp. 1411–1420. doi: 10.1161/01.CIR.97.14.1411.

Carapetis, J. R. et al. (2016) 'Acute rheumatic fever and rheumatic heart disease', *Nature Reviews Disease Primers*, 2(1), p. 15084. doi: 10.1038/nrdp.2015.84.

Chan You, S. et al. (2021) 'Comprehensive comparative effectiveness and safety of first-line β-blocker monotherapy in hypertensive patients', *Hypertension*, 77(5), pp. 1528–1538. doi: 10.1161/HYPERTENSIONAHA.120.16402.

Chandarana, M., Curtis, A. and Hoskins, C. (2018) 'The use of nanotechnology in cardiovascular disease', *Applied Nanoscience*, 8(7), pp. 1607–1619. doi: 10.1007/s13204-018-0856-z.

Chaudhary, M. A. et al. (2016) 'Periadventitial drug delivery for the prevention of intimal hyperplasia following open surgery', *Journal of Controlled Release*, 233, pp. 174–180. doi: 10.1016/j.jconrel.2016.05.002.

Chen, W. et al. (2022) 'Macrophage-targeted nanomedicine for the diagnosis and treatment of atherosclerosis', *Nature Reviews Cardiology*, 19(4), pp. 228–249. doi: 10.1038/s41569-021-00629-x.

Cheng, T.-M. et al. (2022) 'Toxicologic concerns with current medical nanoparticles', *International Journal of Molecular Sciences*, 23(14), p. 7597. doi: 10.3390/ijms23147597.

Choi, K.-A. et al. (2022) 'Current nanomedicine for targeted vascular disease treatment: Trends and perspectives', *International Journal of Molecular Sciences*, 23(20), p. 12397. doi: 10.3390/ijms232012397.

Chopra, H. et al. (2022) 'Nanomaterials: A promising therapeutic approach for cardiovascular diseases', *Journal of Nanomaterials*, pp. 1–25. doi: 10.1155/2022/4155729.

Cicha, I. et al. (2018) 'From design to the clinic: Practical guidelines for translating cardiovascular nanomedicine', *Cardiovascular Research*, 114(13), pp. 1714–1727. doi: 10.1093/cvr/cvy219.

Cid-Conde, L. and López-Castro, J. (2015) 'Hypercholesterolemia — statin therapy — indications, side effects, common mistakes in handling, last evidence and recommendations in current clinical practice', in *Hypercholesterolemia*. InTech. doi: 10.5772/59622.

Dézsi, C. A. and Szentes, V. (2017) 'The real role of β-blockers in daily cardiovascular therapy', *American Journal of Cardiovascular Drugs*, 17(5), pp. 361–373. doi: 10.1007/s40256-017-0221–8.

Fan, C. et al. (2020) 'Nanoparticle-mediated drug delivery for treatment of ischemic heart disease', *Frontiers in Bioengineering and Biotechnology*, 8. doi: 10.3389/fbioe.2020.00687.

Frostegård, J. (2013) 'Immunity, atherosclerosis and cardiovascular disease', *BMC Medicine*, 11(1), p. 117. doi: 10.1186/1741–7015-11–117.

Garcia, M. et al. (2016) 'Cardiovascular disease in women', *Circulation Research*, 118(8), pp. 1273–1293. doi: 10.1161/CIRCRESAHA.116.307547.

George, T. A. et al. (2022) 'Nanocarrier-based targeted therapies for myocardial infarction', *Pharmaceutics*, 14(5), p. 930. doi: 10.3390/pharmaceutics14050930.

Godley, R. W. and Hernandez-Vila, E. (2016) 'Aspirin for primary and secondary prevention of cardiovascular disease', *Texas Heart Institute Journal*, 43(4), pp. 318–319. doi: 10.14503/THIJ-16–5807.

Gorain, B. et al. (2014) 'Nanoemulsion strategy for olmesartan medoxomil improves oral absorption and extended antihypertensive activity in hypertensive rats', *Colloids and Surfaces B: Biointerfaces*, 115, pp. 286–294. doi: 10.1016/j.colsurfb.2013.12.016.

Grace, S. L. et al. (2004) 'Cardiovascular disease', *BMC Women's Health*, 4(Suppl 1), p. S15. doi: 10.1186/1472–6874-4-S1-S15.

Guirguis-Blake, J. M. et al. (2022) 'Aspirin use to prevent cardiovascular disease and colorectal cancer', *JAMA*, 327(16), p. 1585. doi: 10.1001/jama.2022.3337.

Hu, P. P. et al. (2022a) 'Macrophage-targeted nanomedicine for the diagnosis and management of atherosclerosis', *Frontiers in Pharmacology*, 13. doi: 10.3389/fphar.2022.1000316.

Hu, Q. et al. (2022b) 'Nanotechnology for cardiovascular diseases', *The Innovation*, 3(2), p. 100214. doi: 10.1016/j.xinn.2022.100214.

Ichimura, K. et al. (2016) 'A translational study of a new therapeutic approach for acute myocardial infarction: Nanoparticle-mediated delivery of pitavastatin into reperfused myocardium reduces ischemia-reperfusion injury in a preclinical porcine model', *PLoS One*, 11(9), p. e0162425. doi: 10.1371/journal.pone.0162425.

Ishihara, Tomoaki et al. (2015) 'Encapsulation of beraprost sodium in nanoparticles: Analysis of sustained release properties, targeting abilities and pharmacological activities in animal models of pulmonary arterial hypertension', *Journal of Controlled Release*, 197, pp. 97–104. doi: 10.1016/j.jconrel.2014.10.029.

Karimi, M. et al. (2016) 'Nanotechnology in diagnosis and treatment of coronary artery disease', *Nanomedicine*, 11(5), pp. 513–530. doi: 10.2217/nnm.16.3.

Ko, D. et al. (2019) 'Comparative effectiveness of ACE inhibitors and angiotensin receptor blockers in patients with prior myocardial infarction', *Open Heart*, 6(1), p. e001010. doi: 10.1136/openhrt-2019-001010.

Kumar, G. et al. (2022) 'A revolutionary blueprint for mitigation of hypertension via nanoemulsion', *BioMed Research International*, 2022, pp. 1–12. doi: 10.1155/2022/4109874.

Lamptey, R. N. L. et al. (2023) 'Neurogenic hypertension, the blood–brain barrier, and the potential role of targeted nanotherapeutics', *International Journal of Molecular Sciences*, 24(3), p. 2213. doi: 10.3390/ijms24032213.

Lawrence, J. G. et al. (2013) 'Acute rheumatic fever and rheumatic heart disease', *Circulation*, 128(5), pp. 492–501. doi: 10.1161/CIRCULATIONAHA.113.001477.

Li, D. et al. (2023) 'Nanoparticle based cardiac specific drug delivery', *Biology*, 12(1), p. 82. doi: 10.3390/biology12010082.

Liparulo, A. et al. (2020) 'Formulation and characterization of solid lipid nanoparticles loading RF22-c, a potent and selective 5-LO inhibitor, in a monocrotaline-induced model of pulmonary hypertension', *Frontiers in Pharmacology*, 11. doi: 10.3389/fphar.2020.00083.

Mabrouk, M. et al. (2021) 'Nanomaterials for biomedical applications: Production, characterisations, recent trends and difficulties', *Molecules*, 26(4), p. 1077. doi: 10.3390/molecules26041077.

Maddaluno, L. (2022) *Nanoparticle-Based Therapies for the Treatment of Atherosclerosis*. Available at: https://www.powerofparticles.com/nanoparticle-based-therapies-treatment-atherosclerosis.

Martín Giménez, V. M., Kassuha, D. E. and Manucha, W. (2017) 'Nanomedicine applied to cardiovascular diseases: Latest developments', *Therapeutic Advances in Cardiovascular Disease*, 11(4), pp. 133–142. doi: 10.1177/1753944717692293.

Martínez-Milla, J. et al. (2019) 'Role of beta-blockers in cardiovascular disease in 2019', *Revista Española de Cardiología (English Edition)*, 72(10), pp. 844–852. doi: 10.1016/j.rec.2019.04.014.

Martyniak, A. and Tomasik, P. J. (2022) 'A new perspective on the renin-angiotensin system', *Diagnostics*, 13(1), p. 16. doi: 10.3390/diagnostics13010016.

Mills, K. T., Stefanescu, A. and He, J. (2020) 'The global epidemiology of hypertension', *Nature Reviews Nephrology*, 16(4), pp. 223–237. doi: 10.1038/s41581-019-0244-2.

Mirhadi, E. et al. (2023) 'Nanomedicine-mediated therapeutic approaches for pulmonary arterial hypertension', *Drug Discovery Today*, 28(6), p. 103599. doi: 10.1016/j.drudis.2023.103599.

Mitchell, M. J. et al. (2021) 'Engineering precision nanoparticles for drug delivery', *Nature Reviews Drug Discovery*, 20(2), pp. 101–124. doi: 10.1038/s41573-020-0090-8.

Mohamed, N. A. et al. (2022) 'Recent developments in nanomaterials-based drug delivery and upgrading treatment of cardiovascular diseases', *International Journal of Molecular Sciences*, 23(3), p. 1404. doi: 10.3390/ijms23031404.

Möller-Leimkühler, A. M. (2007) 'Gender differences in cardiovascular disease and comorbid depression.', *Dialogues in Clinical Neuroscience*, 9(1), pp. 71–83. doi: 10.31887/DCNS.2007.9.1/ammoeller.

Montarello, N. and Chan, W. P. (Alicia) (2022) 'Coronary artery disease in women', *Australian Prescriber*, 45(6), pp. 193–199. doi: 10.18773/austprescr.2022.065.

Nakamura, K. et al. (2017) 'Nanoparticle-mediated drug delivery system for pulmonary arterial hypertension', *Journal of Clinical Medicine*, 6(5), p. 48. doi: 10.3390/jcm6050048.

Nakano, K. et al. (2009) 'Formulation of nanoparticle-eluting stents by a cationic electrodeposition coating technology', *JACC: Cardiovascular Interventions*, 2(4), pp. 277–283. doi: 10.1016/j.jcin.2008.08.023.

Nakashiro, S. et al. (2016) 'Pioglitazone-incorporated nanoparticles prevent plaque destabilization and rupture by regulating monocyte/macrophage differentiation in ApoE$^{-/-}$ Mice', *Arteriosclerosis, Thrombosis, and Vascular Biology*, 36(3), pp. 491–500. doi: 10.1161/ATVBAHA.115.307057.

Olvera Lopez, E., Ballard, B. D., and Arif, J. (2022) *Cardiovascular Disease, StatPearls*. Available at: https://www.ncbi.nlm.nih.gov/books/NBK535419/.

Pala, R. et al. (2021) 'Nanomaterials as novel cardiovascular theranostics', *Pharmaceutics*, 13(3), p. 348. doi: 10.3390/pharmaceutics13030348.

Patel, S. et al. (2017) 'Renin-angiotensin-aldosterone (RAAS): The ubiquitous system for homeostasis and pathologies', *Biomedicine & Pharmacotherapy*, 94, pp. 317–325. doi: 10.1016/j.biopha.2017.07.091.

Patra, J. K. et al. (2018) 'Nano based drug delivery systems: Recent developments and future prospects', *Journal of Nanobiotechnology*, 16(1), p. 71. doi: 10.1186/s12951-018-0392-8.

Peters, D. et al. (2009) 'Targeting atherosclerosis by using modular, multifunctional micelles', *Proceedings of the National Academy of Sciences*, 106(24), pp. 9815–9819. doi: 10.1073/pnas.0903369106.

Prilepskii, A. Y. et al. (2020) 'Nanoparticle-based approaches towards the treatment of atherosclerosis', *Pharmaceutics*, 12(11), p. 1056. doi: 10.3390/pharmaceutics12111056.

Ranpise, N. S., Korabu, S. S. and Ghodake, V. N. (2014) 'Second generation lipid nanoparticles (NLC) as an oral drug carrier for delivery of lercanidipine hydrochloride', *Colloids and Surfaces B: Biointerfaces*, 116, pp. 81–87. doi: 10.1016/j.colsurfb.2013.12.012.

Rosendorff, C. et al. (2015) 'Treatment of hypertension in patients with coronary artery disease', *Circulation*, 131(19). doi: 10.1161/CIR.0000000000000207.

Rossi, I. et al. (2018) 'Nebulized coenzyme Q 10 nanosuspensions: A versatile approach for pulmonary antioxidant therapy', *European Journal of Pharmaceutical Sciences*, 113, pp. 159–170. doi: 10.1016/j.ejps.2017.10.024.

Roth, G. A. et al. (2020) 'Global burden of cardiovascular diseases and risk factors, 1990–2019', *Journal of the American College of Cardiology*, 76(25), pp. 2982–3021. doi: 10.1016/j.jacc.2020.11.010.

Sahu, T. et al. (2021) 'Nanotechnology based drug delivery system: Current strategies and emerging therapeutic potential for medical science', *Journal of Drug Delivery Science and Technology*, 63, p. 102487. doi: 10.1016/j.jddst.2021.102487.

Schmieder, R. (2005) 'Mechanisms for the clinical benefits of angiotensin II receptor blockers', *American Journal of Hypertension*, 18(5), pp. 720–730. doi: 10.1016/j.amjhyper.2004.11.032.

Segura-Ibarra, V. et al. (2018) 'Nanotherapeutics for treatment of pulmonary arterial hypertension', *Frontiers in Physiology*, 9. doi: 10.3389/fphys.2018.00890.

Seo, J. et al. (2016) 'Therapeutic advantage of inhaled tacrolimus-bound albumin nanoparticles in a bleomycin-induced pulmonary fibrosis mouse model', *Pulmonary Pharmacology & Therapeutics*, 36, pp. 53–61. doi: 10.1016/j.pupt.2016.01.001.

Shah, U., Joshi, G. and Sawant, K. (2014) 'Improvement in antihypertensive and antianginal effects of felodipine by enhanced absorption from PLGA nanoparticles optimized by factorial design', *Materials Science and Engineering: C*, 35, pp. 153–163. doi: 10.1016/j.msec.2013.10.038.

Shi, H. et al. (2022) 'New diagnostic and therapeutic strategies for myocardial infarction via nanomaterials', *eBioMedicine*, 78, p. 103968. doi: 10.1016/j.ebiom.2022.103968.

Smith, B. R. and Edelman, E. R. (2023) 'Nanomedicines for cardiovascular disease', *Nature Cardiovascular Research*, 2(4), pp. 351–367. doi: 10.1038/s44161-023-00232-y.

Soodi, D., VanWormer, J. J. and Rezkalla, S. H. (2020) 'Aspirin in primary prevention of cardiovascular events', *Clinical Medicine & Research*, 18(2–3), pp. 89–94. doi: 10.3121/cmr.2020.1548.

Tai, C. et al. (2017) 'Effect of angiotensin-converting enzyme inhibitors and angiotensin II receptor blockers on cardiovascular events in patients with heart failure: A meta-analysis of randomized controlled trials', *BMC Cardiovascular Disorders*, 17(1), p. 257. doi: 10.1186/s12872-017-0686-z.

Taylor, F. et al. (2013) 'Statins for the primary prevention of cardiovascular disease', *Cochrane Database of Systematic Reviews*, 2021(9). doi: 10.1002/14651858.CD004816.pub5.

Tonelli, M. et al. (2011) 'Efficacy of statins for primary prevention in people at low cardiovascular risk: A meta-analysis', *Canadian Medical Association Journal*, 183(16), pp. E1189–E1202. doi: 10.1503/cmaj.101280.

Tsao, C. W. et al. (2023) 'Heart disease and stroke statistics—2023 update: A report from the American Heart Association', *Circulation*, 147(8). doi: 10.1161/CIR.0000000000001123.

Tu, S. et al. (2022) 'Advances in imaging and treatment of atherosclerosis based on organic nanoparticles', *APL Bioengineering*, 6(4), p. 041501. doi: 10.1063/5.0127835.

Vijan, S. G. (2009) 'Angiotensin-converting enzyme inhibitors (ACEIs), not angiotensin receptor blockers (ARBs), are preferred and effective mode of therapy in high cardiovascular risk patients', *Journal of the Indian Medical Association*, 107(3), pp. 178–82. Available at: https://www.ncbi.nlm.nih.gov/pubmed/19810392.

Wang, D. K., Rahimi, M. and Filgueira, C. S. (2021) 'Nanotechnology applications for cardiovascular disease treatment: Current and future perspectives', *Nanomedicine: Nanotechnology, Biology and Medicine*, 34, p. 102387. doi: 10.1016/j.nano.2021.102387.

WHO (no date) *Cardiovascular diseases (CVDs), 2021*. Available at: https://www.who.int/news-room/fact-sheets/detail/cardiovascular-diseases-(cvds).

Wong, Y. S., Czarny, B. and Venkatraman, S. S. (2019) 'Precision nanomedicine in atherosclerosis therapy: How far are we from reality?', *Precision Nanomedicine*, 2(1), pp. 230–244. doi: 10.33218/prnano2(1).181114.1.

Xu, H., Li, S. and Liu, Y.-S. (2022) 'Nanoparticles in the diagnosis and treatment of vascular aging and related diseases', *Signal Transduction and Targeted Therapy*, 7(1), p. 231. doi: 10.1038/s41392-022-01082-z.

Yajima, S. et al. (2019) 'Prostacyclin analogue–loaded nanoparticles attenuate myocardial ischemia/reperfusion injury in rats', *JACC: Basic to Translational Science*, 4(3), pp. 318–331. doi: 10.1016/j.jacbts.2018.12.006.

Yang, F. et al. (2022) 'Nanoparticle-based drug delivery systems for the treatment of cardiovascular diseases', *Frontiers in Pharmacology*, 13. doi: 10.3389/fphar.2022.999404.

Younis, N. K. et al. (2021) 'Metal-based nanoparticles: Promising tools for the management of cardiovascular diseases', *Nanomedicine: Nanotechnology, Biology and Medicine*, 36, p. 102433. doi: 10.1016/j.nano.2021.102433.

Yusuf, S. et al. (2020) 'Modifiable risk factors, cardiovascular disease, and mortality in 155 722 individuals from 21 high-income, middle-income, and low-income countries (PURE): A prospective cohort study', *The Lancet*, 395(10226), pp. 795–808. doi: 10.1016/S0140–6736(19)32008-2.

Zheng, Z. et al. (2022) 'Scientometric analysis of the relationship between a built environment and cardiovascular disease', *International Journal of Environmental Research and Public Health*, 19(9), p. 5625. doi: 10.3390/ijerph19095625.

Zhou, Q. and Liao, J. (2009) 'Statins and cardiovascular diseases: From cholesterol lowering to pleiotropy', *Current Pharmaceutical Design*, 15(5), pp. 467–478. doi: 10.2174/138161209787315684.

15 Green Synthesis, Characterization, and Application of Nanoparticles for Drug Delivery

Subhankar Das and Manjula Ishwara Kalyani

15.1 INTRODUCTION

Green nanotechnology has acquired significant prominence owing to its ecologically benign method of producing nanoparticles. Professor Norio Taniguchi of Tokyo Science University first used the term "nanotechnology" in 1974. The word "nano" is derived from the Greek word *nanos* meaning extremely small or dwarf. Nanoparticles consist of particles with sizes ranging from 1 to 100 nm (1,2).

Recently, metal and metal oxide nanoparticles have attracted considerable interest due to their wide array of applications in various fields of biotechnology and biomedicine. Metallic nanoparticles have a number of applications in daily products preparation such as medicine, textile, cosmetics and many more. Metallic and metal oxide nanoparticles can be prepared from a variety of metals, such as copper, zinc, gold, silver, palladium, iron, platinum, selenium, cerium, etc. The synthesizing and stabilizing of metallic nanoparticles can be achieved using physical, chemical, and biological methods (3–5).

As shown in Figure 15.1, the physical method of nanoparticle synthesis comprises the approach known as the top-down method, wherein bulk mass is broken down into smaller particles up to nano levels by different physical methods, such as laser ablation, inert gas condensation, pulse wire discharge, mechanical milling, physical vapour condensation, ion implantation, arc discharge lithography, pyrolysis, etching, evaporation, condensation mechanical, and electrochemical techniques. However, the physical methods demand time and energy. On the contrary, the chemical and biological methods imply a bottom-up approach which is also known as building up, whereby methods used to aggregate atoms or molecules to form a uniform structure that is distinct in size and shape. Also, the bottom-up method is mostly administered to produce nanoparticles, as it is the most preferred method among all approaches. Chemical methods, such as emulsion polymerization, electrochemical techniques, photochemical reduction, chemical reduction, photochemical reactions in reverse

DOI: 10.1201/9781003432661-15

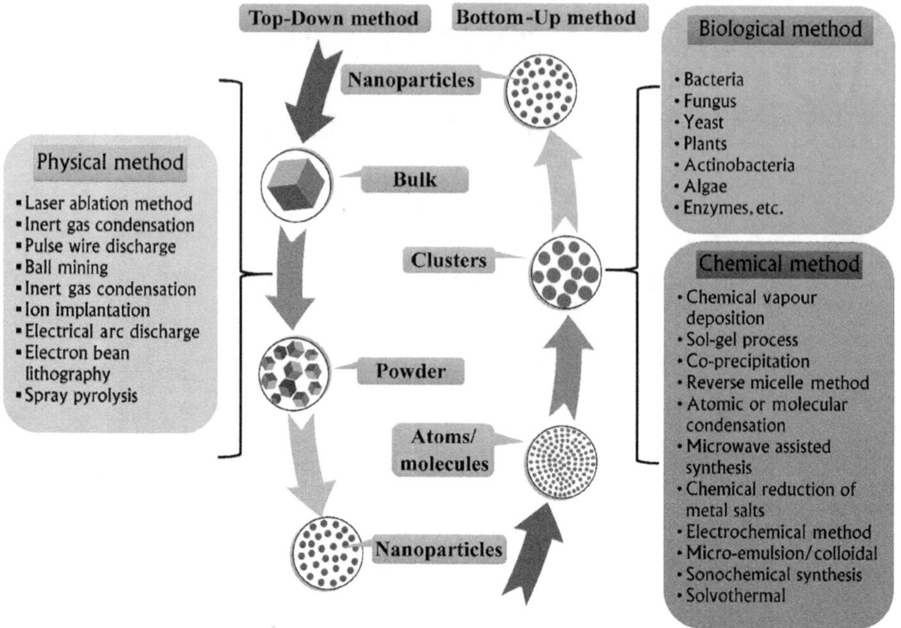

FIGURE 15.1 Schematic illustration of bottom-down and bottom-up method.

micelles, laser-mediated synthesis, sol-gel methods, and chemical precipitation are largely being used for NP synthesis. However, the chemical method leads to the use of toxic, hazardous chemicals and solvents that are not only harmful to the environment but also to human health. Therefore, researchers are looking to develop a noble way of synthesizing metallic nanoparticles that would be eco-friendly as well as non-toxic. Considering all the drawbacks involving chemical as well as physical methods of metallic nanoparticle synthesis, nowadays, emphasis is given to the synthesis of nanoparticles by biological methods, such as bacteria, polysaccharides, proteins, peptides, algae, fungi, plant extracts, etc. The latter has been given utmost importance for its rapidity, cost-effectiveness, less toxic and environment-friendly properties. Moreover, the chemically mediated synthesis of nanoparticles is unsuitable for any biomedical applications due to the concerns related to their toxic nature. The green synthesis approach refers to the implementation of environmentally benign techniques in the synthesis of metallic nanoparticles. The green synthesis of metallic nanoparticles follows the bottom-up approach that includes methods that involve the clustering of atoms and the formation of nanoparticles by reduction or oxidation reactions (6–11).

Moreover, green synthesis of metallic and metal oxide nanoparticles has demonstrated effectiveness in terms of various applications that involve the food packaging industry, catalysis, cosmetics, environmental bioremediation, electronics, textile coating, etc. Furthermore, green nanotechnology has also proven its efficiency in biomedical applications involving wound healing; and properties like antimicrobial, anti-inflammatory, antifungal, antiviral; targeted drug delivery; etc. However, the effectiveness of the nanoparticles lies in their distinct properties, which includes a large surface-to-area volume ratio, size, shape, the nature of the biomaterial, and various other physiochemical characteristics. The pathway involved in the production of nanoparticles varies depending on the biological sources. In terms of microorganisms, they follow both intrinsic and extrinsic pathways, where the reduction and stabilization of the precursor metallic solution are achieved by various intracellular and extracellular biometabolites. Whereas in the case of plant-mediated biosynthesis of metallic nanoparticles, various biometabolites present in the plants are involved in the synthesis process. Furthermore, various parameters also play a significant role in determining the shape, size, and other features of the synthesized metallic nanoparticles. The green-method-inspired synthesis of metallic and metal oxide nanoparticles embodies the promise to revolutionize drug delivery in the field of biomedicine. Green chemistry, which is the nascent branch of green nanotechnology, aims to develop nanoparticles in the absence of any harmful chemicals. The concept of green chemistry has several advantages over traditional chemical approaches, resulting in cleaner, eco-friendly, and low-cost methods (2,5,12–15).

However, the target delivery of medicinal compounds to a specific location is a challenging issue involved in the treatment or diagnosis of a disease. It still concerns scientists and researchers to formulate and design appropriate carriers to specifically deliver drugs to the target site successfully. Furthermore, it is also a deciding factor in lowering the toxicity level and increasing the efficacy of the carrier involved in the drug delivery. In addition, the drawback that involves using traditional large-sized drug delivery systems is their low bioavailability, low absorption or solubility rate, toxicity, etc. (16,17). However, all these limitations can be overcome using the green synthesis of nanoparticles, which has proven to be an appealing alternative in terms of low toxicity, drug dispersion in the body, rate of drug delivery, and bioavailability of the drug. This green-synthesized nanocarrier can be conjugated or loaded with a specific drug of interest or molecular markers that are destined for the timely release of the drug into the predetermined part of the body. Furthermore, the cell-specific target can be achieved by conjugating the cell-specific drug in the synthesis of nanocarriers (18–21). In addition, various metallic and metal oxide nanoparticles are equipped to deliver both hydrophilic and hydrophobic compounds, which include various plant-derived biocompounds, siRNA, biopeptides, chemotherapeutic drugs, etc. The nanoparticles entrap the target drug to protect it from various factors, such as degradation by enzymes, etc., that might impact the drug's ability to reach its target site. The capping and reducing compounds also play an important role in targeting various diseases in terms of antimicrobial activity; the synthesized metallic nanoparticles attack the bacterial cells in multiple locations, distorting their ability to carry on their normal metabolism (14,22,23).

This chapter provides a summarized overview of the green synthesis of metal/metal oxide nanoparticles using various biometabolites derived from biological sources. The synthesized nanoparticles are further loaded with target drugs to treat specific diseases with high efficiency. Moreover, we will explain the characterization techniques involved in the determination of the nature and properties of the nanoparticles. In addition, the application of the nanoparticles in the field of drug delivery will be further addressed.

15.2 GREEN METHODOLOGY INVOLVES IN THE SYNTHESIS OF METALLIC NANOPARTICLES VIA BIOLOGICAL ENTITIES

The green production of nanoparticles offers methods to synthesize nanoparticles by non-toxic and environment-friendly approach. Furthermore, the bottom-up strategy is used in the green synthesis of metal and metal oxide nanoparticles, which utilizes oxidation or reduction reactions to synthesize nanoparticles.

The various biocomponents present in different biological sources, which include enzymes, polyphenols, flavonoids, polysaccharides, carbohydrates, etc., facilitate the reduction and stabilization of the metallic nanoparticles. In addition, these bioactive compounds play a predetermined role in various biological activities. Furthermore, the synthesized metallic nanoparticles are also loaded with or conjugated with specific drugs to deliver them to the target site. However, for the green synthesis of nanoparticles, there are various important parameters that have to be taken into consideration to achieve a desirable shape, size, charge, surface area, and various other properties depending on their application. Therefore, optimization is an important aspect of the biosynthesis of metallic nanoparticles that helps to achieve the desired properties in the synthesized nanoparticles. Furthermore, each biological entity, for instance, plants, fungi, algae, bacteria, etc., requires a separate approach for the synthesis of nanoparticles (as shown in Figure 15.2). The process

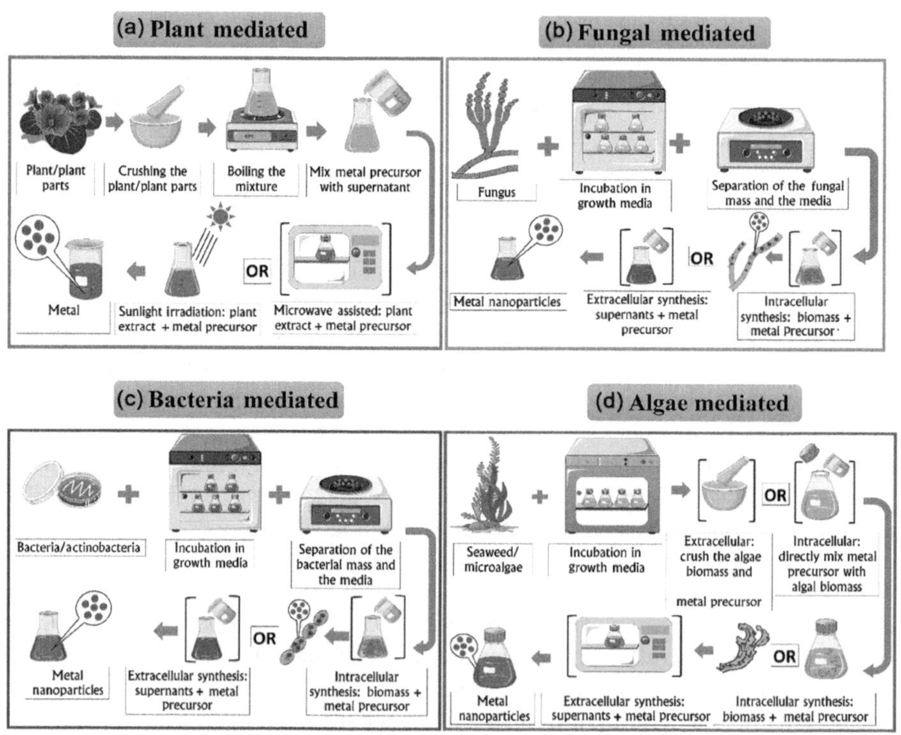

FIGURE 15.2 The process involved in the green synthesis of nanoparticles.

involved in the green biosynthesis of metallic nanoparticles plays a decisive role in the physiochemical characteristics of the synthesized nanoparticles (1,6,9,24). Therefore, we will elucidate the steps involved in the biosynthesis of nanoparticles in the following sections:

15.2.1 Plant-Mediated Green Synthesis of Nanoparticles

Plants are reported to have the ability to reduce ions on their surface as well as in different tissues, including organs that are distant from the entry site and can be useful for synthesizing NPs. This ability of plants to hyper-accumulate and reduce the metal ions is exploited in the field to extract economically important metals that are otherwise not possible to obtain, and the method is also known as phytomining (25,26) Moreover, such potential is also used in bioremediation to remove heavy metal contaminants. A study reports the in vivo presence of silver nanoparticles (AgNPs) in different organs of the *Medicago sativa*, *Brassica juncea*, and *Festuca rubra* plants when exposed to silver nitrate solution (27).

Therefore, this ability of the plants indicates the presence of certain biometabolites necessary to reduce and stabilize metal ions into nanoparticles. According to the literature studies, the generalized procedure involved in the biosynthesis of metallic nanoparticles is to obtain fresh plants or their parts that can be either dried or used fresh to obtain the extract in the presence of distilled water accompanied by boiling and stirring at a certain interval. The precursor metallic solution is then added to the prepared plant extract and incubated to produce the synthesized nanoparticles. Patra et al. (28) biosynthesize gold nanoparticles using onion peels. As reported by the literature, the onion peels were washed, chopped up into pieces, and soaked in boiling distilled water with constant stirring. The prepared extract was brought to room temperature and filtered. Further, the onion peel extract was mixed with the precursor metallic solution (auric chloride) with constant stirring at room temperature. The colour change of the reaction mixture to dark purple further denoted the synthesis of gold nanoparticles in the reaction mixture (28,29). When preparing an extract, it is extremely important to pay attention to both the range of temperature and the duration of time. It is impossible to synthesize nanoparticles during the extraction process if the temperature is high (for example, 80°C–100°C) and the duration is long. It's likely that the denaturation of proteins at higher temperatures and longer extraction time rendered the extract prepared (30).

In a related investigation, Sànchez-Navarro et al. (31) synthesized (AgNPs) using the leaves of *Annona muricata* and loaded them with 5-fluorouracil, a chemotherapeutic drug. The leaf extract was prepared after washing the leaves thoroughly with deionized water and crushing the washed leaves of *Annona muricata* in an electric blender, followed by boiling in the presence of deionized water. The precursor metallic solution, which is silver nitrate, was added to the extract, leading to the onset of the synthesis process for (AgNPs). Later on, a 50 mL solution of (AgNPs) was added to a certain quantity of 5-fluorouracil along with constant sonication, resulting in the absorption of the drug. The synthesis reaction is further assisted by sunlight irradiation, microwaves, and autoclaves that, to some extent, speed up the reaction process in the synthesis of nanoparticles (31).

In a study conducted by Pani et al. (32), an extract from the bark of *Melia azedarach* has been used to synthesize the nanocomposites of Au-Ag. The autoclave process thereby speed up the process, and the synthesis reaction took 1 minute to complete. Furthermore, the autoclave mediated nanoparticles based on the concept of breakdown of the metallic precursor (for instance silver nitrate) in the presence of a reducing agent. The presence of the nanoparticles is further established using various characterization techniques (32,33). Furthermore, in terms of the synthesis of nanoparticles made of copper, nickel, zinc, etc., the basic steps involved in the preparation of plant extracts remain the same (34–36).

Another study conducted by Yusefi et al. (37) reported the synthesis of magnetic iron oxide nanoparticles using the peels of *Punica granatum*. Initially, the fruit peels were washed multiple times to remove any contaminants. The washed fruit peels were then dried and further powdered. For the preparation of an aqueous extract of *Punica granatum* fruit peel, 10 g of the powder was then mixed with 100 mL of distilled water and subjected to heat at 80°C for an hour under continuous stirring. The aqueous extract was then dried in an oven for 14 hours at a temperature of 60°C before being stored at 4°C. The synthesis of the magnetic iron nanoparticles was achieved by the co-precipitation method, where the fruit peel extract as well as sodium hydroxide act as reducing as well as stabilizing components in the synthesis process. A different concentration of the peel extract was mixed with distilled water to make a total volume of 100 mL under continuous stirring for 15 minutes. Later on, Fe^{2+} as well as the Fe^{3+} were added at a 1:2 ratio, and the pH was brought to 11 using 1 M NaOH drop by drop for a duration of 30 minutes. Further, the solution was thrice centrifuged at a speed of 14,000 rpm for 12 minutes, and the precipitate was then heated and oven-dried at 70°C. The predetermined fruit peel sample of 2% weight was then taken for loading of 5-fluorouracil. The drug as well as the selected 2% of magnetic iron oxide nanoparticles were mixed at a ratio of 1:12 with constant stirring for 14 hours at 300 rpm in a stopper bottle. The drug-conjugated nanoparticles were then subjected to centrifugation with repeated washing. Further characterization was undertaken to establish the morphological and physiological characteristics (37). As a result, all plant-based nanoparticle synthesis is accomplished due to the presence of numerous biomolecules that help to reduce and stabilize the synthesized nanoparticles.

15.2.2 Bacteria- and Actinobacteria-Mediated Green Synthesis of Nanoparticles

The bacteria and actinobacteria are the nanobiofactories capable of biosynthesizing nanoparticles. These prokaryotic organisms are however responsible for causing some of the most devastating diseases in the world, but at the same time, they are an excellent source of various biologically active compounds required to produce lifesaving drugs. Both bacteria and actinobacteria are omnipresent and are abundantly found in all types of habitats. Nevertheless, many bacteria and actinobacteria are able to survive extreme environments with high percentages of metallic contaminants due to their evolved biological mechanisms. These inbuilt biological mechanisms ensure the survivability of bacterial strains in hostile environments by metabolizing these heavy metals into non-toxic forms that involve nanoparticle formation. The green synthesis of nanoparticles using bacteria and actinobacteria takes advantage of this capability of bacterial strains to avoid metallic toxicity (38–41).

The actinobacteria phylum is one of the largest phyla in the bacterial domain. However, the bacteria are gram-positive bacteria with high GC content. Morphologically, actinobacteria possess filamentous structure, hence the Greek name "Actinomycetes," which denotes "atkis," meaning "a ray," and "mykes," meaning "fungus." (42,43).

The basic steps involved in biosynthesis using actinobacteria or bacteria, however, remain the same. Both bacteria and actinomycetes are capable of synthesizing nanoparticles intracellularly and extracellularly. For the extracellular synthesis of nanoparticles using bacteria or actinomycetes, the microorganisms are grown in subsequent growth media for a certain period of time, followed by centrifugation and washing of the collected biomass at the bottom of the tube. Upon washing, the biomass is then transferred to distilled water. The biomass immersed in distilled water is then incubated for 24–48 hours at the required growth temperature. After the incubation period, the supernatants are separated from the biomass using centrifugation. The supernatants are then mixed with the metal precursor solution and kept for incubation. The colour change or precipitation formation therefore visually indicates the synthesis of nanoparticles (39,44–47).

In a study reported by Eid et al. (126), the endophytic actinobacteria *Streptomyces laurentii* have been grown in starch nitrate broth for 5 days at around 30°C. Once the biomass was attained, it was centrifuged and washed to separate it from any traces of growth media. The obtained biomass was then resuspended in distilled water for 72 hours at 30±2°C and later filtered to separate the filtrate from the biomass. The obtained filtrate was mixed with the metallic precursor, which is silver nitrate, and the pH of the reaction mixture was adjusted. Further, the reaction mixture was incubated overnight at 35°C. The change in colour of the reaction mixture has confirmed the synthesis of (AgNPs). However, in some literature, it has been stated that after the removal of biomass from the growth media, the growth media and the precursor metallic salt can directly be mixed together to achieve the synthesis of nanoparticles (126).

A similar study conducted by Singh et al. (49) reported the extracellular (AgNP) synthesis using *Pseudomonas* sp. THG-LS1 isolated from the soil. In this study, the growth medium i.e. the nutrient broth was separated from the biomass and was directly mixed with the metal precursor salt, i.e. silver nitrate, and incubated for 48 hours at 28°C. The colour of the solution turned dark brown, indicating the synthesis of (AgNPs) (49).

But when it comes to the intracellular production of nanoparticles, the nanoparticles synthesis takes place inside the cells with the aid of biocompounds present inside the bacteria or actinomycetes. A study conducted by Markus et al. (50) revealed the intracellular synthesis of gold nanoparticles using *Lactobacillus kimchicus* DCY51T strains obtained from kimchi in Korea. The bacterial strain was initially inoculated in de Man, Rogosa, and Sharpe (MRS) broth (growth media) and incubated for 24 hours at 37°C. The biomass was centrifuged, collected, and washed to remove any remnants of the media. It was resuspended in the metallic precursor gold solution and incubated with continuous visual observation to monitor the colour change. Once the colour of the reaction mixture changed to a deep purple, the biomass was separated from the supernatants, and the gold nanoparticles were recovered by ultrasonication (50).

Similar studies were reported by Sukanya et al. (54) where the intracellular biometabolites were released using mortar and pestle for the synthesis of (AgNPs). In this study, the biomass after incubation was separated from the supernatants, and the obtained biomass was washed and later crushed using a mortar and pestle. The crushed biomass was mixed with Milli Q water and further incubated at 37°C for 72 hours. Later, the filtrate was used for the synthesis of nanoparticles. The underlying mechanisms behind the intracellular and extracellular synthesis of nanoparticles are the various biometabolites that are produced intrinsically and extrinsically by the bacterial or actinobacterial community. The biometabolites that are responsible for the bioreduction of the precursor metallic solution include nitrate reductase, proteins, various enzymes, etc. However, the exact mechanisms are still to be uncovered, but the most acceptable mechanism for the intracellular biosynthesis of nanoparticles is that the outer cell wall of the bacteria or actinobacteria is comprised of several binding sites where the metal binds to the cell. Since the heavy metals are toxic to the microbial cells, they try to eliminate the threat by trapping the metal ions in the cell wall using electrostatic interaction. In the later stage, the ions that are trapped by the microbial cells are reduced to elemental atoms by the transfer of an electron from nicotinamide adenine dinucleotide hydrogen (NADH) by the enzyme NADH-dependent reductase present in the plasma membrane of the cell. Then, the formed nuclei slowly grow into nanoparticles and are present inside the cells (3,51–54).

A study reported by Otari et al. (128) reported the biosynthesis of intracellular (AgNPs) using *Rhodococcus* spp. The actinobacterial strains were incubated in M9 growth media for 24 hours at a temperature of 30°C, and later the biomass was collected and mixed with fresh M9 growth media supplemented with silver nitrate at pH 7 for 24 hours. Furthermore, the presence of the 10–30 nm-sized nanoparticles was confirmed in the cytoplasmic region of the actinobacterial strain. Thereby, this study validates the presence of nitrate reductase in the cytoplasmic area of *Rhodococcus* spp. The reduction and stabilization processes in the formation of extracellular nanoparticles are carried out by bioactive molecules, including DNA, sulphur-containing proteins, NADH-dependent nitrate reductase, etc., secreted by bacteria or actinomycetes. Several studies have also reported the nanoparticle synthesis using nitrate reductase to reduce the metallic ions, leading to the production of nanoparticles (15,55–58,128)

15.2.3 Algae-Mediated Green Synthesis of Nanoparticles

Algae are the repositories of various biologically active compounds necessary for the synthesis of nanoparticles. Algae are mostly aquatic, photoautotrophic eukaryotic organisms with the ability to uptake various toxic heavy metals. Algae represent both unicellular and multicellular organisms with microscopic and macroscopic physical features. The harvesting of the algae biomass can easily be achieved on a large scale. Furthermore, the trapped nanoparticles in the algae biomass can be accessible using commercial instruments (59).

Senapati et al. (60) have reported to have synthesized nanoparticles intracellularly using the algal strain *Tetraselmis kochinensis*, where the presence of the gold nanoparticles was found in the cell wall of the algal strain. Compared to the cytoplasm, the presence of the nanoparticles in the cell wall region is beneficial in the extraction process. Algae are also known as the biological factories due to the presence of various biologically active compounds, which include polysaccharides, carbohydrates, vitamins, carotenoids, phenols, proteins, and various other secondary biometabolites that aid in the reduction as well as capping of the nanoparticles. The synthesis of nanoparticles using algae can be achieved both intracellularly and extracellularly. As described by Gürsoy et al. (62), the algal strain *Chlorella sorokiniana* had been cultured at a temperature of 26°C ± 2°C with constant shaking and illuminated in a light environment. The cultured algae were then washed with double distilled water multiple times, and 5 g of biomass was resuspended in 1 mM precursor (HAuCl4) metallic solution. The reaction mixture was then incubated under shaking at a temperature of 26°C ± 2°C. Further, the colour change to pinkish purple confirmed the gold nanoparticle synthesis process. On the other hand, the same investigation has revealed the synthesis procedure for the extracellular synthesis of gold nanoparticles using algal extract. To prepare the extracellular algal extract, the *C. sorokiniana* strain was collected after centrifugation and washed using ultrapure water. The algal biomass was boiled at a temperature of 80°C, followed by filtration. Further, the obtained aqueous extract was mixed with the precursor HAuCl4, and after incubation, a colour change was observed, confirming the synthesis of gold nanoparticles (60–63).

Another study reported by Torabfam et al. (64) synthesized nanoparticles using the microalgal strain *Chlorella vulgaris* with the use of the microwave. The algal strains were cultivated in blue-green (BG11) media, and the biomass was dried and ground. To prepare algal aqueous extract, the dried ground powder was mixed with deionized water under 30°C for around 3 hours and later on for 21 hours at a temperature of 10°C. However, for the synthesis of (AgNPs), 10 mL of algal aqueous extract was mixed with 90 mL of precursor silver nitrate and heated using microwaves at different intervals. The colour change from light green to reddish brown confirmed the synthesis process along with UV spectroscopy analysis (64).

For the loading of therapeutic drug, there are a few additional steps in the synthesis process of nanoparticles, as described by Amina et al. (65) whereby gold nanoparticles were synthesized using the green technique and loaded with doxorubicin. The culture of the algae strain *Dictyosphaerium sp.* DHM2 was initially cultured in bold basal media for the mass production of the algae under white fluorescent lamp with a 24-hour illumination cycle along with constant aeration. The microalgal biomass after 14 days was collected, dried, and powdered. 1 g of algal powder was added to 20 mL of distilled water and was boiled for a duration of 5 minutes. The solution was then cooled and filtered through paper. The solution was further centrifuged, and the surfactants were separated. To the 5 mL of supernatant (algae extract), 1 mM of 45 mL of chloroauric acid was added, and the reaction mixture was then incubated with constant stirring. After 24 hours of incubation, the colour change from light green to ruby red colour determined the completion of the synthesis of gold nanoparticles. After synthesis, gold nanoparticles were centrifuged, and the pellets (gold nanoparticles) were dispersed in distilled water and repeated to remove any remnants that had not reacted. However, to load diosgenin onto the gold nanoparticles, the drug was mixed in distilled water at a concentration of 1 mg/ml and added to the reaction mixture (chloroauric acid and algal extract) and set overnight under continuous stirring. In this case, green colour turns into blue, confirming the completion of the synthesis process (65,66).

15.2.4 Fungi-Mediated Green Synthesis of Nanoparticles

Fungus is an essential biological candidate for the survival of humans and their environment. Fungi take an active role in managing the waste into various beneficial resources. Fungi are also important in various biologically active resources that involve agriculture, medical drug production, pigments, vitamins, etc. However, in terms of fungi-mediated biosynthesis of nanoparticles, the steps involved in the process are more or less the same as those of nanoparticle synthesis using bacteria or actinobacteria. Fungi-mediated nanoparticle synthesis involves both intracellular and extracellular processes. In terms of extracellular synthesis, Mani et al. (70) have stated the extracellular synthesis of copper oxide nanoparticles using endophytic fungus extracellular extract. The fungal inoculum was cultured in minimal growth media at a temperature of $27°C \pm 2°C$ for a period of 96 hours. Later, the culture medium was separated from the biomass, and the culture filtrate was further mixed with copper sulphate precursor solution. After the reaction mixture was incubated for 36–48 hours, a brown precipitate was formed, resulting in the formation of copper oxide nanoparticles.

Similarly, while synthesizing nanoparticles using intracellular methods, two different approaches have been discussed, in which Ahmad et al. (67) mention the biosynthesis of gold nanoparticles using the fungal strain *Trichothecium* sp. where the fungal biomass was grown in malt extract yeast extract glucose peptone (MGYP) medium and was centrifuged later to separate the biomass from the supernatants. The biomass was washed thoroughly and resuspended in 1 mM precursor HAuCl4 solution, which was incubated for 72 hours under continuous shaking at 27°C. The spherically shaped nanoparticles have been reported to be present in large numbers in the cytoplasmic membrane as compared to the cell wall of the fungal strain (67–70). In another method reported by Vetchinkina et al. (71), a slightly different approach was described whereby the biomass after incubation was washed thoroughly and grinded mechanically at 18°C in the presence of a sodium potassium phosphate buffer at pH 6 to release all the intracellular biocomponents from the fungal biomass. The solution was centrifuged, and the supernatants were further subjected to dialysis against water. The filtrate, including the intracellular extract, was then added along with the metallic precursor solutions (71).

Furthermore, the metallic nanoparticles are also reported to have been conjugated with drugs to enhance their functionality. A study conducted by Naimi-Shamel et al.

(72) reported having synthesized gold nanoparticles by the fungal strain *Fusarium oxysporum* loaded with tetracycline drug. It was achieved by adding a few steps to the previously mentioned procedure. The fungal strain was inoculated in a sabouraud dextrose broth medium under continuous agitation at 30°C. After the centrifugation and separation of the biomass, the supernatants were used for the synthesis of gold nanoparticles. Once the synthesis was visually confirmed by change in colour, the gold nanoparticles were washed and added to the 50 μL of tetracycline solution (72).

Studies also suggested the synthesis of (AgNPs) using the macrofungi species *Coriolus versicolor* and *Boletus edulis*, where the sample preparation involves the dried samples of the mushroom species *Coriolus versicolor* and *Boletus edulis* that were further pulverized with the help of a sterile blender. Later, the powdered mushroom was heated in the presence of distilled water at a temperature of 60°C for a duration of 90 minutes. The aqueous extracts of macrofungi strains were then filtered using Whatmann filter paper no. 1, which was followed by centrifugation at 6,000 rpm for 10 minutes. The collected supernatants were used as an aqueous extract for the synthesis of nanoparticles. Both the mushroom strains were separately mixed with silver nitrate for (AgNPs) synthesis (15).

15.3 CHARACTERIZATION TECHNIQUES USED IN GREEN SYNTHESIS OF NANOPARTICLES

The green synthesis of metallic nanoparticles has made significant progress over the past few years. The characterization of the synthesized nanoparticles is an essential part of the process of nanoparticle synthesis to evaluate the size, shape, charge, composition, surface plasmon resonance detection, crystallinity, etc. The characterization process (as shown in Table 15.1) is carried out using various techniques (as shown in Table 15.2), which include UV-vis spectroscopy, Fourier transform infrared spectroscopy (FTIR), scanning electron microscopy (SEM), transmission electron microscopy (TEM), X-ray diffraction (XRD), zeta potential, dynamic light scattering (DLS), etc. During the synthesis of green-mediated nanoparticles, UV-vis spectroscopy plays an important role in understanding the surface plasmon resonance of the synthesized nanoparticles. Furthermore, the metallic or metal oxide nanoparticles possess a distinctive feature, which is the surface plasmon resonance. This strong surface plasmon resonance of the metallic and metal oxide nanoparticles is displayed in the UV region. The true reason behind the surface plasmon resonance of the metallic or metallic oxide nanoparticles is due to the presence of free electrons in the conduction band and also because of the resonance with the light wave that causes the electrons to vibrate among themselves. Furthermore, it also depends on the morphology as well as the composition of synthesized metallic nanoparticles (73–75).

As described by Girón-Vázquez et al. (76), (AgNPs) were synthesized using *Persea americana* seed whereby after the (AgNPs) were synthesized, the reaction mixture that comprised silver nitrate as the precursor metal salt, the aqueous seed extract of *Persea americana*, and ammonium hydroxide changed colour upon incubation for 5 hours at room temperature. The colour change from faint yellow to brown was later

TABLE 15.1
Characterization of Nanoparticles

Instruments	Functions involves in the characterization of nanoparticles	References
Ultraviolet Spectroscopy	The instrument is used to measure surface plasmon resonance, which is a phenomenon caused by the oscillation of electrons on the surface of metallic nanoparticles when a photon strikes them.	(73–75)
Fourier transform infrared spectroscopy (FTIR)	The instrument is used to analyze the presence of various functional groups present in the biological sample used for capping as well as reducing of metallic nanoparticles.	(79,80)
Scanning Electron Microscopy (SEM)	Facilitates to study the morphology of synthesized metallic nanoparticles, including its size, shape as well as its surface characteristics.	(80,86)
Energy-dispersive spectroscopy (EDX)	The analysis is use to reveal the elementary composition of the synthesized nanoparticles.	(86)
Transmission electron microscopy (TEM)	This instrument is used to investigate the shape of nanomaterial and the characteristics of particles.	(81,83,80)
Selected area electron diffraction (SAED)	Along with the TEM analysis, SAED analysis provides information regarding particles' crystallinity.	(81,83)
Atomic force microscopy (AFM)	The AFM analysis is employed to reveal the surface roughness of the nanoparticles.	(81)
X-ray diffraction (XRD)	XRD is an analytical instrument generally used to reveal the phase transition as well as the structure and shape of synthesized metallic nanoparticle.	(85,86)
Zeta potential	Zeta potential is used to measure surface charge potential.	(84)
Dynamic light scattering (DLS)	DLS assays were carried out to figure out hydrodynamic diameters of nanoparticles and particle size.	(82,87)
Thermal gravimetric analysis (TGA)	The instrument assists in analysing thermal stability along with change in mass in relation to temperature and phase transition of synthesized nanoparticles.	(88,89)

measured using UV-vis spectroscopy, which revealed a surface plasmon resonance band at 430 nm that indicated the spherical shape of the synthesized nanoparticles. In some synthesis processes, there are reports where there have been observed multiple surface plasmon resonance peaks due to the presence of multi-shaped nanoparticles, which might be the reason for agglomerations (15,76–78).

In terms of FTIR, the peaks represented by instruments are the functional groups present in the biological components that have been used in the synthesis of nanoparticles. The study conducted by Qian et al. (79) stated the presence of various absorption bands that have been involved in the synthesis of gold nanoparticles. The bands further reveal the presence of various aromatic compounds, proteins, etc. on the surface of the synthesized nanoparticles (79,80). To study the morphological features of the synthesized nanoparticles, microscopic studies are being carried out. The most commonly used microscopic techniques in the nanoparticle synthesis studies involve SEM, TEM, and atomic force microscope (AFM).

TABLE 15.2

Biological Source	Plants/ Parts Used	Metal Salt/Precursor Metal Salt	Loaded/ Conjugated Drug	Types of NPs	Shape/Size (nm)	Application	References
Harpullia pendula	Leaves	Chromium chloride ($CrCl_3.6H_2O$)	5-Fluorouracil	Cr	Spherical; 23 nm and 29 nm	Anticancer: Caco-2 (colorectal cancer)	(18)
Annona muricata	Leaves	Silver nitrate ($AgNO_3$)	5-Fluorouracil	Ag	Quasi-spherical; 10.87 nm	Antibacterial; anticancer: human fibroblasts	(31)
Punica granatum	Peel	Iron (III) chloride hexahydrate ($FeCl_3{\cdot}6H_2O$) and Iron (II) chloride tetrahydrate ($FeCl_2{\cdot}4H_2O$)	5-Fluorouracil	Fe	Spherical shape; 14.38 nm,	Anticancer activity: CCD112 (colon normal cell line;ATCC CRL-1541) and HCT116 (colorectal cancer cell line; ATCC CCL-247)	(37)
Microbial Strain	**Growth Media**	**Metal Salt/Precursor Metal Salt**	**Loaded/ conjugated drug**	**Types of NPs**	**Shape/Size (nm)**	**Application**	**References**
Coriolus versicolor and *Boletus edulis*	-	Silver nitrate ($AgNO_3$)	-	Ag	*Coriolus versicolor* (CV)-AgNPs and BE-AgNPs: 86.0 ± 3.8 nm and 87.7 ± 0.8 nm	Anticancer: MCF-7, HT-29, and HUH-7 cell lines. Antibacterial: *Pseudomonas aeruginosa*, *Klebsiella pneumonia*, *Staphylococcus aureus*, and *Enterococcus faecalis*); Antifungal: *Candida albicans and Candida utilis*; W	(15)
Fusarium oxysporum	Sabouraud dextrose broth	Chloroauric acid (HAuCl4)	Tetracycline	Au	Spherical or hexagonal; 22–30 nm	Antibacterial activity	(72)

(Continued)

TABLE 15.2 (*Continued*)

Microbial Strain	Growth Media	Metal Salt/Precursor metal salt	Loaded/ Conjugated Drug	Types of NPs	Shape/Size (nm)	Application	References
Delftia sp. strain KCM-006	Modified glycerol peptone broth	Hydrogen tetrachloroaurate	Resveratrol	Au	Spherical; and 26.63 nm	Anticancer: human lung cancer cell line (A549)	(163)
Streptomyces antimycoticus L-1	Starch casein broth	$AgNO_3$	-	Ag	Spherical; 13–40 nm	Anticancer; human colorectal adenocarcinoma cells (Caco-2); antibacterial:*Staphylococcus aureus* (ATCC 6538), *Bacillus subtilis* (ATCC 6633), *Escherichia coli* (ATCC 8739), *Pseudomonas aeruginosa* (ATCC 9022), *Salmonella typhimurium* (ATCC 14028), Salem et al. (125)	(125)
Algal Strain	**Growth Media**	**Metal Salt/Precursor Metal Salt**	**Loaded/ Conjugated Drug**	**Types of NPs**	**Shape/Size (nm)**	**Application**	**References**
Chlorella vulgaris	BG11 medium	Silver nitrate ($AgNO_3$)	-	Ag	Allotropic structures: rectangular spheres, decahedral, and polygonal; 24.79 nm.	Antibacterial activity	(64)
Chlorella sorokiniana	-	$HauCl_4$	-	Au	Extracellular synthesis: spherical; 5–15 nm and intracellular synthesis: 20–40 nm	Antifungal activity: *C. tropicalis*, *C. glabrata*, and *C. albicans*	(62)

In the study conducted by Alshehri and Malik (80) in which the (AgNPs) were synthesized using the aqueous extract of the herb *Matricaria chamomilla* L. The synthesized (AgNPs) were then subjected to microscopic analysis, whereby SEM analysis revealed the shape of nanoparticles, which is monodispersed and spherical shaped with presence of some aggregation. Similarly, in TEM analysis, the study conducted by Srinivasan et al. (83) on titanium nanoparticles using leaves of *Sesbania grandiflora* revealed the insightful details of titanium dioxide nanoparticles that showed the scattering of nanoparticles homogenously along with selected area electron diffraction (SAED) to understand the crystallinity as well as the structure of the crystal. The study by Kumar et al. (82) synthesized iron oxide nanoparticles from *Citrus paradise*, where the presence of bright spots in SAED analysis revealed the spherical and polycrystalline nature of the synthesized nanoparticles. The AFM further demonstrates the topography of the surface of nanoparticles and whether any roughness, skewness, kurtosis is present (80–84). Furthermore, XRD is another analytical technique that has been used in the synthesis of nanotechnology to find out the phase distribution of the particles. Moreover, it is also used to establish the crystallinity as well as the purity of nanoparticles. Wu et al. (85), *Cissus vitiginea* mediated copper nanoparticles synthesized were examined to reveal the nanoparticles were crystalline in nature (85,86). DLS is another way to measure the particle size and distribution of synthesized metallic nanoparticles. DLS typically employs focussed, inert, visible laser light on a sample solution to measure the size of particles. Moreover, the zeta potential analysis is conducted to know the surface charge potential present on the surface of the synthesized nanoparticles and is the crucial parameter for establishing the stability of the nanoparticles (84,87). Thermal gravimetric analysis (TGA) is the technique used to study thermal stability as well as annealing temperature of nanoparticles. Sabouri et al. (89) have revealed the TGA analysis of the nanoparticles synthesized using egg white in the presence of oxygen showed an increase in temperature of around 10°C/min minute up to 900°C. The weight loss has occurred at varying temperatures (88,89). Energy-dispersive X-ray analysis, also known as EDS or EDAX, is used to reveal elementary components present in synthesized nanoparticles. The peaks involved in EDS analysis revealed elements that were present in the synthesized nanoparticles (90).

15.4 OPTIMIZATION AND PARAMETERS REGULATING THE SYNTHESIS OF NANOPARTICLES

The optimization step in the green synthesis of nanoparticles determines the morphological fate of the synthesized nanoparticles. The optimization of various parameters, for instance, pH, temperature, concentration of the reactants, concentration of the precursor salts, and reaction time, plays a pivotal role in the synthesis process of nanoparticles:

15.4.1 pH

In the process of nanoparticle synthesis, the pH of reaction mixture is critical in generating the desired properties in terms of shape, size, growth kinetics, reaction aduration, etc. pH has the ability to bring about changes in the biomolecules present in the extract. As per literature, due to the change in charge of the biomolecules in the extract, the synthesis process of nanoparticles is reduced at lower pH (acidic) and speeds up at higher pH (basic). This might be due to the fact that in an acidic pH, the reducibility power of the reactant decreases. Moreover, it has also been reported that at lower pH, biomolecules present in the reactant presumably get distorted, which negatively impacts the synthesis process. As reported in the study conducted by Parthiban et al. (129) the synthesis of (AgNPs) used an aqueous leaf extract of the *Annona reticulate* plant. The study further revealed that the synthesis of (AgNPs) took place at a pH range of 9.8–11. Moreover, when the pH of aqueous leaf extract was in its original range of 6.5–7.3, no formation of nanoparticles was reported. Therefore, this study further stated that pH facilitates the ionization process by facilitating the transfer of electrons in alkaline environment between the compounds present in the aqueous extract and the metallic precursor solution, silver nitrate. Further, the pH facilitates the ionic exchange of the biomolecules present in the extract along with stabilizing the synthesized nanoparticles. Therefore, as stated in the study, the aqueous leaf extract at its initial pH was not able to synthesize nanoparticles due to the presence of protonated molecules in the aqueous extract. By increasing the pH using NaOH, which ionizes the biomolecules in the extract, (AgNPs) were further synthesized. Furthermore, changes in pH also impact the shape as well as the size of the synthesized nanoparticles due to the change in electrical charges among phytoconstituents. In terms of low acidic pH, the synthesis process of nanoparticles becomes slow due to a slow nucleation process that results in the formation of large-sized particles at a low rate of production. On the contrary, with the increase in pH, the reaction occurs fast with rapid nucleation that leads to production of small-sized nanoparticles (92,93,130,131,137,138,139,140,141,142). As described in the study by Haroon et al., whereby (AgNPs) were synthesized using the leaf extract of *Azadirachta indica*, it has been observed that with the increase in the time of reaction at pH 8, the synthesis process of the (AgNPs) enhanced due to the donation of electrons by the leaf extract. The surface plasmon resonance of the reaction mixture was high at pH 8, which revealed the (AgNPs) were smaller in size (91).

15.4.2 Reaction Time

Reaction time in the synthesis of nanoparticles is a critical step in incorporating desired properties into the nanoparticles as well as governing the size, shape, and distribution of the nanoparticles. With the increase in reaction time, the size of synthesized nanoparticles increased. Furthermore, the extended reaction time is essential to complete the regeneration phenomenon, resulting in improved nanoparticle formation (92,94). The study conducted by Nahar et al. (86), where the (AgNPs) have been synthesized using the leaf extract of *Cinnamomum tamala*, revealed that increasing the time of the reaction from 30 to 210 minutes resulted in an increase in the production of nanoparticles. Furthermore, it has been stated that with the increase in the time given, the colour change of reaction mixture gets stronger because of the complete reduction of the metallic salts. In their study, Mankad et al (95) synthesized (AgNPs) using leaf extract of *Azadirachta indica* under the influence of sunlight irradiation.

The study discussed how the extended exposure to the reaction under sunlight resulted in a colour change of the solution from yellow to reddish brown, with the colour change intensifying as the time extended. The increase in the intensity of the colour is due to the further reduction of silver ions into (AgNPs) (95). In a similar study conducted by Khan et al (96) the synthesis of nanoparticles using pullulans under the exposure of sunlight has been further reported. The study indicated that the size, shape, and synthesis process of the nanoparticles can be controlled by regulating the time of the irradiation. It has also been mentioned that longer exposure of silver nitrate in colloidal solution causes (AgNPs) to heat up and break up into smaller-sized particles. This was proved when the irradiation time was increased to 0–96 hours. The particles initially aggregate and later disaggregate, which results in a smaller particle size at the end of the reaction (96). Furthermore, the time parameter of a reaction mixture is essential to determining the morphology of the synthesized nanoparticles. During the synthesis process, the particles may join together to grow and give the particles a different morphology (97). In a study conducted by Balavandy et al. (98) where glutathione-mediated (AgNPs) were prepared, it was reported that after the initial synthesis of nanoparticles, when the time for the incubation of the reaction was extended to 72 hours, the reaction mixture revealed a complete dark brown colour. This also established the fact that by extending the time of reaction mixture, the particle size as well as the aggregation of nanoparticles also increase (98).

15.4.3 Temperature of the Reaction Mixture

The temperature of reaction mixture also plays a crucial role in regulating various morphological features, such as size, shape, reaction kinetics, etc., of the synthesized nanoparticles. In a study conducted by Kim et al (99) where (AgNPs) have been synthesized using algal extract, it has been shown that when the temperature was raised from 90°C to 120°C, the synthesis rate of (AgNPs) further increased. Hence, the temperature serves as a key factor to regulate the synthesis of nanoparticles and accelerate the reaction process (99,140). Kadam et al. (93) synthesized (AgNPs) using the extract of cauliflower waste. The synthesis process was tested at three different temperatures, with the reaction mixture being microwave heated at 600 W for 5 minutes, heated at 100°C for 1 hour, and kept at room temperature for 24 hours. There is significant evidence that by applying temperature, the reaction for the synthesis of nanoparticles is enhanced. Moreover, at room temperature, the synthesis of nanoparticles has not been observed and was further validated by the UV-vis spectra. However, microwave-mediated synthesis had an advantage over heating at 100°C due to its faster heating and sharper peak in the UV-vis spectra compared to the broader peak in heating at 100°C (93). The temperature also influenced the size of synthesized AgNPs nanoparticles, as demonstrated by Rajput et al. (130) by using leaf extract of *Atropa acuminate* and that had reported to exhibited a blue shift in the UV-Vis spectra with the increase in temperature. This, however, implies the fast synthesis of nanoparticles with accelerating kinetic energy. This condition further resulted in the production of small-sized nanoparticles with negligible chances of formation of larger particles (130).

15.4.4 Concentration of the Precursor Metallic Salt

The synthesis of nanoparticles also greatly depends on the precursor metallic salt concentration. As it has been stated in a study conducted by Raza et al. (100), it has been observed that with an increase in the concentration of precursor silver salt, the colour gets intense and imparts a different colour to the reaction mixture. Furthermore, in several studies, it has been stated clearly that with an increase in precursor metallic salt, the colour of the reaction mixture gets darker or the intensity of the UV-vis spectra peak increases due to the increased production of nanoparticles (92,100). However, increasing the concentration of metallic precursor might cause aggregates (99). Further, it has also been evaluated in studies that the increase in the absorbance with regard to the increase in the precursor metal salt concentration might be due to the improved oxidation of hydroxyl groups present in the reactant by the metal ions (62,137). The reduction of the precursor metallic salts is not entirely dependent on their concentration, but also on the amount of reactant required to react with the precursor. Bhatnagar et al. (97) reported that precursor concentration of below 8 mM concentration showed complete conversion and smaller AgNPs than that for the higher precusor concentration (97).

15.4.5 Concentration of the Reactant

The concentration of reactant that will participate in the reduction, capping, and stabilization is important for the proper synthesis of nanoparticles. Furthermore, the concentration as well as the source of reactant or the components of reactant are also critical in regulating the shape and size of synthesized nanoparticles. As per the study reported by Kalpana et al. (30), even though the concentration of the plant extract has been increased for the reduction of silver nitrate, at a certain point, the rate of production of nanoparticles has been lowered, as reflected spectrophotometrically. The reason might be that with the increased plant extraction, silver nitrate gets exhausted and further reduction process becomes slow and ultimately halts (30,139,140). Furthermore, studies conducted by Mosaviniya et al. (131) suggest that using the minimum concentration of the plant extract showed smaller-sized nanoparticles, and the larger-sized nanoparticles might be due to the aggregation of the smaller unconsolidated particles or unconsolidated nuclei on the surface of stable nanoparticles. In contrast, when the concentration of the plant extract gets high, it results in larger-sized nanoparticles. This might be due to the huge quantity of biomolecules in the plant extract, which react faster as well as interact secondarily to give the nanoparticles a larger size (93,95,131).

15.5 APPLICATION OF GREEN-METHOD-INSPIRED NANOPARTICLES IN DRUG DELIVERY

Nanoparticle-mediated drug delivery is designed to deliver the specific drug or pharmaceutical compound intended for that particular disease to its target site. Nanoparticles have been reported to exhibit characteristics that enhance the stability and solubility of the drug that has been encapsulated and assist in its transportation throughout the plasma membrane. Furthermore, nanoparticles enhance the extended circulation periods, thereby increasing safety and effectiveness. Furthermore, the mobility of nanoparticles is limited due to target-specific delivery of the drug, which reduces the chances of any negative impact while at the same time allowing for high concentrations of the drug at the target site. Furthermore, nanoparticle-loaded therapeutic drugs (also mentioned in Table 15.2) can be readily suspended in a liquid medium to deliver to the targeted site (101). The nanoparticles are further able to reach deep into various intended tissues and organs. One more aspect of nanoparticle-mediated drug delivery is their large surface area, which facilitates the loading of the drug at higher concentrations. Thus, the nanoparticles that mediate drug delivery in a controlled and sustainable way have therefore grabbed enormous attention due to their feasibility.

15.5.1 Green-Synthesized Therapeutic Nanoparticles for Cancer Drug Delivery:

Among most of the diseases, cancer is considered one of the most dreaded diseases known to mankind. As per the report of International Cancer Observatory, it had been estimated that approximately 9.9 million people died due to cancer in the year 2020, whereas International Agency for Research on Cancer (GLOBOCAN) has projected 19.3 million cases of 10 million deaths because of cancer. Moreover, by 2040, the number of deaths due to cancer is likely to increase by 16.4 million per year. Cancer is a multifaceted illness that is commonly characterized as the uncontrolled proliferation and growth of cells in tissues, resulting in the formation of tumours. Furthermore, the aggregation of the cells and the tumour formation has the ability to spread to different organs of an individual or travel to other tissues, a process termed metastasis. Today, there are a variety of therapeutics to counter cancer, which include chemotherapy, radiation therapy, target therapy, phototherapy, immune therapy, surgeries, hormone therapies, etc. However, further initiatives are needed to broaden understanding of cancer and its management, including innovative therapeutic approaches. As a result, biocompatible nanomaterials that are continuously expanding hold a huge promise in the field of nanomedicine to combat cancer, among other diseases. An ideal nanomaterial exhibits the following characteristics: superior drug-loading abilities, reduced chances of early drug release, low toxicity, biocompatibility, and planned drug release to the target cancerous cells. However, the toxicity as well as the biocompatibility of a particular nanoparticle depends on its shape, size, surface morphology, presence of functional groups, drug concentration, etc. (102,143,144,145). Furthermore, plant-derived biocompounds are well known for their vast range of protection against various types of cancer. However, using these biologically active compounds as therapeutics poses various disadvantages, including improper targeting of the cancer site, low solubility, etc. Therefore, nanoparticle synthesis using various biological sources imparts these biologically active compounds onto the particles that further enhance their effectiveness and also act as drug cargo for delivering specific drugs along with them (103,104). Several literature studies have reported to conjugate or load metallic/metal oxide nanoparticles with the drug doxorubicin, which is an anthracycline and a chemotherapeutic agent.

The drug doxorubicin is used in a broad variety of cancers like leukaemia, breast cancer, adenocarcinoma, ovarian cancer, bladder cancer, bronchogenic cancer, etc. Nevertheless, the negative impacts associated with doxorubicin are immense and include cardiotoxicity due to excessive reactive oxygen species (ROS) production as well as the inhibitory action of the drug against topoisomerase IIβ inhibition, hair loss, nausea, and developing resistance to the drug. The underlying working mechanisms of the doxorubicin drug involve the intercalation of the drug into the base pairs of double-stranded DNA, which further inhibits the replication and transcription processes in DNA as well as RNA. Furthermore, the drug inhibits the crucial enzyme topoisomerase II, halting DNA replication, transcription, and repairing activity. In addition, the high amount of ROS leads to DNA cleavage and degradation. Moreover, the delivery of the doxorubicin drug can be achieved using a nanocarrier that will specifically deposit the drug in the predetermined diseased site, reducing its spread into healthy tissues, and in this process, it will further increase the efficacy of the drug. Furthermore, target drug delivery can to some extent lower the negative impact on a patient by delivering a specific amount of the drug to the diseased area. As per the study conducted by Yin et al. (105), the gold nanoparticles were synthesised as multifunctional nanoparticles by functionalizing the nuclear localization peptides (NLS), RGD peptides, and doxorubicin drug. However, the conjugation process doesn't alter the action of doxorubicin, and the tumour size of the gold nanoparticles conjugated with NLS, arginine-glycine-aspartate (RGD), and doxorubicin revealed a smaller size compared to the control. Similar studies have also been reported by Devendiran et al. (132) where the gold nanoparticles were synthesized using pectin, which is a polysaccharide found in plants and has an extensive use in various biomedical applications due to its easily biodegradable nature, biocompatibility, and non-toxic nature. The synthesized gold nanoparticles were further loaded with doxorubicin as well as folic acid, which revealed the cytotoxic activity against a breast cancer cell line. Furthermore, the release of doxorubicin drug is slower in the folic acid-pectin-conjugated gold nanoparticles as compared to only doxorubicin, depicting controlled and target delivery. The reason behind this is that the molecules of the drug usually enter cancer cell cytoplasm by passive diffusion pump mechanisms, whereas when the drug is conjugated with the pectin gold nanoparticles, the entry of the drug is carried by endocytosis, which increases the level of drug inside the cell. Further, the pH difference in the tumour microenvironment and the normal tissue guides the proper release of drug into the diseased area (105,146,147,148,149,163). Moreover, over the years, folic acid functionalized drug delivery systems to target the folate receptors on the cell have gained attention among the research community. The folate receptor present on the cell surface is a glycosylphosphatidylinositol-anchored membrane protein that facilitates the intake of folate through the endocytosis process. Studies have also reported that these folate receptors are overexpressed in various types of cancer cells as compared to normal cells. So, functionalizing nanoparticles with folic acids facilitates their entry into cancer cells (106,107). Another study conducted by Al-Dulimi et al. (108) found that gold nanoparticles were conjugated with an amidohydrolase enzyme known as L-asparaginase, which is a popular anticancer drug. The mode of action of L-asparaginase is that it takes part as a catalyst in the degradation of asparagine into L-aspartate and ammonia. As asparagine is dominantly present on the malignant cell surface, it fuels them to proliferate and grow. Another fact is that since the DNA inside malignant cells is damaged, they are unable to synthesize L-asparagine using aspartic and glutamine. As a consequence, the amino acids, which are important for their proliferation and activation, present on the cell surface get depleted, which causes cell death. However, using gold nanoparticles conjugated with the RGD motif within the nanoparticles Gly-Arg-Gly-Asp-Ser-Pro (GRGDSP) that is usually overexpressed in cancer cells is becoming a popular target to deliver specific drugs into the targeted cancer cell by the process of endocytosis. Furthermore, cell-penetrating peptides are conjugated as hydrophilic agents to ensure cellular permeability. Therefore, the study revealed the successful entry of gold nanoparticle-PEG-L-asparaginase-RGD conjugate that showed a high level of cytotoxicity towards breast cancer cells (108,109).

In a similar study by Devi et al. (110), the chemotherapeutic drug epirubicin was loaded onto the synthesized gold nanoparticles by using a leaf extract of *Vitex negundo* for reduction and Arabic gum as a capping agent. The whole process of synthesizing gold nanoparticles functionalized with folic acid and loaded with epirubicin drug was driven by sunlight irradiation. Epirubicin is an anthracycline chemotherapeutic agent that shows toxicity in various normal tissues and further includes cardiotoxicity due to excessive generation of ROS. Furthermore, the fast clearance of drug from the body prevents extravasation of the drug into the tumour microenvironment, lowering its efficiency. However, this study has therefore put forward the possibility of efficiently delivering epirubicin into the target tumour microenvironment. Also, it has been reported that gold nanoparticles are the most commonly used nanoparticles in the field of drug delivery as they exhibit low toxicity when compared to other metal nanoparticles, particularly silver and othernanoparticles (110,144). Among the previously mentioned chemotherapeutic drugs, 5-fluorouracil is a popular chemotherapeutic drug in treating colorectal cancer, which is the third most reported cause of morbidity and mortality. The actual mechanism behind the action of the drug is by inhibiting the synthesis process of DNA by impeding thymidylate synthetase. Nevertheless, the negative effects of drug include increased resistance to it, short half-life of about 10–20 minutes, and negative impact on gastrointestinal tract and bone marrow from its use. Saddik et al. (18) have reported the synthesis of chromium nanoparticles using the leaf extract of *Harpullia pendula* conjugated with 5-fluorouracil. The study further revealed that nanoparticles loaded with 5-fluorouracil lower the IC 50 value in Caco-2 cell line compared to the drug alone. Furthermore, cytotoxicity showed greater toxicity against Caco-2 cells than 5-fluorouracil alone (18,37).

However, not only gold but (AgNPs) also are well equipped to elicit a high extent of cytotoxic activity by various physiochemical mechanisms that involve in destruction of DNA, induction of apoptosis and necrosis cascades, production of ROS and destruction of nucleus components, dehydrogenase lactate leak out, modification of mitochondrial membrane potential, etc. As reported in literature, the metal nanoparticle itself, for instance, (AgNPs), exhibits cell death by releasing silver ions into cellular components that further elevate the synthesis of ROS as well as the generation of oxidative stress that is followed by apoptotic death (as shown in Figure 15.3). Furthermore, it initiates the destruction of cell proteins essential for regular

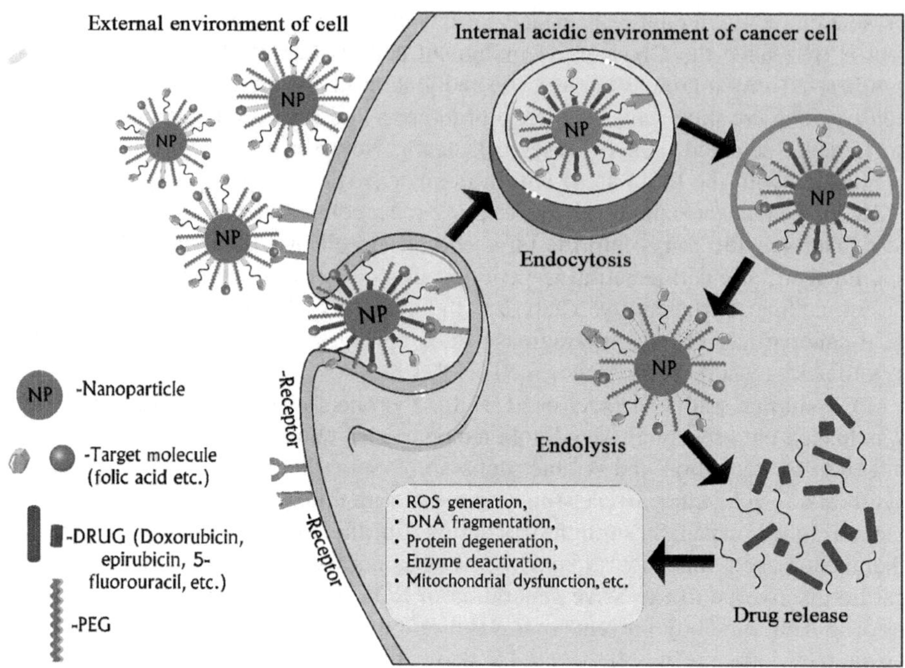

FIGURE 15.3 Representation of the green-synthesized nanoparticle-mediated drug delivery into cancer cells.

metabolism, various enzymes, and halts cell repair mechanisms. One more mechanism exhibited by AgNPs is referred to as Trojan horse mechanism, in which an increased level of silver ions is present after passing through the plasma barrier in the cytoplasmic region of a cell. The increase in toxicity inside cells is due to the high level of silver ions, which leads to apoptosis or necrosis of the cell. In addition, silver ions have the ability to bind themselves to RNA polymerase enzyme, which disrupts its activity. Such reports have been published by Salem et al. (125), where (AgNPs) have been synthesized using the endophytic actinobacterial strain *Streptomyces antimycoticus* L-1 obtained from *Mentha longifolia* L. leaves. The synthesized (AgNPs) exhibit invitro cytotoxicity effects against Caco-2 (human colorectal adenocarcinoma cell line) at which the minimal concentration of 5.6 ± 3.0 μg/mL was reported to eliminate 50% of the Caco-2 as compared to the cell line Vero when exposed to a dose of 511.7 ± 68.5 μg/mL of (AgNPs). Therefore, the observation reported implies that nanoparticles are very much dependent on the amount of their dosage (47,48,111,125,126). Zinc is known as a crucial cofactor in accomplishing various cellular mechanisms and is intended to maintain the cellular haemostasis; Zinc nanoparticles are therefore an excellent candidate for drug delivery to a specific target, especially in terms of cancer, due to its ability to generate ROS that ultimately results in the death of cancer cells. Furthermore, zinc oxides are also recognized by the FDA as "generally recognized as safe" (GRAS). Thereby, zinc nanoparticles can be an excellent nanostructure for target nanodrug delivery (112). Similarly, Akbarian et al. (114) have synthesized zinc oxide nanoparticles to serve as a nanocarrier to deliver a chemotherapeutic drug known as Paclitaxel, which is an antineoplastic drug and an alkaloid derived from plants. However, due to the incomplete solubility of drug, which limits its use, the Cremophor EL (CrEL) formulation is being administered to maintain a decent amount of drug's concentration in a specific tumour and avoid any toxicity. However, CrEL itself is considered a non-inert drug vehicle rather than showing positive effects, for instance, hypersensitivity, erythrocyte aggregation, peripheral neuropathy, etc. Also, it has been reported that CrEL, which is a crucial part of the implications of the chemotherapeutic drug paclitaxel, changes the toxicity of many chemotherapeutic drugs. Therefore, zinc oxide nanoparticles synthesized using the leaves of *Camellia sinesis* L showed to be a suitable nanocarrier for paclitaxel against the cancer cell line MCF-7 (113,114). Nanotechnology has further expanded by using two different metallic oxide nanoparticles to target cancer cells. The bimetallic zinc oxide and copper oxide nanoparticles synthesized using *Sambucus nigra* shoots have thereby induced dose dependent toxicity against cancer cell lines (115). In addition, there have been reports of platinum-based chemotherapeutic agents that include cisplatin, oxaliplatin, and carboplatin, which are popular drugs to treat various types of cancer. However, there are certain side effects associated with the usage of these drugs, which include nephrological toxicity and neurological toxicity. Cai et al. (66) have reported the biosynthesis of gold nanoparticles using the algae species (*Dictyosphaerium* sp. DHM2) and its further conjugation with the drug diosgenin. Diosgenin, which is a steroidal sapogenin, has been cited in various literatures to have been abundantly present in *Trigonella foenum graecum* L. (fenugreek seeds); *Dioscorea villosa* (wild yam); and various other sources, such as *Dioscorea rhizome*, Smilax China, and *Rhizoma polgonati*. Despite the drug's use in the treatment of various diseases, the biological availability of drug is low due to its poorly soluble nature in aqueous medium. The nanoconjugate of diosgenin-loaded gold nanoparticles revealed the antiproliferative action against colorectal cancer cell line HCT116 and breast cancer cell line HCC1954. However, the drug along with diosgenin-conjugated gold nanoparticles is 18 times more potent than simply gold nanoparticles. Thus, it proves the potency of drug-conjugated nanoparticles is more efficient in terms of antiproliferative activity (65,66).

Platinum-based anticancer drugs, which includes cisplatin, carboplatin, and oxaliplatin, have been reported to be widely used in treating various types of cancer, which include colorectal cancer, ovarian cancer, breast cancer, etc. However, the major disadvantage of such drugs is their side effects, which impact one's health. A study was conducted by Alshatwi et al. (116) in which the synthesis of platinum nanoparticles has been reported using tea polyphenols. The functionalized platinum nanoparticles further showed cytotoxic effects on cervical cancer cell lines. The study revealed platinum nanoparticles were further capable of halting the proliferation of cells using an apoptotic pathway leading to cell death. Along with it, platinum nanoparticles induce fragmentation of internucleosomal DNA, cell cycle arrest at the G2/M phase, as well as hypodiploid accumulation (116). A study similar to this has been reported by Jabir et al. (48) where green synthesis of (AgNPs) has been reported using the peel extract obtained from *Annona muricata*. The study further reported that (AgNPs) have the ability to induce antiproliferative as well as pro-apoptotic activity towards the following cell lines: THP-1 (human leukaemia monocytic cell line), AMJ-13 (breast cancer cell line), and HBL (breast epithelial cell line) (48) (Figure 15.4).

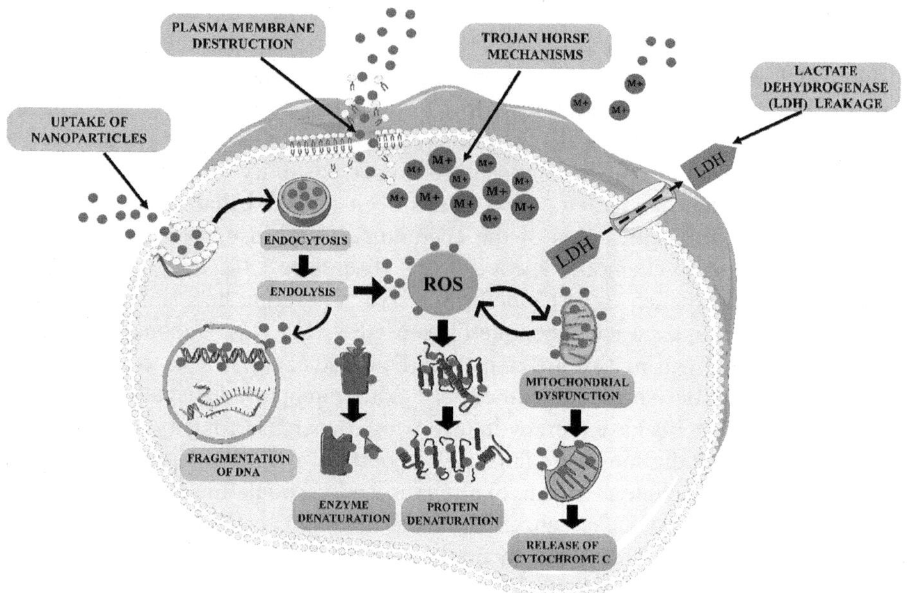

FIGURE 15.4 Schematic representation of proposed mechanisms involved in nanoparticle-mediated anticancer activity.

15.5.2 Green-Synthesized Nanoparticles in Drug Delivery in Other Diseases

Green-synthesized nanoparticles have numerous applications in the treatment of various human diseases through target-oriented delivery of specific drugs to precise locations. Metal or metal oxide nanoparticle-mediated drug delivery has proven to be an effective method to transport drugs for various types of cancer, bacterial infections, wound healing, anti-leishmanial activity, antibacterial and antifungal activity against various resistant strains, etc. (117,133,150). Leishmaniasis is one of the most common and deadliest tropical diseases caused by protozoal infection. The disease is spread by the transmission of parasite into the diseased person by the bite of sandflies (*Phlebotomus spp.*) carrying the parasite. However, there is a constant venture to develop new drugs for these deadly diseases. However, nanoparticles have shown a glimmer of hope in the management of disease and emerged as an antileishmanial agent to target the parasite. In a study reported by Prasanna et al. (133) gold nanoparticles have been synthesised and functionalized with 7,8-dihydroxyflavone. The compound was actively reducing as well as capping the gold nanoparticles at pH of 9. The study further revealed the effect of 7,8-dihydroxyflavone-conjugated gold nanoparticles in inhibiting the enzyme arginase that has led to parasitic cell death. Furthermore, the study has stated that the 7,8-dihydroxyflavone-conjugated gold nanoparticles are active in killing the promastigotes by arginase inhibition. A similar study was reported in 2021 by Awad et al. (134) where (AgNPs) had been synthesized using *Commiphora molmol* resin and were tested to evaluate their cytotoxicity against cutaneous Leishmaniasis major. It has been said that the first line of defence of an infected cell against cutaneous leishmaniasis is by generating ROS. The parasitic pathogen is highly impacted by ROS generation in a cell. However, protozoal parasites have developed enzyme inhibition as a strategy to bypass ROS generation. Therefore, it becomes one of the most important strategies to generate ROS inside cells to overcome the inhibition caused by the parasite. Therefore, the study further emphasized the hypothesis that metallic nanoparticles are well known for their ROS generation inside cells and that, therefore, using metallic nanoparticles does not give leverage to the parasite to inhibit ROS generation due to their non-enzymatic nature. The study has therefore stated that the viability of parasite has been affected by (AgNPs). Furthermore, they have facilitated the healing process of skin lesions (133,134,151,152,153). Metallic nanoparticle-mediated drug delivery has further played a magnificent role in combating multidrug-resistant microbial strains. The onset of multidrug-resistant bacterial strains has raised concerns among researchers as the number of newly discovered antibiotics is very slow. Furthermore, according to WHO, resistance to antibiotics is a threat that is developing globally, and imprudent use of antibiotics has accelerated the issue. On the other hand, nanoparticles provide excellent antimicrobial activity by themselves but also serve as drug carriers of antibiotics as well as other biocompounds to target resistant bacterial as well as fungal species. Furthermore, nanoparticles enter the cell through endocytosis, and upon entry, the drug-loaded nanoparticles carry out a range of mechanisms, including ROS generation, fragmentation or denaturation of DNA, halting protein synthesis, distorting proteins and/or enzymes, etc. (154,155,156). A study conducted by Ansari et al. (2015) (157) showed that the aluminium oxide nanoparticles synthesized using *Cymbopogan citratus* leaves had bactericidal effects on the multi-drug resistant bacterial strain *Pseudomonas aeruginosa*. The clinical isolate used in the study had resistance against an extended spectrum of β-lactamases and metallo β-lactamases. The study has revealed that aluminium oxide nanoparticles were able to penetrate through the outer membrane of bacterial cells, challenging the membrane integrity and leading to cell death. Furthermore, the generation of ROS leads to a cascade of impacts, including DNA destruction, protein damage, deactivation of enzymes, etc., that further impact the survivability of resistant bacteria cell. A similar study performed by Benedec et al. (13) has further demonstrated antimycotic as well as antibacterial effects of biosynthesized gold nanoparticles using the aerial part and its flower extract of *Origanum herba*. As revealed in the study, the antibacterial activity of synthesized gold nanoparticles was tested against *E. coli, Salmonella enteritidis, L. monocytogenes,* and *S. aureus,* and the antifungal activity was tested against *Candida albicans*. The test further showed excellent inhibitory effect against all microbial strains; however, the bacterial strain *S. aureus* and the fungal strain *Candida albicans* revealed the maximum inhibition in the presence of gold nanoparticles. As a result, metallic nanoparticles are a beacon of hope in terms of countering growing resistance among microbial strains and reducing the spread of infection caused by these microorganisms (13,157). Furthermore, in terms of urinary infection, a study by Santhoshkumar et al. (127) where zinc oxide nanoparticles were synthesized using the aqueous leaf extract of *Passiflora caerulea*, showed that those infections are caused by various bacterial strains, which involve *E. coli, Enterococcus sp., Klebsiella sp., Streptococcus* sp. and the study found antibacterial activity and thus proved to be a viable treatment option for urinary tract infections (127). Metallic nanoparticles have been further conjugated for use as a drug vehicle to deliver antibiotics more efficiently. As reported by Naimi-Shamel et al., (72) the study reported to have synthesized gold nanoparticles using culture supernatants of the fungal strain *Fusarium oxysporu*. The synthesized gold nanoparticles were then conjugated with tetracycline antibiotics. The study further revealed that the dosage concentrations of only gold nanoparticles against bacterial strains are high as compared to those of gold nanoparticles conjugated with the antibiotic tetracycline. Therefore, lower dosage in terms of gold nanoparticles conjugated with tetracycline is due to efficient targeting and delivery of the drug to specific bacterial strains. Further, it has been found that these gold nanoparticles with conjugated tetracycline were effective against multidrug-resistant strains, which include *Pseudomonas aeruginosa, S. aureus*, and *E. coli* (72). Another reason bacterial strains develop antibiotic resistance is biofilm. Biofilms are extracellular polymeric substances (EPS) produced by bacteria in an attempt to protect themselves from undesirable pH changes, osmolality, depleted nutrition supplies, antibiotics, effects from host immune responses, etc. This biofilm-mediated resistance of the bacterial cell reduces the efficacy of antibiotics and other drugs in the treatment of infection or disease. However, studies have shown nanoparticles have the ability to disrupt the biofilm barrier and penetrate the bacterial cell, leading to its death. In a study reported by Zimet et al. (135), (AgNPs) were synthesized extracellularly using a cell-free extract of the fungal strain *Phanerochaete chrysosporium*. Synthesized (AgNPs) were stated to have been bioconjugated with nisin, which is a cationic antibacterial peptide that is recognized as GRAS and used as a food additive and is produced by gram-positive bacterial species, such as *Lactococcus* and *Streptococcus*. As a result of the conjugation of such peptides to metallic(AgNPs), the biofilm formation of *S. aureus* has been successfully inhibited, as has antibacterial activity against *E. coli*. Further conjugation of nisin and (AgNPs) has enhanced the efficacy of their activity against the growth of bacteria (135,158,159,160). Furthermore, by delivering precise medicines to specified sites and targets, nanotechnology has the potential to significantly improve the treatment of chronic human diseases.

15.6 TOXICITY INVOLVES WITH METALLIC/METAL OXIDE NANOPARTICLES

Although nanoparticles have been shown to facilitate targeted drug delivery for the treatment of a variety of human diseases, they have also been shown to have deleterious effects on humans, create resistance among microorganisms, and contribute to environmental pollution. The term toxicity can be defined as the potential of a chemical to have an adverse effect on or bring about changes in an organism when that particular chemical is introduced to the organism. Metallic nanoparticles, which comprise various metals, such as silver (Ag), gold (Au), iron (Fe), copper (Cu), platinum (Pt) etc., along with their compounds, such as oxides, fluorides, sulphides, chloride, etc have been used mostly for synthesizing various NPs. When it comes to the ecotoxicity of metal and metal oxide nanoparticles, the stakes are extremely high, which includes toxicity to aquatic as well as terrestrial ecosystems (118). On the other hand, contamination based on ecotoxicology follows potential routes and also raises exposure chances during the manufacturing and fabrication process of the material, handling, usage, and waste disposal. As in the study conducted by Chen et al. (119), three different microalgal strains, viz. *Platymonas subcordiforus*, *Chaetoceros curvisetus*, and *Skeletonema costatum*, were utilised to demonstrate the hazardous impact that cobalt nanoparticles (CoNPs) had on marine algal strains. According to the findings, CoNPs have caused toxic effects on the three different microalgal strains. It was also found that the Co^{2+} produced by CoNPs was a contributing factor in the toxicity of CoNPs to three different species of microalgae. Further, scanning electron microscope analysis revealed that the interaction that took place between CoNPs and the microalgae cell resulted in the formation of agglomeration inside the cells of algae, which led to cell death. CoNPs further enveloped algal cells, blocking their ability to make the most of available light for photosynthesis (119). Antibacterial agents as well as medicinal uses of silver and cerium nanoparticles have contributed to their rise to prominence. As mentioned in the study reported by Sendra et al. (120), two microalgal species, *Chlorella autotrophica* and *Dunaliella salina*, were exposed to ionic and nanoparticle forms of silver and cerium. The toxic impact on these organisms was primarily due to nanoparticle adhesion on the outer cell wall, which then transferred within the cells. Therefore, the study has used two different microalgae strains with different structural morphology, where *D. salina*, lacking a cell wall, and *Chlorella autotrophica*, with a typical cellulosic cell wall, are exposed to nanoparticle toxicity. The study has further reported that the toxicity of cerium and (AgNPs) and their ions has induced toxicity in the microalgal strains and has impacted their reproductive, structural, and physiological systemsThe findings of the study further stated that the toxicity of microalgal strains is higher in their ionic form than in their nanoparticle counterparts (120). In addition, the extent of toxicity of a nanomaterial in a biological system depends on certain properties of the nanomaterial, such as particle size, shape, and propensity to interact with the surrounding tissue. Nanoparticles can cause significant harm to humans due to their toxic properties. There are several reported mechanisms for nanoparticles to reach the human system, including inhalation, absorption through the skin, and gastrointestinal absorption. The toxic effects of (AgNPs) and silver ions have been evaluated and demonstrated cytotoxicity with a potency comparable to that of Ag^+ ions, and the cytotoxicity of AgNPs, like that of Ag^+ ions, was attributable mostly to oxidative stress. The study further emphasized the fact that AgNPs and Ag^+ differentially regulated the expression of oxidative stress-related mRNA species. Also, implying that AgNPs induced toxicity is an intrinsic effect of AgNPs that is independent of free Ag^+ ions (121,160,161,162). A study reported by Park et al. (122) has reported on the cause of cellular damage caused by the inhalation of nanoparticles. The study found that inhalable nanoparticles are able to damage cells directly or indirectly and are dose dependent. The study further showed that nanoparticles, such as n-Zn and n-Ni, had a strong cytotoxic effect on A549 cells (122). It has also been found that nanoparticles have the ability to infiltrate and circulate throughout the human body, eventually accumulating in numerous organs. Also, nanoparticles have the ability to breach the blood brain barrier and penetrate the brain following a specific route (olfactory bulb-olfactory nerve-brain). Upon penetration through the blood brain barrier, the substance remains circulating in blood vessels and releases ions that damage the blood brain barrier with an increase in permeability; however, further intervention is needed to completely understand the impact of nanoparticles on humans (123).

While nanoparticles are well known for their antibacterial properties, studies have also found that chronic or acute exposure of microorganisms to nanoparticles increases the likelihood of developing resistance and mechanisms to bypass the effects of nanoparticles in microorganisms. Furthermore, this resistance gain in microorganisms against nanoparticles also has an impact on treating diseases caused by resistant microorganisms. Study reported by Kotchaplai et al. (136) showed that *Pseudomonas putida* F1 bacteria gained increased tolerance and growth recovery of bacterial cells when exposed to nZVI (nanoscale zerovalent iron) through various mechanisms that induce alteration and modification into the cell. Cell viability was reported to have decreased after exposure to nanoparticles, yet a reversal in cell numbers was detected after prolonged exposure. In addition, cell membrane composition analysis has shown that upon short exposure of the bacterial strain to nZVI, there has been the conversion of cis to trans isomer of unsaturated fatty acids, which gives rise to a more rigid membrane and hence acts against the membrane-fluidizing action of the nZVI (124,136).

However, more extensive research is required to understand and use carbon as a tool for sustainability rather than as a liability for the environment in order to reduce these impacts.

15.7 FUTURE POSSIBILITIES AND CONCLUSION

Since metallic nanoparticles possess a number of desirable qualities, they make an ideal candidate for use as drug carriers. The green synthesis of nanoparticles provide an opportunity to synthesize nanoparticles in a more environmentally benign way. The conventional approach in the synthesis of nanoparticles has various disadvantages, including high cost of production, use of toxic chemicals, and are also harmful towards the environment. The use of nanoparticles as a drug delivery vehicle guarantees that the drug will reach its intended target without harming any of the healthy tissue nearby. However, there are a number of criteria, such as size, shape, texture etc., that must be met for successful drug delivery via nanoparticles to an area of interest. It is also important to remember the toxicity that metal and metal oxide nanoparticles confer. Therefore, we believe that green-synthesized nanoparticles-mediated drug delivery has the potential to significantly impact the biomedical sector as a whole.

REFERENCES

(1) Kargozar, S. and Mozafari, M., 2018. Nanotechnology and Nanomedicine: Start small, think big. *Materials Today: Proceedings*, 5(7), pp. 15492–15500.

(2) Khan, A.K., Rashid, R., Murtaza, G. and Zahra, A.J.T.R., 2014. Gold nanoparticles: Synthesis and applications in drug delivery. *Tropical Journal of Pharmaceutical Research*, 13(7), pp. 1169–1177.

(3) Lee, K.X., Shameli, K., Yew, Y.P., Teow, S.Y., Jahangirian, H., Rafiee-Moghaddam, R. and Webster, T.J., 2020. Recent developments in the facile bio-synthesis of gold nanoparticles (AuNPs) and their biomedical applications. *International Journal of Nanomedicine*, pp. 275–300.

(4) Khanzada, B., Akthar, N., Bhatti, M.Z., Ismail, H., Alqarni, M., Mirza, B., Mostafa-Hedeab, G. and Batiha, G.E.S., 2021. Green synthesis of gold and iron nanoparticles for targeted delivery: An in vitro and in vivo study. *Journal of Chemistry*, 2021, pp. 1–16.

(5) Shafey, A.M.E., 2020. Green synthesis of metal and metal oxide nanoparticles from plant leaf extracts and their applications: A review. *Green Processing and Synthesis*, 9(1), pp. 304–339.

(6) Kurcheti, P.P., Dhayanath, D., Mary, A.J., Jeena, J. and Alim, H., 2020. Biosynthesis of nanoparticles-a new horizon in fish biomedicine. *Journal of Aquaculture & Fisheries*, 4(2), pp. 1–3.

(7) Xu, L., Yi-Yi, W., Huang, J., Chun-Yuan, C., Zhen-Xing, W. and Xie, H., 2020. Silver nanoparticles: Synthesis, medical applications and biosafety. *Theranostics*, 10(20), p. 8996.

(8) Raju, S.K., Karunakaran, A., Kumar, S., Sekar, P., Murugesan, M. and Karthikeyan, M., 2022. Biogenic synthesis of copper nanoparticles and their biological applications: An overview. International Journal of Pharmacy and Pharmaceutical Sciences, 14(3) doi: 10.22159/ijpps.2022v14i3.43842

(9) Dikshit, P.K., Kumar, J., Das, A.K., Sadhu, S., Sharma, S., Singh, S., Gupta, P.K. and Kim, B.S., 2021. Green synthesis of metallic nanoparticles: Applications and limitations. *Catalysts*, 11(8), p. 902.

(10) Khan, I., Saeed, K. and Khan, I., 2019. Nanoparticles: Properties, applications and toxicities. *Arabian Journal of Chemistry*, 12(7), pp. 908–931.

(11) Harish, V., Ansari, M.M., Tewari, D., Gaur, M., Yadav, A.B., García-Betancourt, M.L., Abdel-Haleem, F.M., Bechelany, M. and Barhoum, A., 2022. Nanoparticle and nanostructure synthesis and controlled growth methods. *Nanomaterials*, 12(18), p. 3226.

(12) Soltys, L., Olkhovyy, O., Tatarchuk, T. and Naushad, M., 2021. Green synthesis of metal and metal oxide nanoparticles: Principles of green chemistry and raw materials. *Magnetochemistry*, 7(11), p. 145.

(13) Benedec, D., Oniga, I., Cuibus, F., Sevastre, B., Stiufiuc, G., Duma, M., Hanganu, D., Iacovita, C., Stiufiuc, R. and Lucaciu, C.M., 2018. Origanum vulgare mediated green synthesis of biocompatible gold nanoparticles simultaneously possessing plasmonic, antioxidant and antimicrobial properties. *International Journal of Nanomedicine*, 13, p. 1041.

(14) Kanwar, R., Rathee, J., Salunke, D.B. and Mehta, S.K., 2019. Green nanotechnology-driven drug delivery assemblies. *ACS Omega*, 4(5), pp. 8804–8815.

(15) Kaplan, Ö., Tosun, N.G., Özgür, A., Tayhan, S.E., Bilgin, S., Türkekul, İ. and Gökce, İ., 2021. Microwave-assisted green synthesis of silver nanoparticles using crude extracts of *Boletus edulis* and *Coriolus versicolor*: Characterization, anticancer, antimicrobial and wound healing activities. *Journal of Drug Delivery Science and Technology*, 64, p. 102641.

(16) Patra, J.K., Das, G., Fraceto, L.F., Campos, E.V.R., Rodriguez-Torres, M.D.P., Acosta-Torres, L.S., Diaz-Torres, L.A., Grillo, R., Swamy, M.K., Sharma, S. and Habtemariam, S., 2018. Nano based drug delivery systems: Recent developments and future prospects. *Journal of Nanobiotechnology*, 16(1), pp. 1–33.
(17) Chandrakala, V., Aruna, V. and Angajala, G., 2022. Review on metal nanoparticles as nanocarriers: Current challenges and perspectives in drug delivery systems. *Emergent Materials*, 5(6), pp. 1–23.
(18) Saddik, M.S., Elsayed, M.M., Abdelkader, M.S.A., El-Mokhtar, M.A., Abdel-Aleem, J.A., Abu-Dief, A.M., Al-Hakkani, M.F., Farghaly, H.S. and Abou-Taleb, H.A., 2021. Novel green biosynthesis of 5-fluorouracil chromium nanoparticles using harpullia pendula extract for treatment of colorectal cancer. *Pharmaceutics*, 13(2), p. 226.
(19) Veiseh, O., Gunn, J.W. and Zhang, M., 2010. Design and fabrication of magnetic nanoparticles for targeted drug delivery and imaging. *Advanced Drug Delivery Reviews*, 62(3), pp. 284–304.
(20) Kumar, M., Kumar, U. and Singh, A.K., 2022. Therapeutic nanoparticles: Recent developments and their targeted delivery applications. *Nano Biomedicine & Engineering*, 14(1), pp. 38–52.
(21) Wilczewska, A.Z., Niemirowicz, K., Markiewicz, K.H. and Car, H., 2012. Nanoparticles as drug delivery systems. *Pharmacological Reports*, 64(5), pp. 1020–1037.
(22) Gulia, K., James, A., Pandey, S., Dev, K., Kumar, D. and Sourirajan, A., 2022. Bio-inspired smart nanoparticles in enhanced cancer theranostics and targeted drug delivery. *Journal of Functional Biomaterials*, 13(4), p. 207.
(23) Franco, D., Calabrese, G., Guglielmino, S.P.P. and Conoci, S., 2022. Metal-based nanoparticles: Antibacterial mechanisms and biomedical application. *Microorganisms*, 10(9), p. 1778.
(24) Rahman, A., Chowdhury, M.A. and Hossain, N., 2022. Green synthesis of hybrid nanoparticles for biomedical applications: A review. *Applied Surface Science Advances*, 11, p. 100296.
(25) Makarov, V.V., Love, A.J., Sinitsyna, O.V., Makarova, S.S., Yaminsky, I.V., Taliansky, M.E. and Kalinina, N.O., 2014. "Green" nanotechnologies: Synthesis of metal nanoparticles using plants. *Acta Naturae (англоязычная версия)*, 6(1 (20)), pp. 35–44.
(26) Saim, A.K., Kumah, F.N. and Oppong, M.N., 2021. Extracellular and intracellular synthesis of gold and silver nanoparticles by living plants: A review. *Nanotechnology for Environmental Engineering*, 6, pp. 1–11.
(27) Marchiol, L., Mattiello, A., Pošćić, F., Giordano, C. and Musetti, R., 2014. In vivo synthesis of nanomaterials in plants: Location of silver nanoparticles and plant metabolism. *Nanoscale Research Letters*, 9(1), pp. 1–11.
(28) Patra, J.K., Kwon, Y. and Baek, K.H., 2016. Green biosynthesis of gold nanoparticles by onion peel extract: Synthesis, characterization and biological activities. *Advanced Powder Technology*, 27(5), pp. 2204–2213.
(29) Das, S., Gupta, V., Kalyani, M.I., Kalita, M.C. and Shukla, S., 2019. Biological synthesis and characterization of silver nanoparticles using stem extract of *Langenaria siceraria* and their antibacterial activity against *Escherichia coli* and *Staphylococcus aureus*. *Biomedicine*, 39(4), pp. 580–586.
(30) Kalpana, D., Han, J.H., Park, W.S., Lee, S.M., Wahab, R. and Lee, Y.S., 2019. Green biosynthesis of silver nanoparticles using *Torreya nucifera* and their antibacterial activity. *Arabian Journal of Chemistry*, 12(7), pp. 1722–1732.
(31) Sánchez-Navarro, M.D.C., Ruiz-Torres, C.A., Niño-Martínez, N., Sánchez-Sánchez, R., Martínez-Castañón, G.A., DeAlba-Montero, I. and Ruiz, F., 2018. Cytotoxic and bactericidal effect of silver nanoparticles obtained by green synthesis method using *Annona muricata* aqueous extract and functionalized with 5-fluorouracil. *Bioinorganic Chemistry and Applications*, 2018(1), p. 6506381.

(32) Pani, A., Lee, J.H. and Yun, S.I., 2016. Autoclave mediated one-pot-one-minute synthesis of AgNPs and Au–Ag nanocomposite from *Melia azedarach* bark extract with antimicrobial activity against food pathogens. *Chemistry Central Journal*, 10, pp. 1–11.
(33) Selvi, N.T., Navamathavan, R., Kim, H.Y. and Nirmala, R., 2019. Autoclave mediated synthesis of silver nanoparticles using aqueous extract of *Canna indica* L. rhizome and evaluation of its antimicrobial activity. *Macromolecular Research*, 27, pp. 1155–1160.
(34) Iqbal, J., Abbasi, B.A., Mahmood, T., Hameed, S., Munir, A. and Kanwal, S., 2019. Green synthesis and characterizations of Nickel oxide nanoparticles using leaf extract of *Rhamnus virgata* and their potential biological applications. *Applied Organometallic Chemistry*, 33(8), p. e4950.
(35) Vijayakumar, S., Mahadevan, S., Arulmozhi, P., Sriram, S. and Praseetha, P.K., 2018. Green synthesis of zinc oxide nanoparticles using *Atalantia monophylla* leaf extracts: Characterization and antimicrobial analysis. *Materials Science in Semiconductor Processing*, 82, pp. 39–45.
(36) Shende, S., Ingle, A.P., Gade, A. and Rai, M., 2015. Green synthesis of copper nanoparticles by *Citrus medica* Linn. (Idilimbu) juice and its antimicrobial activity. *World Journal of Microbiology and Biotechnology*, 31, pp. 865–873.
(37) Yusefi, M., Shameli, K., Hedayatnasab, Z., Teow, S.Y., Ismail, U.N., Azlan, C.A. and Rasit Ali, R., 2021. Green synthesis of Fe3O4 nanoparticles for hyperthermia, magnetic resonance imaging and 5-fluorouracil carrier in potential colorectal cancer treatment. *Research on Chemical Intermediates*, 47, pp. 1789–1808.
(38) Bahrulolum, H., Nooraei, S., Javanshir, N., Tarrahimofrad, H., Mirbagheri, V.S., Easton, A.J. and Ahmadian, G., 2021. Green synthesis of metal nanoparticles using microorganisms and their application in the agrifood sector. *Journal of Nanobiotechnology*, 19(1), pp. 1–26.
(39) Alfryyan, N., Kordy, M.G., Abdel-Gabbar, M., Soliman, H.A. and Shaban, M., 2022. Characterization of the biosynthesized intracellular and extracellular plasmonic silver nanoparticles using *Bacillus cereus* and their catalytic reduction of methylene blue. *Scientific Reports*, 12(1), p. 12495.
(40) Raveendran, S., Poulose, A.C., Yoshida, Y., Maekawa, T. and Kumar, D.S., 2013. Bacterial exopolysaccharide based nanoparticles for sustained drug delivery, cancer chemotherapy and bioimaging. *Carbohydrate Polymers*, 91(1), pp. 22–32.
(41) Cheng, Y.J., Luo, G.F., Zhu, J.Y., Xu, X.D., Zeng, X., Cheng, D.B., Li, Y.M., Wu, Y., Zhang, X.Z., Zhuo, R.X. and He, F., 2015. Enzyme-induced and tumor-targeted drug delivery system based on multifunctional mesoporous silica nanoparticles. *ACS Applied Materials & Interfaces*, 7(17), pp. 9078–9087.
(42) Sheik, G.B., Raheim, A.I.A.A., Alzeyadi, Z.A. and AlGhonaim, M.I., 2019. Extracellular synthesis, characterization and antibacterial activity of silver nanoparticles by a potent isolate *Streptomyces* sp. DW102. *Asian Journal of Biological and Life Sciences*, 8(3), p. 89.
(43) Saini, A., Aggarwal, N.K., Sharma, A. and Yadav, A., 2015. Actinomycetes: A source of lignocellulolytic enzymes. *Enzyme Research*, 2015(1), p. 279381.
(44) Pandit, C., Roy, A., Ghotekar, S., Khusro, A., Islam, M.N., Emran, T.B., Lam, S.E., Khandaker, M.U. and Bradley, D.A., 2022. Biological agents for synthesis of nanoparticles and their applications. *Journal of King Saud University-Science*, 34(3), p. 101869.
(45) Kundu, D., Hazra, C., Chatterjee, A., Chaudhari, A. and Mishra, S., 2014. Extracellular biosynthesis of zinc oxide nanoparticles using *Rhodococcus pyridinivorans* NT2: Multifunctional textile finishing, biosafety evaluation and *in vitro* drug delivery in colon carcinoma. *Journal of Photochemistry and Photobiology B: Biology*, 140, pp. 194–204.

(46) Mohd Yusof, H., Abdul Rahman, N.A., Mohamad, R. and Zaidan, U.H., 2020. Microbial mediated synthesis of silver nanoparticles by *Lactobacillus Plantarum* TA4 and its antibacterial and antioxidant activity. *Applied Sciences*, 10(19), p. 6973.
(47) Barabadi, H., Mojab, F., Vahidi, H., Marashi, B., Talank, N., Hosseini, O. and Saravanan, M., 2021. Green synthesis, characterization, antibacterial and biofilm inhibitory activity of silver nanoparticles compared to commercial silver nanoparticles. *Inorganic Chemistry Communications*, 129, p. 108647.
(48) Jabir, M.S., Saleh, Y.M., Sulaiman, G.M., Yaseen, N.Y., Sahib, U.I., Dewir, Y.H., Alwahibi, M.S. and Soliman, D.A., 2021. Green synthesis of silver nanoparticles using *Annona muricata* extract as an inducer of apoptosis in cancer cells and inhibitor for NLRP3 inflammasome via enhanced autophagy. *Nanomaterials*, 11(2), p. 384.
(49) Singh, H., Du, J., Singh, P. and Yi, T.H., 2018. Extracellular synthesis of silver nanoparticles by *Pseudomonas* sp. THG-LS1.4 and their antimicrobial application. *Journal of Pharmaceutical Analysis*, 8(4), pp. 258–264.
(50) Markus, J., Mathiyalagan, R., Kim, Y.J., Abbai, R., Singh, P., Ahn, S., Perez, Z.E.J., Hurh, J. and Yang, D.C., 2016. Intracellular synthesis of gold nanoparticles with antioxidant activity by probiotic *Lactobacillus kimchicus* DCY51T isolated from Korean kimchi. *Enzyme and Microbial Technology*, 95, pp. 85–93.
(51) Bharti, S., Mukherji, S. and Mukherji, S., 2020. Extracellular synthesis of silver nanoparticles by Thiosphaera pantotropha and evaluation of their antibacterial and cytotoxic effects. *3 Biotech*, 10, pp. 1–12.
(52) Ayangbenro, A.S. and Babalola, O.O., 2017. A new strategy for heavy metal polluted environments: A review of microbial biosorbents. *International Journal of Environmental Research and Public Health*, 14(1), p. 94.
(53) Mohd Yusof, H., Mohamad, R., Zaidan, U.H. and Abdul Rahman, N.A., 2019. Microbial synthesis of zinc oxide nanoparticles and their potential application as an antimicrobial agent and a feed supplement in animal industry: A review. *Journal of Animal Science and Biotechnology*, 10, pp. 1–22.
(54) Sukanya, M.K., Saju, K.A., Praseetha, P.K. and Sakthivel, G., 2013. Therapeutic potential of biologically reduced silver nanoparticles from actinomycete cultures. *Journal of Nanoscience*, 2013(1), p. 940719.
(55) Shivaji, S., Madhu, S. and Singh, S., 2011. Extracellular synthesis of antibacterial silver nanoparticles using psychrophilic bacteria. *Process Biochemistry*, 46(9), pp. 1800–1807.
(56) Alshami, H.G.A., Al- Tamimi, W.H. and Hateet, R.R., 2022. Screening for extracellular synthesis of silver nanoparticles by bacteria isolated from Al-Halfaya oil field reservoirs in Missan province, Iraq. *Biodiversitas Journal of Biological Diversity*, 23(7), pp. 3462–3470.
(57) Honary, S., Gharaei-Fathabad, E., Paji, Z.K. and Eslamifar, M., 2012. A novel biological synthesis of gold nanoparticle by *Enterobacteriaceae* family. *Tropical Journal of Pharmaceutical Research*, 11(6), pp. 887–891.
(58) Karthik, L., Kumar, G., Kirthi, A.V., Rahuman, A.A. and Bhaskara Rao, K.V., 2014. *Streptomyces* sp. LK3 mediated synthesis of silver nanoparticles and its biomedical application. *Bioprocess and Biosystems Engineering*, 37, pp. 261–267.
(59) Zhang, Z., Yan, K., Zhang, L., Wang, Q., Guo, R., Yan, Z. and Chen, J., 2019. A novel cadmium-containing wastewater treatment method: Bio-immobilization by microalgae cell and their mechanism. *Journal of Hazardous Materials*, 374, pp. 420–427.
(60) Senapati, S., Syed, A., Moeez, S., Kumar, A. and Ahmad, A., 2012. Intracellular synthesis of gold nanoparticles using alga Tetraselmis kochinensis. *Materials Letters*, 79, pp. 116–118.

(61) Lobus, N.V., 2022. Biogeochemical role of algae in aquatic ecosystems: Basic research and applied biotechnology. *Journal of Marine Science and Engineering*, 10(12), p. 1846.

(62) Gürsoy, N., Öztürk, B.Y. and Dağ, İ., 2021. Synthesis of intracellular and extracellular gold nanoparticles with a green machine and its antifungal activity. *Turkish Journal of Biology*, 45(2), pp. 196–213.

(63) Khan, F., Shahid, A., Zhu, H., Wang, N., Javed, M.R., Ahmad, N., Xu, J., Alam, M.A. and Mehmood, M.A., 2022. Prospects of algae-based green synthesis of nanoparticles for environmental applications. *Chemosphere*, 293, p. 133571. doi: 10.1016/j.chemosphere.2022.133571

(64) Torabfam, M. and Yüce, M., 2020. Microwave-assisted green synthesis of silver nanoparticles using dried extracts of *Chlorella vulgaris* and antibacterial activity studies. *Green Processing and Synthesis*, 9(1), pp. 283–293.

(65) Amina, S.J., Iqbal, M., Faisal, A., Shoaib, Z., Niazi, M.B.K., Ahmad, N.M., Khalid, N. and Janjua, H.A., 2021. Synthesis of diosgenin conjugated gold nanoparticles using algal extract of *Dictyosphaerium* sp. and in-vitro application of their antiproliferative activities. *Materials Today Communications*, 27, p. 102360.

(66) Cai, B., Zhang, Y., Wang, Z., Xu, D., Jia, Y., Guan, Y., Liao, A., Liu, G., Chun, C. and Li, J., 2020. Therapeutic potential of diosgenin and its major derivatives against neurological diseases: Recent advances. *Oxidative Medicine and Cellular Longevity*, 2020(1), p. 3153082.

(67) Ahmad, A., Senapati, S., Khan, M.I., Kumar, R. and Sastry, M., 2005. Extra-/intracellular biosynthesis of gold nanoparticles by an alkalotolerant fungus, *Trichothecium* sp. *Journal of Biomedical Nanotechnology*, 1(1), pp. 47–53.

(68) Copetti, M.V., 2019. Fungi as industrial producers of food ingredients. *Current Opinion in Food Science*, 25, pp. 52–56.

(69) Solomon, L., Tomii, V.P. and Dick, A.A.A., 2019. Importance of fungi in the petroleum, agro-allied, agriculture and pharmaceutical industries. *New York Science Journal*, 12, pp. 8–15.

(70) Mani, V.M., Kalaivani, S., Sabarathinam, S., Vasuki, M., Soundari, A.J.P.G., Das, M.A., Elfasakhany, A. and Pugazhendhi, A., 2021. Copper oxide nanoparticles synthesized from an endophytic fungus *Aspergillus terreus*: Bioactivity and anti-cancer evaluations. *Environmental Research*, 201, p. 111502.

(71) Vetchinkina, E., Loshchinina, E., Kupryashina, M., Burov, A., Pylaev, T. and Nikitina, V., 2018. Green synthesis of nanoparticles with extracellular and intracellular extracts of basidiomycetes. *PeerJ*, 6, p. e5237.

(72) Naimi-Shamel, N., Pourali, P. and Dolatabadi, S., 2019. Green synthesis of gold nanoparticles using *Fusarium oxysporum* and antibacterial activity of its tetracycline conjugant. *Journal de Mycologie Medicale*, 29(1), pp. 7–13.

(73) Supraja, S., Ali, S.M., Chakravarthy, N., Jaya Prakash Priya, A., Sagadevan, E., Kasinathan, M.K., Sindhu, S. and Arumugam, P., 2013. Green synthesis of silver nanoparticles from *Cynodon dactylon* leaf extract. *International Journal of ChemTech Research*, 5(1), pp. 271–277.

(74) Anandalakshmi, K., Venugobal, J. and Ramasamy, V.J.A.N., 2016. Characterization of silver nanoparticles by green synthesis method using *Pedalium murex* leaf extract and their antibacterial activity. *Applied Nanoscience*, 6, pp. 399–408.

(75) Jana, J., Ganguly, M. and PAL, T., 2016. Enlightening surface plasmon resonance effect of metal nanoparticles for practical spectroscopic application. *RSC Advances*, 6(89), pp. 86174–86211.

(76) Girón-Vázquez, N.G., Gómez-Gutiérrez, C.M., Soto-Robles, C.A., Nava, O., Lugo-Medina, E., Castrejón-Sánchez, V.H., Vilchis-Nestor, A.R. and Luque, P.A., 2019. Study of the effect of *Persea americana* seed in the green synthesis of silver nanoparticles and their antimicrobial properties. *Results in Physics*, 13, p. 102142.
(77) Desai, R., Mankad, V., Gupta, S.K. and Jha, P.K., 2012. Size distribution of silver nanoparticles: UV-visible spectroscopic assessment. *Nanoscience and Nanotechnology Letters*, 4(1), pp. 30–34.
(78) Agustina, T.E., Handayani, W. and Imawan, C., 2021, June. The UV-VIS spectrum analysis from silver nanoparticles synthesized using *Diospyros maritima* blume. Leaves extract. In 3rd KOBI Congress, International and National Conferences (KOBICINC 2020) (pp. 411–419). Atlantis Press.
(79) Qian, L., Su, W., Wang, Y., Dang, M., Zhang, W. and Wang, C., 2019. Synthesis and characterization of gold nanoparticles from aqueous leaf extract of *Alternanthera sessilis* and its anticancer activity on cervical cancer cells (HeLa). *Artificial Cells, Nanomedicine, and Biotechnology*, 47(1), pp. 1173–1180.
(80) Alshehri, A.A. and Malik, M.A., 2020. Phytomediated photo-induced green synthesis of silver nanoparticles using *Matricaria chamomilla* L. and its catalytic activity against rhodamine B. *Biomolecules*, 10(12), p. 1604.
(81) Alshamsi, H.A.H. and Jaffer, A.A., 2020. Microwave-assisted synthesis of ZnO nanoparticles and its photocatalytic activity in degradation of Rhodamine B dye. *International Journal of Pharmaceutical Research*, 12(1), pp. 201–210.
(82) Kumar, B., Smita, K., Galeas, S., Sharma, V., Guerrero, V.H., Debut, A. and Cumbal, L., 2020. Characterization and application of biosynthesized iron oxide nanoparticles using Citrus paradisi peel: A sustainable approach. *Inorganic Chemistry Communications*, 119, p. 108116.
(83) Srinivasan, M., Venkatesan, M., Arumugam, V., Natesan, G., Saravanan, N., Murugesan, S., Ramachandran, S., Ayyasamy, R. and Pugazhendhi, A., 2019. Green synthesis and characterization of titanium dioxide nanoparticles (TiO_2 NPs) using *Sesbania grandiflora* and evaluation of toxicity in zebrafish embryos. *Process Biochemistry*, 80, pp. 197–202.
(84) Erdogan, O., Abbak, M., Demirbolat, G.M., Birtekocak, F., Aksel, M., Pasa, S. and Cevik, O., 2019. Green synthesis of silver nanoparticles via *Cynara scolymus* leaf extracts: The characterization, anticancer potential with photodynamic therapy in MCF7 cells. *PLoS One*, 14(6), p. e0216496.
(85) Wu, S., Rajeshkumar, S., Madasamy, M. and Mahendran, V., 2020. Green synthesis of copper nanoparticles using *Cissus vitiginea* and its antioxidant and antibacterial activity against urinary tract infection pathogens. *Artificial Cells, Nanomedicine, and Biotechnology*, 48(1), pp. 1153–1158.
(86) Nahar, K., Aziz, S., Bashar, M.S. and Haque, A., 2020. Synthesis and characterization of silver nanoparticles from *Cinnamomum tamala* leaf extract and its antibacterial potential. *International Journal of Nano Dimension*, 11(1), pp. 88–98.
(87) Falke, S. and Betzel, C., 2019. Dynamic Light Scattering (DLS) principles, perspectives, applications to biological samples. In Alice S. Pereira, Pedro Tavares, Paulo Limão-Vieira. (Eds) *Radiation in Bioanalysis: Spectroscopic Techniques and Theoretical Methods*, pp. 173–193. Springer Nature, Switzerland.
(88) Baig, M.M., Yousuf, M.A., Agboola, P.O., Khan, M.A., Shakir, I. and Warsi, M.F., 2019. Optimization of different wet chemical routes and phase evolution studies of $MnFe_2O_4$ nanoparticles. *Ceramics International*, 45(10), pp. 12682–12690.
(89) Sabouri, Z., Akbari, A., Hosseini, H.A., Khatami, M. and Darroudi, M., 2020. Egg white-mediated green synthesis of NiO nanoparticles and study of their cytotoxicity and photocatalytic activity. *Polyhedron*, 178, p. 114351.

(90) Nasrollahzadeh, M., Sajjadi, M., Komber, H., Khonakdar, H.A. and Sajadi, S.M., 2019. In situ green synthesis of Cu-Ni bimetallic nanoparticles supported on reduced graphene oxide as an effective and recyclable catalyst for the synthesis of N-benzyl-N-aryl-5-amino-1H-tetrazoles. *Applied Organometallic Chemistry*, 33(7), p. e4938.

(91) Haroon, M., Zaidi, A., Ahmed, B., Rizvi, A., Khan, M.S. and Musarrat, J., 2019. Effective inhibition of phytopathogenic microbes by eco-friendly leaf extract mediated silver nanoparticles (AgNPs). *Indian Journal of Microbiology*, 59, pp. 273–287.

(92) Behravan, M., Panahi, A.H., Naghizadeh, A., Ziaee, M., Mahdavi, R. and Mirzapour, A., 2019. Facile green synthesis of silver nanoparticles using *Berberis vulgaris* leaf and root aqueous extract and its antibacterial activity. *International Journal of Biological Macromolecules*, 124, pp. 148–154.

(93) Kadam, J., Dhawal, P., Barve, S. and Kakodkar, S., 2020. Green synthesis of silver nanoparticles using cauliflower waste and their multifaceted applications in photocatalytic degradation of methylene blue dye and Hg^{2+} biosensing. *SN Applied Sciences*, 2, pp. 1–16.

(94) Venil, C.K., Malathi, M., Velmurugan P., and Renuka Devi P., 2021. Green synthesis of silver nanoparticles using canthaxanthin from *Dietzia maris* AURCCBT01 and their cytotoxic properties against human keratinocyte cell line. *Journal of Applied Microbiology*, 130(5), pp. 1730–1744.

(95) Mankad, M., Patil, G., Patel, D., Patel, P. and Patel, A., 2020. Comparative studies of sunlight mediated green synthesis of silver nanoparaticles from *Azadirachta indica* leaf extract and its antibacterial effect on *Xanthomonas oryzae* pv. *oryzae*. *Arabian Journal of Chemistry*, 13(1), pp. 2865–2872.

(96) Khan, M.J., Kumari, S., Shameli, K., Selamat, J. and Sazili, A.Q., 2019. Green synthesis and characterization of pullulan mediated silver nanoparticles through ultraviolet irradiation. *Materials*, 12(15), p. 2382.

(97) Bhatnagar, S., Kobori, T., Ganesh, D., Ogawa, K. and Aoyagi, H., 2019. Biosynthesis of silver nanoparticles mediated by extracellular pigment from Talaromyces purpurogenus and their biomedical applications. *Nanomaterials*, 9(7), p. 1042.

(98) Balavandy, S.K., Shameli, K., Biak, D.R.B.A. and Abidin, Z.Z., 2014. Stirring time effect of silver nanoparticles prepared in glutathione mediated by green method. *Chemistry Central Journal*, 8(1), pp. 1–10.

(99) Kim, D.Y., Saratale, R.G., Shinde, S., Syed, A., Ameen, F. and Ghodake, G., 2018. Green synthesis of silver nanoparticles using Laminaria japonica extract: Characterization and seedling growth assessment. *Journal of Cleaner Production*, 172, pp. 2910–2918.

(100) Raza, Z.A., Bilal, U., Noreen, U., Munim, S.A., Riaz, S., Abdullah, M.U. and Abid, S., 2019. Chitosan mediated formation and impregnation of silver nanoparticles on viscose fabric in single bath for antibacterial performance. *Fibers and Polymers*, 20, pp. 1360–1367.

(101) Gul, A.R., Shaheen, F., Rafique, R., Bal, J., Waseem, S. and Park, T.J., 2021. Grass-mediated biogenic synthesis of silver nanoparticles and their drug delivery evaluation: A biocompatible anti-cancer therapy. *Chemical Engineering Journal*, 407, p. 127202.

(102) Anjum, S., Hashim, M., Malik, S.A., Khan, M., Lorenzo, J.M., Abbasi, B.H. and Hano, C., 2021. Recent advances in zinc oxide nanoparticles (ZnO NPs) for cancer diagnosis, target drug delivery, and treatment. *Cancers*, 13(18), p. 4570.

(103) Saravanakumar, K., Chelliah, R., MubarakAli, D., Oh, D.H., Kathiresan, K. and Wang, M.H., 2019. Unveiling the potentials of biocompatible silver nanoparticles on human lung carcinoma A549 cells and *Helicobacter pylori*. *Scientific Reports*, 9(1), pp. 1–8.

(104) Mariadoss, A.V.A., Vinayagam, R., Xu, B., Venkatachalam, K., Sankaran, V., Vijayakumar, S., Bakthavatsalam, S.R., Mohamed, S.A. and David, E., 2019. Phloretin loaded chitosan nanoparticles enhance the antioxidants and apoptotic mechanisms in DMBA induced experimental carcinogenesis. *Chemico-Biological Interactions*, 308, pp. 11–19.

(105) Yin, H.Q., Shao, G., Gan, F. and Ye, G., 2020. One-step, rapid and green synthesis of multifunctional gold nanoparticles for tumor-targeted imaging and therapy. *Nanoscale Research Letters*, 15, pp. 1–15.

(106) Mariadoss, A.V.A., Saravanakumar, K., Sathiyaseelan, A., Venkatachalam, K. and Wang, M.H., 2020. Folic acid functionalized starch encapsulated green synthesized copper oxide nanoparticles for targeted drug delivery in breast cancer therapy. *International Journal of Biological Macromolecules*, 164, pp. 2073–2084.

(107) Cheung, A., Bax, H.J., Josephs, D.H., Ilieva, K.M., Pellizzari, G., Opzoomer, J., Bloomfield, J., Fittall, M., Grigoriadis, A., Figini, M. and Canevari, S., 2016. Targeting folate receptor alpha for cancer treatment. *Oncotarget*, 7(32), p. 52553.

(108) Al-Dulimi, A.G., Al-Saffar, A.Z., Sulaiman, G.M., Khalil, K.A., Khashan, K.S., Al-Shmgani, H.S. and Ahmed, E.M., 2020. Immobilization of l-asparaginase on gold nanoparticles for novel drug delivery approach as anti-cancer agent against human breast carcinoma cells. *Journal of Materials Research and Technology*, 9(6), pp. 15394–15411.

(109) Asselin, B. and Rizzari, C., 2015. Asparaginase pharmacokinetics and implications of therapeutic drug monitoring. *Leukemia & Lymphoma*, 56(8), pp. 2273–2280.

(110) Devi, P.R., Kumar, C.S., Selvamani, P., Subramanian, N. and Ruckmani, K., 2015. Synthesis and characterization of Arabic gum capped gold nanoparticles for tumor-targeted drug delivery. *Materials Letters*, 139, pp. 241–244.

(111) Saber, M.M., Mirtajani, S.B. and Karimzadeh, K., 2018. Green synthesis of silver nanoparticles using *Trapa natans* extract and their anticancer activity against A431 human skin cancer cells. *Journal of Drug Delivery Science and Technology*, 47, pp. 375–379.

(112) Thomas, S., Gunasangkaran, G., Arumugam, V.A. and Muthukrishnan, S., 2022. Synthesis and characterization of zinc oxide nanoparticles of *Solanum nigrum* and its anticancer activity via the induction of apoptosis in cervical cancer. *Biological Trace Element Research*, 200(6), pp. 2684–2697.

(113) Gelderblom, H., Verweij, J., Nooter, K. and Sparreboom, A., 2001. Cremophor EL: The drawbacks and advantages of vehicle selection for drug formulation. *European Journal of Cancer*, 37(13), pp. 1590–1598.

(114) Akbarian, M., Mahjoub, S., Elahi, S.M., Zabihi, E. and Tashakkorian, H., 2020. Green synthesis, formulation and biological evaluation of a novel ZnO nanocarrier loaded with paclitaxel as drug delivery system on MCF-7 cell line. *Colloids and Surfaces B: Biointerfaces*, 186, p. 110686.

(115) Cao, Y., Dhahad, H.A., El-Shorbagy, M.A., Alijani, H.Q., Zakeri, M., Heydari, A., Bahonar, E., Slouf, M., Khatami, M., Naderifar, M. and Iravani, S., 2021. Green synthesis of bimetallic ZnO–CuO nanoparticles and their cytotoxicity properties. *Scientific Reports*, 11(1), p. 23479.

(116) Alshatwi, A.A., Athinarayanan, J. and Vaiyapuri Subbarayan, P., 2015. Green synthesis of platinum nanoparticles that induce cell death and G2/M-phase cell cycle arrest in human cervical cancer cells. *Journal of Materials Science: Materials in Medicine*, 26, pp. 1–9.

(117) Yugandhar, P., Vasavi, T., Uma Maheswari Devi, P. and Savithramma, N., 2017. Bioinspired green synthesis of copper oxide nanoparticles from *Syzygium alternifolium* (Wt.) Walp: Characterization and evaluation of its synergistic antimicrobial and anti-cancer activity. *Applied Nanoscience*, 7, pp. 417–427.

(118) Egorova, K.S. and Ananikov, V.P., 2017. Toxicity of metal compounds: Knowledge and myths. *Organometallics*, 36(21), pp. 4071–4090.

(119) Chen, X., Zhang, C., Tan, L. and Wang, J., 2018. Toxicity of Co nanoparticles on three species of marine microalgae. *Environmental Pollution*, 236, pp. 454–461.

(120) Sendra, M., Blasco, J. and Araújo, C.V., 2018. Is the cell wall of marine phytoplankton a protective barrier or a nanoparticle interaction site? Toxicological responses of *Chlorella autotrophica* and *Dunaliella* salina to Ag and CeO_2 nanoparticles. *Ecological Indicators*, 95, pp. 1053–1067.

(121) Feng, X., Chen, A., Zhang, Y., Wang, J., Shao, L. and Wei, L., 2015. Central nervous system toxicity of metallic nanoparticles. *International Journal of Nanomedicine*, 10, p. 4321.

(122) Park, S., Lee, Y.K., Jung, M., Kim, K.H., Chung, N., Ahn, E.K., Lim, Y. and Lee, K.H., 2007. Cellular toxicity of various inhalable metal nanoparticles on human alveolar epithelial cells. *Inhalation Toxicology*, 19(1), pp. 59–65.

(123) Sawicki, K., Czajka, M., Matysiak-Kucharek, M., Fal, B., Drop, B., Męczyńska-Wielgosz, S., Sikorska, K., Kruszewski, M. and Kapka-Skrzypczak, L., 2019. Toxicity of metallic nanoparticles in the central nervous system. *Nanotechnology Reviews*, 8(1), pp. 175–200.

(124) Schneider, T., Westermann, M. and Glei, M., 2017. In vitro uptake and toxicity studies of metal nanoparticles and metal oxide nanoparticles in human HT29 cells. *Archives of Toxicology*, 91, pp. 3517–3527.

(125) Salem, S.S., El-Belely, E.F., Niedbała, G., Alnoman, M.M., Hassan, S.E.D., Eid, A.M., Shaheen, T.I., Elkelish, A., and Fouda, A., (2020). Bactericidal and in-vitro cytotoxic efficacy of silver nanoparticles (Ag-NPs) fabricated by endophytic actinomycetes and their use as coating for the textile fabrics. *Nanomaterials*, 10(10), 2082.

(126) Eid, A.M., Fouda, A., Niedbała, G., Hassan, S.E.D., Salem, S.S., Abdo, A.M., F. Hetta, H. and Shaheen, T.I., 2020. Endophytic Streptomyces laurentii mediated green synthesis of Ag-NPs with antibacterial and anticancer properties for developing functional textile fabric properties. *Antibiotics*, 9(10), p. 641.

(127) Santhoshkumar, J., Kumar, S.V. and Rajeshkumar, S., 2017. Synthesis of zinc oxide nanoparticles using plant leaf extract against urinary tract infection pathogen. *Resource-Efficient Technologies*, 3(4), pp. 459–465.

(128) Otari, S.V., Patil, R.M., Ghosh, S.J., Thorat, N.D. and Pawar, S.H., 2015. Intracellular synthesis of silver nanoparticle by actinobacteria and its antimicrobial activity. *Spectrochimica Acta Part A: Molecular and Biomolecular Spectroscopy*, 136, pp. 1175–1180.

(129) Parthiban, E., Manivannan, N., Ramanibai, R., and Mathivanan, N. 2018. Green synthesis of silver-nanoparticles from *Annona reticulata* leaves aqueous extract and its mosquito larvicidal and anti-microbial activity on human pathogens. *Biotechnol Rep (Amst)*, 21, p. e00297. doi: 10.1016/j.btre.2018.e00297

(130) Rajput, S., Kumar, D. and Agrawal, V., 2020. Green synthesis of silver nanoparticles using Indian Belladonna extract and their potential antioxidant, anti-inflammatory, anticancer and larvicidal activities. *Plant cell reports*, 39, pp. 921–939. Doi: https://doi.org/10.1007/s00299-020-02539-7

(131) Mohsen Mosaviniya, Towan Kikhavani, Marjan Tanzifi, Mohammad Tavakkoli Yaraki, Parnian Tajbakhsh, and Aseman Lajevardi, 2019. Facile green synthesis of silver nanoparticles using Crocus Haussknechtii Bois bulb extract: Catalytic activity and antibacterial properties. *Colloid and Interface Science Communications*, 33, p. 100211. https://doi.org/10.1016/j.colcom.2019.100211

(132) Dhinesh Kumar Devendiran, and Valan Arasu Amirtham, 2016. A review on preparation, characterization, properties and applications of nanofluids. *Renewable and Sustainable Energy Reviews*, 60, pp. 21–40. https://doi.org/10.1016/j.rser.2016.01.055

(133) Prasanna P, Kumar P, Mandal S, et al., 2021. 7,8-dihydroxyflavone-functionalized gold nanoparticles target the arginase enzyme of *Leishmania donovani. Nanomedicine (Lond)*, 16(21), pp. 1887–1903. doi: 10.2217/nnm-2021-0161

(134) Manal Ahmed Awad, Ebtesam Mohammed Al Olayan, Muzzammil Iqbal Siddiqui, Nada Mahmmed Merghani, Sarah Saleh Abdu-llah Alsaif, and Abeer S. Aloufi, 2021. Antileishmanial effect of silver nanoparticles: Green synthesis, characterization, in vivo and in vitro assessment. *Biomedicine & Pharmacotherapy*, 137, p. 111294. https://doi.org/10.1016/j.biopha.2021.111294

(135) Zimet, P., Valadez, R., Raffaelli, S., Estevez, M.B., Pardo, H., and Alborés, S., 2021. Biogenic silver nanoparticles conjugated with nisin: Improving the antimicrobial and antibiofilm properties of nanomaterials. *Chemistry*, 3(4), pp. 1271–1285. https://doi.org/10.3390/chemistry3040092

(136) Panaya Kotchaplai, Eakalak Khan, and Alisa S. Vangnai, 2017. Membrane Alterations in Pseudomonas putida F1 Exposed to Nanoscale Zerovalent Iron: Effects of Short-Term and Repetitive nZVI Exposure. *Environmental Science & Technology*, 51(14), pp. 7804–7813. doi: 10.1021/acs.est.7b00736

(137) Saratale, R.G., Shin, H.S., Kumar, G., Benelli, G., Ghodake, G.S., Jiang, Y.Y., Kim, D.S. and Saratale, G.D., 2018. Exploiting fruit byproducts for eco-friendly nanosynthesis: Citrus× clementina peel extract mediated fabrication of silver nanoparticles with high efficacy against microbial pathogens and rat glial tumor C6 cells. *Environmental Science and Pollution Research*, 25, pp. 10250–10263.

(138) Rajeshkumar, S., Malarkodi, C., Paulkumar, K., Vanaja, M., Gnanajobitha, G. and Annadurai, G., 2014. Algae mediated green fabrication of silver nanoparticles and examination of its antifungal activity against clinical pathogens. *International journal of Metals*, 2014, pp. 1–8.

(139) Omran, B.A., Nassar, H.N., Fatthallah, N.A., Hamdy, A., El-Shatoury, E.H. and El-Gendy, N.S., 2018. Waste upcycling of Citrus sinensis peels as a green route for the synthesis of silver nanoparticles. *Energy Sources, Part A: Recovery, Utilization, and Environmental Effects*, 40(2), pp. 227–236.

(140) Kumar, R., Ghoshal, G., Jain, A. and Goyal, M., 2017. Rapid green synthesis of silver nanoparticles (AgNPs) using (Prunus persica) plants extract: exploring its antimicrobial and catalytic activities. *J Nanomed Nanotechnol*, 8(4), pp. 1–8.

(141) Wei, S., Hao, M., Tang, Z., Zhou, T., Zhao, F. and Wang, Y., 2022. Non-medicinal parts of safflower (bud and stem) mediated sustainable green synthesis of silver nanoparticles under ultrasonication: optimization, characterization, antioxidant, antibacterial and anticancer potential. *RSC advances*, 12(55), pp. 36115–36125.

(142) Chutrakulwong, F., Thamaphat, K. and Limsuwan, P., 2020. Photo-irradiation induced green synthesis of highly stable silver nanoparticles using durian rind biomass: Effects of light intensity, exposure time and pH on silver nanoparticles formation. *Journal of Physics Communications*, 4(9), p. 095015.

(143) Khare, S., Singh, R.K. and Prakash, O., 2022. Green synthesis, characterization and biocompatibility evaluation of silver nanoparticles using radish seeds. *Results in Chemistry*, 4, p. 100447.
(144) Wang, J., Liu, N., Su, Q., Lv, Y., Yang, C. and Zhan, H., 2022. Green Synthesis of Gold Nanoparticles and Study of Their Inhibitory Effect on Bulk Cancer Cells and Cancer Stem Cells in Breast Carcinoma. *Nanomaterials*, 12(19), p. 3324.
(145) Vimala, K., Sundarraj, S., Paulpandi, M., Vengatesan, S. and Kannan, S., 2014. Green synthesized doxorubicin loaded zinc oxide nanoparticles regulates the Bax and Bcl-2 expression in breast and colon carcinoma. *Process biochemistry*, 49(1), pp. 160–172.
(146) Gurunathan, S., Jeyaraj, M., Kang, M.H. and Kim, J.H., 2019. Tangeretin-assisted platinum nanoparticles enhance the apoptotic properties of doxorubicin: combination therapy for osteosarcoma treatment. *Nanomaterials*, 9(8), p. 1089.
(147) Norouzi, M., Yathindranath, V., Thliveris, J.A., Kopec, B.M., Siahaan, T.J. and Miller, D.W., 2020. Doxorubicin-loaded iron oxide nanoparticles for glioblastoma therapy: A combinational approach for enhanced delivery of nanoparticles. *Scientific reports*, 10(1), p. 11292.
(148) van der Zanden, S.Y., Qiao, X. and Neefjes, J., 2021. New insights into the activities and toxicities of the old anticancer drug doxorubicin. *The FEBS journal*, 288(21), pp. 6095–6111.
(149) Devendiran, R.M., kumar Chinnaiyan, S., Yadav, N.K., Moorthy, G.K., Ramanathan, G., Singaravelu, S., Sivagnanam, U.T. and Perumal, P.T., 2016. Green synthesis of folic acid-conjugated gold nanoparticles with pectin as reducing/stabilizing agent for cancer theranostics. *RSC advances*, 6(35), pp. 29757–29768.
(150) Anand, K., Tiloke, C., Naidoo, P. and Chuturgoon, A.A., 2017. Phytonanotherapy for management of diabetes using green synthesis nanoparticles. *Journal of Photochemistry and Photobiology B: Biology*, 173, pp. 626–639.
(151) Monzote, L., 2009. Current treatment of leishmaniasis: a review. *The Open Antimicrobial Agents Journal*, 1(1).
(152) Torres-Guerrero, E., Quintanilla-Cedillo, M.R., Ruiz-Esmenjaud, J. and Arenas, R., 2017. Leishmaniasis: a review. F1000Research, 6.
(153) Carneiro, P.P., Conceição, J., Macedo, M., Magalhães, V., Carvalho, E.M. and Bacellar, O., 2016. The role of nitric oxide and reactive oxygen species in the killing of Leishmania braziliensis by monocytes from patients with cutaneous leishmaniasis. *PloS one*, 11(2), p. e0148084.
(154) Basak, S., Singh, P. and Rajurkar, M., 2016. Multidrug resistant and extensively drug resistant bacteria: a study. *Journal of pathogens*, 2016.
(155) Zhang, A.N., Gaston, J.M., Dai, C.L., Zhao, S., Poyet, M., Groussin, M., Yin, X., Li, L.G., van Loosdrecht, M.C., Topp, E. and Gillings, M.R., 2021. An omics-based framework for assessing the health risk of antimicrobial resistance genes. *Nature communications*, 12(1), p. 4765.
(156) https://www.who.int/news-room/fact-sheets/detail/antibiotic-resistance
(157) Ansari, M.A., Khan, H.M., Alzohairy, M.A., Jalal, M., Ali, S.G., Pal, R. and Musarrat, J., 2015. Green synthesis of Al_2O_3 nanoparticles and their bactericidal potential against clinical isolates of multi-drug resistant Pseudomonas aeruginosa. *World Journal of Microbiology and Biotechnology*, 31, pp. 153–164.
(158) Sharma, D., Misba, L. and Khan, A.U., 2019. Antibiotics versus biofilm: an emerging battleground in microbial communities. *Antimicrobial Resistance & Infection Control*, 8(1), pp. 1–10.

(159) Shin, J.M., Gwak, J.W., Kamarajan, P., Fenno, J.C., Rickard, A.H. and Kapila, Y.L., 2016. Biomedical applications of nisin. *Journal of applied microbiology*, 120(6), pp. 1449–1465.

(160) Kim, S., Choi, J.E., Choi, J., Chung, K.H., Park, K., Yi, J. and Ryu, D.Y., 2009. Oxidative stress-dependent toxicity of silver nanoparticles in human hepatoma cells. *Toxicology in vitro*, 23(6), pp. 1076–1084.

(161) Chang, Y.N., Zhang, M., Xia, L., Zhang, J. and Xing, G., 2012. The toxic effects and mechanisms of CuO and ZnO nanoparticles. *Materials*, 5(12), pp. 2850–2871.

(162) Chau, C.F., Wu, S.H. and Yen, G.C., 2007. The development of regulations for food nanotechnology. *Trends in Food Science & Technology*, 18(5), pp. 269–280.

(163) Kumar, C.G., Poornachandra, Y. and Mamidyala, S.K., 2014. Green synthesis of bacterial gold nanoparticles conjugated to resveratrol as delivery vehicles. *Colloids and Surfaces B: Biointerfaces*, 123, pp. 311–317.

16 Recent Advancement in the Use of Nano-Nutraceuticals in Medicine

Chowdhury Mobaswar Hossain, Sabyasachi Choudhuri, Nazmun Lyle, and Sudipto Das

16.1 INTRODUCTION

The medicinal benefits of food have been best known since time immemorial. Ancient civilizations from India, Africa, China, Egypt, Arabia, Japan, and Tibet have been using food-derived products for the treatment of diseases for thousands of years which is also well-documented in the ancient books. However, the concept of nutraceuticals originated long back from the concept of the Greek physician Hippocrates widely known as the "father of the medicine", who first introduced the idea of "let food be thy medicine and medicine be thy food" (Witkamp and Van Norren, 2018).

The word "nutraceutical", was first introduced by Stephen DeFelice in 1989, the founder of the Foundation for Innovation in Medicine, and defined as "a food or parts of food that provide medical or health benefits, including the prevention and/or treatment of disease" (DeFelice, 1995). This is an amalgamation of the two words "nutrition" which refers to food or food components while "pharmaceutical" refers to medicines (DeFelice, 1995). Nutraceuticals are food or parts of food with prospective beneficial effects on health, having the promising ability for the protection against and treatment of the disease—simply put the pharmaceutical nourishment of the body (Kalra, 2003). Foods comprise several dietary ingredients with health benefits that contribute to improving public health and well-being. Hence, the term nutraceuticals comprehensively refers to a broad range of materials including food, herbs, spices, beverages, dietary supplements, antioxidants, prebiotics, probiotics, vitamins, minerals, trace elements, and several other compounds of natural origin, etc. (Khorasani et al., 2018).

This market has been growing rapidly leading to a billion-dollar industry around the world because of the recent trends leaning toward the use of natural products and nutraceutical products, Currently, an increased interest in the intake of nutraceuticals is observed (Zhao, 2007, Nazhand et al., 2022). People are more aware of the correlation between lifestyle diseases, eating habits, and the goodness of natural or

DOI: 10.1201/9781003432661-16

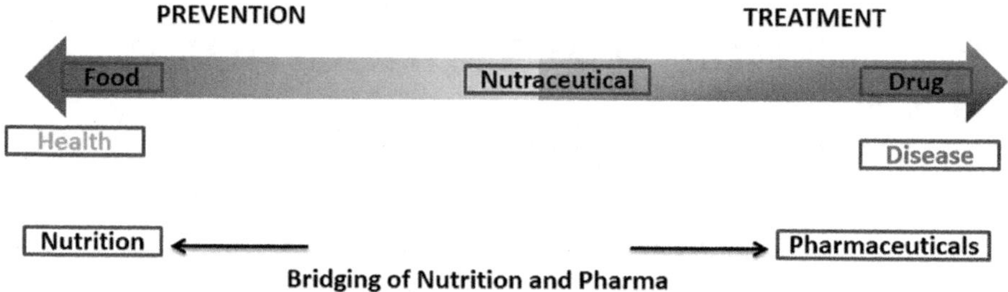

FIGURE 16.1 The bridge between medicinal nutraceuticals and pharmaceuticals.

food-derived compounds increasing the drive for the development of nutraceuticals and nano-nutraceuticals. Nutraceuticals deliver a concentrated form of the potential therapeutic agents derived from food, in a medicine-like package similar to drugs and are used to provide health benefits (Basak and Gokhale, 2022). These are consumed as medicines such as pills, extracts, capsules, tablets, etc. (Figure 16.1).

The term nano-nutraceutical is a combination of the words nanotechnology, nutrition, and pharmaceutical. Nanotechnology is a ground-breaking intervention that has helped scientists to overcome several hindrances associated with the use of nutraceuticals (Jeevanandam et al., 2018; Punia et al., 2019; Niu et al., 2019). Hence, over the last several decades, the amalgamation of nanotechnology and nutraceuticals has increased its importance (Maryana et al., 2016; Dima et al., 2020). However, the utilization and the beneficial effects of numerous nutraceuticals are restricted because of their irrelevant chemico-physical properties, low solubility, low stability, high sensitivity to light and oxygen, slow incorporation, poor bioavailability, etc (Paolino et al., 2021). It is obvious that bioavailability is a significant aspect of nutraceutical products, as their efficacy is purely connected to their bioavailability. However, several factors can alter the bioavailability of nutraceuticals, like physicochemical features, food storage, etc. To overcome these situations, the use of nanotechnology could be a useful intervention to enhance the efficacy of nutraceuticals against some diseases (Mohammad et al., 2015; Sharma et al., 2013; Luo et al., 2017). Nanocarriers are used to improve the pharmacokinetics properties of the nutraceutical components and lower the concentration of drugs needed for biological processes, thereby regulating the nutraceutical application (Buya, 2023). For the better delivery and effectiveness of nutraceuticals, various nanotechnology-based approaches such as polymeric nanoparticles (NPs), dextrin-based, metal and inorganic NPs, magnetic NPs, solid lipid NPs, nanoemulsions, nanospheres, polymeric micelles, nanocapsules, dendrimers, quantum dots, and liposomes are commonly used (Ansari et al., 2012, Patra et al., 2018, Maria Leena et al., 2022, Hoti et al., 2022). Hence, nano-nutraceuticals could emerge as a new frontier of drugs derived from food.

This chapter will focus on the putative role of nutraceuticals, especially nano-nutraceuticals in the promotion of human health, disease prevention, and supportive components of disease treatment. In this chapter modern nanotechnological formulation, and improved bioavailability have been discussed in detail. The bridge between the pharmaceuticals and medical nutraceuticals has been discussed, with a comprehensive discussion on the beneficial effects of medicinal nutraceuticals, providing an overview regarding the use of nano-nutraceuticals to manage pre- and post-COVID-19 outbreak/SARS-CoV-2 infections. Recent updates on NPs for oral delivery, their use as drug delivery platforms, and the associated challenges have also been mentioned. This chapter also tries to shed some light on future trends and prospects, on regulatory and ethical concerns for nano-nutraceuticals.

16.2 BRIDGING PHARMACEUTICALS TO MEDICAL NUTRACEUTICALS

Pharmaceuticals are medicines approved by the US Food and Drug Administration (FDA) and recommended or prescribed by primary care doctors to treat diseases or specific health issues. These are manufactured in pharmaceutical laboratories by pharmaceutical companies. These drugs go through stringent clinical trials with scientific data to support their safety and efficacy. Nutraceutical is a combination of nutrition and pharmaceutical and is not regulated by the FDA. These are components made from whole foods, food products, or natural products and possess health benefits, including the prevention and treatment of diseases (Santini et al., 2018). Presently, nutraceuticals have been defined as "the phytocomplex if they derive from a food of vegetal origin, and as the pool of the secondary metabolites if they derive from a food of animal origin, concentrated and administered in the more suitable pharmaceutical form, which are capable of providing beneficial health effects, including the prevention and/or the treatment of a disease" (Bragazzi et al., 2017; da Costa, 2017; Daliu et al., 2019; Reis et al., 2017). Examples of nutraceuticals include soy protein, garlic, green tea, etc. Therefore, the basic difference between nutraceuticals and pharmaceuticals is that the former are nutrients derived from whole foods while the latter are medicines that contain an isolated nutrient or component. Pharmaceuticals are aimed to treat present problems rather than prevent future problems. Nutraceuticals on the other hand promise to provide overall health benefits and prevention of diseases. Thereby nutraceuticals fill the gaps in symptomatic treatment by modern medicine and in the prevention of the disease (Jha et al., 2020).

Practically, medical nutraceuticals describe a novel concept that bridges the boundary between medicines and food. Nutraceuticals have proven beneficial health effects (Rautiainen et al, 2016, Algan et al., 2022). It possesses the potential to protect the body and is commonly considered as more than just food and if administered before medication may prevent and treat disease conditions. Several studies reported that the regular use of nutraceuticals may be helpful in protecting or delaying the disease (Santini and Novellino, 2017). According to Santini and Novellino, it shows the connection between food and pharmaceuticals (Santini and Novellino, 2018).

However, major concerns related to nutraceuticals are related to their safety profiles. To overcome this, clear regulatory information and particular classification are highly essential. It is highly important to have an accurate and conclusive definition and classification of nutraceuticals with specific guidelines that can be universally used to evaluate the efficacy, mode of action, and safety concerns of nutraceuticals (Kumar and Rajpoot, 2018, Dey et al., 2018). Nevertheless, it would also be necessary to conduct complete clinical trials and evaluate the clinical data related to the effectiveness of nutraceuticals as protection and in the treatment of the disease. Moreover, any probable interactions with drugs should also be reported (Gupta et al., 2021; Santini et al., 2016). To bridge the gap between clinical nutraceuticals and pharmaceuticals, nutraceuticals should have proven pharmacological roles and be safe and effective against disease conditions. Identification of an epidemiological target and epidemiological studies related to efficacy, and toxicity if any is needed to narrow the gap between the two groups. Participation of clinicians in these studies is essential for the right assessment of safety and efficacy (Domínguez Díaz et al., 2020).

16.3 NUTRACEUTICALS ON HUMAN HEALTH/MEDICINAL NUTRACEUTICALS

The therapeutic utilities of foods or food components have been searched and practiced since ancient times (Wildman et al., 2016). Ancient Indians are believed to have made important contributions to the improvement of medical sciences by exploration and utilization of nutraceuticals over 5,000 years back, which is well reported by *Ayurvedic*, *Siddha*, and *Unani* systems of treatment. In *Ayurvedic* medicine, nutraceuticals such as *Chyavanprash* with health promotion properties were used and are being used to date. Nowadays, with the considerable increasing interest and demand of consumers for nutraceuticals, innovative research to discover functions and prospective therapeutic applications of nutraceutical components is also rapidly increasing.

Phytochemicals present in a regular diet with health benefits are terpenoids (phytosterols, carotenoids), glucosinolates, polyphenols (isoflavones, anthocyanins), *Alliaceae*, and different types of polyphenols (flavones, stilbenoids, ellagic acid, etc.). There are enormous nutraceutical compounds like antioxidants, vitamins, probiotics, bioactive peptides, etc. present in food of plant and animal origin and significant scientific information is available to prove their health-promoting effects (Fernandes et al., 2023).

Various epidemiological data have confirmed that plant-origin foods like vegetables, fruits, and dietary fibers prevent and bring down the probability of chronic diseases such as diabetes, cardiovascular diseases, cancer, obesity, etc. (Tsiaka et al., 2022). Researchers across the world have unanimously reported that plant-derived bioactive materials have useful properties (Martínez and Campos, 2023). Various literature indicates that a plant-based diet with vegetables and fruits is able to reduce the risk of cancer (Chandra et al., 2022). The results from different epidemiological studies and preclinical studies reveal that plant-origin diets are substantially effective against cancer of the stomach, lung, oral cavity and pharynx, esophagus, colon, pancreas, etc. (Gul et al., 2016). The origins and the useful components of important nutraceuticals are summarized in Table 16.1

16.3.1 Potential Health Benefits of Nutraceuticals

Nutraceuticals exert different therapeutic effects such as improving health, and protection against chronic diseases. Nutraceuticals also exhibit a protective role against oxidative stress, obesity, diabetes, metabolic syndrome, cancer, atherosclerosis and

TABLE 16.1
Different types of Nutraceutical Substances and their Sources

Plants	Animal	Microbial
Gallic acid	Conjugated Linoleic Acid (CLA)	*Saccharomyces boulardii*
Curcumin	Sphingolipids	*Lactobacillus acidophilus*
β-Glucan	Eicosapentaenoic acid (EPA)	*Bifidobacterium bifidum*
γ-Tocotrienol	Coenzyme Q10	*Streptococcus salvarius*
Indole-3-carbonyl	Docosahexenoic acid (DHA)	*B. longum*
Ascorbic acid	Selenium	*B. infantis*
Quercetin	Creatine	
β-Carotene	Zinc	
α-Tocopherol	Choline	
Luteolin	Minerals	
Glutathione	Lecithin	
Cellulose	Calcium	
Catechins		
Lutein		
Pectin		
MUFA		
Perillyl alcohol		
Lycopene		
Daidzein		
Allicin		
Geraniol		
δ-Limonene		
Capsaicin		
Genistein		
Hemicellulose		
Lignin		
β-Ionone		
Nordihydrocapsaicin		
Selenium		
Potassium		
Zeaxanthin		
Minerals		

cardiovascular diseases, inflammation control, allergies, arthritis, neuronal diseases like aging, Alzheimer's disease, and Parkinson's disease, etc. (Cicero et al., 2019, Paolino et al., 2021, Catalano et al., 2022). The potential benefits and protective properties of nutraceuticals are listed in Table 16.2

16.3.2 Prevention and Treatment of Cancer

To date, conventional cancer treatments are mostly surgery, chemotherapy, and radiation therapy. However, a healthy diet like an antioxidant-rich diet and a healthy lifestyle can act as a preventive measure against cancer. An epidemiological study

TABLE 16.2
Nutraceuticals with their Therapeutic Benefits

Name of Nutraceutical	Therapeutic Benefits	References
Lycopene	Reducing risk of prostate and cervical cancers Promoting cardiovascular health	Grabowska et al. (2019), Holzapfel et al. (2017), Ilic and Misso (2012)
Lutein Esters	Dietary supplement Used as functional foods Antioxidants effects	Muangnoi et al. (2021)
Garlic	Antioxidants Cancer Lowers cholesterol Reduces cardiac diseases Improves diabetes	Kim et al. (2007), Butt et al. (2009), Borek, 2006)
Green Tea	Cancer prevention Weight loss Antioxidant Lowers cholesterol	Khatiwada et al. (2006), Hayat et al. (2015)
Phycocyanin Powder	Antioxidant	Kumar et al. (2022)
Gymnema, Momordica Isoflavones, Omega-3 fatty acids, Psyllium	Diabetic control	Limer and Speirs (2004)
Glucosamine	Arthritis treatment	Reginster et al. (2012)
n-3 PUFAs, Tannins, Anthocyanins, Octacosanol	Cardiovascular disease	Rissanen et al. (2003) Rabanal-Ruiz et al. (2021) Grassi et al. (2021)
Ginkgo Biloba	Allergy treatment	Russo et al. (2009)
Lycopene, Astaxanthin, β-Carotene, Vitamin E, Green tea, Vitamin C	Antioxidant	Wang et al. (2007), Rahimi-Madiseh et al. (2014)
Ginseng	Immunomodulator	Long et al. (2022)
Astragalus, Echinacea angustfolia, Garlic	Immunity problems	Nasri et al. (2014)
β-Carotene, Curcumin, Terpenes, Kaempherol, Moringa oleifera, Saponins, Chitosan	Miscellaneous	Hollman et al. (1996), Chandra et al. (2022), Durazzo et al. (2022)
Quercetin	Allergy	Middha et al. (2015), Nakamura et al. (2020), McCarty et al. (2021)
Probiotics, Prebiotics	Bone and joint health, Metabolic syndrome	Ilesanmi-Oyelere et al. (2021), Nazhand et al. (2022)
Nutritional lipids and oil	Immune system	Al-Khalaifah, 2020)
Green Tea, Capsaicin, Mahuang, Guarana, Psyllium Fiber	Obesity	Watanabe et al. (2020)
Daidzein, Lycopene, β-Carotene, Biochanin	Cancer	Willis and Wians (2003), Limer and Speirs (2004), Thomasset et al. (2007), Cabral et al. (2021)
Glucosamine, Vitamin C, Chondroitin	Inflammation	Kantor et al. (2014)
Lutein, Lycopene, Curcumin, Turmerin	Alzheimer's disease	Iqubal et al. (2022)

has reported that regular consumption of nutraceuticals can help to prevent carcinogenesis. An experimental animal model study of cancer also stated that nutraceutical products can prevent cancer (Zhou et al., 2020).

Nutraceuticals like phytoestrogens can play an important role in chemoprevention in cancer treatments as they are effective and have low or no side effects (Limer and Speirs, 2004). Nutraceuticals of plant origin possess huge amounts of bioactives like curcumin, caffeic acid, gallic acid, isoflavones, and tannins with significant potential roles against various cancers (Li et al., 2003). β-carotene and pectin have potent free-radical scavenging effects so are found to protect against prostate cancers (Jang et al., 1997). A clinical trial reported that nutraceuticals with lycopene, Vitamin D, green tea, and Vitamin E are significantly effective in minimizing prostate cancer. Daily intake of fruits can provide various kinds of nutraceuticals like cysteine, lycopene, ascorbic acid, Vitamin E, etc., and can effectively prevent several kinds of cancer. Few bioactive compounds from glucosinolates have significant protective effects against breast, colon, liver, and lung cancer (Jha et al., 2020). Curcumin is a curcuminoid that originated from turmeric (*Curcuma longa*). It possesses different utilities, such as antioxidant, anticancer, and anti-inflammatory properties (Catalano et al., 2022). It is well reported that nutraceuticals exert their effect against cancer through various mechanisms such as scavenging free radicals, effect on DNA methylation, reduction of N-nitrosamine formation, alteration of estrogen metabolism, through DNA repair, etc. (Paolino et al., 2021).

16.3.3 Cardiovascular Diseases

Cardiovascular diseases (CVDs), heart disease, and stroke are major reasons for mortality in developed countries. In developing countries also CVD plays a major role in 50% of deaths. Recent surveys reported that reactive oxygen species (ROS) and oxidative stress are the pathogenesis of both acute and chronic heart disorders. It is found that the oxidation of low-density lipoproteins (LDL) is the main factor of atherosclerosis and CVD via the initiation of plaque formation (Gul et al., 2016). It is well established that increased serum cholesterol, triacylglyceride concentrations, and decreased high-density lipoprotein (HDL) cholesterol concentrations in turn increase the threat of coronary artery disease as well as CVDs. Some other crucial associated factors for CVD are hyperlipidemia, high blood pressure, obesity, and diabetes.

Several nutraceuticals are utilized in cardiovascular diseases like carnitine, glutathione, N-acetylcysteine, beta-sitosterol, selenium, creatine, resveratrol, and flavonoids. Carnitine is an amino acid derivative synthesized in the liver, kidneys, and brain from lysine and methionine. Two analogs of carnitine, acetyl-L-carnitine and propionyl-L-carnitine, have been used for therapeutic purposes. Carnitine serves an essential role in energy production. Although it is widely used to address primary/secondary carnitine deficiencies, it is also utilized against a variety of cardiovascular conditions (Shindhe et al., 2014). L-carnitine has beneficial effects on cardiovascular functions and it is reported to be cardioprotective due to its antioxidant properties. Various studies have revealed that it considerably lowers plasma triglycerides and increases HDL cholesterol levels. Vitamins, omega-3 fatty acids, antioxidants, minerals, and dietary fibers are developed as nutraceuticals for minimizing CVD management. Vegetables and fruits containing abundant flavonoids are used as nutraceuticals to control CVDs. Dietary indoleamines, Melatonin, tannins, serotonin, etc. have also been explored for use as nutraceuticals for the management of CVDs (Jha et al., 2020). A study has also depicted the efficacy of nutraceuticals like the putative role of coenzyme Q10 in CVDs and the role of polyunsaturated fatty acids (PUFA) in coronary artery disease (Rabanal-Ruiz et al., 2021).

16.3.4 Nutraceuticals Used in the Management of Diabetes

Diabetes is a metabolic disorder and is one of the primary reasons for global deaths as per the World Health Organization. Large numbers of diabetic cases are associated with obesity. Worldwide, about 50% of the population is suffering from diabetes type 2, which is non- insulin-dependent diabetes mellitus, because of changes in lifestyle (Jha et al., 2020). Conventional therapies for diabetes with standard medicines exhibit various harmful side effects so there is an urgent requirement for alternative phytochemical-based therapy. In this context, extensive research is being carried out to develop promising nutraceuticals for the control of diabetes. Several products are in preclinical trial levels as therapeutic drugs for diabetes. The role of isoflavones in type 2 diabetes treatment has shown a significant decrease in mortality rates. Omega-3 fatty acids and n-3 fatty acids are also found to be efficient for diabetes treatment. Lipoic acid and dietary fibers such as psyllium are included in nutraceuticals in order to decrease diabetic neuropathy, and hyperlipidemia, and control blood sugar levels (Behradmanesh and Nasri, 2013, Shahbazian, 2013). Besides these, several medicinal plants are documented as having anti-diabetic properties. In addition, tomato peel, nectarines, and olive leaves are used as components of nutraceuticals. A recent study stated that polyphenolic components from these sources exhibit a potential effect on insulinemia and post-prandial glycemia. Another study depicted that the phenolic compound of citrus peels (Citrus maxima), also exerts repressive action toward α-amylase and α-glucosidase, thus confirming their effectiveness against type-2 diabetes (Oboh and Ademosun, 2011, Tenore et al., 2020).

16.3.5 Nutraceuticals Against Obesity Complications

Obesity is now becoming a serious health problem throughout the world, especially in Asia, parts of Africa, and the Americas. In the European countries, the occurrence of obesity has been noticeably higher. Due to lifestyle changes, sedentary routines, and low physical activity energy consumption, overweight and obesity are the obvious outcomes and cause major social and health impacts. It is a pathological state defined by the acquisition of extra body fat, connected with a short life span and enhanced disease condition (Gul et al., 2016).

To attenuate the situation excessive energy intake should be avoided together with an increase in energy expenditure. These include a balanced diet, practicing healthy eating habits, and regular physical activities (International Obesity Task Force, 2005). Many studies have documented that fiber-enriched foods can have encouraging effects in attenuating obesity. High fiber is considered to help in weight reduction and aids in lowering obesity (Pereira and Ludwig, 2001, Rayalam et al., 2008).

16.3.6 Nutraceuticals in Alzheimer's Disease

Alzheimer's disease is a progressive neurodegenerative disorder, and about 26 million people around the world are affected by this disease. It is characterized by the onset of early dementia, followed by Alzheimer's disease and finally leads to death. This disease mostly affects elderly people and to date it is incurable. Certain nutraceutical products such as β-carotene, curcumin, lycopene, and lutein are found to be useful in the attenuation of Alzheimer's disease. Some research claims that several phytochemical extracts such as *Zizyphus jujube* and *Lavandula officinalis* were able to ameliorate memory, and were found active against Alzheimer's disease (Akhondzadeh and Abbasi, 2006, Rabiei et al., 2014).

16.3.7 Nutraceuticals Beneficial in Ophthalmic Disorders

Age-related Macular Degeneration (AMD) is a disease that commonly affects aged people and concomitantly may lead to blindness. AMD can be protected against by the consumption of vitamins and other medicinal plant-origin components like lutein, zeaxanthin, and n-3 fatty acids. Moreover, some strong antioxidants like polyphenolic flavonoids and carotenoids are found active in preventing AMD Astaxanthin, a carotenoid originating from marine animals like salmons, shrimps, and sea bream has the potential for slowing age-related ophthalmic diseases. Another carotenoid namely lutein found in vegetables and fruits, etc. can also be utilized against visual disorders (Nashine et al., 2017, Chew et al., 2022).

16.3.8 Benefits of Nutraceuticals on Gut Microbiome

A few probiotic microorganisms can utilize creatinine, urea, uric acid, and other toxins as nutrients for their growth. They help a higher diffusion of uremic toxins from the blood through the intestine into the bowel. With the help of microbes, enteric toxins can be directly removed from the system. To maintain an effective kidney function, the oral use of probiotics has been clinically tested and reported to be safe, efficient, and with no side effects (Choudhuri et al., 2022).

16.3.9 Nutraceuticals in Allergic Disorders

Allergy is a disorder that occurs because of hypersensitivity in the immune system. This is responsible for various problems in the body extending from irritation to fatal acute respiratory distress. Quercetin is a plant-derived bioactive compound frequently used in nutraceuticals in the control of allergies because of its role in low-density lipoproteins. Eucalyptus essential oil is another putative plant derivative often used as a nutraceutical in attenuating allergic disorders (Nakamura et al., 2020, McCarty et al., 2021).

16.4 REGULATORY AND ETHICAL CONCERNS FOR NANO-NUTRACEUTICALS

A Greek pharmacist, Galen who practiced medicine from 129 to 200 AD, was the first person to recognize the medicinal advantages of herbals, a traditional medical practice (Cheng and Zhen, 2004). Stephen L. DeFelice first used the phrase nutraceuticals in 1989, combining the words "nutrition" and "pharmaceutical" (Kalra, 2003). Nutraceuticals are foods or food components with clearly documented advantageous physiological effects. Contrary to functional foods, which must remain classified as foods (Gulati and Ottaway, 2006), nutraceutical items sometimes straddle the line between the legal classifications of food and drugs.

Because of their higher surface-to-mass ratio compared to bulk materials, nanomaterials (NMs) exhibit distinct functional characteristics. Because of their unique features, NMs are extensively utilized in an array of application domains, providing novel and inventive products for everyday usage. Nanotechnology is being used in the food and agriculture industries, and an increasing proportion of NM-containing commodities are already in the marketplace (Bouwmeester et al., 2014). In recent years, new technical breakthroughs have already created a multibillion-dollar sector, and the worldwide market is predicted to reach $1 trillion by 2015, engaging approximately 2 million people (Roco and Bainbridge, 2001).

The creation of lead compounds for treating various ailments required the use of natural products. In fact, natural products account for 60% of the drugs that are currently on the market. In addition, 80% of people in Asian and African nations rely on phyto drugs for primary health care (Khare, 2004).

Compared to allopathic medicines, the use of phytomedicines has skyrocketed due to their superior efficacy and lack of side effects. Nonetheless, low bioavailability and poor dissolvability in water are the central points, which prevent them from being used to treat and prevent a variety of diseases. Therefore, the issues of phytomedicine's toxicity, solubility, degradation, absorption, and biological response are solved by material nanoscience in the form of nano phytomedicine. Nano phytomedicines are typically made from active phytoconstituents or standard extracts. By combining nanotechnology techniques and transforming them into nano phytomedicine, the biological and therapeutic properties of a number of phytomedicines have been enhanced to new heights (Newman and Cragg, 2007).

Food and food-related applications of nanotechnology aim to (i) enhance sensory perceptions through flavor/color enhancement and texture modification, (ii) boost absorption and targeted delivery of bioactive compounds and nutrients, (iii) stabilize active ingredients like nutraceuticals in food materials, (iv) extend shelf life with packaging technologies, (v) enhance food safety through the use of nano-based sensors and tracers, and (vi) eradicate pathogens. Nanotechnology is being used in food and food-related applications to destroy dangerous microorganisms in food.

The field of nanoscience has undergone rapid growth in recent years. This sector's research and development expenditures are rising in every nation. In addition to posing significant risks to human well-being, life, and the environment, nanotechnology also offers opportunities for technological development and human growth, earning it the title "technology of dual use". Nanomaterials, such as proteins and DNA miRNAs, can enhance both the reactivity of high molecular weight bioactive molecules and the biological activity of drugs containing them, as they can swiftly permeate biological membranes. As a result, NPs may possess toxic properties that pose a threat to animals and humans. Although the European Union (EU) has adopted regulations regarding nanotechnology since 2004, there is still no appropriate regulation. The EU legislation should inform the public of innovative nanotechnology technologies, especially those related to privacy, health, and environmental protection. In addition, the ethics of nanoscience and nanotechnologies are a constant topic of discussion. Due to the relative complexity and cross-talk mechanism of various disorders, as well as the limited clinical efficacy of synthetic drugs, there was justification to use a variety of plants as there is a long and storied history of medical evidence of different communities across human development using them to treat ailments despite not being documented in scholarly texts. Throughout human development, various populations have known about and used plants as herbal medicines (Pottoo et al., 2019).

Also, this approach has the potential to improve novel pharmaceuticals by enhancing selectivity and potency, protecting molecules from thermal or photo-degradation, minimizing adverse effects, and testing the development of active compounds prior to their commercialization or therapeutic application. Due to the advantages they bring, such as altered release strategies and the opportunity to develop novel formulations that were previously unrealistic due to a variety of questions relevant to the active ingredients, the pharmaceutical industry has demonstrated a growing interest in nanotechnological advancements. Despite the benefits of nanotechnology for a number of drugs, there are some drawbacks that must be highlighted. Some other factors, like huge costs and scaling issues, have been discussed by clinical experts. Inhaling simple NPs can cause dangerous lung disorders and other diseases that may shift homeostasis or even lead to death.

16.4.1 Regulatory and Ethical Considerations of Nano-Nutraceuticals

While there have been many new breakthroughs in nanobiotechnology, it may also raise legal concerns. There are no specific laws as yet in place regarding nanotechnology. There is a concern that in the future the general public will disagree and raise concerns due to safety concerns over NP exposure in the workplace, in the surrounding environment, as well as in implementation in human health care. It is, therefore, critical to follow current rules that have been successful in regulating the use of medications and treatments. Nonetheless, this technological field needs clear regulations because there will be many problems that haven't been addressed and will need to be in the near future.

Additionally, human safety must be guaranteed as the primary objective, and it may be done by way of significant judicial rulings. REACH, which refers to registration, evaluation, assessment, authorization, and restrictions on chemicals, is the new EU chemical policy. Some people are concerned that it will be used as a model for monitoring nanotechnology. If this occurs, there may be a shift in the burden of proving safety from the government to the manufacturer. A comparison of EU and US regulatory frameworks for nanotechnology has been published in a summary of present and future EU regulations. The European Medicines Agency's (EMEA) current thinking and actions, which have been prompted by the recent development of nanotechnology-based phytomedicines, highlight the range of phytomedicines based on nanotechnology for human use.(Resnik and Tinkle, 2007).

Under the current regulatory regimes, pharmaceuticals using NPs have already received authorization in the EU and the US. The FDA regulates a variety of goods, including those that may use nanotechnology or include nanomaterials, such as foods, cosmetics, pharmaceuticals, electronics, and veterinary items; nevertheless, the FDA has not yet created an official definition for the term. Clinical uses of novel technologies require FDA approval, and significant regulatory issues may arise during the approval of goods based on nanotechnology. Furthermore, the FDA has a Nanotechnology Working Group whose job is to decide on regulatory tactics to promote the continuous development of unique, secure, and effective FDA-regulated goods that use nanotechnology components (Jain and Jain, 2008).

The FDA asserts that alterations to a food substance's physical and chemical qualities can have an impact on its bioavailability through altered absorption, distribution, metabolism, and excretion. This claim is outlined in the draft for nanotechnology for food guidance. In addition, they concur that such alterations to the substance's biological interactions may have an effect on how severe any negative consequences may potentially be. In the recently issued New Dietary Ingredient (NDI) drafting guideline, the FDA uses nanotechnology as an illustration of a method that could produce a new dietary ingredient that requires notifying the FDA. This is because the FDA may require notice if the procedure causes the ingredient's chemical properties to change or makes it appear as new, which has regulatory repercussions (Javeri, 2016).

Clinical research using nano phytomedicines must generally be conducted in accordance with international and national ethical standards and regulations to advance the development of any products. The study strategy and methodology must follow ethical standards. All ethical issues must be properly discussed, identified, and addressed in accordance with ethical regulations and guidelines, particularly those pertaining to nano phytomedicine's cognition and inherent characteristics. There are different moral issues to be tended to no matter the progression or advancement in research in nanotechnology. Morals are driven by science leading to certain events in which moral perplexity emerges. As moral and administrative perspectives are critical in rehearsing medication, the equivalent is material to nano phytomedicine. Nanobiotechnology products are the subject of clear regulations being developed by the FDA. The FDA will control the improvement of drugs that contain NPs and procedures of medication conveyance as it does for other biopharmaceutical items. It is extremely challenging to address all of the ethical issues associated with novel technologies like nano phytomedicine. However, it would be beneficial to address many of these in advance. The particle size, how it affects human health, how safe it is in the environment, the possibility of unanticipated side effects, and the negative effects of using nano phytomedicine are all common ethical concerns (Sayamov, 2021).

Since, NPs are complicated multi-component 3D structures, meticulous design development, engineering methods, reproducible scaling-up, and manufacturing processes are required to produce a consistent and uniform product. Hence, even a small modification in different borders might have an effect on the security profile.

Also, the effectiveness of NP-based medications necessitates careful evaluation in preclinical and clinical tests. Furthermore, compared to conventional pharmaceuticals, NP-based medications may face more challenging regulatory issues and development challenges (Peng et al., 2018).

Moreover, clinical trials of nanomedicine products have unique challenges in terms of risk management due to the lack of knowledge on the physicochemical properties of nanoscale materials in biological systems, and human-subject communication. On the other hand, products based on nanotechnology are able to get around the limits of traditional approaches. Significant difficulties remain regarding its harmfulness, natural perils, creation cost, and availability to unreachable faraway regions (Benetti et al., 2016).

16.4.2 Regulatory Structure

There is no global regulatory structure for ensuring the safety of food. For food safety and the usage of nanomaterials in food, there are three main qualities that are essential.

The first aspect of the regulation is the "market placement", which can be authorized after a premarket authorization, notification, or direct commercialization, with different safety information standards and made publicly available to consumers. The choice available is typically based on whether to use "novel" foods or components vs. "classic" and already-approved things. In every circumstance, national authorities monitor the post-market situation.

Analyzing a product's effectiveness is the second step. To ensure the safety of food meant for human consumption, every country has put in place a regulatory framework. There is a general agreement regarding the information requirements and approval processes, even if regulations may vary from country to country (including the separation of risk assessment and risk management) (Magnuson et al., 2013) released a review of the regulatory framework for food and the status of NMs regulation in the major industrialized countries, including the EU, USA, Canada, and Australia. The review highlights the definition of NMs, the New Foods rule, the procedures for licensing the commercialization of foods and dietary supplements, and the nanolabeling requirements. Authorization is referred to as both notification and registration.

16.5 NANO-NUTRACEUTICALS TO MANAGE PRE- AND POST-COVID-19 OUTBREAK OR SARS-COV-2 INFECTION

Severe Acute Respiratory Syndrome Coronavirus-2 (SARS-CoV-2) is responsible for the rapid and deadliest pandemic of Coronavirus Disease 2019 (COVID-19). Worldwide, human society experienced the devastating effects of COVID-19 on morbidity, healthcare systems, and the economy. The clinical severity range of SARS-CoV-2 may vary from asymptomatic to severe conditions. Most COVID-19-infected patients suffer mild to acute respiratory distress syndromes with symptoms such as fever, cough, and dyspnea, and in severe cases might lead to multi-organ failure and even death. It is unanimously observed and reported that there is a direct correlation between inflammatory response, the presence of comorbidities, and mortality in COVID-19 patients (Farheen et al., 2021, Scarcella, et al., 2022).

Immune therapy, antiviral, and antimicrobial therapies have been used according to the guidelines for the treatment of the COVID-19 disease. A number of vaccines were used across the world to prevent the disease. However, because of the continuous mutation of COVID-19 and the emergence of new variants, the pandemic is still continuing and spreading. Therefore, there is an urgent need for updated therapeutic strategies. To manage the COVID-19 pandemic, application of bio-nanotechnology is essential to make nano-nutraceuticals against the SARS-CoV-2. In this aspect, rising interest and interventions are established in nutraceutical products, with vitamins (C, D, and E), minerals, prebiotics and probiotics, natural origin products like flavonoids and curcumin, etc. (Dubey et al., 2022).

A large number of patients have suffered from the various post-COVID-19 syndromes. The long COVID syndrome includes diverse clinical manifestations leading to multi-system disease that attacks the central nervous system (CNS), the peripheral nervous system (PNS), and other organs, such as the pulmonary, gastrointestinal, cardiovascular, immunological, endocrine, and renal systems (Carfì et al, 2020, Taquet et al., 2021, Ahamed and Laurence, 2022, Phillips and Williams, 2021, Gholami et al., 2021, Zubair et al., 2020). Among these neurological complications are included prolonged fatigue, cognitive impairments, decline in memory, depression, anosmia, headache, anxiety, myalgias, etc. that can remain for several months or may last for years (Bratosiewicz-Wąsik., 2022, Edinoff et al., 2022, Maury et al., 2021). It is well reported that neurons are highly susceptible to inflammation and (ROS) mediated oxidative stress. Disorders of the cholinergic systems, neuroinflammation, and oxidative stress played a pivotal role in the pathophysiological mechanisms of the post-COVID syndrome (Kopańska et al., 2022, Pliss et al., 2022, Akanchise and Angelova, 2023). Therefore, antioxidant treatment is believed to diminish and prevent oxidative stress. In addition to protection against viral components, a number of antioxidants such as polyphenols showed the potential to prevent the entry of the coronavirus, and are recognized as potent agents to control the SARS-CoV-2 infection (De Flora et al., 2021). Numerous studies have proposed that flavonoids, such as luteolin, quercetin, baicalin, gallocatechin gallate, hesperetin, epigallocatechin gallate, naringenin, taxifolin, catechin, cyanidin, genistein, luteolin-7- glucoside, kaempferol, rutin, and apigenin-7-glucoside, etc. can exhibit a restrictive action against SARS-CoV-2 by binding to essential proteins engaged in the coronavirus infection series such as Mpro, PLpro, 3CLpro, and NTPase /helicase. Therefore, nano-nutraceuticals with antioxidant properties may be useful in decreasing and attenuating complications that appear due to the post-COVID-19 syndrome (Khaerunnisa et al., 2020, Sekiou et al., 2020, Utomo et al., 2020, Tallei et al., 2020, Adem et al., 2022).

Nonetheless, numerous antioxidants have poor bioavailability, instability, and problems of specific delivery on the target area, restricting their medical efficacy. These are major problems of antioxidant agents for controlling and preventing various disorders as consequences of the long COVID-19 disease. To overcome these problems, NPs-based delivery systems, lipid-based NPs, and new nanostructured combinations are employed for better drug delivery, higher pharmacokinetics, and for accurate targeting (Puttasiddaiah et al., 2022). Various nanocarriers, e.g., liposomes, dendrimers, cubosomes, micelles, solid lipid NPs, carbon-based nanostructures, nanoceria, and other inorganic NPs, may be used as promising tools to enhance antioxidant bioavailability (Rakotoarisoa et al., 2022, Satoh et al., 2022). Further, the utilization of specific ligands on the outer surface of NPs to identify receptors of the targeted areas is a novel and innovative approach to enhancing their efficacy (Yayehrad et al., 2021).

Many studies reported that curcumin nanocarriers can control SARS-CoV-2 by the transfer of curcumin to adhere to the S protein, ACE2 receptor, and Mpro of the virus, thus preventing virus replication. Moreover, curcumin nanocarriers can affect the inflammatory response by altering the ER stress and removing ROS (Valizadeh et al., 2020, Dourado et al., 2021). Nanosized natural origin medications have been widely recognized as nano-nutraceuticals. Innovation of highly precise nanoformulations to treat the COVID-19 infection significantly is feasible through the approach of nanotechnology and nanomedicine (Mal'tseva et al., 2022; Akanchise and Angelova, 2023). The potential nutraceuticals are loaded with nanocarriers to facilitate the delivery, thereby significantly contributing to the treatment against the pandemic such as COVID-19 (Yang et al., 2020, Dubey et al., 2022, Ulker et al., 2022).

This chapter summarizes the COVID-19 manifestations and the therapeutic approaches of nutraceuticals in the protection and therapy of the COVID-19 disease and long COVID complications (Catalano et al., 2022). Specific attention is drawn to the potential role of NP-mediated drug-delivery systems involving nano-antioxidants and nanomedicine-based therapies against pre and post-COVID-19 syndromes. The potential NPs and nanoconjugates that can ameliorate COVID-19-induced manifestations are mentioned in Table 16.3

TABLE 16.3
Potential Nanoparticles and Nanoconjugates to Ameliorate COVID-19-Induced Manifestations

Nanosystem	Neurological Condition	Outcome	References
Curcumin-loaded Nanocapsules	Alzheimer's disease	Decreased Ameloid β mediated oxidative stress in the brain. Increased antioxidant SOD and CAT enzymes.	Fidelis et al. (2019)
Sinacurcumin, Curcuminoid Nano micellar	COVID-19	Helps curcuminoids' oral absorption Exert antiviral properties against different viruses	Saber-Moghaddam et al. (2021)
Glycyrrhizic acid (GA) Nanoparticles (GANPs)	COVID-19	Works on the specific target regions of inflammation, in the mouse model of COVID-19 damage Provides significant survival support to sick mice Exerts GANP accumulation and therapeutic efficacy	Zhao et al. (2021)

(*Continued*)

TABLE 16.3 (*Continued*)
Potential Nanoparticles and Nanoconjugates to Ameliorate COVID-19-Induced Manifestations

Nanosystem	Neurological Condition	Outcome	References
Chitosan Nanoparticles	COVID-19	It is used to treat COVID-19-associated digestive problems because of their mucoadhesive characteristics	Cavalcanti et al. (2020), Zuo et al. (2020)
Squalene Nanoparticles,	COVID-19	It reduced pro-inflammatory cytokines and augmented IL-10 and controlled inflammation	Campos et al. (2020)
PLGA-PEG/ Curcumin Nanoparticle Conjugate with B6 Peptide	Alzheimer's disease	Enhanced spatial learning and memory ability of mice model Decreased Ameloid β production as well as accumulation in the hippocampus Decreased tau hyperphosphorylation	Dourado et al. (2021)
Solid Lipid Curcumin	Dysfunctional cognition and mood	Improved cognition and mood	Cox et al. (2015)
Nanostructured Lipid Carriers containing Resveratrol	Ischemic stroke	Diminished infarct volume Increased motor and cognitive function Attenuated neuro-inflammatory and oxidative stress markers Increased antioxidant enzyme activities and Na+, K+, ATPase Inhibited caspases 3 and 9, IL-1β, IL−6, and TNF-α activities	Ashafaq et al. (2021)
Dendrimer-based N-acetylcysteine (NAC)	Neuroinflammation	Decreased neuroinflammation Improved motor function Enhanced myelination and reduced neuronal injury Reduced pro-inflammatory microglia.	Kannan et al. (2012)
Edaravone-loaded Nanoparticles	Cerebral hemorrhage	Enhanced neurological function Decreased edema Attenuated formation and secretion of interleukin and tumor necrosis factor	Dang et al. (2021)
Edaravone-loaded ceria Nanoparticles (E-A/P-CeO_2)	Stroke	Effective blood-brain barrier (BBB) crossing Removal of reactive oxygen species (ROS)	Bao et al. (2018)
Nanoceria	Cytokine storm, mild brain injury	Inhibited inflammatory pathways to protect the multi-organ impairment Improved cognitive recovery and motor function Protected neuronal death and calcium dysregulation	Bailey et al. (2020), Ulker et al. (2022)

16.6 NANOPARTICLES AS A DRUG DELIVERY PLATFORM AND CHALLENGES

Due to their distinctive qualities, such as their large surface area, high stability, and capacity to penetrate cellular barriers, NPs have attracted a lot of attention in the field of medication administration (Bernela et al., 2018). NPs have a number of benefits over traditional drug transport methods, including increased drug solubility, better pharmacokinetics, and decreased toxicity. The use of NPs as medication delivery platforms and the challenges involved will be discussed in the concurrent topics.

NPs can be used as drug delivery platforms by encapsulating drugs within their structures or by attaching drugs onto their surfaces. This makes it possible to transport drugs specifically to the body's target cells or regions (Bertero et al., 2021). Liposomes, dendrimers, and polymeric NPs are just a few of the kinds of NPs that have been considered drug-delivery vehicles.

16.6.1 Current Drug Delivery Systems

i. **Liposomes:** Liposomes are spherical NPs composed of a lipid bilayer that can encapsulate both hydrophilic and hydrophobic drugs. Due to their biocompatibility, capacity to contain a broad variety of medications, and ability to target particular cells or tissues in the body, liposomes have been thoroughly researched as drug delivery platforms (van der Koog et al., 2022, Mishra et al., 2013). Drugs for cancer, infectious illnesses, and circulatory conditions have all been delivered using liposomes.

ii. **Dendrimers:** Dendrimers are highly twisted, resembling trees, NPs that can be created with a great deal of control over their surface characteristics, size, and form. Dendrimers can be functionalized with targeting ligands to increase their selectivity for particular cells or regions and have a high drug-loading capacity. Dendrimers have been investigated for medication administration in neurological conditions, infectious diseases, and malignancy (Yamamoto et al., 2019).

iii. **Polymeric nanoparticle:** Polymeric NPs can be created with a high degree of control over their size, form, and surface characteristics and are made of biocompatible polymers. Polymeric NPs have been investigated for drug transport in cancer, infectious illnesses, and neurodegenerative conditions (Banik et al., 2016). They can be functionalized with targeting ligands.

16.6.2 Lipid-based Nanoparticle System

Lipid-based nanoparticles (LNPs) have emerged as a versatile platform for drug delivery due to their biocompatibility, biodegradability, and ability to encapsulate a wide range of therapeutic payloads. The lipid bilayer that makes up LNPs can be functionalized with targeting molecules to allow the transport of medicines, nucleic acids, and vaccines to particular sites (Tenchov et al., 2021). LNPs' lipid makeup can be adjusted to modify their physical characteristics, such as size, surface charge, and stability, which can affect how well they are absorbed by cells and distributed throughout the body (Javeri, 2016). LNPs have been thoroughly researched for the treatment of cancer because they can be functionalized with targeting ligands to transport chemotherapy drugs to tumor cells only. LNPs have also shown promise for the delivery of gene therapeutics, including small interfering RNA (siRNA) and messenger RNA (mRNA), which can be encapsulated in LNPs to enhance their stability and facilitate their intracellular delivery (Kauffman et al., 2016). LNPs have also been used to create vaccines against infectious illnesses like COVID-19, where they can transport viral antigens to cells that present antigens in order to trigger an immune reaction. The ongoing development of LNPs, a potential drug delivery technology with many biomedical uses, is anticipated to enhance therapeutic results for a variety of illnesses.

16.6.3 Nanoliposome Formulation

Nanoliposomes are lipid-based vesicles that can contain both hydrophilic and hydrophobic molecules. Their typical width ranges from 10 to 100 nm. Among other things, they have been used for the creation of vaccines, gene therapy, and drugs delivery (Hallaj-Nezhadi and Hassan, 2015). One benefit of the nanoliposome formulation is its capacity to shield the molecules it encapsulates from immune system degradation and removal. This makes the drug more bioavailable and less toxic, improving its therapeutic efficacy and safety. Additionally, compared to other delivery methods, nanoliposomes have a high loading capability, which means they can hold more of the substance. By prolonging the period that drugs are in circulation in the body, the nanoliposome formulation can also enhance the pharmacokinetics of medications (Bilal et al., 2021). The concentration of the drug at the target location can be increased and the amount required for successful therapy can be decreased when the nanoliposomes gather in particular tissues or cells. Additionally, nanoliposomes are safe and impermanent, making them well-tolerated by the body and less likely to build up in tissues over time. They are therefore a desirable choice for long-term therapy plans.

i. Solid-core Micelles

   Amphiphilic block copolymers that assemble themselves into a core-shell form in aqueous liquids give rise to solid-core micelles. The micelle's center is made up of the copolymer's hydrophobic block, and its exterior is made up of its hydrophilic block (Rapoport, 2007). Hydrophobic medications can be distributed to specific bodily locations by being enclosed in solid-core micelles.

ii. Nanoemulations

   Another form of colloidal dispersion is a nanoemulsion, which is made of two immiscible substances (typically oil and water) and is stabilized by one or more surfactants (Fernandez et al, 2004). They have a wide range of uses, including manufacturing makeup, medicines, and foods and beverages.

Drugs that are lipophilic can be delivered using nanoemulsions in the setting of nanoliposome composition. While the nanoliposomes can be distributed in the water phase of the nanoemulsion, the lipophilic substance can be dissolved in the oil phase. The nanoemulsion is stabilized and the nanoliposomes are prevented from clustering by the surfactant or a combination of surfactants (Bernela et al., 2018).

iii. Cholecalciferol (vitamin D3) mini-tablets

This is a fat-soluble vitamin that is essential for the metabolism of calcium and bones. The process of formulating cholecalciferol as nanoliposomes is one method to increase its absorption and effectiveness. Cholecalciferol's solubility and uptake can be improved, and nanoliposomes can be used to transport the substance specifically to certain cells or organs.

Cholecalciferol nanoliposomes mini-tablets are prepared by first creating a phospholipid and cholesterol lipid combination. The lipid combination is then used to dissolve cholecalciferol, and the resulting fluid is either sonicated or extruded to create the nanoliposome structure (Liu, 2019). By mixing the nanoliposomes with an appropriate excipient, such as microcrystalline cellulose or lactose, and compressing the resulting combination into tablets of the desired size and form, the nanoliposomes can be further processed to formulate mini-tablets.

iv. Protein-based nanocarriers

Protein-based nanocarriers are a class of drug transport devices made of proteins or peptides that have the capacity to self-assemble into nanoscale structures. A broad variety of medicinal agents, including medications, genes, and sensing agents, can be delivered using these nanocarriers (Delfi et al., 2021).

Protein-based nanocarriers can be integrated into the liposome framework during the formulation of nanoliposomes to produce hybrid nanocarriers with enhanced characteristics. For instance, the protein-based nanocarrier can offer better payload loading, improved targeting, and increased durability.

The first stage in creating protein-based nanocarriers in a nanoliposome formulation is to create the protein or peptide that will act as the nanocarrier's building component. Usually, the self-assembling abilities of this protein or peptide are designed, such as the capacity to create a stable nanoscale structure in solution. Then, to formulate the hybrid nanocarrier, the protein-based nanocarrier is mixed with the phospholipids and other materials needed to make the nanoliposome structure. This mixture is then exposed to high-energy techniques like sonication or extrusion (Assadpour, 2019).

The durability, particle size, and drug release rates of the final protein-based nanocarrier nanoliposome formulation can be assessed. Targeting ligands or other functional groups can be added to the protein-based nanocarrier to allow transport to particular cells or regions. By changing the lipid bilayers or the protein-based nanocarrier's makeup, the drug release rates can be tailored.

16.6.4 Polysaccharide-Based Nanoparticles

Polysaccharide-based NPs are nanosized particles composed of naturally occurring carbohydrates, such as chitosan, cellulose, starch, and hyaluronic acid, which have gained considerable interest in the field of nanotechnology due to their biocompatibility, biodegradability, and low toxicity (Allawadhi et al., 2022). Among other things, these NPs can be applied to tissue engineering, gene therapy, and targeted medication transport.

One of the polymers that has been the subject of the most research is chitosan, which is used to make nanomaterials. Chitosan, a naturally occurring biopolymer is found in the exoskeleton of crustaceans. It has been demonstrated that chitosan NPs have strong mucoadhesive qualities, making them ideal for the transport of drugs to mucosal surfaces (Elieh-Ali-Komi and Hamblin, 2016).

Cellulose is another commonly used polysaccharide for the preparation of NPs. It has been demonstrated that cellulose-based NPs have excellent mechanical resilience and the ability to load drugs, making them ideal for prolonged drug release (Svagan et al., 2007).

Starch-based NPs have also been extensively studied for drug delivery applications. Several techniques, including liquid extraction, emulsification, and nanoprecipitation, can be used to create starch NPs (Wang et al., 2021).

Hyaluronic acid is a natural polysaccharide that is extensively used in tissue engineering and drug delivery. It has been demonstrated that hyaluronic acid NPs have excellent biocompatibility and can be used to transport drugs to cancer cells with precision (Oliveira and Reis, 2011).

16.6.5 Challenges Associated with the Use of Nanoparticles as Drug Delivery Platforms

NPs as drug delivery systems have many benefits, but there are still a number of disadvantages that need to be resolved before they are widely used in therapeutic settings. Following are some of the disadvantages:

i. **Toxicity:** Due to their tiny dimension, large surface area, and propensity to accumulate in specific tissues or systems, NPs can cause toxicity. The physical characteristics of NPs, such as size, form, and surface charge, have a significant impact on their toxicity. Before using NPs for therapeutic uses, researchers must closely consider how toxic they are.
ii. **Biocompatibility:** To prevent tissue injury or negative immune responses, NPs must be safe. To make NPs more biocompatible and less poisonous, the surface composition can be changed.
iii. **Stability:** In physiological settings, NPs can degrade or aggregate, which can impact the effectiveness and timing of drug release. To guarantee NPs' long-term effectiveness, meticulous consideration must be given to their durability.

16.7 NANOPARTICLES FOR ORAL DELIVERY

Oral administration is still the recommended method of administration for the majority of drugs, despite the availability of other routes of administration. Given its ease, ability to be administered by the patient themselves, and extensive flexibility in the dosing schedule, the oral route is associated with the best level of patient compliance, particularly for chronic conditions. Since they don't have to be made in sterile conditions, oral goods are less expensive to make. Oral pharmaceuticals accounted for 38% of the market for drug delivery in North America in 2012, according to data from the sector. By 2018, the market for oral medication delivery is expected to grow to $100 billion from its 2013 forecast of $64.3 billion (Chenthamara et al., 2019).

A medicine is dissolved, entrapped, contained, or coupled to the NP matrix in NPs, which are colloidal particles. Depending on the medication to be enclosed and the qualities of the polymers, NPs can be made using a variety of approaches. NPs have been used frequently in oral drug administration because they can prevent the medication from being broken down by enzymatic and hydrolytic processes in the gastrointestinal (GI) tract, prolong the time the medication spends in the gut through mucoadhesion, and significantly increase drug absorption and bioavailability. Because these medication-entrapped NPs were taken orally, their bioavailability increased. When it comes to cancer treatments, for instance, it was noted that the infamously insoluble medicine paclitaxel was ten times more bioavailable in vivo than Taxol when used in combination with other cancer medications. The best combination of properties can be found in polymer materials: They govern the kinetics of drug release, can be easily changed to display a range of surface-attached ligands, and many polymers have a long history of human safety. They are stable and allow numerous compounds to be loaded to high concentrations (Soppimath et al., 2001).

Oral drug delivery will consequently continue to rule the market and pharmaceutical research. For physiological reasons as well, the oral route is intriguing. The absorptive epithelial cells known as enterocytes have a large surface area (between 300 and 400 m^2) in the GI tract that they use to absorb medicines. Additional GI tract cell types, such as goblet cells that secrete mucin, endocrine cells, Paneth cells, and specialist M cells associated with Peyer's patches that transmit antigen through dendritic cells are all possible candidates for involvement in medicine absorption. The poor bioavailability of taxanes, aminoglycosides, polyene antibiotics, and other medications with these features when taken orally is caused by their lack of physicochemical (solvency, strength), biopharmaceutical (penetrability, metabolic solidity), and hydrophobic and hydrophilic properties (Soppimath et al., 2001).

16.7.1 BIODEGRADABLE NANOPARTICLES FOR ORAL DRUG DELIVERY

Polysaccharides are typical biodegradable hydrophilic polymers that have great biocompatibility for the delivery of oral drugs, including chitosan (CS), alginate, gelatin, dextran, and others. The most common natural polysaccharide, CS, has mucoadhesive properties that enable it to bond with anionic sialic corrosive deposits of the digestive mucosa and reduce transepithelial electrical obstruction by advancing the section of small electrolytes and momentarily opening tight combination between epithelial cells. CS has undergone synthetic alteration to enhance its physicochemical properties, such as watery dissolvability and mucoadhesive and digesting saturation capacities. Chitosan which has been trimethylated (TMC) and also thiolated (CS) has been used in the delivery of oral drugs and has undergone thorough evaluation (Sonia and Sharma, 2012).

The delivery of a variety of pharmacophores, including small atoms like leuprolide, peptide medicines, and anticancer treatments, has been done using these CS and CS subordinate-based frameworks. After this medicine captured NPs were administered orally, and increased gastrointestinal pervasion and bioavailability were achieved. To combine the effects of digestive mucoadhesion as well as penetration enhancement for oral insulin delivery, trimethyl chitosan-cysteine form (TMC-Cys) was added.

The disulfide that forms between TMC-Cys and mucin is mostly responsible for the 2.1–4.7-fold increase in mucoadhesion of TMC-Cys/insulin NPs' compared to TMC/insulin NPs. On the other hand, when combined with insulin administration and TMC NPs, TMC-Cys NPs significantly increased the amount of insulin that reached the mouse digestive system. TMC-Cys NPs were not harmful, according to a biocompatibility analysis. Self-gathered NPs between TMC-Cys and negatively charged protein medicines may be a potential oral delivery system. For the delivery of oral medications, CS is additionally combined with other polysaccharides such as dextran and alginate. Ionotropic polyelectrolyte pre-gelation produced insulin-loaded CS/alginate NPs (Sheng et al., 2015).

16.7.2 Drug Delivery Using Non-Biodegradable Nanoparticles

Oral medication delivery can be carried out using non-biodegradable polymers such as polystyrene, poly (cyanoacrylates), polyethyleneimine, poly(methyl methacrylate) (Eudragit), and poly(methyl methacrylate) (PMMA). Cyclosporin A (CyA)-loaded Eudragit RS and RL NPs were created by Ubrich et al. for the study of oral medication administration (Zhang et al., 2012). They tested in rabbits and compared the oral absorption of CyA from these polymeric NPs to that from the Neoral capsule. In comparison to the 3% achieved after orally administering purified CyA nanospheres to dogs, their bioavailability data showed a considerably higher absorption (Ubrich et al., 2005). Solid lipid nanoparticles (SLNs) are a safe and effective alternative to traditional polymeric NPs since they are made from physiologically acceptable lipids. They also have extra benefits over polymeric NPs and are free of any potential toxicities. SLNs are more stable than other lipid nanocarriers and can tolerate the conditions in the upper GI. In order to increase the oral absorption and bioavailability of hydrophilic medications like insulin and poorly soluble pharmaceuticals like bufalin, risperidone, and puerarin, SLNs have been widely researched. Study findings suggest that the incorporation of weakly hydrophilic medicines into SLNs can increase their oral bioavailability (Ganesan and Narayanasamy, 2017).

16.7.3 Current Approaches in Lipid-Based Nanocarriers for Oral Drug Delivery

Lipid-based nanocarriers represent a substantial advancement in the medication delivery process. Research on lipid-based nanocarriers led to the development of Doxil®, the first nanocarrier approved by the FDA. Among other applications, it is advancing quickly in peptide delivery and malignant development. One of the reasons why these nanocarriers have attracted so much attention over the past few years is due to the exceptional qualities of their lipid components, which include remarkable flexibility, biocompatibility, and low toxicity. Lipid-based nanocarriers can be used to improve the clinical effectiveness of medications with biological constraints like low watery solvency or dependability and to offer alternatives to the parental course. The investigation of oral lipid-based nanocarriers has been boosted by the benefits and accommodations of the oral route, such as its simplicity of organization and high consistency of acceptability (Liu, 2015, Zohuri and Behgounia, 2023).

16.7.4 Oral Medication Delivery Using Polymeric Micelles

Above the critical micellar concentration, surfactants and amphiphilic polymers may combine in colloidal dispersions with aggregates of molecules of 20–100 nm known as micelles. Polymeric micelles offer a lot of opportunities as drug delivery systems for substances with limited bioavailability and hydrophobicity. The stability and bioavailability of poorly soluble drugs are increased when they are integrated into the inner hydrophobic core of micelles (Coimbra et al., 2012). Micelles have drawn a lot of interest as a potential drug carrier for intravenous administration due to their ability to bypass the biological membranes in the human body, such as minimal absorption through the GI tract and a high hepatic first-pass effect (Huang, 2012).

16.7.5 Antioxidant Potential of Nanoparticles

A food or food extract that has been shown to have a positive impact on human health is referred to as a nutraceutical. This is how Western culture has responded to the drawbacks of commonly eaten diets. The term "nutraceuticals" combines the words "nutrition" and "pharmaceutical". It refers to the group of dietary supplements comprising food ingredients, which are considered foods and to which an active therapeutic material has been added in order to have an influence on an individual's health, and food supplements, which are enriched with active substances from a particular food. It is significant to note that, in accordance with an EFSA judgment, it includes those foods that have been labeled with health claims. According to studies, these qualify as nutraceuticals. Several classes of substances, including minerals, trace elements, vitamins, alkaloids, oligo- and polysaccharides, fiber, amino acids, compounds with a proteinaceous composition, fatty acids, lipids, and probiotics are included in the category of nutraceuticals.

All of these substances affect different bodily organs and systems, either directly (by replacing deficient or essential molecules) or indirectly (by interacting with cells and tissues). They frequently function as disease-preventing agents or as supplements for elements that are challenging to receive from regular nourishment. The immunological, gastrointestinal, urogenital, cardiovascular, and central neurological systems, as well as body weight, can all be impacted by nutraceuticals. They can also delay the onset of hormonal imbalances or premature aging (Dini, 2022).

16.7.5.1 Vitamin C

Vitamin C, or l-ascorbic acid, is a water-soluble substance required for survival and preserving physical health. It is extremely sensitive to oxidation and thermolabile and sensitive to light also. Albert Szent-Györgyi, a Hungarian scientist and recipient of the 1937 Nobel Prize in Physiology and Medicine, discovered vitamin C in 1928. People must consume this vitamin, which is synthesized by the majority of animals and plants. The vitamin C content of several fruits and vegetables is high. Vitamin C is not stored by the body; rather, the kidneys remove any extra. The amount of vitamin C in food decreases significantly when it is heated (Gonzalez et al., 2014). Moreover, it encourages the generation of white blood cells, the growth of bones, teeth, and cartilage, as well as the assistance of iron absorption. Moreover, it helps the cell's antioxidant defense by lowering the tocopheryl radical; but, in some circumstances, it might have a prooxidative effect. A daily intake of 90 mg of vitamin C is advised. Scurvy, anemia, hemorrhage, joint swelling, brittle bones, infertility, infections, atrophy, and stomach ulcers are all brought on by avitaminosis. Vitamin C and folic acid (FA)-co-laden liposomes (100–150 nm) were distinguished by improved stability, better entrapment efficiency (EE), and antioxidant characteristics when compared to liposomes loaded with individual vitamins. Vitamin C proliposome powder boosted ex vivo antioxidant activity in brain and hepatic cells and released 90% of the vitamin in 2 hours (Downs et al., 2021).

16.7.5.2 Vitamin B12

The intricate interaction between the central cobalt atom and the four nitrogen atoms of the pyrrole nuclei, which are connected by a corrin ring, forms the basis of the vitamin B12 molecule. Vitamin B12 is required for hematopoiesis, the creation of DNA and ATP, and the efficient operation of the nervous system. Eggs, milk, cheese, and meat are the primary food sources of this vitamin in the diet. Sources of plant food do not contain it. B12 helps the body function properly and lessens the risk of heart disease while also improving memory and concentration (Jampilek, 2020).

16.7.5.3 Phenolic Compounds

Phenolic chemicals have the power to control skin inflammation, wound healing, and barrier homeostasis by scavenging metal ions, inhibiting dangerous free radicals, and promoting the expression of genes that protect against oxidative stress. However, the low levels of solubility, poor gastrointestinal stability, minimal absorption, and lack of target selectivity in the human body limit their application.

To improve the transport and bioavailability of polyphenols, a variety of nanosystems are used, such as nanocapsules, solid lipid NPs, niosomes, and microemulsions. For instance, polymeric nanocapsule suspensions are employed as a component in semisolid formulations or topical formulations that are applied directly to the skin.

Epigallocatechin-3-gallate is enclosed in chitosan-tripolyphosphate NPs, whereas curcumin is loaded into chitosan particles and methoxyPEG-palmitate nanocapsules (Pisoschi and Pop, 2015).

16.7.5.4 Coenzyme Q10 (CoQ10)

Humans may produce the antioxidant coenzyme Q10 (CoQ10), which is utilized in cosmetics to stop photoaging. It has been demonstrated to serve as a radical scavenger and protect DNA and lipids from oxidative damage. Liposomes, lipid NPs, and solid NPs have all been used to increase the product's penetration into the skin's deeper layers. CoQ10 has been added to SLNs, nanoemulsions, and hydrogels in a number of trials to enhance skin elasticity and hydration and lessen the impacts of UVB radiation. It has also been demonstrated that vitamin E and CoQ10 caprolactone nanocapsules can lessen the effects of UVB radiation (Vinardell and Mitjans, 2015).

16.7.5.5 Terpenoids (Isoprenoids)

Terpenes, tocopherols, tocotrienols, retinol-encapsulated chitosan NPs, alpha-tocopherol and tocopherol acetate, and fullerene nanocapsules are just a few of the substances that are covered in this section along with their properties and applications. Terpenes are supposed to partition into fatty membranes in response to free radicals. Because of their ability to condition the skin and act as antioxidants, tocopherols are employed in cosmetic compositions. Tocopherol is a skin irritant and light-sensitive liquid; thus, it is combined with nanocarriers to create a formulation that is aesthetically pleasing. Tocotrienols are employed in skincare and oral care, and the most common form of vitamin E found in commercial sunscreen and skin-care products is tocopherol acetate. Both alpha-tocopherol and tocopherol acetate are used to create supplements and are generally accepted as safe dietary components. Fullerene nanocapsules containing vitamin E and ascorbic acid are used to improve skin protective activity against premature aging.

16.7.5.6 Carotenoids (Alpha-Carotene, Beta-Carotene, Lycopene, Phytoene, and Phytofluene)

It has been demonstrated that carotenoids, such as astaxanthin, beta-carotene, zeaxanthin, phytoene, and phytofluene, offer protection against cancer, cardiovascular illnesses, and eye and skin conditions. The differentiation and proliferation of skin cells is another function of retinoic acid and its derivatives. Carotenoids function as UV photoprotective agents, enhancing skin health and reducing hyperpigmentation. To enhance its anti-wrinkle properties, astaxanthin was incorporated into NPs, where it particularly boosts antioxidant enzyme activity and inhibits tyrosinase activity. Beta-carotene shields the skin against wrinkling and flaccidity while defending against sunlight. Zeaxanthin increases the hydration and flexibility of the skin, while phytoene and phytofluene lighten the skin. Generally, carotenoid intake reduces skin pigmentation and yellowness (Meléndez-Martínez et al., 2019).

Amino acid N-acetylcysteine (NAC) is a powerful antioxidant and free radical scavenger. It acts as a starting point for the production of glutathione (GSH), which controls intracellular levels of the antioxidant GSH. NAC can suppress the NF-B pathway and the release of inflammatory cytokines, as well as interact with other free radicals to lower ROS levels. NAC has been proven to be able to suppress the mitogen-activated protein kinase (MAPK) pathway and reverse CoNP-induced cell death, and in vivo, experiments on rats have shown that it can repair the harm that TiO_2-NPs have caused to testicular tissue, as well as raise GSH and testosterone levels while lowering lipid peroxidation. NAC has a lot of potential to be an antioxidant in conditions of oxidative stress brought on by NPs.

L-arginine (Arg), a different amino acid that is classified as conditionally necessary, can be used to relieve NP-induced toxicities. Rats were used as a model organism in a recent in vivo investigation by (Abdelhalim et al., 2013). They received treatment with gold nanoparticles (AuNPs), and measurements of important indicators (ALP, ALT, GGT, total protein, MDA, and GSH) allowed for the assessment of the degree of oxidative stress. Significant hepatotoxicity was brought on by the administration of AuNP, and oxidative stress levels rose. The usage of arginine was found to be very effective in reducing all oxidative stress indices, acting as a protective mechanism against the impact of AuNPs.

16.7.5.7 Organosulfur Compounds

Sulfur atoms are present in a variety of functional groups in organic molecules known as organosulfur compounds. These substances have a variety of biological actions, such as anti-atherosclerotic, antifungal, antimicrobial, immunostimulatory, and antithrombotic properties. As skin conditioners and antioxidants, they are utilized in cosmetic compositions. It is known that certain organosulfur compounds can improve the glutathione/glutathione disulfide ratio in B16 cells by inhibiting the production of melanin and tyrosinase. These substances can be supplied using NPs and pegylated liposomes, and they have been utilized in anti-dandruff shampoos. Moreover, it has been demonstrated that sulforaphane and broccoli extract, which are high in glucosinolates, reduce the risk of skin lesions brought on by UV radiation, while allicin inhibits leukocyte elastase and delays the onset of premature aging (Dini, 2022).

16.7.6 Applications of Nanoparticles in Medicine

Nanomedicine is a branch of nanotechnology that applies nanomaterials and nanoscale electronic biosensors to the study of health and medicine. It has the potential to treat a number of complex disorders, such as diabetes, cancer, Parkinson's disease, Alzheimer's disease, cardiovascular diseases, and multiple sclerosis. It provides advantages like enhanced diagnosis, appropriate treatment, and follow-up of diseases, as well as early detection and prevention. For quick and accurate biological testing, NPs can be utilized as labels and tags. Gene sequencing can be done using gold nanoparticles. The advancement of tissue engineering, which may revolutionize organ transplantation and artificial implants, is made possible by the ability of nanotechnology to help heal and replicate damaged tissue.

The use of nanotechnology to interact with biological molecules at the micro size is the basis of the relatively young scientific and technological subject known as nanomedicine. Both inside human cells and in the extracellular media, this contact is possible. Using nanodevices enables the exploitation of physical characteristics, such as the volume/surface ratio, that are distinct from those seen at the micro size. The use of gold nanoshells to diagnose and treat cancer and the use of liposomes as vaccine adjuvants and drug delivery vehicles are two examples of nanomedicine that have already been tested in mice and are awaiting human trials. Rats that were being drug-detoxified were successfully treated with nanomedicine.

16.7.6.1 Application in Drug Delivery

By enhancing treatment efficacy and lowering their hazardous side effects, NPs have changed medicine delivery. One of the best examples of a medicine made with NPs is Abraxane, which is used to treat breast cancer. Several studies have shown that NPs have the ability to deliver medications to tumors more precisely and effectively. For instance, in a mouse study conducted at Rice University and the University of Texas MD Anderson Cancer Center, carbon NPs were employed to increase the delivery of paclitaxel to head and neck cancer cells by displacing the hazardous Cremophor EL. Similar to this, Case Western Reserve University delivered doxorubicin to breast cancer cells via a chain of NPs. This made it possible to release the medicine selectively using a radiofrequency field, which led to more efficient tumor growth inhibition with less damage to healthy cells. These studies demonstrate how NPs may enhance medicine delivery for the treatment of cancer.

Targeting certain bodily regions and minimizing negative effects are achieved through the use of nanotechnology in medicine delivery. Small medicinal molecules are transported using a variety of NPs, including dendrimers and micelles. For the release of active drugs, nano-electromechanical systems are also utilized. Targeted medicine lowers medication costs and drug usage. Nanoengineered tools, such as nanorobots, are used for molecular targeting in order to administer medications with cellular accuracy. Another application for NPs as a contrast for magnetic resonance imaging (MRI) and ultrasound is in vivo imaging. The creation of biocompatible nanotechnology can identify malignant cells, assess the severity of the condition, and create reports that can guide appropriate treatment. Self-assembling nanodevices can be developed to treat ailments and diseases like cancer thanks to breakthroughs in nanotechnology.

In order to minimize side effects and lower treatment costs, site-specific drug delivery utilizes NPs such as dendrimers, nanoporous materials, and micelles. Drug bioavailability can be increased and medications can be delivered to cells precisely by employing molecular targeting on nanoengineered devices, such as nanorobots. NP contrast for in vivo imaging is also being developed. Self-assembling biocompatible nanodevices can be made to identify and treat malignant cells as well as generate reports thanks to breakthroughs in nanotechnology. In general, nanotechnology is transforming the practice of medicine by offering patients efficient treatment alternatives while also lowering patient expenditures and discomfort.

16.7.6.2 Use in DNA Sequencing DNA

This can be swiftly and precisely sequenced using nanopores. Low copy number DNA can be distinguished by the passage of DNA through nanopores. This idea was first demonstrated using a collection of cylindrical gold nanotubules.

Both pyrimidine and purine nucleotide bases along a single RNA molecule, as well as DNA strands of equal length and composition that differ only in base pair sequence, can be distinguished using nanopores. Furthermore, DNA nanopores can be used to discriminate between individual DNA strands that are up to 30 nucleotides long and differ only by a single base substitution. This technique has been utilized to push RNA and DNA polymers via a protein channel called alpha-hemolysin placed in a core nanopore of a lipid bilayer, even in electric fields (Yezdani et al., 2018).

16.7.6.3 Applications in Stem Cell Biology and Medicine

Modern biosensors with unique properties can be made using carbon nanotubes. These biosensors are useful for astrobiology and can shed light on the origins of life. Furthermore, sensors for cancer diagnostics are being developed using this technology.

CNT (carbon nanotube) is latent, but a test particle may very likely functionalize it at the tip.

Fantastic progress has been achieved in the study of undifferentiated cells thanks to nanotechnology. For instance, magnetic nanoparticles (MNPs) have been employed (Nikalje, 2015) for many cellular biotechnology related applications.

In tracking and visualizing stem cells for research purposes, nanotechnology can be used. Both translational medicine and basic science can benefit from using it. By combining biological molecules with nanocarriers, stem cells can be altered. Nanotechnology can be employed for intracellular access, intelligent biomolecule delivery, and biomolecule sensing. These innovations significantly influence research on the stem cell microenvironment and tissue engineering, and they have a lot of potential for use in biological applications (Ricardo and Lino, 2010).

16.7.6.4 Use in Cancer Therapy

NPs, especially in imaging, can be very useful in oncology because of their small size. MRI can be combined with NPs like quantum dots that have quantum confinement qualities like size-tunable light emission to create outstanding images of tumor locations. NPs are significantly brighter than organic colors and only require one light source to be excited. Hence, using fluorescent quantum dots as contrast media could result in a stronger contrast image at a lesser cost than using organic dyes. However, the materials used to make quantum dots are frequently highly hazardous. Due to their unusually high surface area to volume ratio, NPs can attach a variety of functional groups, which then bind to specific tumor cells. Additionally, because tumors lack a functional lymphatic drainage system, NPs with a size of 10–100 nm can preferentially aggregate at tumor locations (Nikalje, 2015).

Future cancer treatments may make use of multifunctional NPs that can photograph, detect, and then treat tumors. With the help of radio waves that only heat the NPs and the nearby (cancerous) cells, Kanzius RF therapy "cooks" tumors inside the body by attaching small NPs to cancer cells (Yezdani et al., 2018).

16.7.6.5 Use in Parkinsonism

Parkinson's disease (PD) is a widespread neurological condition that impairs movement, but current treatments merely enhance functional capability and do not slow the disease's progression. The development of innovative technologies for directed axon growth and active signaling signals for neuroprotection are the main goals of nanotechnology research (Wong et al., 2012). An approach being investigated involves using an intracranial nano-enabled scaffold device (NESD) for site-specific dopamine delivery to the brain, which may reduce the peripheral side effects of traditional medication. Further being researched for CNS illnesses are peptides and peptidic NPs (Yezdani et al., 2018).

Application to Alzheimer's Disease: Early detection and treatment of Alzheimer's disease, which affects over 35 million people globally, have been made possible through the application of nanotechnology. To target circulating amyloid forms and create a "sink effect" to alleviate the disease, NPs with great selectivity for brain capillary endothelial cells have been developed. With the development of immunological sensors, scanning tunneling microscopy techniques, and ultrasensitive NP-based bio-barcodes that can detect A1–40 and A1–42, in vitro diagnostics for AD have made significant strides. NPs may be useful in the therapy of Alzheimer's disease, according to recent studies (Brambilla et al., 2011, Nikalje, 2015).

16.7.6.6 Use in Operative Dentistry

Nanotechnology is the process of making and using objects at the atomic and molecular level, and it is thought that materials made of nano-filled composite resin have outstanding wear resistance, strength, and aesthetics for use in dentistry. By increasing the load of the inorganic phase and improving its mechanical properties, nanofillers are used (Sivaramakrishnan and Neelakantan, 2014). In terms of operational dentistry, nano-filled micro hybrid composites are the greatest alternative. Non-agglomerated discrete NPs are evenly dispersed in resins or coatings to produce nanocomposites with better hardness, flexural strength, modulus of elasticity, decreased polymerization shrinkage, and excellent handling properties. Aluminosilicate powder, which has an alumina-to-silica ratio of 1:4 M and a refractive index of 1.508, is the nanofiller used (Nikalje, 2015).

16.7.6.7 Use in Tuberculosis

Due to the lengthy period of therapy and heavy pill load, which has resulted in the establishment of multi-drug-resistant (MDR) strains, tuberculosis (TB) is a deadly infectious illness that poses considerable hurdles.

The absence of first-line drugs in pediatric formulations further exacerbates the issue, necessitating the development of novel antibiotics that can surmount drug resistance, shorten treatment duration, and minimize interactions with antiretroviral therapies. Nanotechnology offers a promising avenue for the creation of more efficient and user-friendly medications. Recent advancements in nanotechnology-based drug delivery systems that encapsulate and dispense anti-TB drugs have the potential to enhance the effectiveness and accessibility of TB pharmacotherapy while being affordable (Yezdani et al., 2018).

16.7.6.8 Use in Ophthalmology

With the aid of nanodevices and nanostructures, the discipline of nanomedicine seeks to enhance human biological systems at the molecular level. Nanotechnology can be used in ophthalmology to produce prosthetics and regenerative medicine, as well as to treat a number of disorders including oxidative stress, glaucoma, and retinal degenerative disease. For the treatment of severe evaporative dry eye, a novel nanoscale-dispersed eye ointment (NDEO) that is stable and safe for ocular use has been effectively created (Zhang et al., 2014). Recent studies have demonstrated the potential for ocular drug administration and therapy using diverse nanoparticulate systems. Nanotechnology can also be employed for nanodiagnostics and nanoimaging. The application of nanotechnology in ophthalmology is anticipated to revolutionize drug delivery and postoperative scarring and may offer a treatment option for people with blindness by recovering their vision from retinal degenerative disease (Sahoo et al., 2008)

16.7.6.9 By Visualization

The distribution of drugs and their metabolism can be studied by monitoring mobility. Scientists used colored cells to follow how they moved around the body. These dyes are energized by light to shine at a certain wavelength. Different numbers of cells were colored using luminescent tags. These tags are proteins with attached quantum dots that can cross cell membranes. There were different-sized specks made of bio-inert material. As a result, sizes are chosen so that one set of quantum dots fluoresces while another group incandesces at the same light frequency. As a result, a single source of light can illuminate both groups (Yezdani et al., 2018).

16.7.6.10 Use in Tissue Engineering

Nanotechnology can be used in tissue engineering to create new tissues or repair damaged ones. In organ transplants or artificial implantation therapy, the use of appropriate scaffolds and growth factors based on nanomaterials can artificially increase cell multiplication and lengthen life (Nikalje, 2015).

16.8 FUTURE TRENDS AND PROSPECTS

The main advantages of nano-nutraceuticals are that they can enhance the bioavailability and efficacy of bioactive compounds. Additionally, the weakly soluble bioactive substances' stability and solubility can be greatly improved by nano-nutraceuticals, which can improve their delivery and absorption in the body (Puttasiddaiah et al., 2022, Bhatia and Bhatia, 2016). Furthermore, nano-nutraceuticals may be created to discharge bioactive substances gradually, which may enhance their therapeutic benefits.

Nano-nutraceuticals' potential applications in health are numerous and exciting. The following are some possible uses for nano-nutraceuticals:

i. **Cancer treatment:** Chemotherapy can be made more effective and less harmful by delivering medicinal substances directly to tumor cells using nano-nutraceuticals.
ii. **Cardiovascular health:** Bioactive substances, such as omega-3 fatty acids and polyphenols, can be delivered using nano-nutraceuticals to lower the chance of arterial illnesses.

iii. **Neurodegenerative illnesses:** Bioactive substances, such as curcumin and resveratrol, can be delivered using nano-nutraceuticals to enhance brain health and lower the chance of neurodegenerative diseases.
iv. **Diabetes management:** Bioactive substances like berberine and quercetin can be delivered using nano-nutraceuticals to enhance insulin sensitivity and glucose metabolism.
v. **Immune system modulation:** Bioactive substances like probiotics and prebiotics can be delivered via nano-nutraceuticals to regulate the immune system and enhance general health.

Although there is a lot of potential for using nano-nutraceuticals in medicine, more study is needed to completely grasp their efficacy and safety. The following list includes some of the present study gaps concerning nano-nutraceuticals in medicine:

I. Dearth of standardized methods for the production and classification of nano-nutraceuticals: The synthesis and characterization of nano-nutraceuticals differ greatly, and there is a dearth of standardized methods for these processes. This can produce erratic findings and make it difficult to compare various research.
II. Limited knowledge of the metabolism and biodistribution of nano-nutraceuticals: The body's processes for absorbing, dispersing, metabolizing, and excreting nano-nutraceuticals are poorly understood. This is important to know in order to administer nano-nutraceuticals at the proper dose and time.
III. Insufficiency of long-term safety statistical data: Despite the fact that nano-nutraceuticals are usually regarded as safe, their safety must be assessed over an extended period of time in order to identify any possible side effects.
IV. Limited knowledge of the mechanism of action of nano-nutraceuticals: At the molecular and cellular levels, it is important to comprehend the mode of action of nano-nutraceuticals. This will make it easier to pinpoint their precise targets and maximize their use in various therapy contexts.
V. Inconsistencies in reporting and data analysis: Studies employing nano-nutraceuticals have inconsistent reporting and data analysis. As a result, comparing the findings of various research and coming to useful conclusions may be challenging.

Addressing these research gaps will be crucial to further advance the development and application of nano-nutraceuticals in medicine.

16.9 CONCLUSIONS

NPs have the potential to revolutionize drug delivery by improving drug solubility, pharmacokinetics, and reducing toxicity. Before being widely used in therapeutic uses, drug delivery platforms like liposomes, dendrimers, and polymeric NPs have undergone significant research and development. Before using NPs for therapeutic uses, researchers must closely consider the toxicity, biocompatibility, and stability of those particles. NPs continue to be a hopeful instrument for targeted medication delivery in a variety of illnesses despite these difficulties.

The biological efficacy of biologically active compounds and nutraceuticals, as well as their advantageous action for keeping a healthy lifestyle, were the primary topics of this chapter. Natural-source nutraceutical substances can cure a variety of maladies, including inflammation, cancer, and cardiovascular conditions. We also discussed the hopeful role that food technology could play in the sustained release and tailored delivery of nutraceuticals and bioactive substances, as well as their protection from harsh environments through the use of different nanofabricated delivery systems. Numerous delivery methods, including those involving proteins, lipids, nanoemulsions, and liposome-mediated transport systems, have attracted scientific attention and helped researchers overcome many of the drawbacks associated with the use of nutraceuticals. However, regulatory agencies like the EFSA, EMA, and FDA require companies to conduct extensive safety testing on nanofabricated materials and to provide detailed information about the properties of these materials. This information helps regulators evaluate the safety of new products and technologies and ensures that they benefit humanity and keep a standard level of living. It is also important for preserving or enhancing dietary components, flavor, and taste as well as for curing different diseases.

REFERENCES

Abdelhalim, M.A., Moussa, S.A., 2013. The biochemical changes in rats' blood serum levels exposed to different gamma radiation doses. *African Journal of Pharmacy and Pharmacology*, *7*(15), pp. 785–92.

Adem, Ş., Eyupoglu, V., Ibrahim, I.M., Sarfraz, I., Rasul, A., Ali, M. and Elfiky, A.A., 2022. Multidimensional in silico strategy for identification of natural polyphenols-based SARS-CoV-2 main protease (Mpro) inhibitors to unveil a hope against COVID-19. *Computers in Biology and Medicine*, *145*, p. 105452.

Ahamed, J. and Laurence, J., 2022. Long COVID endotheliopathy: Hypothesized mechanisms and potential therapeutic approaches. *The Journal of Clinical Investigation*, *132*(15), e161167.

Akanchise, T. and Angelova, A., 2023. Potential of nano-antioxidants and nanomedicine for recovery from neurological disorders linked to long COVID syndrome. *Antioxidants*, *12*(2), p. 393.

Akhondzadeh, S. and Abbasi, S.H., 2006. Herbal medicine in the treatment of Alzheimer's disease. *American Journal of Alzheimer's Disease & Other Dementias®*, *21*(2), pp. 113–118.

Algan, A.H., Gungor-Ak, A. and Karatas, A., 2022. Nanoscale delivery systems of lutein: An updated review from a pharmaceutical perspective. *Pharmaceutics*, *14*(9), p. 1852.

Al-Khalaifah, H., 2020. Modulatory effect of dietary polyunsaturated fatty acids on immunity, represented by phagocytic activity. *Frontiers in Veterinary Science*, *7*, p. 569939.

Allawadhi, P., Singh, V., Govindaraj, K., Khurana, I., Sarode, L.P., Navik, U., Banothu, A.K., Weiskirchen, R., Bharani, K.K. and Khurana, A., 2022. Biomedical applications of polysaccharide nanoparticles for chronic inflammatory disorders: Focus on rheumatoid arthritis, diabetes and organ fibrosis. *Carbohydrate Polymers*, *281*, p. 118923.

Ansari, S.H., Islam, F. and Sameem, M., 2012. Influence of nanotechnology on herbal drugs: A Review. *Journal of Advanced Pharmaceutical Technology & Research*, *3*(3), p. 142.

Ashafaq, M., Alam, M.I., Khan, A., Islam, F., Khuwaja, G., Hussain, S., Ali, R., Alshahrani, S., Makeen, H.A., Alhazmi, H.A. and Al Bratty, M., 2021. Nanoparticles of resveratrol attenuates oxidative stress and inflammation after ischemic stroke in rats. *International Immunopharmacology*, *94*, p. 107494.

Assadpour, E. and Mahdi Jafari, S., 2019. A systematic review on nanoencapsulation of food bioactive ingredients and nutraceuticals by various nanocarriers. *Critical Reviews in Food Science and Nutrition*, *59*(19), pp. 3129–3151.

Bailey, Z.S., Nilson, E., Bates, J.A., Oyalowo, A., Hockey, K.S., Sajja, V.S.S.S., Thorpe, C., Rogers, H., Dunn, B., Frey, A.S. and Billings, M.J., 2020. Cerium oxide nanoparticles improve outcome after in vitro and in vivo mild traumatic brain injury. *Journal of Neurotrauma*, *37*(12), pp. 1452–1462.

Banik, B.L., Fattahi, P. and Brown, J.L., 2016. Polymeric nanoparticles: The future of nanomedicine. *Wiley Interdisciplinary Reviews: Nanomedicine and Nanobiotechnology*, *8*(2), pp. 271–299.

Bao, Q., Hu, P., Xu, Y., Cheng, T., Wei, C., Pan, L. and Shi, J., 2018. Simultaneous blood–brain barrier crossing and protection for stroke treatment based on edaravone-loaded ceria nanoparticles. *ACS Nano*, *12*(7), pp. 6794–6805.

Basak, S. and Gokhale, J., 2022. Immunity boosting nutraceuticals: Current trends and challenges. *Journal of Food Biochemistry*, *46*(3), p. e13902.

Behradmanesh, S. and Nasri, H., 2013. Association of serum calcium with level of blood pressure in type 2 diabetic patients. *Journal of Nephropathology*, *2*(4), p. 254.

Benetti, F., Micheletti, C. and Manodori, L., 2016. Regulatory perspectives on nanotechnology in nutraceuticals. In *Nutraceuticals* (pp. 183–230). Available at: https://doi.org/10.1016/b978-0-12-804305-9.00006-3.

Bernela, M., Kaur, P., Ahuja, M. and Thakur, R., 2018. Nano-based delivery system for nutraceuticals: The potential future. In: Suresh Kumar Gahlawat, Joginder Singh Duhan, Raj Kumar Salar, Priyanka Siwach, Suresh Kumar, and Pawan Kaur (eds.) *Advances in Animal Biotechnology and Its Applications* (pp. 103–117). Springer Nature, Singapore.

Bertero, A., Fossati, P., Coccini, T., Spicer, L.J. and Caloni, F., 2021. Application of "nano" nutraceuticals in medicine. In: Ramesh C. Gupta, Rajiv Lall, and Ajay Srivastava (eds.) *Nutraceuticals* (pp. 263–270). Academic Press, WI, United States.

Bhatia, S. and Bhatia, S., 2016. Nanoparticles types, classification, characterization, fabrication methods and drug delivery applications. In *Natural Polymer Drug Delivery Systems: Nanoparticles, Plants, and Algae* (pp. 33–93). Springer International Publishing, Switzerland.

Bilal, M., Qindeel, M., Raza, A., Mehmood, S. and Rahdar, A., 2021. Stimuli-responsive nanoliposomes as prospective nanocarriers for targeted drug delivery. *Journal of Drug Delivery Science and Technology*, *66*, p. 102916.

Borek, C., 2006. Garlic reduces dementia and heart-disease risk. *The Journal of Nutrition*, *136*(3), pp. 810S–812S.

Bouwmeester, H., Brandhoff, P., Marvin, H.J., Weigel, S. and Peters, R.J., 2014. State of the safety assessment and current use of nanomaterials in food and food production. *Trends in Food Science & Technology*, *40*, pp. 200–210.

Bragazzi, N.L., Martini, M., Saporita, T.C., Nucci, D., Gianfredi, V., Maddalo, F., Di Capua, A., Tovani, F. and Marensi, L., 2017. Nutraceutical and functional food regulations in the European Union. In: Debasis Bagchi and Sreejayan Nair (eds.) *Developing New Functional Food and Nutraceutical Products* (pp. 309–322). Academic Press, WI, USA.

Brambilla, D., Le Droumaguet, B., Nicolas, J., Hashemi, S.H., Wu, L.P., Moghimi, S.M., Couvreur, P. and Andrieux, K., 2011. Nanotechnologies for Alzheimer's disease: Diagnosis, therapy and safety issues. *Nano Medicine: Nanotechnology, Biology and Medicine*, *7*, pp. 521–540.

Bratosiewicz-Wąsik, J., 2022. Neuro-COVID-19: An insidious virus in action. *Neurologia i Neurochirurgia Polska*, *56*(1), pp. 48–60.

Butt, M.S., Sultan, M.T., Butt, M.S. and Iqbal, J., 2009. Garlic: Nature's protection against physiological threats. *Critical Reviews in Food Science and Nutrition*, *49*(6), pp. 538–551.

Buya, A., 2023. Nanosystems trends in nutraceutical delivery. In: Raj K. Keservani, Rajesh Kumar Kesharwani, and Anil K. Sharma (eds.) *Advances in Novel Formulations for Drug Delivery* (pp. 97–125). Scrivener Publishing LLC, Beverly, MA.

Cabral, E.M., Mondala, J.R.M., Oliveira, M., Przyborska, J., Fitzpatrick, S., Rai, D.K., Sivagnanam, S.P., Garcia-Vaquero, M., O'Shea, D., Devereux, M. and Tiwari, B.K., 2021. Influence of molecular weight fractionation on the antimicrobial and anticancer properties of a fucoidan rich-extract from the macroalgae *Fucus vesiculosus*. *International Journal of Biological Macromolecules*, *186*, pp. 994–1002.

Campos, E.V., Pereira, A.E., De Oliveira, J.L., Carvalho, L.B., Guilger-Casagrande, M., De Lima, R. and Fraceto, L.F., 2020. How can nanotechnology help to combat COVID-19? Opportunities and urgent need. *Journal of Nanobiotechnology*, *18*(1), pp. 1–23.

Carfì, A., Bernabei, R. and Landi, F., 2020. Gemelli against COVID-19 post-acute care study group. Persistent symptoms in patients after Acute COVID-19. *JAMA*, *324*(6), pp. 603–605.

Catalano, A., Iacopetta, D., Ceramella, J., Maio, A.C.D., Basile, G., Giuzio, F., Bonomo, M.G., Aquaro, S., Walsh, T.J., Sinicropi, M.S. and Saturnino, C., 2022. Are nutraceuticals effective in COVID-19 and post-COVID prevention and treatment? *Foods*, *11*(18), p. 2884.

Cavalcanti, I.D.L. and Cajuba de Britto Lira Nogueira, M., 2020. Pharmaceutical nanotechnology: Which products are been designed against COVID-19? *Journal of Nanoparticle Research*, *22*(9), p. 276.

Chandra, S., Saklani, S., Kumar, P., Kim, B. and Coutinho, H.D., 2022. Nutraceuticals: Pharmacologically active potent dietary supplements. *BioMed Research International*, *2022*, p. 2051017.

Cheng, Z. and Zhen, C., 2004. *The Cheng Zhi-Fan Collectanea of Medical History*. Peking University Medical Press, Beijing.

Chenthamara, D., Subramaniam, S., Ramakrishnan, S.G., Krishnaswamy, S., Essa, M.M., Lin, F.H. and Qoronfleh, M.W., 2019. Therapeutic efficacy of nanoparticles and routes of administration. *Biomaterials Research*, *23*(1), pp. 1–29.

Chew, E.Y., Clemons, T.E., Agrón, E., Domalpally, A., Keenan, T.D., Vitale, S., Weber, C., Smith, D.C., Christen, W., SanGiovanni, J.P. and Ferris, F.L., 2022. Long-term outcomes of adding lutein/zeaxanthin and ω-3 fatty acids to the AREDS supplements on age-related macular degeneration progression: AREDS2 report 28. *JAMA Ophthalmology*, *140*(7), pp. 692–698.

Choudhuri, S., Panda, J. and Maitra, S., 2022. Influence of gut microbial flora in body's serotonin turnover and associated diseases. In: Debasis Bagchi and Bernard William Downs (eds.) *Microbiome, Immunity, Digestive Health and Nutrition* (pp. 245–264). Academic Press, Oxford.

Cicero, A.F.G., Fogacci, F., Bove, M., Giovannini, M. and Borghi, C., 2019. Three-arm, placebo-controlled, randomized clinical trial evaluating the metabolic effect of a combined nutraceutical containing a bergamot standardized flavonoid extract in dyslipidemic overweight subjects. *Phytotherapy Research*, *33*(8), pp. 2094–2101.

Coimbra, M., Rijcken, C.J.F., Stigter, M., Hennink, W.E., Storm, G. and Schiffelers, R.M., 2012. Antitumor efficacy of dexamethasone-loaded core-crosslinked polymeric micelles. *Journal of Controlled Release*, *163*(3), pp. 361–367.

Cox, K.H., Pipingas, A. and Scholey, A.B., 2015. Investigation of the effects of solid lipid curcumin on cognition and mood in a healthy older population. *Journal of Psychopharmacology*, *29*(5), pp. 642–651.

Da Costa, J.P., 2017. A current look at nutraceuticals–Key concepts and future prospects. *Trends in Food Science & Technology*, *62*, pp. 68–78.

Daliu, P., Santini, A. and Novellino, E., 2019. From pharmaceuticals to nutraceuticals: Bridging disease prevention and management. *Expert Review of Clinical Pharmacology*, *12*(1), pp. 1–7.

Dang, L., Dong, X. and Yang, J., 2021. Influence of nanoparticle-loaded edaravone on post-operative effects in patients with cerebral hemorrhage. *Journal of Nanoscience and Nanotechnology*, *21*(2), pp. 1202–1211.

De Flora, S.I.L.V.I.O., Balansky, R. and La Maestra, S.E.B.A.S.T.I.A.N.O., 2021. Antioxidants and COVID-19. *Journal of Preventive Medicine and Hygiene*, *62*(1 Suppl 3), p. E34.

DeFelice, S.L., 1995. The nutraceutical revolution: Its impact on food industry R&D. *Trends in Food Science & Technology*, *6*(2), pp. 59–61.

Delfi, M., Sartorius, R., Ashrafizadeh, M., Sharifi, E., Zhang, Y., De Berardinis, P., Zarrabi, A., Varma, R.S., Tay, F.R., Smith, B.R. and Makvandi, P., 2021. Self-assembled peptide and protein nanostructures for anti-cancer therapy: Targeted delivery, stimuli-responsive devices and immunotherapy. *Nano Today*, *38*, p. 101119.

Dey, P., Jain, N. and Nagaich, U., 2018. Nutraceuticals: An overview of regulations. *International Journal of Pharmacy & Life Sciences*, *9*(3), p. 5762.

Dima, C., Assadpour, E., Dima, S. and Jafari, S.M., 2020. Bioavailability of nutraceuticals: Role of the food matrix, processing conditions, the gastrointestinal tract, and nanodelivery systems. *Comprehensive Reviews in Food Science and Food Safety*, *19*(3), pp. 954–994.

Dini, I., 2022. Contribution of nanoscience research in antioxidants delivery used in nutricosmetic sector. *Antioxidants*, *11*(3), p. 563.

Domínguez Díaz, L., Fernández-Ruiz, V. and Cámara, M., 2020. The frontier between nutrition and pharma: The international regulatory framework of functional foods, food supplements and nutraceuticals. *Critical Reviews in Food Science and Nutrition*, *60*(10), pp. 1738–1746.

Dourado, D., Freire, D.T., Pereira, D.T., Amaral-Machado, L., Alencar, É.N., de Barros, A.L.B. and Egito, E.S.T., 2021. Will curcumin nanosystems be the next promising antiviral alternatives in COVID-19 treatment trials? *Biomedicine & Pharmacotherapy*, *139*, p.111578.

Downs, B.W., Banik, S.P., Bagchi, M., Morrison, B.S., Kushner, S.W., Piacentino, M. and Bagchi, D., 2021. Design of a novel bioflavonoid and phytonutrient enriched formulation in boosting immune competence and sports performance: A product development investigation. *American Journal of Biopharmacy and Pharmaceutical Sciences*, *1*, p. 2.

Dubey, A.K., Chaudhry, S.K., Singh, H.B., Gupta, V.K. and Kaushik, A., 2022. Perspectives on nano-nutraceuticals to manage pre and post COVID-19 infections. *Biotechnology Reports*, *33*, p. e00712.

Durazzo, A., Arcanjo, D.D.R. and Lucarini, M., 2022. The health effects of dietary supplements. *Evidence-Based Complementary and Alternative Medicine*, *2022*, p. 9851048.

Edinoff, A.N., Chappidi, M., Alpaugh E.S., Turbeville, B.C., Falgoust, E.P., Cornett, E.M., Murnane, K.S., Kaye, A.M., and Kaye, A.D., 2022. Neurological and Psychiatric Symptoms of COVID-19: A Narrative Review. *Psychiatry International*, *3*(2), pp. 158–68.

Elieh-Ali-Komi, D. and Hamblin, M.R., 2016. Chitin and chitosan: Production and application of versatile biomedical nanomaterials. *International Journal of Advanced Research*, *4*(3), p.411.

Farheen, S., Agrawal, S., Zubair, S., Agrawal, A., Jamal, F., Altaf, I., Kashif Anwar, A., Umair, S.M. and Owais, M., 2021. Patho-physiology of aging and immune-senescence: Possible correlates with comorbidity and mortality in middle-aged and old COVID-19 patients. *Frontiers in Aging*, *2*, p. 748591.

Fernandes, E., Lopes, C.M. and Lúcio, M., 2023. Bioactive lipids: Pharmaceutical, nutraceutical, and cosmeceutical applications. In: Manuela Pintado, Manuela Machado, and Luís Miguel Rodríguez-Alcalá (eds.) *Bioactive Lipids* (pp. 349–409). Academic press, Oxford OX5 1GB, United Kingdom.

Fernandez, P., André, V., Rieger, J. and Kühnle, A., 2004. Nano-emulsion formation by emulsion phase inversion. *Colloids and Surfaces A: Physicochemical and Engineering Aspects*, *251*(1–3), pp. 53–58.

Fidelis, E.M., Savall, A.S.P., da Luz Abreu, E., Carvalho, F., Teixeira, F.E.G., Haas, S.E., Sampaio, T.B. and Pinton, S., 2019. Curcumin-loaded nanocapsules reverses the depressant-like behavior and oxidative stress induced by β-amyloid in mice. *Neuroscience*, *423*, pp. 122–130.

Ganesan, P. and Narayanasamy, D., 2017. Lipid nanoparticles: Different preparation techniques, characterization, hurdles, and strategies for the production of solid lipid nanoparticles and nanostructured lipid carriers for oral drug delivery. *Sustainable Chemistry and Pharmacy*, 6, pp. 37–56.

Gholami, M., Safari, S., Ulloa, L. and Motaghinejad, M., 2021. Neuropathies and neurological dysfunction induced by coronaviruses. *Journal of Neurovirology*, *27*(3), pp. 380–396.

Gonzalez, M.J., Miranda-Massari, J.R. and Jorge, R., 2014. *New Insights on Vitamin C and Cancer*. Springer, New York.

Grabowska, M., Wawrzyniak, D., Rolle, K., Chomczyński, P., Oziewicz, S., Jurga, S. and Barciszewski, J., 2019. Let food be your medicine: Nutraceutical properties of lycopene. *Food & Function*, *10*(6), pp. 3090–3102.

Grassi, D., Necozione, S., Desideri, G., Abballe, S., Mai, F., De Feo, M., Carducci, A. and Ferri, C., 2021. Acute and long term effects of a nutraceutical combination on lipid profile, glucose metabolism and vascular function in patients with dyslipidaemia with and without cigarette smoking. *High Blood Pressure & Cardiovascular Prevention*, *28*, pp. 483–491.

Gul, K., Singh, A.K. and Jabeen, R., 2016. Nutraceuticals and functional foods: The foods for the future world. *Critical Reviews in Food Science and Nutrition*, *56*(16), pp. 2617–2627.

Gulati, O.P. and Berry Ottaway, P., 2006. Legislation relating to nutraceuticals in the European Union with a particular focus on botanical-sourced products. *Toxicology*, *221*(1), pp. 75–87. Available at: https://doi.org/10.1016/j.tox.2006.01.014.

Gupta, R.C., Lall, R. and Srivastava, A. eds., 2021. *Nutraceuticals: Efficacy, Safety and Toxicity*. Academic Press, London.

Hallaj-Nezhadi, S. and Hassan, M., 2015. Nanoliposome-based antibacterial drug delivery. *Drug Delivery*, *22*(5), pp. 581–589.

Hayat, K., Iqbal, H., Malik, U., Bilal, U. and Mushtaq, S., 2015. Tea and its consumption: Benefits and risks. *Critical Reviews in Food Science and Nutrition*, *55*(7), pp. 939–954.

Hollman, P.C., Hertog, M.G., and Katan, M.B., 1996. Role of dietary flavonoids in protection against cancer and coronary heart disease. *Biochemical Society Transactions*, *24*, pp. 785–9.

Holzapfel, N.P., Shokoohmand, A., Wagner, F., Landgraf, M., Champ, S., Holzapfel, B.M., Clements, J.A., Hutmacher, D.W. and Loessner, D., 2017. Lycopene reduces ovarian tumor growth and intraperitoneal metastatic load. *American Journal of Cancer Research*, *7*(6), p. 1322.

Hoti, G., Matencio, A., Rubin Pedrazzo, A., Cecone, C., Appleton, S.L., Khazaei Monfared, Y., Caldera, F. and Trotta, F., 2022. Nutraceutical concepts and dextrin-based delivery systems. *International Journal of Molecular Sciences*, *23*(8), p. 4102.

Huang, J., Zhang, K., Wang, K., Xie, Z., Ladewig, B., and Wang, H., 2012. Fabrication of polyethersulfone-mesoporous silica nanocomposite ultrafiltration membranes with antifouling properties. *Journal of Membrane Science*, *423*, pp. 362–70.

Ilesanmi-Oyelere, B.L., Roy, N.C. and Kruger, M.C., 2021. Modulation of bone and joint biomarkers, gut microbiota, and inflammation status by synbiotic supplementation and weight-bearing exercise: Human study protocol for a randomized controlled trial. *JMIR Research Protocols*, *10*(10), p. e30131.

Ilic, D. and Misso, M., 2012. Lycopene for the prevention and treatment of benign prostatic hyperplasia and prostate cancer: A systematic review. *Maturitas*, *72*(4), pp. 269–276.

International Obesity Task Force, 2005. Obesity in Europe: EU Platform Briefing Paper. https://ec.europa.eu/health/ph_determinants/life_style/nutrition/documents/iotf_en.pdf

Iqubal, A., Iqubal, M.K., Fazal, S.A., Pottoo, F.H. and Haque, S.E., 2022. Nutraceuticals and their derived nano-formulations for the prevention and treatment of Alzheimer's disease. *Current Molecular Pharmacology*, *15*(1), pp. 23–50.

Jampilek, J., and Kralova, K., 2020. Potential of nanonutraceuticals in increasing immunity. *Nanomaterials*, *10*(11), p. 2224.

Jain, K.K. and Jain, K.K., 2008. Ethical, safety, and regulatory issues of nanomedicine. In: Kewal K. Jain (ed.) *The Handbook of Nanomedicine*. Humana Press, Totowa, NJ.

Jang, M., Cai, L., Udeani, G.O., Slowing, K.V., Thomas, C.F., Beecher, C.W., Fong, H.H., Farnsworth, N.R., Kinghorn, A.D., Mehta, R.G. and Moon, R.C., 1997. Cancer chemopreventive activity of resveratrol, a natural product derived from grapes. *Science*, *275*(5297), pp. 218–220.

Javeri, I., 2016. Application of "nano" nutraceuticals in medicine. In *Nutraceuticals* (pp. 189–192). Academic Press.

Jeevanandam, J., Barhoum, A., Chan, Y.S., Dufresne, A. and Danquah, M.K., 2018. Review on nanoparticles and nanostructured materials: History, sources, toxicity and regulations. *Beilstein Journal of Nanotechnology*, *9*(1), pp. 1050–1074.

Jha, S.K., Roy, P. and Chakrabarty, S., 2020. Nutraceuticals with pharmaceuticals its importance and their application. *International Journal of Drug Development and Research*, *13*(S3), p. 002.

Kalra, E.K., 2003. Nutraceutical-definition and introduction. *AAPS PharmSci*, 5(3), pp. 27–28. Available at: https://doi.org/10.1208/ps050325.

Kannan, S., Dai, H., Navath, R.S., Balakrishnan, B., Jyoti, A., Janisse, J., Romero, R. and Kannan, R.M., 2012. Dendrimer-based postnatal therapy for neuroinflammation and cerebral palsy in a rabbit model. *Science Translational Medicine*, *4*(130), p. 130ra46.

Kantor, E.D., Lampe, J.W., Navarro, S.L., Song, X., Milne, G.L. and White, E., 2014. Associations between glucosamine and chondroitin supplement use and biomarkers of systemic inflammation. *The Journal of Alternative and Complementary Medicine*, *20*(6), pp. 479–485.

Kauffman, K.J., Webber, M.J. and Anderson, D.G., 2016. Materials for non-viral intracellular delivery of messenger RNA therapeutics. *Journal of Controlled Release*, *240*, pp. 227–234.

Khaerunnisa, S., Kurniawan, H., Awaluddin, R., Suhartati, S. and Soetjipto, S., 2020. Potential inhibitor of COVID-19 main protease (Mpro) from several medicinal plant compounds by molecular docking study. *Preprints*, 2020, p. 2020030226.

Khare, C.P., 2004. *Indian Herbal Remedies: Rational Western Therapy, Ayurvedic, and Other Traditional Usage*. Springer, New York.

Khatiwada, J., Verghese, M., Walker, L.T., Shackelford, L., Chawan, C.B. and Sunkara, R., 2006. Combination of green tea, phytic acid, and inositol reduced the incidence of azoxymethane-induced colon tumors in Fisher 344 male rats. *LWT-Food Science and Technology*, *39*(10), pp. 1080–1086.

Khorasani, S., Danaei, M. and Mozafari, M.R., 2018. Nanoliposome technology for the food and nutraceutical industries. *Trends in Food Science & Technology*, *79*, pp. 106–115.

Kim, Y.A., Xiao, D., Xiao, H., Powolny, A.A., Lew, K.L., Reilly, M.L., Zeng, Y., Wang, Z. and Singh, S.V., 2007. Mitochondria-mediated apoptosis by diallyl trisulfide in human prostate cancer cells is associated with generation of reactive oxygen species and regulated by Bax/Bak. *Molecular Cancer Therapeutics*, *6*(5), pp. 1599–1609.

Kopańska, M., Batoryna, M., Bartman, P., Szczygielski, J. and Banaś-Ząbczyk, A., 2022. Disorders of the cholinergic system in COVID-19 era—a review of the latest research. *International Journal of Molecular Sciences*, *23*(2), p.672.

Kumar, H. and Rajpoot, A.K., 2018. Nutraceuticals: Today's need for health care. *European Journal of Pharmaceutical and Medical Research*, *5*, pp. 255–262.

Kumar, S., Saxena, J., Srivastava, V.K., Kaushik, S., Singh, H., Abo-EL-Sooud, K., Abdel-Daim, M.M., Jyoti, A., Saluja, R., 2022. The interplay of oxidative stress and ROS scavenging: antioxidants as a therapeutic potential in sepsis. *Vaccines*, *10*(10), p. 1575.

Leena, M.M., Anukiruthika, T., Moses, J.A. and Anandharamakrishnan, C., 2022. Co-delivery of curcumin and resveratrol through electrosprayed core-shell nanoparticles in 3D printed hydrogel. *Food Hydrocolloids*, *124*, p. 107200.

Li Y, Qian Q, Zhou Y, Yan M, Sun L, Zhang M, Fu Z, Wang Y, Han B, Pang X, Chen M, and Li J. 2003. BRITTLE CULM1, which encodes a COBRA-like protein, affects the mechanical properties of rice plants. *Plant Cell, 15*(9), pp. 2020–31. doi: 10.1105/tpc.011775

Limer, J.L. and Speirs, V., 2004. Phyto-oestrogens and breast cancer chemoprevention. *Breast Cancer Research*, *6*, pp. 1–9.

Liu, G., Jingqi Yang, Yixiang Wang, Xinghai Liu, Le Luo Guan, and Lingyun Chen, 2019. Protein-lipid composite nanoparticles for the oral delivery of vitamin B12: Impact of protein succinylation on nanoparticle physicochemical and biological properties. *Food Hydrocolloids*, *92*, pp. 189–197.

Liu, L., Zhang, K., Sandoval, H., Yamamoto, S., Jaiswal, M., Sanz, E., Li, Z., Hui, J., Graham, B.H., Quintana, A., and Bellen, H.J., 2015. Glial lipid droplets and ROS induced by mitochondrial defects promote neurodegeneration. *Cell*, *160*(1), pp. 177–90.

Long, Z., Phillips, B., Radtke, D., Meyer-Hermann, M., and Bannard, O., 2022. Competition for refueling rather than cyclic reentry initiation evident in germinal centers. *Science immunology*, *7*(69), p. eabm0775.

Luo, X., Zhou, Y., Bai, L., Liu, F., Deng, Y. and McClements, D.J., 2017. Fabrication of β-carotene nanoemulsion-based delivery systems using dual-channel microfluidization: Physical and chemical stability. *Journal of Colloid and Interface Science*, *490*, pp. 328–335.

Madiseh, M.R., Heidarian, E., and Rafieian-kopaei, M., 2014. Biochemical components of Berberis lycium fruit and its effects on lipid profile in diabetic rats. *Journal of HerbMed Pharmacology*, *3*(1), pp. 15–9.

Magnuson, B., Munro, I., Abbot, P., Baldwin, N., Lopez-Garcia, R., Ly, K., Mcgirr, L., Roberts, A., Socolovsky, S., 2013. Review of the regulation and safety assessment of food substances in various countries and jurisdictions. *Food Additives & Contaminants: Part A*, *30*, p. 1147–1220.

Mal'tseva, V.N., Goltyaev, M.V., Turovsky, E.A. and Varlamova, E.G., 2022. Immunomodulatory and anti-inflammatory properties of selenium-containing agents: Their role in the regulation of defense mechanisms against COVID-19. *International Journal of Molecular Sciences*, *23*(4), p. 2360.

Martínez, J.P.Q. and Campos, M.R.S., 2023. Bioactive compounds and functional foods as coadjuvant therapy for thrombosis. *Food & Function*, *14*(2), pp. 653–674.

Maryana, W., Rachmawati, H. and Mudhakir, D., 2016. Formation of phytosome containing silymarin using thin layer-hydration technique aimed for oral delivery. *Materials Today: Proceedings*, *3*(3), pp. 855–866.

Maury, A, Lyoubi, A, Peiffer-Smadja, N, De Broucker, T, and Meppiel, E., 2021. Neurological manifestations associated with SARS-CoV-2 and other coronaviruses: A narrative review for clinicians. *Revue Neurologique*, *177*(1–2), pp. 51–64.

McCarty, M.F., Lerner, A., DiNicolantonio, J.J. and Benzvi, C., 2021. Nutraceutical aid for allergies–strategies for down-regulating mast cell degranulation. *Journal of Asthma and Allergy*, *14*, pp. 1257–1266.

Meléndez-Martínez, A.J., Stinco, C.M. and Mapelli-Brahm, P., 2019. Skin carotenoids in public health and nutricosmetics: The emerging roles and applications of the UV radiation-absorbing colourless carotenoids phytoene and phytofluene. *Nutrients*, 11(5), p. 1093.

Middha, S.K., Goyal, A.K., Lokesh, P., Yardi, V., Mojamdar, L., Keni, D.S., Babu, D. and Usha, T., 2015. Toxicological evaluation of *Emblica officinalis* fruit extract and its anti-inflammatory and free radical scavenging properties. *Pharmacognosy Magazine*, *11*(Suppl 3), p. S427.

Mishra, D., Hubenak, J.R. and Mathur, A.B., 2013. Nanoparticle systems as tools to improve drug delivery and therapeutic efficacy. *Journal of Biomedical Materials Research Part A: An Official Journal of the Society for Biomaterials, The Japanese Society for Biomaterials, and The Australian Society for Biomaterials and the Korean Society for Biomaterials*, *101*(12), pp. 3646–3660.

Mohammad, Khalid, Rai, D.C. and Andhare, B.C. 2015. Effect of different nutraceuticals on physico-chemical quality of flavoured milk. *Research Journal of Animal Husbandry and Dairy Science, 6*(1), pp. 61–65.

Muangnoi, C., Phumsuay, R., Jongjitphisut, N., Waikasikorn, P., Sangsawat, M., Rashatasakhon, P., Paraoan, L. and Rojsitthisak, P., 2021. Protective effects of a lutein ester prodrug, lutein diglutaric acid, against H_2O_2-induced oxidative stress in human retinal pigment epithelial cells. *International Journal of Molecular Sciences*, *22*(9), p. 4722.

Nakamura, T., Yoshida, N., Yamanoi, Y., Honryo, A., Tomita, H., Kuwabara, H. and Kojima, Y., 2020. Eucalyptus oil reduces allergic reactions and suppresses mast cell degranulation by downregulating IgE-FcεRI signalling. *Scientific Reports*, *10*(1), p. 20940.

Nashine, S., Cohen, P., Chwa, M., Lu, S., Nesburn, A.B., Kuppermann, B.D. and Kenney, M.C., 2017. Humanin G (HNG) protects age-related macular degeneration (AMD) transmitochondrial ARPE-19 cybrids from mitochondrial and cellular damage. *Cell Death & Disease*, *8*(7), pp. e2951–e2951.

Nasri, H., Baradaran, A., Shirzad, H. and Rafieian-Kopaei, M., 2014. New concepts in nutraceuticals as alternative for pharmaceuticals. *International Journal of Preventive Medicine*, *5*(12), p. 1487.

Nazhand, A., Durazzo, A., Lucarini, M., Guerra, F., Souto, S.B., Souto, E.B. and Santini, A., 2022. Nutraceuticals and functional beverages: Focus on prebiotics and probiotics active beverages. In: Rajeev Bhat (ed.) *Future Foods* (pp. 251–258). Academic Press, London, United Kingdom.

Newman, D.J. and Cragg, G.M. (2007) Natural products as sources of new drugs over the last 25 years. *Journal of Natural Products*, *70*(3), pp. 461–477.

Nikalje, A.P., 2015. Nanotechnology and its applications in medicine. *Medicinal Chemistry*, *5*(2), pp. 81–89.

Niu, B., Ping Shao, and Peilong Sun, (2020) Ultrasound-assisted emulsion electrosprayed particles for the stabilization of β-carotene and its nutritional supplement potential, *Food Hydrocolloids, 102*, p. 105634. https://doi.org/10.1016/j.foodhyd.2019.105634

Oboh, G. and Ademosun, A.O., 2011. Shaddock peels (Citrus maxima) phenolic extracts inhibit α-amylase, α-glucosidase and angiotensin I-converting enzyme activities: A nutraceutical approach to diabetes management. *Diabetes & Metabolic Syndrome: Clinical Research & Reviews*, *5*(3), pp. 148–152.

Oliveira, J.T. and Reis, R.L., 2011. Polysaccharide-based materials for cartilage tissue engineering applications. *Journal of Tissue Engineering and Regenerative Medicine*, *5*(6), pp. 421–436.

Paolino, D., Mancuso, A., Cristiano, M.C., Froiio, F., Lammari, N., Celia, C. and Fresta, M., 2021. Nanonutraceuticals: The new frontier of supplementary food. *Nanomaterials*, *11*(3), p.792.

Patra, J.K., Das, G., Fraceto, L.F., Campos, E.V.R., Rodriguez-Torres, M.D.P., Acosta-Torres, L.S., Diaz-Torres, L.A., Grillo, R., Swamy, M.K., Sharma, S. and Habtemariam, S., 2018. Nano based drug delivery systems: Recent developments and future prospects. *Journal of Nanobiotechnology*, *16*(1), pp. 1–33.

Peng, C., Zheng, J., Chen, D., Zhang, X., Deng, L., Chen, Z. and Wu, L., 2018. Response of hPDLSCs on 3D printed PCL/PLGA composite scaffolds in vitro. *Molecular Medicine Reports*, *18*(2), pp. 1335–1344. https://doi.org/10.3892/mmr.2018.9076.

Pereira, M.A. and Ludwig, D.S., 2001. Dietary fiber and body-weight regulation: Observations and mechanisms. *Pediatric Clinics of North America*, *48*(4), pp. 969–980.

Phillips, S. and Williams, M.A., 2021. Confronting our next national health disaster—long-haul Covid. *New England Journal of Medicine*, *385*(7), pp. 577–579.

Pisoschi, A.M. and Pop, A., 2015. The role of antioxidants in the chemistry of oxidative stress: A review. *European Journal of Medicinal Chemistry*, *97*, pp. 55–74.

Pliss, A., Kuzmin, A.N., Prasad, P.N. and Mahajan, S.D., 2022. Mitochondrial dysfunction: A prelude to neuropathogenesis of SARS-CoV-2. *ACS Chemical Neuroscience*, *13*(3), pp. 308–312.

Pottoo, F.H., Barkat, M.A., Ansari, M.A., Javed, M.N., Jamal, Q.M. and Kamal, M.A., 2019. Nanotechnologoical based miRNA intervention in the therapeutic management of neuroblastoma. *Seminars in Cancer Biology*. https://doi.org/10.1016/j.semcancer.2019a.09.017

Punia, S., Sandhu, K.S., Kaur, M. and Siroha, A.K., 2019. Nanotechnology: A successful approach to improve nutraceutical bioavailability. In: Prasad, R., Kumar, V., Kumar, M., and Choudhary, D. (eds.) *Nanobiotechnology in Bioformulations. Nanotechnology in the Life Sciences*. Springer, Cham. https://doi.org/10.1007/978-3-030-17061-5_5

Puttasiddaiah, R., Lakshminarayana, R., Somashekar, N.L., Gupta, V.K., Inbaraj, B.S., Usmani, Z., Raghavendra, V.B., Sridhar, K. and Sharma, M., 2022. Advances in nanofabrication technology for nutraceuticals: New insights and future trends. *Bioengineering*, *9*(9), p. 478.

Rabanal-Ruiz, Y., Llanos-González, E. and Alcain, F.J., 2021. The use of coenzyme Q10 in cardiovascular diseases. *Antioxidants*, *10*(5), p. 755.

Rabiei, Z., Rafieian-Kopaei, M., Mokhtari, S., Alibabaei, Z. and Shahrani, M., 2014. The effect of pretreatment with different doses of *Lavandula officinalis* ethanolic extract on memory, learning and nociception. *Biomedicine & Aging Pathology*, *4*(1), pp. 71–76.

Rakotoarisoa, M., Angelov, B., Drechsler, M., Nicolas, V., Bizien, T., Gorshkova, Y.E., Deng, Y. and Angelova, A., 2022. Liquid crystalline lipid nanoparticles for combined delivery of curcumin, fish oil and BDNF: In vitro neuroprotective potential in a cellular model of tunicamycin-induced endoplasmic reticulum stress. *Smart Materials in Medicine*, *3*, pp. 274–288.

Rapoport, N., 2007. Physical stimuli-responsive polymeric micelles for anti-cancer drug delivery. *Progress in Polymer Science*, *32*(8–9), pp. 962–990.

Rautiainen, S., Manson, J.E., Lichtenstein, A.H. and Sesso, H.D., 2016. Dietary supplements and disease prevention—a global overview. *Nature Reviews Endocrinology*, *12*(7), pp. 407–420.

Rayalam, S., Della-Fera, M.A. and Baile, C.A., 2008. Phytochemicals and regulation of the adipocyte life cycle. *The Journal of Nutritional Biochemistry*, *19*(11), pp. 717–726.

Reginster, J.Y., Neuprez, A., Lecart, M.P., Sarlet, N. and Bruyere, O., 2012. Role of glucosamine in the treatment for osteoarthritis. *Rheumatology International*, *32*, pp. 2959–2967.

Reis, F.S., Martins, A., Vasconcelos, M.H., Morales, P. and Ferreira, I.C., 2017. Functional foods based on extracts or compounds derived from mushrooms. *Trends in Food Science & Technology*, *66*, pp. 48–62.

Resnik, D.B. and Tinkle, S.S., 2007. Ethical issues in clinical trials involving nanomedicine. *Contemporary Clinical Trials*, *28*(4), pp. 433–441.

Ricardo, P.N. and Lino, F., 2010. Stem cell research meets nanotechnology. *Revista Da Sociedade Portuguesa D Bioquimica, CanalBQ*, *7*, pp. 38–46.

Rissanen, T.H., Voutilainen, S., Virtanen, J.K., Venho, B., Vanharanta, M., Mursu, J. and Salonen, J.T., 2003. Low intake of fruits, berries and vegetables is associated with excess mortality in men: the Kuopio Ischaemic Heart Disease Risk Factor (KIHD) Study. *The Journal of Nutrition*, *133*(1), pp. 199–204.

Roco, M.C. and Bainbridge, W.S., 2001. *Societal Implications of Nanoscience and Nanotechnology*. Kluwer Academic Publishers, Boston.

Russo, V., Stella, A., Appezzati, L., Barone, A., Stagni, E., Roszkowska, A.M. and Noci, N.D., 2009. Clinical efficacy of a Ginkgo biloba extract in the topical treatment of allergic conjunctivitis. *European Journal of Ophthalmology*, *19*(3), pp. 331–336.

Saber-Moghaddam, N., Salari, S., Hejazi, S., Amini, M., Taherzadeh, Z., Eslami, S., Rezayat, S.M., Jaafari, M.R. and Elyasi, S., 2021. Oral nano-curcumin formulation efficacy in management of mild to moderate hospitalized coronavirus disease-19 patients: An open label nonrandomized clinical trial. *Phytotherapy Research*, *35*(5), pp. 2616–2623.

Sahoo, S.K., Dilnawaz, F. and Krishnakumar, S., 2008. Nanotechnology in ocular drug delivery. *Drug Discovery Today*, *13*(3–4), pp. 144–151.

Santini A, Novellino E. 2017. To nutraceuticals and back: Rethinking a concept. *Foods*, *6*(9), p. 74. https://doi.org/10.3390/foods6090074

Santini, A. and Novellino, E., 2018. Nutraceuticals-shedding light on the grey area between pharmaceuticals and food. *Expert Review of Clinical Pharmacology* 11(6), pp. 545–547.

Santini, A., Cammarata, S.M., Capone, G., Ianaro, A., Tenore, G.C., Pani, L. and Novellino, E., 2018. Nutraceuticals: Opening the debate for a regulatory framework. *British Journal of Clinical Pharmacology*, *84*(4), pp. 659–672.

Santini, A., Tenore, G.C., and Novellino, E., 2017. Nutraceuticals: A paradigm of proactive medicine. *European Journal of Pharmaceutical Sciences, 96*, pp. 53–61. doi: 10.1016/j.ejps.2016.09.003

Satoh, T., Trudler, D., Oh, C.K. and Lipton, S.A., 2022. Potential therapeutic use of the rosemary diterpene carnosic acid for Alzheimer's disease, Parkinson's disease, and long-COVID through NRF2 activation to counteract the NLRP3 inflammasome. *Antioxidants*, *11*(1), p. 124.

Sayamov, Y.N., 2021. Bioethics in international relations. *International Journal of Foresight and Innovation Policy*, *15*(1–3), pp. 120–130.

Scarcella, M., Scarpellini, E., Ascani, A., Commissari, R., Scorcella, C., Zanetti, M., Parisi, A., Monti, R., Milic, N., Donati, A. and Luzza, F., 2022. Effect of whey proteins on malnutrition and extubating time of critically Ill COVID-19 patients. *Nutrients*, *14*(3), p. 437.

Sekiou, O., Bouziane, I., Bouslama, Z., and Djemel, A., 2020. In-silico identification of potent inhibitors of COVID-19 main protease (Mpro) and Angiotensin Converting Enzyme 2 (ACE2) from Natural Products: Quercetin, Hispidulin, and Cirsimaritin Exhibited Better Potential Inhibition than Hydroxy-Chloroquine Against COVID-19 Main Protease Active Site and ACE2. ChemRxiv, doi:10.26434/chemrxiv.12181404.v1.

Shahbazian, H, and Rezaii, I., 2013. Diabetic kidney disease; review of the current knowledge. *Journal of Renal Injury Prevention*, 2(2), p. 73.

Sharma, N., Mishra, S., Sharma, S., Deshpande, R.D. and Sharma, R.K., 2013. Preparation and optimization of nanoemulsions for targeting drug delivery. *International Journal of Drug Development and Research*, *5*(4), pp. 37–48.

Sheng, J., Han, L., Qin, J., Ru, G., Li, R., Wu, L., Cui, D., Yang, P., He, Y. and Wang, J., 2015. N-trimethyl chitosan chloride-coated PLGA nanoparticles overcoming multiple barriers to oral insulin absorption. *ACS Applied Materials & Interfaces*, *7*(28), pp. 15430–15441.

Shindhe, V.M, Shindhe, M.M, Kammar, K.F, and Siddapur, P.R., 2015. A comparative study of PEFR and MVV between Indian born Tibetan youths and Indian youths. *Journal of Evolution of Medical and Dental Sciences Predatory*, *15*(4), pp. 748–54.

Sivaramakrishnan, S.M. and Neelakantan, P., 2014. Nanotechnology in dentistry-what does the future hold in store. *Dentistry*, *4*(2), p. 1.

Sonia, T.A. and Sharma, C.P., 2012. An overview of natural polymers for oral insulin delivery. *Drug Discovery Today*, *17*(13–14), pp. 784–792.

Soppimath, K.S., Aminabhavi, T.M., Kulkarni, A.R. and Rudzinski, W.E., 2001. Biodegradable polymeric nanoparticles as drug delivery devices. *Journal of Controlled Release*, *70*(1–2), pp. 1–20.

Svagan, A.J., Azizi Samir, M.A. and Berglund, L.A., 2007. Biomimetic polysaccharide nanocomposites of high cellulose content and high toughness. *Biomacromolecules*, *8*(8), pp. 2556–2563.

Tallei, T.E., Tumilaar, S.G., Niode, N.J., Kepel, B.J., Idroes, R., Effendi, Y., Sakib, S.A. and Emran, T.B., 2020. Potential of plant bioactive compounds as SARS-CoV-2 main protease (M pro) and spike (S) glycoprotein inhibitors: A molecular docking study. *Scientifica*, *2020*, p. 6307457.

Taquet, M., Dercon, Q., Luciano, S., Geddes, J.R., Husain, M. and Harrison, P.J., 2021. Incidence, co-occurrence, and evolution of long-COVID features: A 6-month retrospective cohort study of 273,618 survivors of COVID-19. *PLoS Medicine*, *18*(9), p. e1003773.

Tenchov, R., Bird, R., Curtze, A.E. and Zhou, Q., 2021. Lipid nanoparticles— from liposomes to mRNA vaccine delivery, a landscape of research diversity and advancement. *ACS Nano*, *15*(11), pp. 16982–17015.

Tenore, G.C., Caruso, D., D'Avino, M., Buonomo, G., Caruso, G., Ciampaglia, R., Schiano, E., Maisto, M., Annunziata, G. and Novellino, E., 2020. A pilot screening of agro-food waste products as sources of nutraceutical formulations to improve simulated postprandial glycaemia and insulinaemia in healthy subjects. *Nutrients*, *12*(5), p. 1292.

Thomasset, S.C., Berry, D.P., Garcea, G., Marczylo, T., Steward, W.P. and Gescher, A.J., 2007. Dietary polyphenolic phytochemicals—promising cancer chemopreventive agents in humans? A review of their clinical properties. *International Journal of Cancer*, *120*(3), pp. 451–458.

Tsiaka, T., Kritsi, E., Tsiantas, K., Christodoulou, P., Sinanoglou, V.J. and Zoumpoulakis, P., 2022. Design and development of novel nutraceuticals: Current trends and methodologies. *Nutraceuticals*, *2*(2), pp. 71–90.

Ubrich, N., Schmidt, C., Bodmeier, R., Hoffman, M. and Maincent, P., 2005. Oral evaluation in rabbits of cyclosporin-loaded Eudragit RS or RL nanoparticles. *International Journal of Pharmaceutics*, *288*(1), pp. 169–175.

Ulker, D., Abacioglu, N. and Sehirli, A.O., 2022. Cerium oxide (CeO2) nanoparticles could have protective effect against COVID-19. *Letters in Applied NanoBioScience*, *12*(1), p. 12.

Utomo, R.Y., Ikawati, M. and Meiyanto, E., 2020. Revealing the potency of citrus and galangal constituents to halt SARS-CoV-2 infection. *Preprints*, https://doi.org/10.20944/preprints202003.0214.v1

Valizadeh, H., Abdolmohammadi-Vahid, S., Danshina, S., Gencer, M.Z., Ammari, A., Sadeghi, A., Roshangar, L., Aslani, S., Esmaeilzadeh, A., Ghaebi, M. and Valizadeh, S., 2020. Nano-curcumin therapy, a promising method in modulating inflammatory cytokines in COVID-19 patients. *International Immunopharmacology*, *89*, p. 107088.

van der Koog, L., Gandek, T.B. and Nagelkerke, A., 2022. Liposomes and extracellular vesicles as drug delivery systems: A comparison of composition, pharmacokinetics, and functionalization. *Advanced Healthcare Materials*, *11*(5), p. 2100639.

Vinardell, M.P. and Mitjans, M., 2015. Nanocarriers for delivery of antioxidants on the skin. *Cosmetics*, 2(4), pp. 342–354.

Wang, C.Z., Mehendale, S.R. and Yuan, C.S., 2007. Commonly used antioxidant botanicals: Active constituents and their potential role in cardiovascular illness. *The American Journal of Chinese Medicine*, *35*(4), pp. 543–558.

Wang, H., Hu, H., Yang, H. and Li, Z., 2021. Hydroxyethyl starch based smart nanomedicine. *RSC Advances*, *11*(6), pp. 3226–3240.

Watanabe, M., Risi, R., Masi, D., Caputi, A., Balena, A., Rossini, G., Tuccinardi, D., Mariani, S., Basciani, S., Manfrini, S. and Gnessi, L., 2020. Current evidence to propose different food supplements for weight loss: A comprehensive review. *Nutrients*, *12*(9), p.2873.

Wildman, R.E., Wildman, R. and Wallace, T.C., 2016. *Handbook of Nutraceuticals and Functional Foods*. CRC Press, Boca Raton.

Willis, M.S., and Wians, Jr. F.H., 2003. The role of nutrition in preventing prostate cancer: a review of the proposed mechanism of action of various dietary substances. *Clinica Chimica Acta*, *330*(1–2), pp. 57–83.

Witkamp, R.F. and van Norren, K., 2018. Let thy food be thy medicine.... when possible. *European Journal of Pharmacology*, *836*, pp. 102–114.

Wong, H.L., Wu, X.Y. and Bendayan, R., 2012. Nanotechnological advances for the delivery of CNS therapeutics. *Advanced Drug Delivery Reviews*, *64*(7), pp. 686–700.

Yamamoto, K., Imaoka, T., Tanabe, M. and Kambe, T., 2019. New horizon of nanoparticle and cluster catalysis with dendrimers. *Chemical Reviews*, *120*(2), pp. 1397–1437.

Yang, F., Zhang, Y., Tariq, A., Jiang, X., Ahmed, Z., Zhihao, Z., Idrees, M., Azizullah, A., Adnan, M. and Bussmann, R.W., 2020. Food as medicine: A possible preventive measure against coronavirus disease (COVID-19). *Phytotherapy Research*, *34*(12), pp. 3124–3136.

Yayehrad, A.T., Siraj, E.A., Wondie, G.B., Alemie, A.A., Derseh, M.T. and Ambaye, A.S., 2021. Could nanotechnology help to end the fight against COVID-19? Review of current findings, challenges and future perspectives. *International Journal of Nanomedicine*, *16*, p. 5713.

Yezdani, U., Khan, M.G., Kushwah, N., Verma, A. and Khan, F., 2018. Application of nanotechnology in diagnosis and treatment of various diseases and its future advances in medicine. *World Journal of Pharmaceutical Sciences*, *7*(11), pp. 1611–1633.

Zhang, W., Wang, Y., Lee, B.T.K., Liu, C., Wei, G. and Lu, W., 2014. A novel nanoscale-dispersed eye ointment for the treatment of dry eye disease. *Nanotechnology*, *25*(12), p. 125101.

Zhang, Y., Wu, X., Meng, L., Zhang, Yu, Ai, R., Qi, N., He, H., Xu, H. and Tang, X., 2012. Thiolated Eudragit nanoparticles for oral insulin delivery: Preparation, characterization and in vivo evaluation. *International Journal of Pharmaceutics*, *436*(1–2), pp. 341–350.

Zhao, J., 2007. Nutraceuticals, nutritional therapy, phytonutrients, and phytotherapy for improvement of human health: A perspective on plant biotechnology application. *Recent Patents on Biotechnology*, *1*(1), pp. 75–97.

Zhao, Z., Xiao, Y., Xu, L., Liu, Y., Jiang, G., Wang, W., Li, B., Zhu, T., Tan, Q., Tang, L. and Zhou, H., 2021. Glycyrrhizic acid nanoparticles as antiviral and anti-inflammatory agents for COVID-19 treatment. *ACS Applied Materials & Interfaces*, *13*(18), pp. 20995–21006.

Zhou, Y., Zhang, J., Wang, K., Han, W., Wang, X., Gao, M., Wang, Z., Sun, Y., Yan, H., Zhang, H. and Xu, X., 2020. Quercetin overcomes colon cancer cells resistance to chemotherapy by inhibiting solute carrier family 1, member 5 transporter. *European Journal of Pharmacology*, *881*, p. 173185.

Zohuri, B. and Behgounia, F., 2023. Application of artificial intelligence driving nano-based drug delivery system. In: Anil Philip, Aliasgar Shahiwala, Mamoon Rashid, and Md. Faiyazuddin (eds.). *A Handbook of Artificial Intelligence in Drug Delivery* (pp. 145–212). Academic Press, Oxford.

Zubair, A.S., McAlpine, L.S., Gardin, T., Farhadian, S., Kuruvilla, D.E. and Spudich, S., 2020. Neuropathogenesis and neurologic manifestations of the coronaviruses in the age of coronavirus disease 2019: A review. *JAMA Neurology*, *77*(8), pp. 1018–1027.

Zuo, T., Zhang, F., Lui, G.C., Yeoh, Y.K., Li, A.Y., Zhan, H., Wan, Y., Chung, A.C., Cheung, C.P., Chen, N., and Lai, C.K., 2020. Alterations in gut microbiota of patients with COVID-19 during time of hospitalization. *Gastroenterology*, *159*(3), pp. 944–55.

17 Nutraceuticals Delivery System Using Nano-Based Formulations

Kazi Asraf Ali, Chowdhury Mobaswar Hossain, Amlan Bishal, Sourav Maji, Puja Mandal, and Bikram Biswas

17.1 INTRODUCTION

Nutraceuticals have the dual purpose of providing nutrition, serving as medicine, and providing health benefits above and beyond fundamental nutrition. Such products are substances that offer physiological advantages or safeguard against chronic ailments. Nutraceuticals are substances found in food or food components that have therapeutic or health benefits and may be used to treat or prevent illness. Aside from different kinds of food like genetically modified foods (genetic engineering is a specific form of gene technology that changes the genetic code of living things like plants, animals, and microbes), and processed goods like cereals, soups, and drinks, they can also include isolated nutrients, herbal products, dietary supplements, and beverages. There is no denying that many of these products perform essential physiological processes and contribute to healthy cellular processes (Dureja et al., 2003; Karami and Mahasti Shotorbani, 2018). However, the poor oral bioavailability of many nutraceuticals considerably reduces their effectiveness as medicines that fight disease. Drug oral bioavailability refers to the proportion of the administered drug dose that ultimately reaches the desired site of action for therapeutic purposes. Utilizing engineered nanoparticle (EN)-based delivery systems is an efficient approach to increasing the oral bioavailability of nutraceuticals (Yao et al., 2015). The design and development of novel functional food ingredients with enhanced water solubility, thermal stability, oral bioavailability, sensory attributes, and physiological performance is a significant application of nanotechnology in food and nutrition (Huang et al., 2010). Nanotechnology is the field of engineering and science that focuses on studying, creating, and utilizing materials and devices at the nanometer scale. By manipulating matter at this tiny scale, researchers gain control over the fundamental molecular structure, enabling them to influence the macroscopic physical and chemical properties of the material or device. So carefully examining individual molecules and their interactions is necessary, as they directly affect the overall

DOI: 10.1201/9781003432661-17

characteristics of the bulk material or device (Saini et al., 2010). Early disease detection and prevention, better disease diagnosis, appropriate treatment, and follow-up are all made feasible with the aid of nanotechnology. Damaged tissue can also be replicated or repaired. These so-called artificially stimulated cells in tissue engineering could revolutionize artificial implants or organ donation (Nikalje, 2015).

17.2 HISTORICAL DEVELOPMENT

Dr. Stephen DeFelice, the founder and leader of the Foundation for Innovation in Medicine (FIM), coined the term "nutraceutical" by blending the words "nutriceutical" and "pharmaceutical" together in 1989 (Brower, 1998). The integrity of the food supply has long been of great interest to and worry to civilized societies. Before nutrition became a separate science field, philosophers and later doctors focused on how one's daily diet affected personal and societal health. It's interesting to note that there wasn't much of a distinction between food and drugs over the last 2000 years, from the time of Hippocrates (460–377 BC) to the advent of contemporary medicine. Selecting healthy natural foods was a key component of treatment (Andlauer and Fürst, 2002).

Nutraceuticals' and functional foods' formulation, production, and methods have used some nanoscale phenomena. To increase product usefulness and delivery effectiveness, new ideas based on nanotechnology are being investigated (Scott and Chen, 2012). A wealth of novel information can be found in systems with large interfacial areas, such as emulsion, dispersion, and bicontinuous structured fluid. A better grasp of these structures' functionality and a better ability to visualize them in nanometer resolution are made possible by recently developed capabilities in nanoscale characterization (Chen et al., 2006).

Michael Faraday spent much time in 1857 studying the creation and characteristics of colloidal solutions containing "Ruby" gold nanoparticles (GNPs). These nanoparticles' (NPs) distinctive optical and electrical features make them especially attractive. Faraday showed that, depending on the illumination circumstances, gold NPs could produce various colored solutions (Bayda et al., 2019). The Japanese scientist Norio Taniguchi coined the word "nanotechnology" in a 1974 paper on production technology that makes objects and features on the scale of a nanometer. The American physicist Richard Feynman is credited with systematically discussing nanotechnology for the first time in a lecture in 1959. There's Plenty of Room at the Bottom was the theme. Richard Zsigmondy, a science Nobel Prize winner from 1925, was the one who first coined the term "nanometer" (VJoy et al., 2020).

17.3 BIOAVAILABILITY CONCERNS OF NUTRACEUTICALS

Bioavailability refers to the portion of a bioactive ingredient in a nutrient utilized and absorbed by the body for essential physiological functions. Their bioavailability decreases following oral ingestion when derived from bioactive compounds like vitamins (A, D, and E), carotenoids, curcumin, conjugated linoleic acids, omega-3 fatty acids, and coenzyme Q10. Various physiochemical and physiological factors, including absorption and transformation, contribute to this decrease in bioavailability (Rein et al., 2013).

While creating pharmaceutical forms of food bioactives (tablets, powders, capsules, suppositories, etc.) may be straightforward for a formulator, it may be challenging to achieve an appropriate bioavailability for such nutraceuticals (Zhang et al., 2016). Bioavailability is typically compromised by a bioactive's low solubility, stability, and permeability in the gastrointestinal tract (GIT). Curcumin's deficient serum levels, restricted tissue distribution, apparent fast metabolism, and short circulation half-life are the leading causes of its limited oral bioavailability. However, the poor water solubility and slow dissolution rate in GI fluids of the highly lipophilic antioxidant coenzyme Q10 posed a barrier to the substance's bioavailability (log P = 21) (Suárez-Rivero et al., 2021). Further limiting factors for permeability include the high molecular weight (863), P-glycoprotein efflux, and active transport by several transporters, including peptide transporters (PEPT1), cation/carnitine transporters (OCT1, OCTN1, OCTN2, and OCT3), and organic anion transporters (MCTl and AE2) (Anand et al., 2007). The "Probiotics" subcategory of nutraceuticals has recently grown in popularity. Low GIT bacterial stability and the resulting loss of viability due to excessive acidity and bile salt concentrations make oral probiotic delivery difficult. Formulators have attempted to address the issue of oral verbalization nutraceuticals at acceptable bioavailability with varying degrees of success. For the distribution of probiotics, one approach involves immobilizing the bacteria within a polymer matrix, creating an enteric system that remains intact in the stomach but dissolves and degrades in the gut. A new development is the Probiotics Encapsulation Technology, or "PET," which aims to protect and safely formulate and transport the living probiotic cell. The selection of biomaterials, the kind and toxicity of solvents, and the use of appropriate technologies are all factors that sustain cell viability. Researchers utilize both natural and artificial polymers in the biomaterial, requiring careful considerations-

i. Physical and chemical characteristics (chemical make-up, morphology, mechanical strength, and stability in GI fluids) (Palamakula, 2004);
ii. Toxicity estimation;
iii. Manufacturing and sterilization procedures (Zaki, 2014).

Researchers are experimenting with various methods, including extrusion, freeze-drying, fluidized bed drying, spray-drying, and emulsification. Before establishing a standardized methodology that mimics the conditions of the GIT, it is essential to confirm the release of gastro-protected encapsulated probiotics in vitro using simulated intestinal fluid (SIF) (Abuhassan et al., 2021).

17.4 METHODS FOR IMPROVING NUTRACEUTICAL ORAL BIOAVAILABILITY

17.4.1 Labile Compounds

The body must digest nutraceuticals after being consumed directly. Oral medications must go through liver first-pass metabolism and intestinal absorption (Olivares-Morales et al., 2014). Digestion is a complicated process that takes place in a variety of physiochemical and physiological settings. The GI system undergoes various environmental alterations between the mouth and the colon that alter these active ingredients' chemical structures. The variables include ionic strength, pH changes, enzyme degradations, and mechanistic motilities. All of these elements significantly speed up the deterioration of nutraceuticals. As a result, delivery methods built with defense mechanisms may help improve the gastric stability of labile bioactive nutrients and the effectiveness of oral dosing (Asghar et al., 2018).

17.4.2 Extension of Gastric Retention Time

The typical length of the mammalian GIT in humans is about 5 m, extending from the mouth to the anus (Helander and Fändriks, 2014). During digestion, nutrients are dynamic as they are transported to different sites for digestion and absorption within the GIT. The critical stage for nutraceutical effectiveness is oral bioavailability, which involves several steps:

- The release of nutraceuticals from food matrices or nanocarriers in GI fluids
- Their solubilization and interaction with other components in the GI fluids
- Their absorption through the epithelial layer
- Their subsequent chemical and biochemical transformations within epithelial cells (Dima et al., 2020).

Insufficient nutritional absorption, excessive compound excretion, and reduced effectiveness of therapeutic dosage receptivity result from a short gastric retention time. To extend the time bioactives spend in the GIT, researchers are developing thicker delivery methods that can slow down the movement of compounds in the stomach. This approach increases the number of bioactives taken before gastric discharge (Asghar et al., 2018).

17.4.3 Intonation of Metabolic Activities

The first barrier to bioavailability is absorption, and the second is first-pass metabolic processes, which lower the systemic dose levels of nutraceuticals. Adding chemical or physical metabolic enzyme inhibitors to delivery systems can significantly enhance our understanding of the story of bioactives in the circulatory system. However, consuming such enzyme inhibitors may need more careful consideration to prevent toxicity due to the resulting impairment in detoxification activity (Asghar et al., 2018). Figure 17.1 represents the metabolic activity of nutraceuticals given through the oral route.

17.5 ROUTES OF DELIVERY OF NUTRACEUTICALS

17.5.1 Oral Delivery

The oral route of drug delivery is the most convenient delivery system of all. Simplicity and affordability in formulation make it a widely accepted method of administration. Many elements, including therapeutic impact, physicochemical stability, and bioavailability, contribute to the efficacy of nutraceutical substances. Limited intestinal

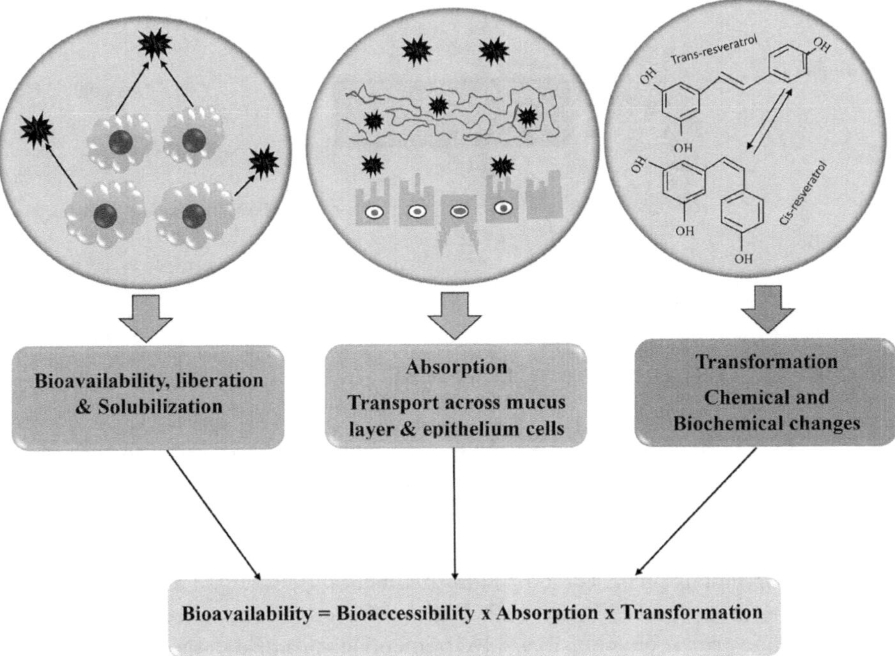

FIGURE 17.1 Diagrammatic representation of drugs administered through the oral route.

permeability, poor GI solubility, and hepatic first-pass metabolism are the leading causes of the low bioavailability of many bioactive compounds. A bioactive chemical must dissolve in gastric fluid and be stable before entering the bloodstream to be absorbed effectively. However, lipophilic bioactive compounds frequently have limited bioavailability and insufficient absorption because they have poor water solubility (Arzani et al., 2015). The second component significantly reducing bioavailability is metabolism, specifically enteric and first-pass breakdown. One of the primary formulation research studies that directly benefit health through experimental and marketable advances is a delivery system based on nanotechnology (Dabholkar et al., 2021). Polymers, metals, and lipids have all been utilized to create nanocarriers, among other materials (Ragelle et al., 2017). These nanocarriers could result in the same site-specific targeted distribution of medicinal substances, exact release completed in short or extended periods, and enhanced half-life. It includes liposomes, niosomes, solid lipid nanoparticles (SLNs), nanostructured lipid carriers (NLCs), self-emulsifying drug delivery systems (SEDDS), etc. (Koh and Wong, 2019).

- **Nanoemulsion:**
  In order to address the significant issues associated with traditional drug delivery systems, researchers have developed a cutting-edge method of drug delivery. As delivery methods for nutraceuticals, nanoemulsions (NEs) are produced (Koh and Wong, 2019) in nanometer sizes to improve the supply of pharmacologically active ingredients.

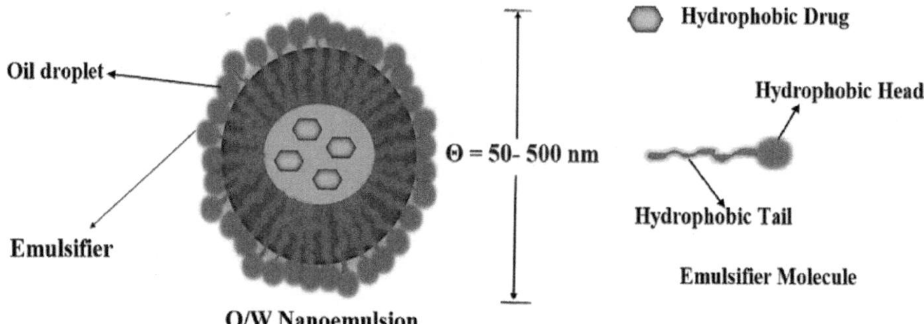

FIGURE 17.2 Diagrammatic representation of NE.

Thermodynamically stable isotropic systems can be produced by combining two immiscible liquids into a single phase with an emulsifying agent, such as a surfactant and a co-surfactant. NE typically has droplet sizes between 20 and 200 nm. The size and shape of the particles scattered in the continuous phase is the primary distinction between an emulsion and a NE, as presented in Figure 17.2. With improved functionality and durability, nanostructured emulsions have tremendous promise in the fields of food and medicinal applications. Along with many other bioactive compounds, they can encapsulate, transport, and deliver both hydrophilic and lipophilic nutraceuticals. Recent studies have shown that many common bioactive are enclosed in nanoscale delivery, including essential fatty acids (EFA) and essential oils (EO), antioxidants, vitamins, minerals, probiotics, prebiotics, and coenzymes, to prevent degradation during processing and storage and to escalation bioavailability after consumption.

- **Nanosuspension:** Solubility issue is one of the major significant sues with nutraceuticals. For nutraceuticals that are practically insoluble or can't be formulated or incorporated in any vehicles, like liposomes, niosomes, etc., nanosuspension can be the breakthrough. Nanosuspensions are made up of poorly water-soluble nutraceuticals dispersed in a dispersion without any polymeric matrix (Koh and Wong, 2019). They can be used to improve the solubility of medications that are ineffective in lipid and water-based media. A faster maximum plasma level is obtained as a result of higher solubility, which also increases the pace of flooding of the active chemical. The size of the nutraceuticals can be achieved in the nanorange through suitable size reduction methods existing.
- **Liposomes:** These phospholipid bilayered vesicular systems have a concentric water core that is surrounded by one (unilamellar) or multiple (multilamellar) phospholipid membranes. It was designed to distribute nutrients at the ideal, desired spot. As a means of providing nutrients to our bodily cells, liposomes serve as nutraceutical delivery vehicles; therefore, scientists named it "Liposomal delivery is biologically intelligent" (Dabholkar et al., 2021).

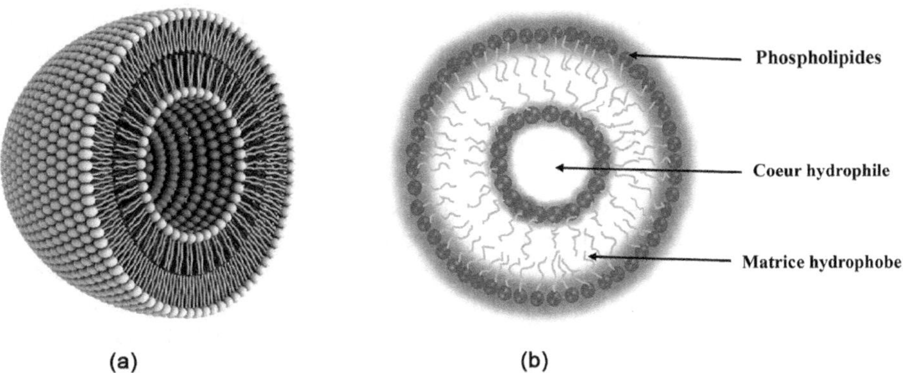

FIGURE 17.3 Structural view of liposome.

Liposomes offer a number of significant advantages. Hydrophobic, hydrophilic, and amphiphilic bioactive chemicals may be incorporated into liposomes, which enhances the pharmacokinetics of nutraceuticals and makes integration easier. Localized delivery can be done using it. Simple to market for various nutraceutical compositions. The structures of liposomes are represented in Figure 17.3.

- **Niosomes:** Identical to liposomes, the only difference is that here the bilayers are made up of nonionic surfactants. Like liposomal formulation, it also has some unique salient features, i.e., easily biodegradable, very much compatible with biological systems, and vesicle's characteristics. Less expensive formulation than the liposomes. Even if it is made so precisely, it can achieve the delivery of nutraceuticals through blood–brain barrier (Dabholkar et al., 2021).
- **Solid lipid nanoparticles (SLNs):** The SLNs are created by substituting solid lipids for liquid lipids in an emulsion recipe. SLNs provide some advantages over liposomes and niosomes and almost overcome their limitations, like diminishing leakage of integrated nutraceutical compounds and shielding the entrapped compound from adverse GI conditions. It is possible to avoid the use of organic solvents while formulating large-scale production with low production costs. In order to get around the pharmacokinetic restrictions of nutraceuticals and boost the nutraceutical potential, SLNs are better as oral delivery vehicles (Dabholkar et al., 2021).

17.5.2 Transdermal Delivery of Nutraceuticals

Nutraceuticals have acquired considerable recognition globally due to their effectiveness in treating chronic diseases, low toxicity, cheap cost, and simplicity of accessibility, among other factors. Another vital factor in the commercialization of nutraceuticals is their efficacy as well as safety. The efficacy and bioavailability of medications derived from herbal sources have been continually improved via the study of several revolutionary enhanced drug delivery systems. The traditional method of ingesting nutraceuticals can be effectively replaced by transdermal medication delivery technology. The development of transdermal system-based nutraceuticals may provide advantages such as improved solubility, bypassing first-pass metabolism, and targeted drug delivery in conditions connected to the brain. It also has the advantage of not being intrusive (Chauhan et al., 2020).

- **Nanostructured lipid carriers (NLCs):** The second generation of lipid nanoparticles is a revolutionary pharmacological formulation of physiological and biocompatible lipids. Surfactants and co-surfactants are the main ingredients of NLCs. Because of their numerous positive properties, including skin hydration, occlusion, increased bioavailability, and skin targeting, NLCs have a significant promise in the nutraceutical medicines and cosmetic markets. Advantages include greater loading capacity, less water required to disperse, minimum drug expulsion during storage, control release and targeted drug release possible, avoidance of organic solvents possible, inexpensive, more physical stability, easy preparation and scale-up, improved benefit/risk ratio, increased skin hydration and elastic property, small size confirms intimate contact with the horney layer of the skin and faster drug release, enhanced drug stability (Chauhan et al., 2020).
- **Nanoemulsion:** As delivery vehicles for nutraceuticals, NEs are made up of nanoscale droplets that are distributed in either an oil-in-water (O/W) or a water-in-oil (W/O) biphasic configuration. An active surfactant stabilizes these droplets. The development of NE-based medication delivery, particularly for cutaneous and transdermal administration, is the subject of ongoing study. The objective is to identify the best semi-solid dosage form for certain NE types (O/W, W/O, and others), as well as to look into how particle size and zeta potential affect drug delivery through the dermal or transdermal route. Notably, W/O NEs display excellent spreadability and make it simple for nutraceuticals to penetrate the skin thanks to the oil phase and the skin's favorable lipophilicity (Lushchak et al., 2020).

17.5.3 Ophthalmic Delivery of Nutraceuticals

Eye health is crucial since diseases that begin to develop can shorten patients' lifespans and result in vision loss. Progressive and irreversible vision loss is primarily brought on by a number of pathologies, including cataracts, ocular atrophy, corneal opacity, age-related macular degeneration (AMD), uncorrected refractive error, posterior capsular opacification, uveitis, glaucoma, diabetic retinopathy, retinal detachment, undetermined disease, and other conditions involving oxidative stress and inflammation. Because they are constantly exposed to the environment, the eyes need to be protected from external harm. Oral administration of nutraceuticals has been shown to be effective in treating a variety of ocular disorders, including presbyopia, cataracts, dry eye disease (DED), glaucoma, AMD, and diabetic retinopathy. Nevertheless, oral administration loses potency due to first-pass metabolism and issues of low bioavailability. Ocular surface epithelium, tear film, and other barriers, as well as internal blood-aqueous and blood-retina barriers, pose a problem for administering nutraceuticals. Additionally, choroidal, conjunctival, and lymphatic barriers, as well as eye clearance rates, affect how effective drugs are distributed to the eye (Zhang et al., 2021; Zhou et al., 2013).

The use of NPs and liposomes in the treatment of eye conditions has drawn a lot of interest. NPs, among them, have demonstrated great potential as a local delivery system. The distribution of NPs inside the eye is substantially influenced by their size and surface properties. Ocular tissue has a long retention duration for NPs between 200 and 2,000 nm, sometimes even up to 2 months. NPs stick to the mucosa, allowing them to stay in the anterior corneal tissue for a longer period of time. These NPs have the potential to increase the therapeutic value of pharmaceuticals by encapsulating, conjugating, or adsorbing them. For the formation of NPs, biodegradable polymers, including alginate, chitosan, gelatin, polycaprolactone, polylactic acid, and polylactic co-glycolic acid (PLGA), are frequently utilized (Zhou et al., 2013).

- **Nanosuspensions:** In contrast to conventional matrix-framework nanosystems, they do not need carrier materials. A nanosuspension is a flexible composition that combines traditional and cutting-edge elements. It is made up of 100% pure medicine NPs with diameters in the nanometer range, usually stabilized with polymers or surfactants. Reducing the drug's particle size after it has been synthesized in a nanosuspension enhances the drug's contact area and time spent in contact with the cornea, and raising the drug's concentration in the infected tissue and the solubility of a poorly soluble medication boosts bioavailability (Zhang et al., 2021).
- **Nanomicelles:** Nanosuspensions, in contrast to conventional matrix-framework nanosystems, do not need carrier materials. A nanosuspension is a flexible composition that combines traditional and cutting-edge elements. It is made up of 100% pure medicine, nutraceuticals NPs with diameters in the nanometer range, usually stabilized with polymers or surfactants. Reducing the drug's particle size after it has been synthesized in a nanosuspension enhances the drug's contact area and time spent in contact with the cornea, and raising the drug's concentration in the infected tissue and the solubility of a poorly soluble medication boosts bioavailability. It has been shown that polymeric micelles can increase a medication's bioavailability in the anterior eye tissues, aid in spreading the drug across the sclera, and have a sustained drug delivery effect in ophthalmic applications (Zhang et al., 2021).
- **Microemulsions/nanoemulsions:** Research on drug delivery has used a variety of other nanotechnology-based carriers, including NEs and microemulsions (MEs). Moreover, because of their high surfactant/co-surfactant concentrations, they have the ability to solubilize drugs and improve penetration. NEs have a high degree of stability, minimal levels of toxicity and irritation, a high capacity for drug loading, and significantly increased drug bioavailability. In the area of local drug delivery to the eyes, NEs are among the most investigated and used nanocarriers. NEs are primarily absorbed through the cornea after local administration to the eye. The emulsion also contains an emulsifier, a co-emulsion, an oil phase, and a water phase. The emulsion increases the amount of time that the drug is in touch with the corneal epithelial cells, encourages drug absorption by the cornea, sclera,

or conjunctiva, and enhances emulsion adhesion. Despite the fact that NEs offer numerous physical, chemical, and physiological benefits, the composition of the corneal layers has an impact on how they are absorbed and distributed.

- ***In situ* gelling drug delivery systems:** Over the past 10 years, *in situ* gelling drug delivery methods have attracted a lot of attention in the field of ophthalmology. Drug delivery systems with *in situ* gelling are capable of producing gels in response to various endogenous cues when in a sol state prior to administration. Such systems can successfully be employed as carriers for drug-loaded nano- and micro-particles to treat ocular illnesses and can be supplied through various ways to accomplish ocular medication delivery. To further increase the retention period of medications on the ocular surface and increase their bioavailability, composite systems made of other nano-preparations, such as liposomes and NPs, have been created. The nanocomposite gel technique has extensive quality control. The quality of the entire system must be taken into account, including the stability of the gel and the in situ gel's ability to gel at a macro level. Because the nano-gel composite system makes extensive use of auxiliary materials, safety must come first (Zhang et al., 2021).

17.6 NANOCARRIERS AS DELIVERY PLATFORM FOR NUTRACEUTICALS

17.6.1 Nanoparticles

NPs are often used in drug delivery systems and can be constructed of various materials, including proteins (Jain et al., 2018), lipids (Desfrançois et al., 2018), and polymers (poly-D, L-lactide-co-glycolide, lactic acid polymer, and polycaprolactone). In particular, food-grade materials must be employed to create NPs if they are to be used in the food and nutraceutical industries (Wei et al., 2020). Zein, a protein derived from maize, chitosan, and gelatin, are a few examples of the food-grade materials used (Yuan et al., 2020). Soy proteins have caught the attention of researchers to be employed in the creation of nanocarriers for the transport of bioactive substances, nutraceuticals included, due to their ability to degrade, bioavailability, and the potential to encapsulate hydrophobic chemicals (DeFrates et al., 2018; Verma et al., 2018). In order to encapsulate insoluble curcumin, a polyphenol known for its antioxidant and anticancer properties, researchers employed soy-conglycinin (a preserved globulin) to create NPs. In 2021, there were a total of 5,11,792 occurrences of 19 inflammatory behaviors (Basnet and Skalko-Basnet, 2011). The vicilin storage amino acids of soybeans, -conglycinin, was disassembled, and then reassembly was carried out via urea and without the addition of any other organic solvent; the resulting NPs appear to be more organic and are distinguished by an adequate solubility and efficiency of encapsulation (around 80%) higher than that acquired in previous works. Curcumin was shown to have a bioaccessibility of about 40% (as opposed to 20% for free curcumin). For hydrophobic chemicals, conglycinin nanostructures offer promising biocompatible delivery strategies (Liu et al., 2019). Two citrus fruit flavonoids, hesperidin and naringin, were enclosed in gold and silver NPs stabilized using plant cellulose, tragacanth, and acacia gum, respectively. Jain and his colleagues created beta-carotene-loaded NPs of zein to investigate their potential application in breast cancer. Both *in vitro* (MCF-7 lymphocytes) as well as *in vivo* (induced carcinoma of the breast in rats), the acquired system demonstrated better anticancer efficacy in relation to free beta-carotene; this is likely because there was a higher cellular uptake of zein NPs. Another nutrient, resveratrol, when encapsulated into NPs, has shown increased antitumor effectiveness against MCF-7. Different anti-inflammatory, antioxidant, and anticancer effects are displayed by this polyphenolic molecule. Because of this, encapsulation into cyclodextrins (CDs) has recently been proposed (Venuti et al., 2014). In particular, it was shown that association produced an ongoing increase in the soluble state of resveratrol in water and, as a result, a substantial boost in the anticancer effects of resveratrol in multiple cell lines. However, it is nearly insoluble in water (0.03 mg/mL at 25°C). In the study conducted by Poonia and coworkers, mimetic folate receptor-specific NPs were employed to encapsulate resveratrol, with an encapsulation effectiveness of roughly 90%. Due to the overexpression of folate receptors in the MCF-7 cancer line, the acquired system demonstrated favorable *in vitro* anticancer characteristics. The *in vivo* results were more significant; in fact, the authors demonstrated that when given intravenously to Wistar rats, resveratrol in capsule form circulated for more than 48 hours, compared to 6 hours for free medication, thanks to the aforementioned NPs. The combined effect of *in vitro* and *in vivo* properties allows us to think of the mimetic folate channel targeted NP as a viable resveratrol delivery method, and this result validated the capacity of NPs to shield the encapsulated medication from environmental stimuli (Poonia et al., 2020).

The synergistic combination of the two separate nutraceuticals, piperine and curcumin, was a recent method that was suggested. These nutraceuticals were enclosed in chitosan-coated core-shell NPs consisting of zein and hyaluronic acid. The unique and intricate makeup of the particles enables the co-encapsulation of multiple nutritional supplements with distinct physicochemical properties, yielding an encapsulation efficiency for curcumin and piperine of 90% and 86%, respectively. The experimental digestion investigation was carried out by simulating the GI situation; the findings show that piperine is released from NPs more quickly than curcumin. For the simultaneous delivery as well as defense of nutraceuticals with various chemical properties, the food-grade formulated formulation emerged as a potential nanocarrier method (Chen et al., 2019). In order to shield them from exposure to heat and light deterioration and improve their bioavailability through the mouth by permitting an extended absorption at the GI threshold, the identical nutraceutical, curcumin, was encapsulated together with piperine through NPs made of a mixture of zein (core) and carrageenan (shell). This was shown by *in vitro* experiments. Additionally, it was discovered that piperine as well as curcumin-loaded NPs had an *in vitro* antioxidant ability of about 70% compared to 20% for free medicines (Chen et al., 2020). Finally, the nanoprecipitation method was used by Sanna and associates to create polymeric NPs loaded with white tea extract using a combination of poly(-caprolactone) and alginate. The results obtained demonstrate how this polymeric structure enables polyphenolic extract protection, regulated distribution in the intestines, and the preservation of antioxidant function (Sanna et al., 2015).

TABLE 17.1
Chitosan-Based Surface Modification of SLN Delivery Systems for the Bioavailability of Phytocompounds to the Target Organs

Types of Chitosan-Modified Solid Lipid Nanoparticles	Bioactive Compounds	Disease Models	References
Solid lipid nanoparticles with chitosan coating	Curcumin	Pancreatic cancer model	Chen et al. (2019)
	Resveratrol	Studies on brain bioavailability	Chen et al. (2020)
	Caffeic acid	Study on oral bioavailability	Sanna et al. (2015)
	Tea polyphenols	Cancer	Chen et al. (2019)
	Ferulic acid	Model for pancreatic cancer	Chen et al. (2019)
	EGCG	Bioavailability	Chen et al. (2019)
SLNs with a trimethyl chitosan coating	Curcumin	Studies on brain bioavailability	Chen et al. (2020)
	Resveratrol	Studies on brain bioavailability	Poonia et al. (2020)
SLNs with a surface modified by N-trimethyl chitosan-g-palmitic acid	Resveratrol	Studies on brain bioavailability	Sanna et al. (2015)
Nanoliposomes	Quercetin	Cancer Therapy	Thakkar et al. (2015)
NPs with polymeric mucoadhesion	Extract of Red Grape Seeds	Coronary artery disease	Ramalingam and Ko (2016b)
NPs of silver	Fruit extract of Piper Longum	Pathogenic bacteria	Fathi et al. (2013)

17.6.2 Solid Lipid Nanoparticles

A first-generation nano-SLN form of delivery called a SLN has been extensively employed to administer phytocompounds orally for sustained release in the treatment of many chronic disorders. Many brand-new oral nanodelivery techniques have recently been created. A reduced manufacturing cost, long-term stability, and tolerability, biodegradability with less harmful effects, as well as improved oral administration of phyto-bioactive chemicals, are SLN's main advantages in bulk production (Table 17.1).

17.6.3 Mesoporous Nanoparticles of Silica

Due to their outstanding biological compatibility, excellent stability, stiff structure, established pore structure, easily adjustable shape, and variable surface chemistry, mesoporous nanoparticles of silica (MSNs) are of particular relevance for protein delivery. Thus, using MSNs as carriers of delivery, better stability of proteins, improved action, responsive release, intracellular delivery, extracellular distribution, antimicrobial protein delivery, enzyme mobilization, and catalysis have all been accomplished (Ramalingam and Ko, 2015).

17.6.3.1 Application of MSNs for Delivery of Intracellular Proteins

Protein therapies have a high level of target specificity, which makes them the future medications for more precise cell function treatments. Additionally, since there is no change in genes, they are thought to be safer than gene treatments. Protein treatments must function inside cells in many applications, including cancer therapy and immunological therapy, but bare proteins cannot cross cell membranes on their own (Ramalingam and Ko, 2016a).

17.6.3.2 Application of MSNs for Delivery of Extracellular Protein

MSNs also offer a platform to safeguard their activity and accomplish responsive release for protein therapies that operate outside of cells. For instance, insulin is frequently used to control diabetes. However, the several daily insulin injections are highly uncomfortable, and for many patients, this discomfort can prevent them from using the medication. The significant drug-loading ability, strong biocompatibility, and simple surface modification provided by MSNs have led to the development of a variety of MSN-based glucose-sensitive insulin release devices (Veiseh et al., 2015).

17.6.3.3 Utilization of MSNs in Catalysis and Enzyme Mobilization

By addressing the inherent problems of the native enzymes, MSNs are also very important for enzyme immobilization and catalysis. A variety of MSNs with pore diameters ranging from 2 to 40 nm were utilized for the immobilization of numerous enzymes, namely, peroxidase, cytochrome C, and catalase. After insertion inside MSNs, the enzyme activity was prominent in different pH ranges and also after exposure to reagents that degrade enzymes, such as proteases. It should be emphasized that after 25 batches of subsequent reactions, the MSN enzyme preserved 70% of its initial activity. The use of branching mesoporous organosilica nanomaterials containing benzene chains as a structure for an enzyme, lipase, and immobilization was also recently reported. It's noteworthy to note that lipase has shown improved pH and heat stability as well as increased activity when packed into organosilica NPs relative to free lipase. Additionally, after five cycles, the lipase packed in MSNs still had 94% of its original catalytic activity, demonstrating the benefit of reusability (Shikinaka et al., 2018).

17.6.3.4 Application of MSNs for Delivery of Antibacterial Proteins

The delivery of antimicrobial proteins via NPs has considerable promise for the cure of bacterial illnesses. As an illustration, the surface of MSN-41 was covered with lysozyme, a naturally occurring protein that may catalyze the degradation of bacterial walls, which improved the interaction with *E. coli*, a popular Gram-negative bacterium, and increased the local levels of lysozyme. In comparison to free lysozyme, the minimal inhibitory concentration was five times lower following conjugation with MSNs. Song et al. (2016) created MSNs with large pores that had the potential to load lysozyme inside in order to address the issue of lysozyme exposure on the exterior surface. They then demonstrated the enhanced ability to mitigate the effects of *E. coli in vitro* in addition to an *ex vivo* intestinal infection model. Produced branching MSNs for lysozyme loading, with pore diameters ranging from 2.7 to 22.4 nm. The researchers discovered that MSNs with wide porosity had a high capacity for lysozyme loading (244.5 mg/g) and displayed a profile of sustained release. The minimum inhibitory concentration, or MIC, of free lysozyme was reduced from 2,500 mg/mL to 500 g/mL when lysozyme was loaded inside MSNs, demonstrating a superior antibacterial action against *E. coli* (Li and Wang, 2013).

17.6.4 Niosomes and their Use in the Administration of Nutritional Supplements

In order to regulate their absorption by the body and improve the nutritional value of food and dairy goods with which these goods can be enriched, niosomes have recently been used as dietary supplement vehicles of functional elements helpful in avoiding the development of many diseases triggered by oxidative stress. Although niosomes have been studied for almost 20 years, it is only recently that food scientists have started to use them to fortify dairy products with controlled ingestion of functional ingredients like peptides, enzymes, vitamins, along with flavors. This increases the dairy products' nutraceutical as well as organoleptic qualities and makes niosomes a great hope for the avoidance of numerous illnesses in which oxidative damage plays a significant role. Tween 60 niosomes may be attractive candidates for the development of prolonged-release dosage forms that can be taken orally for the administration of antioxidants as individual molecules or in combination. A novel nutrient delivery system in the prevention of diseases caused by oxidative stress (Subramanian, 2021).

17.6.5 Nanoliposomes

Nanoscale lipid bilayers, also known as nanoliposomes, are typically spherical vesicles created when phospholipid molecules are energetically dispersed in a water-based media. The tocosome, the other nanoscale substance covered in this post, is a recently developed bioactive carrier consisting primarily of tocopheryl phosphates. These nanocarriers may transport hydrophilic and hydrophobic substances independently or simultaneously because of their bi-compartmental framework, which is composed of lipidic as well as aqueous compartments. Sensitive food-grade bioactive compounds can be protected and released over time using nanoliposomes and tocosomes. They are used to produce functional products, enrich and fortify various food and nutraceutical formulations, and encapsulate various types of bioactive substances (such as medications, minerals, antioxidants, and preservatives). Lipid vesicles, such as nanoliposomes, have several uses in the cosmetics and pharmaceutical industries. Their use in the food systems has been constrained, nevertheless, by concerns about cost-effectiveness and food safety. However, these issues might be resolved by using specialized methods for the mass production of lipid-based vesicles using commercially available, reasonably priced lecithin components (Zarrabi et al., 2020).

17.6.5.1 Applications in the Food and Nutraceutical Industry

Scientists are now using nanoliposomes to facilitate the encapsulation as well as controlled delivery of nutraceuticals as well as functional food components such as antioxidants, proteins, polysaccharides, digestive enzymes, vitamins, flavors, additives, and EFAs. This is based on the effective utilization of liposomes in the biomedical and pharmaceutical industries (Table 17.2) (Mohan et al., 2015). One of the main benefits of using nanoliposomes in the food and nutraceutical industries is that they frequently escape our sensory perception, making it possible to fortify foods and beverages with bioactive ingredients (like omega fatty acids derived from fish) without impairing the sensory qualities of the original product. Nanoliposomes are apparently undetectable to the naked eye due to their nanometric size. They scarcely scatter visible light and preserve transparency if kept below 80 nm in size (and not at extremely high concentrations or if the particle refractive index is not significantly distinct from the rest of the solution). Such covert vesicles can be used, for example, to add hydrophobic nutraceuticals or substances with unpleasant flavors or odors to clear liquids. The graphic shows a few advantages of using nanoliposomes in the fields of food and nutraceuticals. The fact that safe substances from organic sources, like eggs, soy, or milk, can be used to make nanoliposomes is another distinguishing benefit of this technology. As a result, they might be granted approval from regulators to be utilized in goods that are fit for human consumption (Malik et al., 2017).

Humans can benefit from the phospholipid components of liposomes as well as nanoliposomes in a number of ways, including protection of the liver and improved memory. Sphingolipids, on the other hand, are necessary for cellular signaling and have been linked to the regulation of inflammation, cancer, cancer cell proliferation, and apoptosis (Huwilera, 2000). Another component used to make nanoliposomes, sphingomyelin (SM), has the ability to reduce the amount of fat and cholesterol absorbed through the intestinal tract, while milk SM is becoming more efficient than egg SM (Peel, 1999). As a result, nanoliposomes provide significant medical advantages to consumers in addition to protecting and delivering the items they carry.

TABLE 17.2
Some Examples of Utilization of Nanoliposomes for Combination Therapy and Synergistic Bioactive Delivery

Therapeutic Agents Carrier	Indication/Health Benefit	System Targeting	Mode/Administration Route
Vitamin E and glutathione	Oxidative stress and immediate lung damage	Nanoliposome	Endotracheal tube-based pulmonary delivery
Vitamin E, ascorbic acid, and ascorbyl palmitate	Scurvy, immune system booster, and antioxidant	Nanoliposome	Oral (Mishra et al., 2018)

The dairy food business has shown a great deal of interest in liposomes and nanoliposomes. Law and King (1985) utilized bilayer lipid vesicles to encapsulate cheese-ripening enzymes, aiming to resolve this problem. (Law and King, 1985). By adding edible enzymes like proteinases before separating the curds, time and, subsequently, expenses can be cut during dairy ripening and hardening. Free (unencapsulated) enzyme addition, however, has several drawbacks, such as quick casein proteolysis leading to unfavorable curd quality and low yields. Bilayer lipid vesicles were used by Law and King (1985) for encapsulating cheese-ripening enzymes in order to solve this issue (Kheadr et al., 2002). They found that adding liposome-encapsulated proteinases to cheese curd caused the development of hard cheese by limiting the proteolytic breakdown of casein and preserving the curd form by preventing any unfavorable enzymatic activity. Investigations into the use of lipase to enhance cheese production (Kheadr et al., 2002). According to some reports, using liposome-encapsulated lipase allowed cheddar cheese to become more cohesive and stretchy while also reducing its stiffness. The important thing to remember is that adding proteinases and lipases to cheese made with cheddar should be properly monitored for better ripening and acceleration to prevent adverse effects on overall food quality. One of the most important regulatory criteria that manufacturers must take into account is the composition of the nanoliposome in order to prevent the formation of undesirable flavors and to guarantee the release of materials in a controlled but predictable way (Taylor et al., 2005). The effectiveness of liposomes and nanoliposomes in the encapsulation and distribution of carotenoids has also been investigated (Livney, 2015). In a different investigation, nanoliposomes were used to encapsulate hydrophilic substances like green tea catechins (Rashidinejad et al., 2014). To examine the simultaneous encapsulation of lipophilic and hydrophilic nutritional supplements in nanoliposomes composed of soy phospholipids, two distinct commercial plant sterols were employed. The impact of a hydrophilic as well as water-resistant plant sterol on ascorbic acid's stability and capacity to be effectively encapsulated. At pH 7.0, nanoliposomes were created utilizing the high-pressure homogenization technique. The initial size distribution for each nanoliposome formulation was monomodal, with an average size between 115 and 150 nm. While dilution demonstrated an extended profile of release over time, the addition of plant sterols improved the average size of nanoliposomes. The study demonstrated that the existence of plant sterols impacts the stability of colloidal particles and the encapsulation effectiveness of nanoliposomes produced by high-pressure homogenization. Another type of nutraceutical that would greatly benefit from the encapsulating process in terms of enhancing its nutritional value is antioxidant chemicals. One such is the dual-functional nanoliposomal antioxidant composition that contains both vitamin C and vitamin E, ascorbic acid (Kirby, 1993). Figure 17.4 describes the flowchart of advantages of nanoliposomes in the nutraceutical industries.

17.6.6 Nanofibers

A polymer mixture and a strong electric field are used in the effective and affordable technique of electrospinning to create nanofibers. These can be used for a variety of biological and medicinal purposes. Electrospun nanofibers are regarded as potential materials for the production of drug delivery systems because of their significant

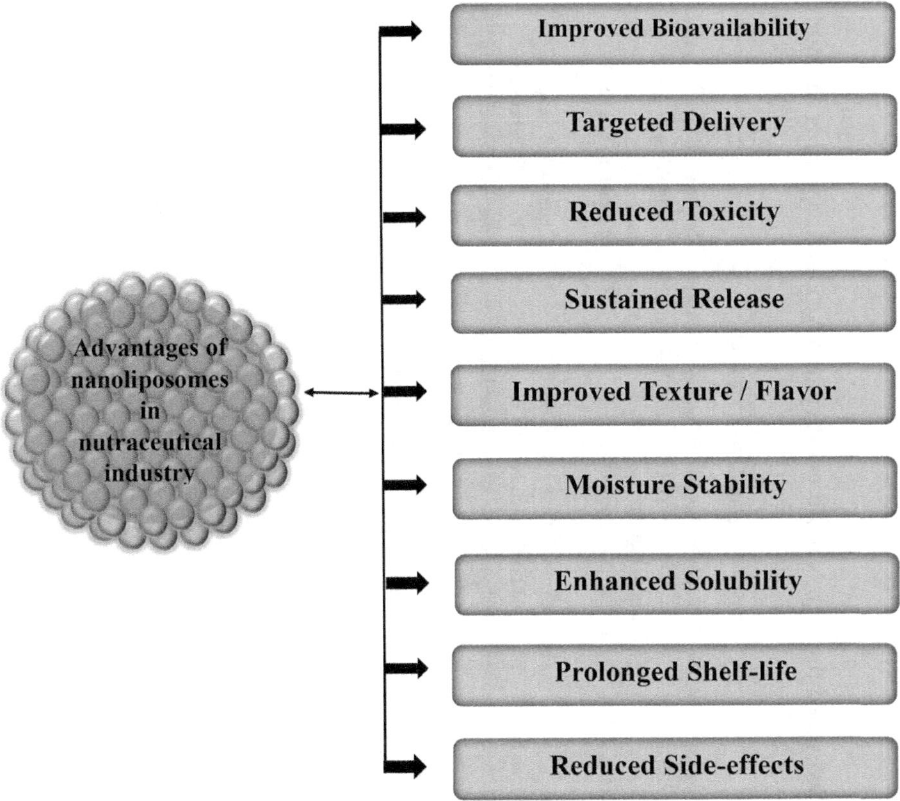

FIGURE 17.4 Nanoliposomes in nutraceutical industries.

surface area, adjustable surface functionalization and characteristics, and typically high biocompatibility. Poorly soluble pharmaceuticals may be converted into amorphous solid dispersions by electrospinning, which may improve solubility, bioavailability, and drug release targeting. It works well for the encapsulation of nutritional supplements as well. Nutraceuticals are dietary supplements generated from food that may help in illness prevention and treatment. They consist of prebiotics, omega-3 fatty acids and organized fatty acids, phytochemicals, as well as extracts of plants, carbohydrates, carotenoids and antioxidants, peptides, amino acids, vitamins, minerals, and proteins. Probiotics are living bacteria thought to have a positive effect on health. To help protect delicate molecules from extremes during processing, minimize undesirable interactions that occur between nutritional supplements and food matrix, and avoid degradation before releasing them at the target site, precise strategies for nutraceutical delivery are required. Encapsulation offers a solution to these problems (Bhavaniramya et al., 2019). Probiotic microcapsules can be used to functionalize foods like meat (fermented sausage), dairy (cheese and yogurt), juices (from vegetables and fruits), bakery goods (biscuits, baked goods, and bread), and other things (fermented drinks, mayonnaise, and ice cream) (Table 17.3) (Mutlu-Ingok et al., 2020).

TABLE 17.3
Selected Nutraceuticals of Interest to the Food Industry Delivered through Nanofibers Prepared by Electrospinning Methods and their Associated Health Benefits

Category	Food Source	Examples	Some Associated Health Benefits	Ref.
Probiotics	Bread, milk, cheese, sourdough, kimchi, sauerkraut, organic whey, and yoghurt	Lactic acid bacteria, a kind of lactobacilli, Lactobacillus casei, Bifidobacterium	Immune system improvement, intestinal health, and modification of microbial disease and health markers	Giraffa et al. (2010); Mattarelli et al. (2017)
The bioactive peptides	Fish, milk, meat, and plants	Peptides found in sardines, milk, and eggs	Antihypertensive properties	Marques et al. (2012)
Dietary lipids	Fish, the seeds of flax, calamari, krill, the algae, and seeds and plants that have been genetically modified	Docosahexaenoic acid, eicosapentaenoic acid, and alpha-linoleic acid	Fewer chances of atherosclerosis increased heart function enhanced mental focus and brain health decreased risk of some malignancies	Augustin and Sanguansri (2015); Elizabeth Lane and Derbyshire (2013)
	Milk fat	Alkyl linolenic acid conjugate	Reduced chance of atherosclerosis characteristics that are anti-inflammatory, immunomodulatory, and anti-carcinogenic	Augustin and Sanguansri (2015); Bassaganya-Riera et al. (2002)
Vitamins	Vegetables, dairy products, fruits, and meat	Vitamin A, C, D, E, K, B1, B3, B6, B9, and B12	Numerous health advantages, including the antioxidant properties of vitamins A, C, and E and the role of vitamin K in blood clotting	Augustin and Sanguansri (2015); Ghani et al. (2019)
Minerals	Typically, accessible as salts	Iron, magnesium, phosphorus, calcium, zinc, and iron	Several health advantages (for instance, zinc is necessary for cell reproduction)	Augustin and Sanguansri (2015); Ghani et al. (2019)
Inorganic phenols and polyphenols	Fruits and vegetables, olive trees, tea, pomegranate chocolate, grapeseed, and seeds	Catechins, curcuminoids, resveratrol, flavones, flavanols, and phenolic acidS	Decrease in oxidative stress protection from cancer, metabolic, cardiovascular, and neurological disorders	Augustin and Sanguansri (2015); Y Aboul-Enein et al. (2013)
Carotenoids	Marigolds, carrots, tomatoes, microalgae, and green leafy veggies	Lutein, lycopene, -carotene, and astaxanthin	Protection from macular degeneration due to age. Macular eye disease, cancer, heart disease, and cataracts	Augustin and Sanguansri (2015); Estrada-Gil et al. (2021)

Small molecules are present in several nutraceuticals. Antifungal, antioxidant, and antiseptic activities can be found in several bioactive substances, such as vitamins and EOs (Mutlu-Ingok et al., 2020). Electrospinning nanofibers can effectively address the issue of low aqueous solubility. Making fibers from complexes of inclusion of the desired substance combined with CD has garnered a lot of interest in the field of nutraceuticals. Both the inclusion complex plus a polymer, as well as extremely concentrated forms of the addition complex alone, can be used to create fibers (Balusamy et al., 2020; Coban et al., 2021). In several experiments, fast-dissolving fibers with complex inclusions containing curcumin (Celebioglu and Uyar, 2020a), the acid ferulic (Celebioglu and Uyar, 2020b), and lipoic acids (Celebioglu and Uyar, 2019), among others, were effectively electrospun. In addition to solubility problems, fiber production can assist in solving them. One natural antioxidant with weak thermal as well as oxidative stability and limited solubility is lipoic acid. The dissolution rate can be accelerated by electrospun nanofibers of lipoic acid-CD complexes while also aiding in the preservation of their antioxidant properties (McClements and Rao, 2011). Similar outcomes have been noted for the antioxidant vitamin E, where fibers made from CD complexes of inclusion could boost photostability and extend shelf life.

17.6.7 Nanoemulsion

The use of consumable NEs to encapsulate, protect, and transport lipophilic nutrients, such as volatile ingredients, polyphenols, flavors, pigments, vitamins, proteins, oil-soluble flavor, preservatives, etc., which are currently needed globally, is receiving increasing attention in the modern food industry. The transmission of both hydrophilic and hydrophobic substances, higher stability, stronger antibacterial properties, good taste, higher affinity, a longer shelf life, and an improvement in the bioavailability of components are just a few of the potential benefits of NEs over conventional emulsions. They are also very effective at increasing the ability to dissolve and/or solubility of inadequately water-soluble substances, which may lead to improved pharmacokinetic and pharmacodynamic aspects of nutraceutical substances.

The oil phase, the surfactant used, co-surfactant, ingredients, water phase, and functional chemicals make up the majority of food NEs.

The nanoemulsification technique is the most renowned of the several emulsification technologies that have emerged quickly in recent years. There are numerous ways to make NEs (Figure 17.5). Due to varying preparation techniques, operational settings, and system compositions, the generated NE droplet sizes may change. The preparation techniques can be roughly divided into extremely energetic and low-energy techniques based on the underlying operating principles (Bai et al., 2016).

17.6.7.1 The Uses of Nanoemulsions

Leaders in the food industry are currently putting a lot of effort into creating NEs from nutritious components to help new foods suit people's dietary needs. In the food business, emulsion is a brand-new class of nutrition delivery technologies with outstanding performance. The successful study on the use of NEs as food carriers for bioactive substances and wholesome foods is summarized in Table 17.4.

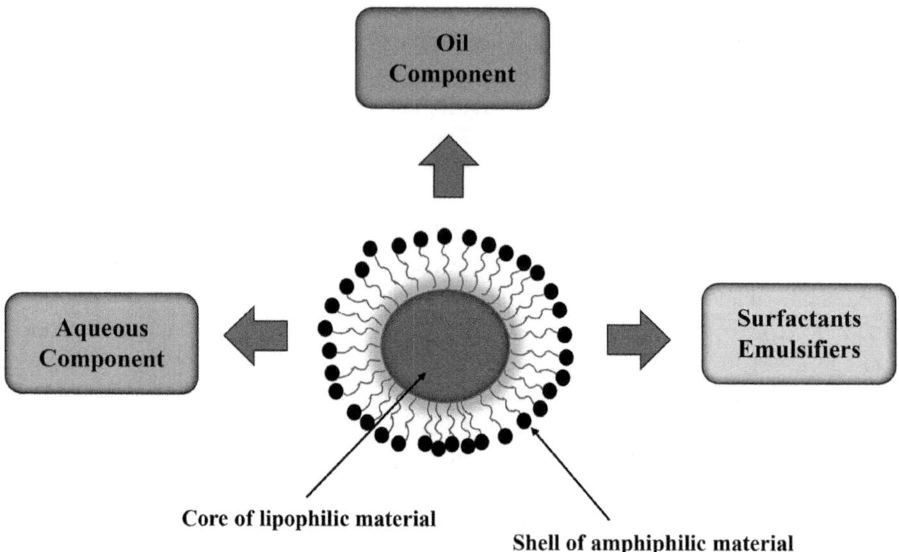

FIGURE 17.5 Core-shell framework of nanodroplets in NEs and other NE components is shown schematically.

17.6.8 Nanocapsules

Nanocapsules are extremely small particles that range in size from one tenth nanometer up to a nanometer. They are made up of a liquid or solid core with a cavity in which the medication is deposited, encircled by a unique polymer membrane comprised of organic or synthetic polymers. Due to the barrier coating, which is often pyrophoric, rapidly oxidized, and delays the dissolution of active substances, they have drawn a lot of attention. The production of nanocapsules involves a number of technical techniques, but the ones that are most frequently used include interfacial polymerization for monomers and nano-deposition for premade polymers. Particle size and size distribution are the most crucial aspects of their preparation, and these properties can be assessed using a variety of methods, including X-ray diffraction, scanning electron microscopes, transmitted electron microscopy, high-resolution transmission electron microscopes, X-ray photoelectron spectroscopy, superconductive quantum interference instruments, multi-angle laser light scattering, and other spectroscopic methods. A wide range of biological applications exist for nanocapsules with exceedingly high repeatability. They can be used in radiotherapy, liposomal nanocapsules for nutritional science, agricultural chemicals, genetic engineering, cosmetics, products for cleaning, wastewater procedures, binding component applications, strategic drug delivery in malignancies, nanocapsule dressings to fight infections, and nutraceuticals. They can also function as materials that can mend themselves (Kothamasu et al., 2012).

TABLE 17.4
The Use of Nanoemulsions as Food Carriers for Bioactive Substances and Wholesome Foods

Functional Compound	Emulsification Method	Objectives	Outcome of the Study	Ref.
Vitamin D_3	Homogenization under high pressure	By modeling the digestive system, the physical characteristics and in vitro availability of the Vit D3 NP emulsion were investigated.	NEs can not only improve the bioavailability of VD3 but also reduce the risk of some people being exposed to VD3	Guttoff et al. (2015)
Vitamin E	Phase inversion	Emulsified phase inversion approach is used to create a food-grade NE that is abundant in vitamin E acetate.	The EPI technique may generate smaller droplets at greater surfactant concentrations for sealing oil-soluble micronutrients in food, beverages, cosmetics, and pharmaceutical items as opposed to the high-energy method.	Mayer et al. (2013)
Fish oil	High speed homogenization/ ultrasonication	O/W NE as well as conventional emulsions (CE) have been created using fish fat oil including EPA and DHA as raw ingredients, and how they were absorbed in the small intestinal tract of rats was studied.	In rats, NE dramatically increases the uptake of lipids in the small intestine's emulsion system.	kumar Dey et al. (2012)
β-Carotene	High pressure homogenization	Researchers looked at how modified starch stabilization affected the stability and bioavailability of -carotene in NE.	After embedding, the bioaccessibility of the -carotene NE clearly improves.	Liang et al. (2013)
Curcumin	Ultrasonication	Orally given new curcumin natural gel NEs were utilized to examine its bioavailability and broaden its use in food.	When compared to unformulated curcumin, curcumin NE has a greater dissolving rate and a 9 times higher oral bioavailability.	Yu and Huang (2012)
	Ultrasonication	The use of nanotechnology to address curcumin's volatility and bioavailability issues	Curcumin's stability is increased when it is encapsulated as an emulsion. Curcumin NE's gradual release can increase bioavailability.	Sari et al. (2015)
Lycopene	Emulsification as a means of evaporation	To preserve the antioxidant properties of the lycopene extracts and increase its biological accessibility, the lycopene nano dispersion was created using the emulsification-evaporation process.	The best in vitro bioavailability was found in NEs having droplets smaller than 100 nm.	Ha et al. (2015); Kim et al. (2014)

(*Continued*)

TABLE 17.4 (*Continued*)
The Use of Nanoemulsions as Food Carriers for Bioactive Substances and Wholesome Foods

Functional Compound	Emulsification Method	Objectives	Outcome of the Study	Ref.
Lemongrass essential oil (LEO)	Microfluidization	Researchers looked at the impact of a NE coating film containing EOs of lemongrass (LEO) on the security and freshness of freshly cut red Fuji apples after storage.	NEs provide potential benefits over conventional emulsions for enhancing the freshness and safety of fresh fruit.	Salvia-Trujillo et al. (2015)
Coenzyme Q10	Homogenization under high pressure	To compare the pharmacokinetics of three orally given formula of CoQ10.	An improved method for increasing Coenzyme Q10's bioavailability is to use NEs.	Belhaj et al. (2012); Shin et al. (2015)
Resveratrol	Homogenization under high pressure	To maximize the effectiveness of orally taken resveratrol capsules, several O/W NEs were created.	A food-grade NE containing resveratrol enhanced their stability and bioavailability.	Sessa et al. (2014)
5Demethyltangeretin (5DT)	Homogenization under high pressure	To increase the effectiveness of 5DT and its absorption in intestinal cancer cells, use an emulsion-based delivery strategy.	An increase in cell absorption and a decrease in cancer cell survival rat can result from wrapping 5DT in NE.	Zheng et al. (2014)
Capsaicin (CAP)	Method of self-assembly	In order to improve the bioavailability and solubility of CAP and lessen its irritability, an edible NE was created.	Organogel CAP NE's biological accessibility and dissolution rate also increased. It had a stronger calming impact. on the irritation of the gastric mucosa	Choi et al. (2013)
Ellagic acid	Method of spontaneous emulsification	Create a food-grade nanoemulsification method to enhance ellagic acid absorption and solubility.	In comparison to suspensions and pomegranate extract, the rate of absorption of ellagic acid in the NE is 6.5-fold and 3.2-fold higher, respectively.	Wang et al. (2017)
Quercetin	Homogenization under high pressure	The instability and poor ingestion rate of quercetin were improved by using a rice bran protein nano particles carrier.	Quercetin's bioavailability was enhanced via NE, which also decreased quercetin's harm to cells and raised its cell permeability.	Karadag et al. (2013)
Clove oil	Ultrasonication	to achieve stable NEs of clove oil with droplet sizes smaller than 50 nm by optimizing critical preparation factors	Oil in a water-based solution is stabilized and given a better antibacterial effect using NE.	Shahavi et al. (2016)
Ginger essential oil (GEO)	Ultrasonication	A NE-based food-grade coating comprising GEO was studied for its antimicrobial and antioxidant effectiveness.	GEO NE improved the sturdiness of chicken breast more than standard emulsion.	Noori et al. (2018)

17.6.9 Nanocrystal

The demand to supplement daily nutrition with additives or nutraceuticals is rising along with nutritional health consciousness. The notion of a healthy population places a lot of emphasis on diet. The market for nutraceuticals is expanding, and many of these substances, such as antioxidants, are not very soluble. Coenzyme Q10 capsules are now the most popular molecules, yet Q10 has poor oral bioavailability. There are solutions on the market that advertise "nano Q10" as being 100% bioavailable and only requiring a tenth of the usual dose in conventional solutions (e.g., containing surfactants for solubilization). Additionally, poorly soluble nutraceuticals, including coenzyme Q10, and apigenin, can benefit from using nanocrystals as a formulation method (Jahangir et al., 2020).

17.6.10 Nanocomplexation

Due to consumers' growing health consciousness and a desire to combat the high frequency of chronic diseases around the world, there has been an increase in fascination with the creation of functional foods during the past few decades. Numerous bioactives or nutraceuticals, including polyphenols, flavonoids, phytosterols, and curcuminoids, have been discovered and isolated from food and have been shown to have a significant role in the connection between diet and health. However, many nutritional supplements or bioactives with well-known health advantages have very poor water solubility and are physically and chemically unsustainable in aqueous conditions (or during digestion), resulting in extremely low bioaccessibility/bioavailability. The development of food-grade delivery systems is one of the methods that have been suggested to increase the water dispersion as well as the bioaccessibility/bioavailability of poorly soluble nutraceuticals. Due to their biodegradability, biocompatibility, and renewability, protein-based nanocarriers have been identified as one of the most promising and efficient nanotechnologies for the delivery of poorly soluble drugs or nutraceuticals among all the stated nanoencapsulation techniques (Tang, 2020). It's interesting to note that many proteins, including milk proteins, act as natural nanocarriers for hydrophobic or poorly soluble nutraceuticals. In this instance, these nutraceuticals are capable of binding to proteins on their own through hydrophobic interactions, leading to the formation of nanocomplexes.

17.7 APPLICATION OF NANOCOMPLEXES IN NUTRACEUTICAL DELIVERY

Several poorly soluble nutraceuticals, including turmeric (Tang, 2020), resveratrol, vitamin D, folic acid (FA), omega-3 polyunsaturated fatty acids, coenzyme Q10, carotene, quercetin, and epigallocatechin gallate, have demonstrated significant enhancements in water dispersibility, stability, and bioactivities.

17.7.1 Carbon Nanotubes

Carbon nanotubes (CNTs), which are nanostructures formed of wrapped graphene planes, offer a variety of fascinating chemical and physical properties. CNTs can be combined with a variety of biological substances, including hormones, proteins, and nucleic acids, to achieve biofunctionalities. CNTs come in single-walled nanotube (SWNT) and multi-walled nanotube (MWNT) varieties. A few of their noteworthy qualities include their enormous aspect ratio, ultra-lightweight, durability, high heat conductivity, and electrochemical properties that range from metallic to semiconductor. Thermal synthesis, chemical vapor deposition, arc discharge evaporation, laser ablation, plasma-based synthesis, and plasma-enhanced vapor deposition are a few processes that can be used to create CNTs. CNTs are helpful in a variety of applications, including medication delivery, cancer treatment, immunological therapy, bioimaging, biosensing, and tissue engineering (Kaur et al., 2019).

17.7.2 Application of CNTs in Nutraceutical Delivery

We employed SWCNTs, a significant class of synthetic nanomaterials with unique physicochemical characteristics, as novel carriers for curcumin. Curcumin-loaded SWCNT structures for utilizing the anticancer properties of curcumin by overcoming the traditional constraints of extremely low solubility in water and unpredictability under physiological circumstances, and blending SWCNTs photothermal therapy made possible by the elevated optical absorption of SWCNTs in the 0.8–1.4 m that causes excessive local heating. SWCNTs that had been functionalized had been coupled with curcumin (SWCNT-Cur).

Numerous modern antioxidant assays have been created as a result of the active research being done on the measurement of antioxidants in various diets. Since many antioxidants are naturally electroactive, using electrochemical techniques to assess the total antioxidant efficacy of a nutraceutical matrix without the addition of reactive species may be a viable option. Due to its numerous medicinal advantages, green tea is thought to be an antioxidant-rich beverage. One of its components, catechin, is a significant antioxidant and has the capacity to scavenge free radicals. The first screen-printed electrode (SPE) is centered on CNTs, the second one is based on gold NPs (GNPs), and the third one is designed on CNTs with GNPs (CNTs-GNPs). The electrochemical characteristics of these three SPEs are described in the current research. The laccase (Lac) enzymes were used to modify all three electrodes, and glutaraldehyde was used to create a cross-link among the groups of amino acids on the lactic acid and the groups of aldehydes of the reticulation substance. The efficiency of the biological sensors has been substantially enhanced because this particular enzyme is a thermally stable catalyst. Using cyclic voltammetry (CV) as well as differential pulse voltammetry, also known as DPV, the electro-oxidative characteristics of catechin were examined, and these results showed that the combination of CNTs-GNPs considerably increased both the selectivity and sensitivity of the biosensor.

Worldwide, herbal food nutritional supplements (HFS) are becoming more and more popular, with a sizeable population turning to these items for the management of various health issues and/or to supplement vitamin and mineral shortages (Xu et al., 1999). However, due to the fact that a lot of them are still not tested and are being improperly managed, public health worries about their safety have surfaced. Inadequate quality control, inaccurate labeling, and a lack of adequate user information frequently compromise safety (Meng et al., 2008). As a result, there are relatively few recognized potential side effects for them, making it challenging to ascertain the safest and most efficient manner to use them. Additionally, some HFS have been found to contain heavy metals, according to some research (Nguyen et al., 2014; Pham-Huy et al., 2008). It is crucial to identify any potential contamination of heavy metals in HFS. The graphite electrodes were altered with bismuth NP (BiNP), MWCNT, and Nafion by using the drop coating technique. A reasonably priced and environmentally friendly sensor for detecting heavy metal contamination is the modified graphite electrode made of BiNP/MWCNT/Nafion (Pham-Huy et al., 2008).

17.8 APPLICATION OF NANO-BASED NUTRACEUTICALS

Delivery systems for nutraceuticals and bioactive natural goods with low water solubility are frequently made using nanotechnology platforms. Here, we discuss some of the commonly studied nanomaterials used in nutraceuticals. Figure 17.6 demonstrates possible uses for nutraceuticals to which nanotechnology can be applied. Table 17.5 summarizes the potential applications of nutraceutical delivery systems with nano-based

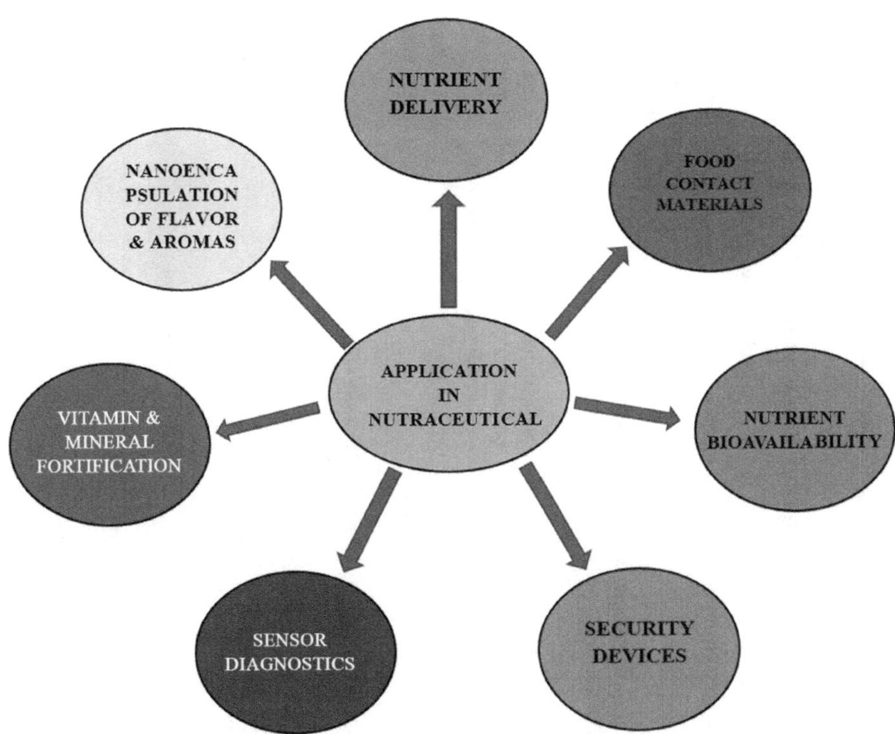

FIGURE 17.6 Applications of nanotechnology in nutraceutical formulation.

TABLE 17.5
The Potential Applications of Nutraceuticals Delivery System Nano-Based Formulation

Components	Delivery System	Applications	Reference
Hydrophobins (Hyd)- Vitamin D_3	Nanoencapsulation	The hydrophobic nutraceutical hydrod was discovered to be a potential nanocarrier for food and beverage enrichment. Hyd provides superior protection for vitamin D3 against deterioration.	Israeli-Lev and Livney (2014)
Milk protein, commercial-resistant flour, and folic acid	Nanoencapsulation	Greater encapsulation efficiency Improved folic acid stability Increase bioactive stabilization	Patel (2015)
DL-α-tocopheryl acetate and β-carotene	Emulsification-diffusion technique, pluronic-127, and polycaprolactone encapsulate nanocapsules (EDM)	EDM is a promising method to prepare NPs for food materials.	Papas (2021)
Vitamin D_3 entrapped with whey protein NPs with different calcium concentrations	Encapsulation	High vitamin D3 stability can be used as an enriching ingredient in both transparent and opaque beverages.	Gopi and Amalraj (2016)
Calcium and Folic acid	Duel nutraceutical nanomaterial	To make sure proper levels of vital nutrients for human health.	Fogacci et al. (2020)
Curcumin, ergocalciferol, folic acid, and beta-carotene	soluble protein-polysaccharide nano compound	To increase the antioxidant activity.	Manocha et al. (2022)
Carotenoids	Lipid nanocarriers	Excellent practical application possibilities for the new method of lipophilic plant extract distribution.	Jaswir et al. (2011)
CoQ10	Lipid-free nanoformulation	Effective vehicle for improving oral bioavailability of CoQ10	Zhou et al. (2013)
Long-chain fatty acids and CoQ10	NE	Lipophilic nutraceuticals have improved oral bioavailability thanks to NE-based delivery methods.	Cho et al. (2014)

(Continued)

TABLE 17.5 (*Continued*)
The Potential Applications of Nutraceuticals Delivery System Nano-Based Formulation

Components	Delivery System	Applications	Reference
Oil-soluble micronutrients and omega-3 fatty acids	Biopolymericnanogels	• Encapsulate and safeguard bioactive • Use only components that are fit for human consumption. • The manufactured system raises the standard of foods and drinks.	Sanguansri and Augustin (2007)
Curcumin	Organogel-based NE	• NE digests remarkably quickly and completely. • Curcumin's oral absorption improved. • Can be applied to the pharmaceutical, nutritional supplement, and functional food sectors.	Kharat and McClements (2019)
Alpha -Tocopherol	supercritical nanosuspension with assistance	• Increases the dissolution rate • Increases the bioavailability • Increases the stability	Blondeau (2016)
(Negative)epigalocatechin-3-gallate	Protein-polyphenol co-assemblies: LF-based NPs	• EGCG can be protected by LF-EGCG-nano and submicrometer particles, which can also be used to regulate the discharge of other bioactive substances. • Food formulations based on LF as a container of bioactive substances may be developed using LF-EGCG.	Roy et al. (2005)
Clove oil and Eugenol	Oil titration–precipitation of COM and EM	A homogenous, water-based, thermodynamically stable dosage of clove oil can be administered orally using the mixture in ME.	Al-Okbi et al. (2014)
Dextran and isoflavonegenistein	Enzymatic-assisted inclusion complexation method	• Increased the output of including nutraceuticals by 11 to 141 times as a result of the interplay between van der Walls and newly formed H-bonds. • Genistein inclusion in the enzyme dextran has been discovered to work better with the DMSO-water inclusion procedure.	Semyonov et al. (2014)

formulations. The use of hydrophobins (Hyd) to encapsulate nutraceuticals for food fortification is very intriguing because they compete with hydrophobic substances like vitamin D3 (VD3). VD3 was well protected against deterioration by Hyd. Hyd was also discovered to be a potential nanobase of hydrophobic nutraceuticals for enhancing foods and drinks (Israeli-Lev and Livney, 2014). Two different matrices (whey protein concentrate (WPC) and an industrial-resistant starch) and two different encapsulation processes (spray drying and electrospraying) were used to contain FA. Using WPC as the enclosing material resulted in greater encapsulation effectiveness. In the food business, electrospraying holds promise for encapsulation uses (Patel, 2015).

An ideal substitute for creating nanocapsules from food ingredients is the emulsification-diffusion technique (EDM). Under ideal circumstances, the EDM (Electrohydrodynamic atomization) has demonstrated versatility and reproducibility in forming nanocapsules containing DL-tocopheryl acetate and beta-carotene when different materials are utilized in the samples (Papas, 2021). Whey protein isolate (WPI) NPs made with various calcium amounts contained VD3. The combination of calcium NPs can produce a compact shape that reduces the breakdown of VD3 over the course of storage. WPI NPs with VD3 can be added to transparent or opaque liquids like herbal teas, fruit juices, or low-fat foods to make them taste better (Gopi and Amalraj, 2016). The exfoliation-reassembly hybridization method was employed to create dual nutraceutical nanohybrids based on the layered double hydroxide (LDH) structure using FA and calcium. Because FA/LDH nanohybrids contained more essential nutrients for human health, they could be regarded as dual nutraceutical nanomaterials (Fogacci et al., 2020).

The possible use of protein-polysaccharide soluble nanocomplexes as nutraceutical delivery methods in liquid meals was investigated. Under various experimental circumstances, the complexation of four nutraceutical models —carotene, FA, curcumin, and ergocalciferol with lactoglobulin (BLG) was studied. The low water-soluble nutraceuticals were effectively trapped inside electrostatically stable nanocomplexes (Manocha et al., 2022). Investigators looked into the possibility of simultaneously encapsulating and releasing the plant extract high in carotenoids using nanocarriers derived from hempseed oil or a combination of amaranth and hempseed oils. The nanocarriers have a great deal of promise for therapeutic uses as a fresh method of delivering other bioactive-rich lipophilic plant extracts (Jaswir et al., 2011). A novel lipid-free nano-CoQ10 system was developed and stabilized using a variety of detergents. To evaluate the bioavailability of CoQ10, Sprague-Dawley rats were administered an oral dose of the CoQ10 mixture. The formulation showcased its potential to enhance the oral bioavailability of CoQ10, as researchers confirmed a significant increase in both the peak plasma concentration and the area under the plasma concentration-time curve (Sanguansri and Augustin, 2007).

An animal feeding study was used to examine the effects of droplet size and oil solubility on the bioavailability of heptadecanoic acid and CoQ10. The oral bioavailability of lipophilic nutraceuticals has improved with the NE-based delivery method (Cho et al., 2014). Omega-3 fatty acids, conjugated linoleic acid, oil-soluble vitamins, flavors, colorants, and nutraceuticals are just a few examples of the lipophilic functional components that can be delivered using a variety of food-grade biopolymers, proteins, and polysaccharides (Sanguansri and Augustin, 2016). Improved organogel-based NEs were created to transport curcumin orally and increase its absorption. According to *in vitro* lipolysis profiles, the NE digested substantially more quickly and thoroughly than the organogel. The oral transport of weakly soluble nutraceuticals with high loading capacity can be accomplished using organogel-based NE, which has important implications for the pharmaceutical, nutritional supplement, and functional food sectors (Kharat and McClements, 2019).

α-Tocopherol NP suspensions were created using the liquid antisolvent method with supercritical assisted injection, and the resulting NPs can be used in the food, cosmetics, and pharmaceutical sectors as an antioxidant and a nutritional supplement (Blondeau, 2016). It was looked into whether natural and thermally modified lactoferrin (LF) could co-assemble into delivery systems for (-)-epigallocatechin-3-gallate (EGCG). The creation of regulated releases of other bioactive substances may benefit from the use of LF-EGCG nano and submicrometer particles, which could serve as EGCG's protective carriers (Roy et al., 2005). On obese livers and dyslipidemia in high-fructose-fed rodents, the effects of clove essential oil (CO) and one of its main components, eugenol, were investigated. CO and eugenol microemulsion (EM) caused a significant improvement in fatty liver and dyslipidemia, providing protection against cardiovascular disease and other complications related to fatty liver (Al-Okbi et al., 2014). For the enzymatic production of dextran NPs, two nutraceutical induction techniques-DMSO diffusion in water and acidification —were used to entrap the hydrophobic nutraceutical genistein. The DMSO technique produced a high genistein load and a high proportion of NPs, making it more appropriate for genistein inclusion in dextran (Semyonov et al., 2014). Table 17.6 represents the types of nano-based delivery systems and applications.

17.9 REGULATORY ISSUES

The development and commercialization of nano-based nutraceuticals face several regulatory challenges, as these compounds are subject to a complex regulatory framework that involves multiple agencies and jurisdictions. The regulation requirements for medicinal goods with respect to safety, effectiveness, quality testing, and marketing clearance processes would apply to nutraceutical products asserting medicinal advantages (Santini et al., 2018). Although it has become popular to use nanodelivery systems to create food that is both fresh and healthy, too many of them can pose significant risks to people's safety (Singh and Sinha, 2012). A number of regulatory bodies, such as the Food Safety and Standards Authority of India (FSSAI), European Food and Safety Authority (EFSA), Environmental Protection Agency (EPA), and Food & Drug Administration (FDA), regulate the use of nanosystems in food by the National Institute for Occupational Safety and Health (NIOSH), the Occupational Safety and Health Administration (OSHA), the US Department of Agriculture (USDA), the Consumer Product Safety Commission (CPSC), and the US Patent and Trademark Office (USPTO) (the Government Regulatory acts and Regulatory issues, Table 17.7).

The FDA published two preliminary guideline papers on nanotechnology in 2012. The papers cover the categories of food and makeup, but none of them explicitly mention nutritional supplements because, according to the FDA, they are regarded as a type of food. A dietary substance's bioavailability changes if its physical or chemical

TABLE 17.6
Types of Nano-Based Delivery Systems and Applications

Description	Size (nm)	Applications	Limitations	Reference
Nanoemulsions A colloidal dispersion of two immiscible liquids (oil and aqueous) with particles that are less than one nanometer in size	10–100	Amphiphilic and lipophilic substances are encapsulated	Thermodynamic-Cally unstable	Dizaj et al. (2016)
Nanomicelles Include surfactant molecules with an outer hydrophilic coating and a hydrophobic center.	Less than 100	Amphiphilic and lipophilic substances are encapsulated	The use of a lot of detergents	Rahimi et al. (2016)
Solid-Lipid Nanoparticles Consist of solid lipid core	100–200	• Increased stability • Controlled release of bioactive compounds	• Crystallization of fat globules • Particle size cannot be controlled	Paliwal et al. (2020)
Nanoliposomes A lipid membrane surrounds small compartments. Consists of cholesterol and phospholipids.	10–300	• Lipophilic and hydrophilic substances are encapsulated • emission of bioactive substances under control	• Physical instability • Chemical degradation	Walait et al. (2022)
Nanocochelates A thin lipid bilayer surrounds the small compartments.	50–500	• Lipophilic and hydrophilic substances are encapsulated • Increased mechanical stability • improved encapsulation security for compounds	Expensive	Nayak et al. (2022)
NanoCocervates Electrostatic reactions between two oppositely charged proteins and/or polysaccharides to form biopolymer compounds	10–600	• Very small lipophilic compounds, such as flavoring oils, are encapsulated • emission under control of useful substances	• Complex procedure and structure • Expensive	Rangan et al. (2016)

TABLE 17.7
List of Regulatory Act and Regulatory issues

Country	Regulatory Act	Regulatory Issues	References
India	• In 2006, the Food Safety and Standards Act (FSSA) was passed. • In 2008, the Food Safety and Standard Authority of India (FSSAI) • In 2011, the Food Safety and Standards Rules & Regulations. • In 2020, the Food Safety and Standard Authority of India (FSSAI).	• The production, distribution, or importation of new foods, GMF, irradiated foods, organic foods, foods for specific dietary purposes, functional foods, nutraceuticals, and dietary supplements. • A single point of reference for all issues regarding standards and food safety. • Applying more of a focus on evidence-based and democratic decisions. • Describe the prescribed food labeling standards and the key information that must be displayed on the sites where food is produced, processed, served, and stored.	FSSAI (n.d.)
European Union	• In 1996, Functional food science in Europe (FUFOSE). • n 2010, Regulation (EU) No 383/2010 • In 2017, Regulation (EU) 2017/745	• Create a scientific methodology for topics in functional food science. • Authorize foods that improve children's health and disease risk. • Clinical investigation and sale of medical devices for human use.	FUFOSE – ILSI Europe (n.d.)
USA	• In 1990, Nutrition Labeling and Education Act (NLEA) • In 1997, the Food and Drug Administration Modernization Act (FDAMA) • In 2011, Food Safety Modernization Act (FSMA) • In 2022, Food Safety Modernization Act (FSMA)	• Most food nutrition labels are subject to Agency regulation. • Regulation of food, pharmaceuticals, gadgets, and biological products under the Federal Food, Drug, and Cosmetic Act • protect the US food supply against contamination to ensure its safety • *Implement*	U.S. Food and Drug Administration, Center for Food Safety and Applied Nutrition (2023)
Japan	• In 1991, Food for specified health (FOSHU) • In 2015, Foods with Nutrient Function Claims" (FNFC)	• Focuses on particular product health claims. • *Implement nutritional or health functions.*	FOSHU (2023)
China	• In 2005, the State Food and Drug Administration (SFDA) • In 2021, State Food and Drug Administration(SFDA)	• A registration guideline for functional foods was released. • Efforts to improve the safety of food and drugs	Commissioner (2023)

characteristics change, according to FDA guideline documentation. Additionally, such modifications may have an impact on the degree of toxicity. The FDA used nanotechnology as an example of a process that produces a new dietary ingredient and thus necessitates notice to the FDA in its preliminary new dietary ingredient (NDI) guidelines. However, because they are not subject to regulation, nano-nutraceuticals can be put on the market with little to no safety testing. The FDA expects that the Office of Combination Goods should have authority over these nanotechnology goods (Singh and Sinha, 2012). According to the EC Food Law Regulation, several factors must be taken into account when developing nanomaterials for food uses, such as the use of toxic and heavy metals and mycotoxin-free nanomaterials. As per Directive 89/107/EEC, NPs designed for use in food containers must first be assessed as a straight food additive (Fogacci et al., 2020).

17.10 CONCLUSIONS AND FUTURE PROSPECTS

Delivery of bioactives is essential for showing the efficacy and therapeutic value of nutraceuticals. Out of the various tools and technologies, researchers have proven nanotechnology to be the most efficient method for delivering bioactives and nutraceuticals. Nanotechnology-based formulations produce nanocarriers like NE NPs, nanosuspensions, polymeric micelles, and liposomes, each with unique physicochemical properties. Different functional attributes have opened new possibilities for delivering nutraceuticals, food production, and processing. Advancement in the field has created a broad potential for nanotechnology, particularly in improving nutraceuticals' solubility, bioavailability, permeability, and efficacy.

Along with these advantages, the targeting of bioactives has also been reported. In brief, nanotechnology is crucial to the advent of nutraceutical delivery tools. However, challenges associated with this technology, such as toxicity, cost, and others, also need to be considered.

We can easily incorporate nutraceuticals into food products to create a range of valuable meals that meet customers' requirements regarding health and well-being. The efficacy of nutraceuticals, however, depends on maintaining their bioavailability. It is possible to modify the bioaccessibility, absorption, or transformation characteristics of nutraceuticals in the GIT using delivery methods, increasing their bioavailability and, as a result, their health advantages. Experts are transferring their expertise from pharmaceutical uses, including utilizing nanodelivery systems, absorption enhancers, or excipient foods that have demonstrated increased solubility, stability, and permeability of nutraceuticals. Future research should concentrate on enhancing the physical properties of the delivery systems by meticulously considering each delivery system's composition.

REFERENCES

Abuhassan, Q., Khadra, I., Pyper, K., Halbert, G.W., 2021. Small scale in vitro method to determine a bioequivalent equilibrium solubility range for fasted human intestinal fluid. *European Journal of Pharmaceutics and Biopharmaceutics* 168, 90–96.

Al-Okbi, S.Y., Mohamed, D.A., Hamed, T.E., Edris, A.E., 2014. Protective effect of clove oil and eugenol microemulsions on fatty liver and dyslipidemia as components of metabolic syndrome. *Journal of Medicinal Food* 17, 764–771. https://doi.org/10.1089/jmf.2013.0033.

Anand, P., Kunnumakkara, A.B., Newman, R.A., Aggarwal, B.B., 2007. Bioavailability of curcumin: Problems and promises. *Molecular Pharmaceutics* 4, 807–818.

Andlauer, W., Fürst, P., 2002. Nutraceuticals: A piece of history, present status and outlook. *Food Research International* 35, 171–176.

Arzani, G., Haeri, A., Daeihamed, M., Bakhtiari-Kaboutaraki, H., Dadashzadeh, S., 2015. Niosomal carriers enhance oral bioavailability of carvedilol: Effects of bile salt-enriched vesicles and carrier surface charge. *International Journal of Nanomedicine* 10, 4797.

Asghar, A., Randhawa, M.A., Masood, M.M., Abdullah, M., Irshad, M.A., 2018. Nutraceutical formulation strategies to enhance the bioavailability and efficiency: An overview, in: Alexandru Mihai Grumezescu, Alina Maria Holban (eds.) *Role of Materials Science in Food Bioengineering*, Academic Press, Oxford, United Kingdom. pp. 329–352.

Augustin, M.A., Sanguansri, L., 2015. Challenges and solutions to incorporation of nutraceuticals in foods. *Annual Review of Food Science and Technology* 6(1), 463–77.

Bai, L., Huan, S., Gu, J., McClements, D.J., 2016. Fabrication of oil-in-water nanoemulsions by dual-channel microfluidization using natural emulsifiers: Saponins, phospholipids, proteins, and polysaccharides. *Food Hydrocolloids* 61, 703–711.

Balusamy, B., Celebioglu, A., Senthamizhan, A., Uyar, T., 2020. Progress in the design and development of "fast-dissolving" electrospun nanofibers based drug delivery systems-A systematic review. *Journal of Controlled Release* 326, 482–509.

Basnet, P., Skalko-Basnet, N., 2011. Curcumin: An anti-inflammatory molecule from a curry spice on the path to cancer treatment. *Molecules* 16, 4567–4598.

Bassaganya-Riera, J., Hontecillas, R., Wannemuehler, M., 2002. Nutrition impact of conjugated linoleic acid: A model functional food ingredient. *In Vitro Cellular & Developmental Biology-Plant* 38, 241–246.

Bayda, S., Adeel, M., Tuccinardi, T., Cordani, M., Rizzolio, F., 2019. The history of nanoscience and nanotechnology: from chemical–physical applications to nanomedicine. *Molecules* 25(1), 112.

Belhaj, N., Dupuis, F., Arab-Tehrany, E., Denis, F.M., Paris, C., Lartaud, I., Linder, M., 2012. Formulation, characterization and pharmacokinetic studies of coenzyme Q10 PUFA's nanoemulsions. *European Journal of Pharmaceutical Sciences* 47, 305–312.

Bhavaniramya, S., Vishnupriya, S., Al-Aboody, M.S., Vijayakumar, R., Baskaran, D., 2019. Role of essential oils in food safety: Antimicrobial and antioxidant applications. *Grain & Oil Science and Technology* 2, 49–55.

Blondeau, N., 2016. The nutraceutical potential of omega-3 alpha-linolenic acid in reducing the consequences of stroke. *Biochimie* 120, 49–55. https://doi.org/10.1016/j.biochi.2015.06.005

Brower, V., 1998. Nutraceuticals: poised for a healthy slice of the healthcare market?. *Nat Biotechnol* 16(8), 728–731. doi:10.1038/nbt0898-728.

Celebioglu, A., Uyar, T., 2019. Encapsulation and stabilization of α-lipoic acid in cyclodextrin inclusion complex electrospun nanofibers: Antioxidant and fast-dissolving α-lipoic acid/cyclodextrin nanofibrous webs. *Journal of Agricultural and Food Chemistry* 67, 13093–13107.

Celebioglu, A., Uyar, T., 2020a. Fast-dissolving antioxidant curcumin/cyclodextrin inclusion complex electrospun nanofibrous webs. *Food Chemistry* 317, 126397.

Celebioglu, A., Uyar, T., 2020b. Development of ferulic acid/cyclodextrin inclusion complex nanofibers for fast-dissolving drug delivery system. *International Journal of Pharmaceutics* 584, 119395.

Chauhan, I., Yasir, M., Verma, M., Singh, A.P., 2020. Nanostructured lipid carriers: A groundbreaking approach for transdermal drug delivery. *Advanced Pharmaceutical Bulletin* 10, 150–165. https://doi.org/10.34172/apb.2020.021

Chen, J., Jonoska, N., 2006. *Nanotechnology: science and computation.* Rozenberg G, (ed.) Berlin: Springer.

Chen, S., Li, Q., McClements, D.J., Han, Y., Dai, L., Mao, L., Gao, Y., 2020. Co-delivery of curcumin and piperine in zein-carrageenan core-shell nanoparticles: Formation, structure, stability and in vitro gastrointestinal digestion. *Food Hydrocolloids* 99, 105334.

Chen, S., McClements, D.J., Jian, L., Han, Y., Dai, L., Mao, L., Gao, Y., 2019. Core–shell biopolymer nanoparticles for co-delivery of curcumin and piperine: Sequential electrostatic deposition of hyaluronic acid and chitosan shells on the zein core. *ACS Applied Materials & Interfaces* 11, 38103–38115.

Cho, H.T., Salvia-Trujillo, L., Kim, J., Park, Y., Xiao, H., McClements, D.J., 2014. Droplet size and composition of nutraceutical nanoemulsions influences bioavailability of long chain fatty acids and Coenzyme Q10. *Food Chemistry* 156, 117–122. https://doi.org/10.1016/j.foodchem.2014.01.084

Choi, A.Y., Kim, C.-T., Park, H.Y., Kim, H.O., Lee, N.R., Lee, K.E., Gwak, H.S., 2013. Pharmacokinetic characteristics of capsaicin-loaded nanoemulsions fabricated with alginate and chitosan. *Journal of Agricultural and Food Chemistry* 61, 2096–2102.

Coban, O., Aytac, Z., Yildiz, Z.I., Uyar, T., 2021. Colon targeted delivery of niclosamide from β-cyclodextrin inclusion complex incorporated electrospun Eudragit® L100 nanofibers. *Colloids and Surfaces B: Biointerfaces* 197, 111391.

Dabholkar, N., Waghule, T., Krishna Rapalli, V., Gorantla, S., Alexander, A., Narayan Saha, R., Singhvi, G., 2021. Lipid shell lipid nanocapsules as smart generation lipid nanocarriers. *Journal of Molecular Liquids* 339, 117145. https://doi.org/10.1016/j.molliq.2021.117145

DeFrates, K., Markiewicz, T., Gallo, P., Rack, A., Weyhmiller, A., Jarmusik, B., Hu, X., 2018. Protein polymer-based nanoparticles: Fabrication and medical applications. *International Journal of Molecular Sciences* 19, 1717.

Desfrançois, C., Auzély, R., Texier, I., 2018. Lipid nanoparticles and their hydrogel composites for drug delivery: A review. *Pharmaceuticals* 11, 118.

Dima, C., Assadpour, E., Dima, S., Jafari, S.M., 2020. Bioavailability of nutraceuticals: Role of the food matrix, processing conditions, the gastrointestinal tract, and nanodelivery systems. *Comprehensive Reviews in Food Science and Food Safety* 19, 954–994.

Dizaj, S.M., Yaqoubi, S., Adibkia, K., Lotfipour, F., 2016. Nanoemulsion-based delivery systems: Preparation and application in the food industry, in: Alexandru Mihai Grumezescu (ed.) Emulsions. Elsevier, Cambridge, pp. 293–328.

Dureja, H., Kaushik, D., Kumar, V., 2003. Developments in nutraceuticals. *Indian Journal of Pharmacology* 35, 363–372.

Elizabeth Lane, K., Derbyshire, E., 2013. Systematic review of omega-3 enriched foods and health. *British Food Journal* 116, 165–179.

Estrada-Gil, L.E., Contreras-Esquivel, J.C., Mata-Gómez, M.A., Flores-Gallegos, A.C., Zugasti-Cruz, A., Rodríguez-Herrera, R., Govea-Salas, M., Ascacio-Valdés, J., 2021. Functional foods and ingredients, supplements, nutraceuticals, and superfoods uses and regulation, in: Elizabeth Carvajal-Millan, Abu Zahrim Yaser, A. K. Haghi (eds.) *Natural Food Products and Waste Recovery*. Apple Academic Press, New York, pp. 51–67.

Fathi, M., Mirlohi, M., Varshosaz, J., Madani, G., 2013. Novel caffeic acid nanocarrier: Production, characterization, and release modeling. *Journal of Nanomaterials* 2013, 434632.

Fogacci, S., Fogacci, F., Cicero, A.F., 2020. Nutraceuticals and hypertensive disorders in pregnancy: The available clinical evidence. *Nutrients* 12, 378.

FOSHU, 2023. [WWW Document]. URL https://www.mhlw.go.jp/index.html (accessed 6.6.23).

FSSAI, n.d. [WWW Document]. URL https://www.fssai.gov.in/cms/food-safety-and-standards-regulations.php (accessed 6.6.23).

FUFOSE – ILSI Europe, n.d. [WWW Document]. URL https://ilsi.eu/eu-projects/past-projects/fufose/ (accessed 6.6.23).

Ghani, U., Naeem, M., Rafeeq, H., Imtiaz, U., Amjad, A., Ullah, S., Rehman, A., Qasim, F., 2019. A novel approach towards nutraceuticals and biomedical applications. *Scholars International Journal of Biochemistry* 2, 245–252.

Giraffa, G., Chanishvili, N., Widyastuti, Y., 2010. Importance of lactobacilli in food and feed biotechnology. *Research in Microbiology* 161, 480–487.

Gopi, S., Amalraj, A., 2016. Introduction of nanotechnology in herbal drugs and nutraceutical: A review. *Journal of Nanomedicine & Biotherapeutic Discovery* 6. https://doi.org/10.4172/2155-983X.1000143

Guttoff, M., Saberi, A.H., McClements, D.J., 2015. Formation of vitamin D nanoemulsion-based delivery systems by spontaneous emulsification: factors affecting particle size and stability. *Food chemistry* 171, 117–22.

Ha, T.V.A., Kim, S., Choi, Y., Kwak, H.-S., Lee, S.J., Wen, J., Oey, I., Ko, S., 2015. Antioxidant activity and bioaccessibility of size-different nanoemulsions for lycopene-enriched tomato extract. *Food Chemistry* 178, 115–121.

Helander, H.F., Fändriks, L., 2014. Surface area of the digestive tract–revisited. *Scandinavian Journal of Gastroenterology* 49, 681–689.

Huang, Q., Yu, H., Ru, Q., 2010. Bioavailability and delivery of nutraceuticals using nanotechnology. *Journal of Food Science* 75, R50–R57.

Huwilera, A., 2000. Physiology and pathophysiology of sphingolipid metabolism and signaling. *Biochimica et Biophysica Acta* 1485, 63–99.

Israeli-Lev, G., Livney, Y.D., 2014. Self-assembly of hydrophobin and its co-assembly with hydrophobic nutraceuticals in aqueous solutions: Towards application as delivery systems. *Food Hydrocolloids* 35, 28–35. https://doi.org/10.1016/j.foodhyd.2013.07.026

Jahangir, M.A., Imam, S.S., Muheem, A., Chettupalli, A., Al-Abbasi, F.A., Nadeem, M.S., Kazmi, I., Afzal, M., Alshehri, S., 2020. Nanocrystals: Characterization overview, applications in drug delivery, and their toxicity concerns. *Journal of Pharmaceutical Innovation* 17, 237–248.

Jain, A., Singh, S.K., Arya, S.K., Kundu, S.C., Kapoor, S., 2018. Protein nanoparticles: Promising platforms for drug delivery applications. *ACS Biomaterials Science & Engineering* 4, 3939–3961.

Jaswir, I., Noviendri, D., Hasrini, R.F., Octavianti, F., 2011. Carotenoids: Sources, medicinal properties and their application in food and nutraceutical industry. *Journal of Medicinal Plants Research* 5, 7119–7131. https://doi.org/10.5897/JMPRX11.011

Karadag, A., Yang, X., Ozcelik, B., Huang, Q., 2013. Optimization of preparation conditions for quercetin nanoemulsions using response surface methodology. *Journal of Agricultural and Food Chemistry* 61, 2130–2139.

Karami, F., Mahasti Shotorbani, P., 2018. Genetically modified foods: Pros and cons for human health. *Food & Health* 1(2), 18–23.

Kaur, J., Gill, G.S., Jeet, K., 2019. Applications of carbon nanotubes in drug delivery: A comprehensive review, in: *Characterization and Biology of Nanomaterials for Drug Delivery*, pp. 113–135.

Kharat, M., McClements, D.J., 2019. Recent advances in colloidal delivery systems for nutraceuticals: A case study–delivery by design of curcumin. *Journal of Colloid and Interface Science* 557, 506–518.

Kheadr, E., Vuillemard, J., El-Deeb, S., 2002. Acceleration of Cheddar cheese lipolysis by using liposome-entrapped lipases. *Journal of Food Science* 67, 485–492.

Kim, S.O., Ha, T.V.A., Choi, Y.J., Ko, S., 2014. Optimization of homogenization–evaporation process for lycopene nanoemulsion production and its beverage applications. *Journal of Food Science* 79, N1604–N1610.

Kirby, C., 1993. Controlled delivery of functional food ingredients: Opportunities for liposomes in the food industry. *Liposome Technology* 2, 215–232.

Koh, K.S., Wong, V.L., 2019. *Nanoemulsions: Properties, Fabrications and Applications*. BoD–Books on Demand, United Kingdom.

Kothamasu, P., Kanumur, H., Ravur, N., Maddu, C., Parasuramrajam, R., Thangavel, S., 2012. Nanocapsules: The weapons for novel drug delivery systems. *BioImpacts: BI* 2(2), 71–81.

kumar Dey, T., Ghosh, S., Ghosh, M., Koley, H., Dhar, P., 2012. Comparative study of gastrointestinal absorption of EPA & DHA rich fish oil from nano and conventional emulsion formulation in rats. *Food Research International* 49, 72–79.

Law, B.A., King, J.S., 1985. Use of liposomes for proteinase addition to Cheddar cheese. *Journal of Dairy Research* 52, 183–188.

Li, L., Wang, H., 2013. Antibacterial agents: Enzyme-coated mesoporous silica nanoparticles as efficient antibacterial agents in vivo (Adv. Healthcare Mater. 10/2013). *Advanced Healthcare Materials* 2, 1298–1298.

Liang, R., Shoemaker, C.F., Yang, X., Zhong, F., Huang, Q., 2013. Stability and bioaccessibility of β-carotene in nanoemulsions stabilized by modified starches. *Journal of Agricultural and Food Chemistry* 61, 1249–1257.

Liu, L.-L., Liu, P.-Z., Li, X.-T., Zhang, N., Tang, C.-H., 2019. Novel soy β-conglycinin core–shell nanoparticles as outstanding ecofriendly nanocarriers for curcumin. *Journal of Agricultural and Food Chemistry* 67, 6292–6301.

Livney, Y.D., 2015. Nanostructured delivery systems in food: Latest developments and potential future directions. *Current Opinion in Food Science* 3, 125–135.

Lushchak, O., Strilbytska, O., Koliada, A., Zayachkivska, A., Burdyliuk, N., Yurkevych, I., Storey, K.B., Vaiserman, A., 2020. Nanodelivery of phytobioactive compounds for treating aging-associated disorders. *Geroscience* 42, 117–39.

Malik, B., Pirzadah, T.B., Kumar, M., Rehman, R.U., 2017. Biosynthesis of nanoparticles and their application in pharmaceutical industry, in: *Metabolic Engineering for Bioactive Compounds: Strategies and Processes*, pp. 331–349.

Manocha, S., Dhiman, S., Grewal, A.S., Guarve, K., 2022. Nanotechnology: An approach to overcome bioavailability challenges of nutraceuticals. *Journal of Drug Delivery Science and Technology* 72, 103418.

Marques, C., Manuela Amorim, M., Odila Pereira, J., Estevez Pintado, M., Moura, D., Calhau, C., Pinheiro, H., 2012. Bioactive peptides-Are there more antihypertensive mechanisms beyond ACE inhibition? *Current Pharmaceutical Design* 18, 4706–4713.

Mattarelli, P., Biavati, B., Holzapfel, W.H., Wood, B.J., 2017. *The Bifidobacteria and Related Organisms: Biology, Taxonomy, Applications*. Academic Press, Oxford.

Mayer, S., Weiss, J., McClements, D.J., 2013. Behavior of vitamin E acetate delivery systems under simulated gastrointestinal conditions: Lipid digestion and bioaccessibility of low-energy nanoemulsions. *Journal of Colloid and Interface Science* 404, 215–222.

McClements, D.J., Rao, J., 2011. Food-grade nanoemulsions: Formulation, fabrication, properties, performance, biological fate, and potential toxicity. *Critical Reviews in Food Science and Nutrition* 51, 285–330.

Meng, J., Meng, J., Duan, J., Kong, H., Li, L., Wang, C., Xie, S., Chen, S., Gu, N., Xu, H., 2008. Carbon nanotubes conjugated to tumor lysate protein enhance the efficacy of an antitumor immunotherapy. *Small* 4, 1364–1370.

Mishra, S.S., Behera, P.K., Kar, B., Ray, R.C., 2018. Advances in probiotics, prebiotics and nutraceuticals, in: Sandeep Kumar Panda, Prathapkumar Halady Shetty *Innovations in Technologies for Fermented Food and Beverage Industries*, Springer Cham. pp. 121–141.

Mohan, A., Rajendran, S.R., He, Q.S., Bazinet, L., Udenigwe, C.C., 2015. Encapsulation of food protein hydrolysates and peptides: A review. *Rsc Advances* 5, 79270–79278.

Mutlu-Ingok, A., Devecioglu, D., Dikmetas, D.N., Karbancioglu-Guler, F., Capanoglu, E., 2020. Antibacterial, antifungal, antimycotoxigenic, and antioxidant activities of essential oils: An updated review. *Molecules* 25, 4711.

Ray, S., and Nayak, A.K., (eds.), 2022. *Design and Applications of Theranostic Nanomedicines*. Woodhead Publishing, Oxford.

Nguyen, D.T., Barham, W., Zheng, L., Shillinglaw, B., Tzou, W.S., Neltner, B., Mestroni, L., Bosi, S., Ballerini, L., Prato, M., 2014. Carbon nanotube facilitation of myocardial ablation with radiofrequency energy. *Journal of Cardiovascular Electrophysiology* 25, 1385–1390.

Nikalje, A.P., 2015. Nanotechnology and its applications in medicine. *Med Chem* 5, 081–089.

Noori, S., Zeynali, F., Almasi, H., 2018. Antimicrobial and antioxidant efficiency of nanoemulsion-based edible coating containing ginger (*Zingiber officinale*) essential oil and its effect on safety and quality attributes of chicken breast fillets. *Food Control* 84, 312–320.

Olivares-Morales, A., Hatley, O.J., Turner, D., Galetin, A., Aarons, L., Rostami-Hodjegan, A., 2014. The use of ROC analysis for the qualitative prediction of human oral bioavailability from animal data. *Pharmaceutical Research* 31, 720–730.

Palamakula, A., 2004. *Biopharmaceutical Classification and Development of Limonene-Based Self-Nanoemulsified Capsule Dosage Form of Coenzyme Q10*. Texas Tech University. Lubbock, USA.

Paliwal, R., Paliwal, S.R., Kenwat, R., Kurmi, B.D., Sahu, M.K., 2020. Solid lipid nanoparticles: A review on recent perspectives and patents. *Expert Opinion on Therapeutic Patents* 30, 179–194.

Papas, A.M., 2021. Vitamin E TPGS and its applications in nutraceuticals, in: Ramesh C. Gupta, Rajiv Lall and Ajay Srivastava (eds.) *Nutraceuticals*. Elsevier, Academic Press, Oxford. pp. 991–1010.

Patel, S., 2015. Emerging trends in nutraceutical applications of whey protein and its derivatives. *Journal of Food Science and Technology* 52, 6847–6858. https://doi.org/10.1007/s13197-015-1894-0

Peel, M., 1999. Liposomes produced by combined homogenization/extrusion. *GIT Laboratory Journal* 3, 37–38.

Pham-Huy, L.A., He, H., Pham-Huy, C., 2008. Free radicals, antioxidants in disease and health. *International Journal of Biomedical Science* 4, 89–96.

Poonia, N., Lather, V., Narang, J.K., Beg, S., Pandita, D., 2020. Resveratrol-loaded folate targeted lipoprotein-mimetic nanoparticles with improved cytotoxicity, antioxidant activity and pharmacokinetic profile. *Materials Science and Engineering: C* 114, 111016.

Ragelle, H., Danhier, F., Préat, V., Langer, R., Anderson, D.G., 2017. Nanoparticle-based drug delivery systems: A commercial and regulatory outlook as the field matures. *Expert Opinion on Drug Delivery* 14, 851–864.

Rahimi, H.R., Nedaeinia, R., Shamloo, A.S., Nikdoust, S., Oskuee, R.K., 2016. Novel delivery system for natural products: Nano-curcumin formulations. *Avicenna Journal of Phytomedicine* 6, 383.

Ramalingam, P., Ko, Y.T., 2015. Enhanced oral delivery of curcumin from N-trimethyl chitosan surface-modified solid lipid nanoparticles: Pharmacokinetic and brain distribution evaluations. *Pharmaceutical Research* 32, 389–402.

Ramalingam, P., Ko, Y.T., 2016a. Improved oral delivery of resveratrol from N-trimethyl chitosan-g-palmitic acid surface-modified solid lipid nanoparticles. *Colloids and Surfaces B: Biointerfaces* 139, 52–61.

Ramalingam, P., Ko, Y.T., 2016b. Validated LC–MS/MS method for simultaneous quantification of resveratrol levels in mouse plasma and brain and its application to pharmacokinetic and brain distribution studies. *Journal of Pharmaceutical and Biomedical Analysis* 119, 71–75.

Rangan, A., Manjula, M.V., Satyanarayana, K.G., 2016. 17- Trends and methods for nanobased delivery for nutraceuticals, in: Grumezescu, A.M. (Ed.), *Emulsions, Nanotechnology in the Agri-Food Industry*. Academic Press, pp. 573–609. https://doi.org/10.1016/B978-0-12-804306-6.00017-9

Rashidinejad, A., Birch, E.J., Sun-Waterhouse, D., Everett, D.W., 2014. Delivery of green tea catechin and epigallocatechin gallate in liposomes incorporated into low-fat hard cheese. *Food Chemistry* 156, 176–183.

Rein, M.J., Renouf, M., Cruz-Hernandez, C., Actis-Goretta, L., Thakkar, S.K., da Silva Pinto, M., 2013. Bioavailability of bioactive food compounds: A challenging journey to bioefficacy. *British Journal of Clinical Pharmacology* 75, 588–602.

Roy, A.M., Baliga, M.S., Katiyar, S.K., 2005. Epigallocatechin-3-gallate induces apoptosis in estrogen receptor–negative human breast carcinoma cells via modulation in protein expression of p53 and Bax and caspase-3 activation. *Molecular Cancer Therapeutics* 4, 81–90.

Saini, R., Saini, S., Sharma, S., 2010. Nanotechnology: The future medicine. *Journal of Cutaneous and Aesthetic Surgery* 3, 32.

Salvia-Trujillo, L., Rojas-Graü, M.A., Soliva-Fortuny, R., Martín-Belloso, O., 2015. Use of antimicrobial nanoemulsions as edible coatings: Impact on safety and quality attributes of fresh-cut Fuji apples. *Postharvest Biology and Technology* 105, 8–16.

Sanguansri, L., Augustin, M.-A., 2007. Microencapsulation and delivery of Omega-3 fatty acids, in: John Shi (ed.) *Functional Food Ingredients and Nutraceuticals - Processing Technologies*, CRC Press, Boca Raton, pp. 297–327.

Sanguansri, L., Augustin, M.A., 2016. Microencapsulation and delivery of omega-3 fatty acids. *Funct Food Ingredients Nutraceuticals* 13, 373–407.

Sanna, V., Lubinu, G., Madau, P., Pala, N., Nurra, S., Mariani, A., Sechi, M., 2015. Polymeric nanoparticles encapsulating white tea extract for nutraceutical application. *Journal of Agricultural and Food Chemistry* 63, 2026–2032.

Santini, A., Cammarata, S.M., Capone, G., Ianaro, A., Tenore, G.C., Pani, L., Novellino, E., 2018. Nutraceuticals: Opening the debate for a regulatory framework. *British Journal of Clinical Pharmacology* 84, 659–672.

Sari, T., Mann, B., Kumar, R., Singh, R., Sharma, R., Bhardwaj, M., Athira, S., 2015. Preparation and characterization of nanoemulsion encapsulating curcumin. *Food Hydrocolloids* 43, 540–546.

Scott, N., Chen, H., 2012. Nanoscale science and engineering for agriculture and food systems. *Industrial Biotechnology* 8(6), 340–3.

Semyonov, D., Ramon, O., Shoham, Y., Shimoni, E., 2014. Enzymatically synthesized dextran nanoparticles and their use as carriers for nutraceuticals. *Food & Function*. 5, 2463–2474. https://doi.org/10.1039/C4FO00103F

Sessa, M., Balestrieri, M.L., Ferrari, G., Servillo, L., Castaldo, D., D'Onofrio, N., Donsì, F., Tsao, R., 2014. Bioavailability of encapsulated resveratrol into nanoemulsion-based delivery systems. *Food Chemistry* 147, 42–50.

Shahavi, M.H., Hosseini, M., Jahanshahi, M., Meyer, R.L., Darzi, G.N., 2016. Clove oil nanoemulsion as an effective antibacterial agent: Taguchi optimization method. *Desalination and Water Treatment* 57, 18379–18390.

Shikinaka, K., Funatsu, Y., Kubota, Y., Tominaga, Y., Nakamura, M., Navarro, R.R., Otsuka, Y., 2018. Tuneable shape-memory properties of composites based on nanoparticulated plant biomass, lignin, and poly (ethylene carbonate). *Soft Matter* 14, 9227–9231.

Shin, G.H., Kim, J.T., Park, H.J., 2015. Recent developments in nanoformulations of lipophilic functional foods. *Trends in Food Science & Technology* 46, 144–157.

Singh J, Sinha S, 2012. Classification, regulatory acts and applications of nutraceuticals for health. *International Journal of Pharma and Bio Sciences* 2, 177–87.

Song, B., Thompson, D., Fiorino, A., Ganjeh, Y., Reddy, P., Meyhofer, E., 2016. Radiative heat conductances between dielectric and metallic parallel plates with nanoscale gaps. *Nature nanotechnology* 11(6), 509–14.

Suárez-Rivero, J.M., Pastor-Maldonado, C.J., Povea-Cabello, S., Álvarez-Córdoba, M., Villalón-García, I., Munuera-Cabeza, M., Suárez-Carrillo, A., Talaverón-Rey, M., Sánchez-Alcázar, J.A., 2021. Coenzyme q10 analogues: Benefits and challenges for therapeutics. *Antioxidants* 10, 236.

Subramanian, P., 2021. Lipid-based nanocarrier system for the effective delivery of nutraceuticals. *Molecules* 26, 5510.

Tang, C.-H., 2020. Nanocomplexation of proteins with curcumin: From interaction to nanoencapsulation (A review). *Food Hydrocolloids* 109, 106106. https://doi.org/10.1016/j.foodhyd.2020.106106

Taylor, T.M., Weiss, J., Davidson, P.M., Bruce, B.D., 2005. Liposomal nanocapsules in food science and agriculture. *Critical Reviews in Food Science and Nutrition* 45, 587–605.

Thakkar, A., Chenreddy, S., Wang, J., Prabhu, S., 2015. Ferulic acid combined with aspirin demonstrates chemopreventive potential towards pancreatic cancer when delivered using chitosan-coated solid-lipid nanoparticles. *Cell & Bioscience* 5, 1–14.

U.S. Food and Drug Administration, Center for Food Safety and Applied Nutrition, 2023. Food [WWW Document]. FDA. URL https://www.fda.gov/food (accessed 6.6.23).

Veiseh, O., Tang, B.C., Whitehead, K.A., Anderson, D.G., Langer, R., 2015. Managing diabetes with nanomedicine: challenges and opportunities. *Nature Reviews Drug Discovery* 14(1), 45–57.

Venuti, V., Cannavà, C., Cristiano, M.C., Fresta, M., Majolino, D., Paolino, D., Stancanelli, R., Tommasini, S., Ventura, C.A., 2014. A characterization study of resveratrol/sulfobutyl ether-β-cyclodextrin inclusion complex and in vitro anticancer activity. *Colloids and Surfaces B: Biointerfaces* 115, 22–28.

Verma, D., Gulati, N., Kaul, S., Mukherjee, S., Nagaich, U., 2018. Protein based nanostructures for drug delivery. *Journal of Pharmaceutics* 2018, 9285854.

VJoy, N., Gupta, P., Jyothikiran, H., Raghunath, N., 2020. Nanotechnology in Orthodontics-An Update. *Nanotechnology* 7(9).

Walait, M., Mir, H.R., Anees, K., 2022. Edible biofilms and coatings; its characterization and advanced industrial applications. *NRFHH* 3, 28–37. https://doi.org/10.53365/nrfhh/149622

Wang, S.-T., Chou, C.-T., Su, N.-W., 2017. A food-grade self-nanoemulsifying delivery system for enhancing oral bioavailability of ellagic acid. *Journal of Functional Foods* 34, 207–215.

Wei, Y., Yang, S., Zhang, L., Dai, L., Tai, K., Liu, J., Mao, L., Yuan, F., Gao, Y., Mackie, A., 2020. Fabrication, characterization and in vitro digestion of food grade complex nanoparticles for co-delivery of resveratrol and coenzyme Q10. *Food Hydrocolloids* 105, 105791.

Xu, D., Guo, G., Gui, L., Tang, Y., Shi, Z., Jin, Z., Gu, Z., Liu, W., Li, X., Zhang, G., 1999. Controlling growth and field emission property of aligned carbon nanotubes on porous silicon substrates. *Applied Physics Letters* 75, 481–483.

Y Aboul-Enein, H., Berczynski, P., Kruk, I., 2013. Phenolic compounds: The role of redox regulation in neurodegenerative disease and cancer. *Mini Reviews in Medicinal Chemistry* 13, 385–398.

Yao, M., McClements, D.J., Xiao, H., 2015. Improving oral bioavailability of nutraceuticals by engineered nanoparticle-based delivery systems. *Current Opinion in Food Science* 2, 14–19.

Yu, H., Huang, Q., 2012. Improving the oral bioavailability of curcumin using novel organogel-based nanoemulsions. *Journal of Agricultural and Food Chemistry* 60, 5373–5379.

Yuan, Y., Li, H., Zhu, J., Liu, C., Sun, X., Wang, D., Xu, Y., 2020. Fabrication and characterization of zein nanoparticles by dextran sulfate coating as vehicles for delivery of curcumin. *International Journal of Biological Macromolecules* 151, 1074–1083.

Zaki, N.M., 2014. Progress and problems in nutraceuticals delivery. *Journal of Bioequivalence & Bioavailability* 6, 75.

Zarrabi, A., Alipoor Amro Abadi, M., Khorasani, S., Mohammadabadi, M.-R., Jamshidi, A., Torkaman, S., Taghavi, E., Mozafari, M., Rasti, B., 2020. Nanoliposomes and tocosomes as multifunctional nanocarriers for the encapsulation of nutraceutical and dietary molecules. *Molecules* 25, 638.

Zhang, Z., Zhang, R., McClements, D.J., 2016. Encapsulation of β-carotene in alginate-based hydrogel beads: Impact on physicochemical stability and bioaccessibility. *Food Hydrocolloids* 61, 1–10.

Zhang, J., Jiao, J., Niu, M., Gao, X., Zhang, G., Yu, H., Yang, X., Liu, L., 2021. Ten years of knowledge of nano-carrier based drug delivery systems in ophthalmology: Current evidence, challenges, and future prospective. *International Journal of Nanomedicine* 16, 6497.

Zheng, J., Li, Y., Song, M., Fang, X., Cao, Y., McClements, D.J., Xiao, H., 2014. Improving intracellular uptake of 5-demethyltangeretin by food grade nanoemulsions. *Food Research International* 62, 98–103.

Zhou, H.-Y., Hao, J.-L., Wang, S., Zheng, Y., Zhang, W.-S., 2013. Nanoparticles in the ocular drug delivery. *International Journal of Ophthalmology* 6, 390–396. https://doi.org/10.3980/j.issn.2222-3959.2013.03.25

18 Potential Use of Nanomaterials in Dietary Supplements and Medical Purpose Food

*Sreemoyee Chakraborty,
Somashree Bandyopadhaya, Debabrata Bera,
Chandan Kumar Ghosh, and Lakshmishri Roy*

18.1 INTRODUCTION

Food choices and lifestyle over the years have been shaped by a range of factors, including technological advancements, changes in work and leisure patterns, social and cultural shifts, and increased awareness of the importance of health and wellness. One significant trend in food choices and lifestyle is the increasing emphasis on healthy eating and nutrition. Availability of technological infrastructure is one of the guiding factors impacting food choices and lifestyle in the new millennia. The rise of social media has led to a greater awareness of different cuisines and food cultures, awareness regarding the potential functional benefits of foods and food therapy, while food tracking apps and wearable technology have made it easier for people to monitor their diet and physical activity levels.

In the 21st century, food choices and lifestyle are complex and multifaceted, reflecting a range of social, cultural, economic, and technological factors. It is important to be mindful of these factors and make conscious choices about how to navigate the rapidly changing landscape of modern life. There has been a huge paradigm shift toward healthier lifestyle choices which can promote health and decrease the risk of long-term diseases such as obesity, cardiovascular disease (CVD) and high blood sugar. These choices may include eating an optimal balanced diet, engaging in regular physical exercise, maintaining healthy daily routine, decreasing reliability on medicines and increasing dependency on food therapy and nutraceuticals. While medication is often necessary to treat and manage various health conditions, prolonged use of medication can have several drawbacks and potential negative effects on the body. The application of food therapy in conjunction with medicine can help to supplement the effectiveness of medical treatments, reduce side effects, and improve overall health outcomes. For example, in patients with diabetes, combining medication with a carefully planned diet can help to regulate blood sugar levels, control weight, and prevent complications associated with the disease.

DOI: 10.1201/9781003432661-18

Food therapy can also be used to control the onset of certain health conditions, such as heart disease, diabetes, osteoporosis and cancer. Food therapy and medicine are complementary approaches to treating and preventing health conditions. While medicine and pharmaceutical drugs are used to control symptoms and address the underlying causes of disease, food therapy uses a balanced and structured diet plan and nutrition to promote optimal health of an individual. The core of food-based therapeutic approach constitutes functional or medical purpose foods and dietary supplements. These functional foods, also known as nutraceuticals, are food products that are fortified with targeted bioactive compounds that are thought to provide health benefits above and beyond basic nutrition. They are usually derived from natural sources, such as animals, plants and marine sources, and are formulated to provide specific health benefits. Examples of nutraceuticals include probiotics, polyphenols, omega-3 fatty acids, and fiber (Krause, 1979).

Nutraceuticals are often marketed as dietary supplements or medical purpose foods, and are available in a variety of forms, including capsules, powders, and fortified foods. However, it is crucial to note that the health benefits of nutraceuticals are not always backed by scientific evidence, and some products may be marketed with exaggerated or false health claims. Products that include one or more dietary elements, such as herbs, vitamins, minerals, amino acids or additional substances used to complement the diet, are referred to as dietary supplements. These items are primarily used orally and available in a variety of forms, including capsules, pills, liquids, and powders. The intended use of dietary supplements is to provide additional nutrients that may not be obtained in sufficient quantities through the diet alone. Medical purpose foods, however, are products that are intended to be consumed as part of a dietary management plan for a specific medical condition or disease. These products are formulated to provide specific nutrients, such as vitamins, minerals, and other substances that are beneficial for managing certain medical conditions. Medical purpose foods are typically used as part of a comprehensive medical treatment plan, under the guidance of a healthcare professional. They may be prescribed for conditions such as malnutrition, gastrointestinal (GI) disorders, metabolic disorders, and other medical conditions that require specific nutrient requirements. In summary, dietary supplements are products intended to supplement the diet and provide additional nutrients, while medical purpose foods are formulated to provide specific nutrients for managing medical conditions (Paul and Dewangan, 2016).

The key to optimize or enhance the effectivity of nutraceuticals is by increasing the bioavailability and biosorptibility of the nutrient components. The easiest way to achieve this is by employing nanotechnology to develop particles having distinct characteristics that are different from the ones at the macroscopic or even microscale level in this size range. In order to attain certain features and purposes that are not achievable with bigger materials, scientists and engineers construct and manipulate nanoscale materials using a variety of approaches. The study of this manipulation of materials at the scale between 1 and 100 nm constitutes the field of research known as nanotechnology. A nanoparticle (NP) is a tiny particle with measurements on the order of a nanometre. A broad variety of substances, including metals, semiconductors, ceramics, and polymers, can be used to create these particles. NPs are helpful for a range of applications because they might have distinctive physico-chemical and surface characteristics that are different from those of their bulk counterparts (Arshad et al. 2021).

NPs have the potential to revolutionize food engineering by improving food quality, safety, and functionality. NPs such as silver and zinc oxide can be incorporated into packaging materials to provide antimicrobial properties that help to prevent bacterial contamination and other harmful microorganisms that can spoil food and cause foodborne illnesses.

NPs can also be used to enrich the nutritional content of the food matrix by encapsulating vitamins, minerals, and other bioactive compounds. This can help to improve the bioavailability and bioabsorption of these nutrients by the body. The versatility of NPs can be explored to improve the processing and preservation of food by enhancing the stability of emulsions, suspensions, and foams. For example, NPs can be used to stabilize oil-in-water emulsions, which are commonly used in salad dressings, mayonnaise, and other food products. NPs have a significant application in detection and monitoring of food quality and safety by detecting contaminants such as microorganisms, toxins, and other adulterants that can be present in food. NPs can be used to improve the flavor and aroma of food by encapsulating and releasing volatile compounds that add to the taste and smell of food. This can help to enhance the sensory quality of food and enhance the overall consumer experience. Overall, the utilization of nanoscale materials in food processing has the criteria to improve versatility, safety, quality, and functionality of the developed product. However, the application of NPs in food and food grade materials also raises major concerns about their implications on environment and public health, as well as their potential for unintended consequences. Therefore, it is important to conduct careful research and regulation of the use of NPs to minimize budding risks and maximize their benefits (Powell and Colin, 2008).

In recent years, nanotechnology has a great potential to transform food products in many ways, such as improving functionality, enhancing shelf life, optimizing their safety with quality, and promoting good health. Because of its promising performance, several food corporations are eager to design products utilizing this developing technology. Manufacturers are developing unique products with appealing attributes in accordance with consumer demands and interests. Nanotechnology is frequently seen as a "double-edged sword". NPs hold characteristics that render them potentially useful, yet these same traits may lead to interplay with biological systems, causing potential harm. Critical knowledge of the safety and effects of nanoformulations on population health, and their toxicity in the environment falls under ongoing nanotoxicology research. The application of nanotechnology in the food and pharmaceutical industries is classified into several categories, covering dietary supplements, additives, packaging materials, and sensor or detector systems. In contrast to achieving maximum functionality, nanomaterials are anticipated to have no negative effects on consumer health environment throughout their life cycle. Safety measures define the conditions of exposure to a nanomaterial in taking into account both safety hazards, which is the potential for a nanomaterial to pose a health risk, and exposure over time. Hence, it is important to consider any potential risks and hazards that could arise both during the manufacture itself and during the use or disposal of nanoproducts in order to ensure their safe application (He et al., 2019).

18.2 DIETARY SUPPLEMENTS AND MEDICAL PURPOSE FOODS: CURRENT SCENARIO

Non-communicable diseases (NCDs) are a significant contributor to the community's health issues following the epidemiological change (Karimi et al., 2012). The primary categories of NCDs, as defined by World Health Organization (WHO, n.d.), are chronic respiratory diseases, CVDs, malignancies, and diabetes, which account for about 70% of all fatalities globally. By 2030, this group expects that NCDs will be to blame for 75% of all deaths worldwide (Mathers, 2008). A significant global trend in health is the use of dietary supplements, such as vitamins, antioxidants, fiber, trace minerals, and amino acids (Stickel et al., 2011). Nowadays, pharmacists sell many different kinds of nutritional supplements (Stickel et al., 2011; Radimer et al., 2004). According to estimates from Henderson et al. (2003), more than 50% of adults in the UK consume at least one dietary supplement every day.

Over 70% of Americans regularly consume dietary supplements, and the sector as a whole generates over $28 billion in revenue (Martin et al., 2018).

The estimated size of the international market for dietary supplements and food intended for medical purposes in 2021 was USD 151.9 billion, and it is projected to increase at a rate of 8.9% from 2022 to 2030. Rising consumer awareness of the health and well-being of consumers is likely to be an important market driver for nutraceutical market over the forecast timeframe. The working population globally struggles to get enough daily nutrition due to bustling schedules and changing lifestyles. Due to supplements' high degree of convenience, the sector is predicted to become more dependent on them to satisfy nutritional demands.

Therapeutic foods are substances that resemble regular meals yet have been proven to provide health benefits. Nutraceuticals, however, are goods created from food that are used medicinally and exhibit physiological benefits. They can be taken as pills, capsules or liquids. This category includes nutraceuticals, herbal supplements, and other organic products. Nutraceuticals and functional foods, however, are occasionally used interchangeably. However, improving health and decreasing the risk of disease via prevention are the main objectives of such products. This group differs significantly from pharmaceuticals in that the former are multifunctional mixes present at low concentrations, while the latter are pure compounds used at high levels that only operate on one particular region (Paul and Dewangan, 2016).

These food groups can be classified into the following types (Figure 18.1):

Nutraceuticals: In the media and literature, the terms nutraceuticals and functional foods are commonly used interchangeably. Actually, the term "nutraceutical", which combines the terms "nutrition" and "pharmaceutical", was made by Stephen DeFelice, M.D., the founder of the Foundation for Innovation in Medicine in Cranford, New Jersey. There are many different products included in it, such as foods with a variety of nutrients, fortified foods, dietary supplements, functional ingredients, and foods with medicinal applications. Nutraceuticals would therefore better be described as "food components or whole foods that have a medical or health benefit, including the prevention and treatment of disease". The U.S. Food Drug and

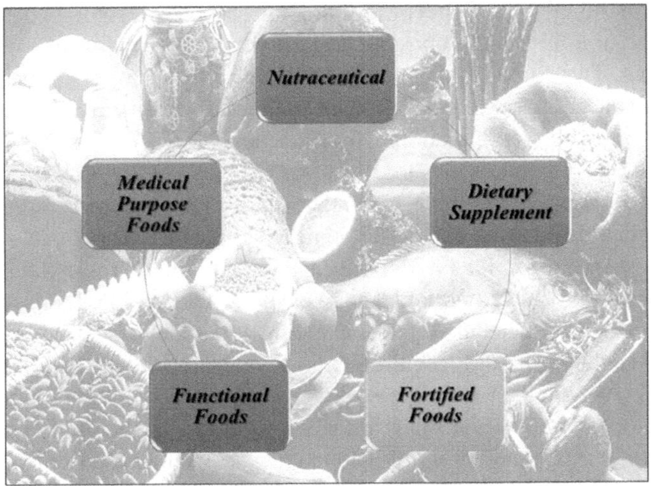

FIGURE 18.1 Classes of foods with functional properties.

Administration (USFDA) has traditionally categorized any kind of food/consumable used for sickness control or treatment as drugs.

Dietary supplements: A dietary supplement is any consumable ingredient that is intended to complement the diet and contains at least one of the substances listed below: a vitamin or mineral, herb or other botanical extract, amino acid or metabolite, or any combination thereof. According to USFDA, dietary supplements may be distributed in food form as long as they are clearly labelled as such and are not "represented" as ordinary foods. Specific health or functional claims on dietary supplements are allowed if the USFDA decides there is enough scientific evidence to support the claim.

Fortified foods: The recommended daily allowance (RDA), sometimes referred to as the dietary reference intake (DRI), for each vitamin and mineral is normally between 50% and 100% of the amount added to fortified foods. As in the instance of adding B vitamins to many baked goods, fortification of these products is usually mandated by law to restore nutrients lost during manufacture. Breakfast cereals have been fortified as a food category since the 1940s.

Functional foods: A meal or food item is considered to be functional if it has the potential to be healthy in addition to the typical nutrients it provides. This idea is challenging to grasp because the only "traditional nutrients" are vitamins and minerals. The justification is that these are thought to be required for eating and/or to treat a disease brought on by a nutritional deficiency; for instance, vitamin C treats scurvy. In contrast to soy, which includes soy protein associated with a drop in CVD, sardines, which contain vitamin D and help prevent rickets, are not an example of a functional food. This is due to the fact that soya protein is not thought of as a necessary nutrient like oat bran (for the fiber content), red grapes, cranberry juice, and oligomeric proanthocyanidins (OPCs) which are other foods with functional qualities. These foods all have wholesome benefits attributed to "non-nutrient" components as described by the term's recognized meaning. The "super-fortified" foods, or those that have been fortified with more than the recommended DRI or with extra botanicals or supplements, are also considered functional foods. The latter includes salad toppings with omega-3 polyunsaturated fatty acids (PUFAs) and orange juice with Echinacea. Functional foods may make claims about their structure or function or health if there is enough scientific support for them.

Medical purpose foods: Foods with a medical function are those that are intended to be consumed under medical supervision. The food item is purposed for the exact nutritional balancing for a sickness or deficiency for which specific dietary requirements have been established by medical experts. Although, strictly speaking, medical purpose foods are only given by doctors and not via ordinary retail shops, they may be used to control illnesses like high blood pressure, blood glucose level, obesity or heart disease and may make specific claims.

Although there is a large market for nutraceuticals and other functional meals, it can be difficult to produce them since they must address the issue of organoleptic acceptability, which is not a concern for pharmaceutical or nutraceutical goods. These foods or dietary supplements can only be referred to as such if they have one or more functional components that can either improve food quality or address health concerns.

The following list includes some examples of the mentioned functional components:

Omega-3 fatty acid: Omega-3 fatty acids, included in fatty fish, flaxseeds, and other foods, have been demonstrated to enhance cognitive function, lower inflammation, and improve heart health. Protein, long-chain PUFA, dietary fiber, vitamins, and minerals are all key components found in seaweeds. Additionally, they are known as edible sea algae. Numerous studies have recently focused on the possible health benefits of marine algae and the components that make them up as nutraceuticals and functional meals. Its omega-3 fatty acids, antioxidants, and other bioactives are mostly to blame for this. Omega-3 fatty acids are passed on to marine fish and animals farther down the food chain despite coming from phytoplanktons or algae. The lipids in the bodies of fishes like mackerel, salmon, cod, herring and halibut, and the bladder of marine creatures like sharks, seals and whales are rich in long-chain omega-3 fatty acids (Shahidi, 2012). Omega-3 fatty acids are found in a variety of ready-to-eat foods, such as baked goods, extruded products, dairy products, table spreads, and juices, and they are important for boosting health and preventing and treating a number of chronic disorders. They can also be consumed as liquid or tablet dietary supplements. Long-chain omega-3-PUFA are of significant interest due to their efficacy in the prevention and control of malignancies, hypertension, diabetes, arthritis and other inflammatory conditions, autoimmune diseases and neurological function, such as depression, schizophrenia, and coronary heart disease (Shahidi, 2008; Schmidt et al., 2000; Howe, 1997; Krishna Mohan & Das, 2001; Babcock et al., 2000; Kelly, 2001; Rose and Connolly, 1999; Akihisa et al., 2004). In particular, for the brain and retina, they are essential for the upkeep and aid in normal growth (Anderson et al., 1990). Though the specific molecular mechanism behind the cardioprotective properties of omega-3 fatty acids is unknown, ideas contend that they may be a result of a convergence of their antiarrhythmic, antiatherogenic, and antithrombotic activity and thrombostatic qualities. Eicosanoids can be produced from long-chain PUFA to reduce thrombosis, improve membrane fluidity, and reduce blood triacylglycerol levels. They conduct certain physiological duties to avoid thrombosis, cholesterol accumulation, and allergies (Howell et al., 1998; Kinsella, 1986; Kimoto et al., 1994).

Antioxidants: These are substances that assist in defending against damage from free radicals and may lower the risk of chronic illnesses like cancer and heart disease. They may be found in foods like berries, dark chocolate, and green tea. Plant meals are rich in phenolic and polyphenolic compounds. Fruit peel and seeds have the highest levels of phenolics and polyphenolics, despite the fact that leaves are normally a better source of phenolics. Although phenolic and polyphenolic compounds are frequently referred to as antioxidants, their ability to scavenge free radicals, chelate pro-oxidant metal ions or act as reducing agents does not entirely explain how these effects are produced (Kunwar and Priyadarsini, 2011).

The processes by which polyphenolic compounds function are as follows (Shahidi, 2012):

- Modifying the environment or metabolism of oestrogen in the colon.
- Directly eliminating reactive oxygen species (ROS)/reactive nitrogen species (RNS) or cellular antioxidant capacity enhancement.
- Changing the differentiation of cells.
- Increasing the activity of the enzymes that detoxify carcinogens.
- Preventing the synthesis of N-nitrosamines.
- Increasing the death of cancer cells and/or decreasing their growth.
- Interfering with deoxyribonucleic acid (DNA) methylation and/or DNA maintenance and repair.
- Preserving the intracellular matrices

Fiber: Fiber is essential for maintaining digestive health and has been linked with a decreased risk of heart disease, diabetes, and other chronic illnesses. Fiber may be found in whole grains, fruits, and vegetables.

Probiotics: These are living microorganisms that are present in several fermented foods, including yogurt and kefir, and are thought to enhance immune function and digestive health.

Due to their potential health advantages, probiotics and prebiotics are two categories of nutraceuticals that have grown in popularity recently. Probiotics are living microorganisms that, when taken in adequate quantities, boost immunity. These bacteria can be found in dietary supplements as well as fermented foods like yogurt, kefir, and kimchi. By reestablishing the balance of helpful bacteria in the gut microbiome, which can be upset by things like antibiotic usage, diet, and stress, probiotics are considered to promote gut health. However, prebiotics are non-digestible fibers that are present in several foods, including whole grains, onions, garlic, and bananas. Prebiotics provide nourishment for the good bacteria in the gut microbiome, fostering their activity and growth. Prebiotics can thereby promote immune function while also enhancing gut health. Synbiotics are a term used to describe probiotics and prebiotics that act together to support gut health. Dietary supplements and functional foods like yogurt and granola bars include synbiotics. Probiotics and prebiotics are generally regarded as safe for the majority of people to eat, while research on their potential health benefits is ongoing. However, due to the danger of illness from specific bacterial strains, those with weakened immune systems should speak with a doctor before taking probiotics. Additionally, some persons who consume probiotics or prebiotics may have digestive symptoms like gas or bloating; however, these symptoms are often moderate and go away on their own (Damián et al., 2022).

Vitamins and minerals: Vitamins and minerals are essential components that our bodies need to function at their peak. It makes sense to consider whether the many different vitamin and mineral supplements on the market may aid in preventing CVD. A prospective study on arterial hypertension by Rautiainen et al. (2016) revealed no association between vitamin supplementation and a woman's chance of getting hypertension. Wang et al.'s (2009) randomized study on obese women at risk for CVD found that supplementing with a vitamin–mineral preparation for 26 weeks significantly lowered blood pressure compared to the placebo-controlled group.

Although it was determined that vitamin–mineral supplements did not lower the risk of developing hypertension, researchers also argued that they could be beneficial for those who already have the condition (Li et al., 2018). Supplemental potassium has been demonstrated to provide a number of benefits. Experts claim that potassium supplementation is beneficial for treating hypertension people and may be suggested (Poorolajal et al., 2017; Filippini et al., 2020).

18.3 TYPES OF NANOMATERIALS WITH POTENTIAL FOOD USE

Although nanotechnology is employed extensively across a wide range of sectors, including farming, biochemistry, health care, and a number of other fields, it is still a relatively new field that lends itself better than other technologies to creative and complicated applications in food systems. It offers a practical strategy for using novel technology for a range of operations related to the manufacture of food, growth, production, shipment, storage, and distribution. The most fundamentally advanced technology in nano-based food science is NPs, which deal with a wide range of nanostructured materials and nano-methods. This method was developed to increase the shelf life and fluidity of food, to increase the accessibility of bioactive molecules, to safeguard food components, to offer dietary guidance, to fortify meals, and to distribute food or component parts. Due to their bigger surface areas and mass transfer rates, NPs appear to have better chemical and biological functions, catalytic behavior, penetrability, proteolytic activation, and quantum characteristics than larger particles (with the same makeup) (Avella et al., 2007). Depending on their size, properties, and structures, different types of nanomaterials are categorized. These physiochemical properties of these NPs with a high surface volume ratio include solubility, bioaccessibility, diffusivity, imaging, color, strength, impairment, magnetism, and thermodynamics (Sahoo et al., 2021).

Better uniformity, taste, and texture are promised by the food components made using nanostructures. Currently, food additives are incorporated into food products utilizing nanocarriers without changing their basic structure. Size of the particle may directly affect the flow of any bioactive chemical to different locations inside the body, as it has been demonstrated that in some cell lines, only the submicron NPs may be effectively absorbed compared to the larger size micro-particles. An optimal system for distribution should be able to efficiently keep the active ingredients at the correct levels for lengthy periods of duration (in storage), ensure availability at the required time and rate, and transport the active component exactly to the intended place. NPs are more successful in enveloping and releasing compounds than conventional encapsulation procedures (Ezhilarasi et al., 2013). Nanoencapsulations can control relations of the active substances with the food framework, control the release of the substances, ensure access at a target time at a particular rate, and mask smells or tastes along with safeguarding active ingredients from heat, moisture, chemical or biological breakdown during preparation, preservation, and use (Ubbink and Kruger, 2006). According to Weiss et al. (2006), they also show compatibility with other substances in the system. Furthermore, due to their smaller size and ability to make it deeper into tissues, these forms of delivery can effectively distribute active compounds to certain regions of the body (Lamprecht et al., 2004).

Assessing the significance of nanotechnology in food manufacturing may also be done by looking at how they affect food products' (i) appearance, (ii), form, (iii), aroma, (iv) nutrient density, and (v) shelf life. Nanotechnology makes many improvements to food safety and flavor possible. Nanoencapsulation methodologies have been widely used to enhance flavor release and retention and to offer culinary harmony (Nakagawa, 2014). Zhang et al. (2014) nanoencapsulated anthocyanins, an extremely reactive and fragile plant-based dye with a range of biological roles. The majority of bioactive compounds are susceptible to the extremely acidic surroundings and enzymatic activity of the duodenum and stomach. These bioactive compounds are poorly water-soluble in non-capsulated form, making it difficult for them to easily integrate into food products. However, by being encapsulated, these bioactive compounds can withstand such extreme conditions. Small edible capsules made from NPs have been developed to improve the dispersion of drugs, vitamins or sensitive micronutrients in daily meals (Yan and Gilbert, 2004; Koo et al., 2005). Nanoencapsulation allows these bioactive components to prolong the shelf life of therapeutic foods where bioactive components often become deteriorated and ultimately led to deactivation due to the adverse conditions by halting the steps of degradation or stopping decline until the product has arrived at the target site. Aside from providing tastes, colors, digestive enzymes, and anti-browning agents, edible nanocoatings on various food components may also operate as an impediment to moisture and gas exchange, prolong the freshness of processed foods regardless of whether the packaging has been opened, and function as a wall to moisture and gas exchange (Renton, 2006; Weiss et al., 2006). By employing nanocomposites as an active component for wrapping and coating, food packaging may be improved (Pinto et al., 2013). Many researchers like Gálvez et al. (2007) and Schirmer et al. (2009) were interested in learning more about the antimicrobial properties of organic substances such as bacterial antibiotics, organic acids, and essential oils as well as how they may be used in polymeric substrates for antimicrobial packaging. However, these compounds cannot be employed in the many food processing methods that need high temperatures and pressures due to their severe reactivity to these physical conditions. Inorganic NPs can be used to provide a potent antibacterial activity in modest concentrations and greater durability in challenging settings. Hence, there has recently been an abundance of interest in using these NPs in antimicrobial food packaging. Nanomaterials provide an elevated degree of responsiveness and other cutting-edge properties for application in biosensor fabrication. Nanosensors or nanobiosensors are used in the field of food microbiology, according to Cheng et al. (2006) and Helmke and Minerick (2006), to measure the different elements of food that are now accessible, identify pathogens in food or processing plants, and inform distributors and consumers of the food's safety status. The nanosensor serves as an indication that reacts to changes in environmental parameters like percentage relative humidity or temperature in storage spaces, contamination by bacteria or product deterioration, claim Bouwmeester et al. (2009).

18.4 NANOFORMULATIONS AND THEIR APPLICATIONS IN DESIGNING FUNCTIONAL FOODS

Because of their poor solubility, several minerals and phytochemicals have lower bioavailability. As a result, functional components are frequently included in the delivery method, and vitamins, minerals, and phytochemicals are rarely employed in their purest form. The delivery technique affects the flavor, texture, and shelf life of the supplement in addition to moving the nutrient to the target location (Tarver, 2006). Theoretically, nanotechnology solves this problem by offering a more effective delivery mechanism through the use of various nanoformulations, e.g. nanoemulsion (NE) (Figure 18.2).

NE was one such variation that was effectively employed to increase the functioning of a bioactive chemical. A kind of extremely tiny emulsion droplets known as NEs range in size from 50 to 200 nm. The size of earlier emulsions varied from 1 to 100 m. By encapsulating curcumin and evaluating its anti-inflammation effectiveness in vivo in mice, a team of researchers investigated the possibilities of utilizing NEs. The antioxidant, anti-inflammatory, and anticancer properties of curcumin, the turmeric-derived yellow pigment, have not yet been shown in human clinical studies. Because it is insoluble in water, relatively little curcumin taken as a supplement enters the circulation after digestion (Wang et al., 2008).

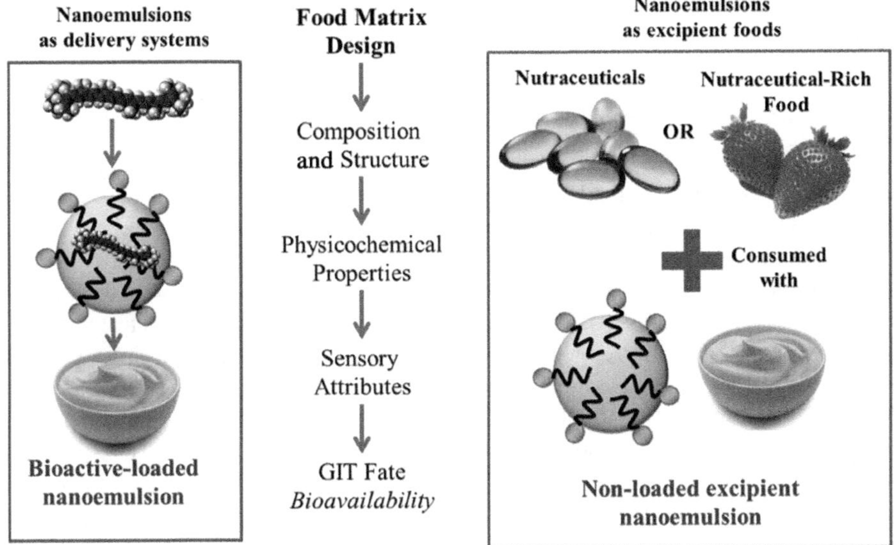

FIGURE 18.2 Schematic representation of NE-based delivery system and NE-based food product. (Salvia-Trujillo et al., 2016.)

Researchers at Rutgers University developed oil-in-water NEs of various sizes to encapsulate curcumin to boost its anti-inflammation action in an effort to solve this problem. With the use of a mouse ear inflammation model, the activity was assessed. With mean droplet diameters ranging from 618.6 to 79.5 nm, the emulsions were created using medium-chain triglycerols and Tween 20 (the brand name for polysorbate 20, a standard molecular-biology-grade detergent). When evaluated on mice, the injection of 1% curcumin encapsulated in oil-in-water emulsions measuring 618.6–79.5 nm reduced the mice's ears' and caused oedema by 43% and 85%, respectively. Giving 1% curcumin in a Tween 20 water solution to patients revealed little to no reduction in inflammation. This shows increasing the bioavailability of curcumin by encapsulating it in NEs (Ilkay, 2010).

Goncalves et al. (2018) provided a summary of the design of nanonutraceuticals with the aim of ensuring effective preservation or maximum of their bioactivity and safety inside the human body. Arora and Jaglan (2016) provided an overview of current advances in the field of nanocarrier-based nutraceutical delivery for the prevention and treatment of cancer. Katouzian and Jafari (2016) summarized recent findings concerning improvements made in the nanoencapsulation of lipophilic and hydrophilic vitamins, safety concerns, and health risks associated with the consumption of these products, which would lead to the widespread use of nanoencapsulated vitamins in the food and beverage products in the future. Chai et al. (2018) discussed the intelligent delivery methods for bioactive chemicals in food that are intended to increase their low solubility, poor stability, and low permeability in the GI tract (GIT) and improve their oral bioavailability, considering physico-chemical and physiological circumstances, absorption pathways, barriers, and response techniques.

Numerous nanoformulations have the potential to be used in the production of foods with medicinal purposes, nutritional supplements, and other functional foods.

18.4.1 Engineered Nanoparticles

Several critical nutraceuticals have a severely reduced potential to promote health due to their poor oral bioavailability. Engineered NPs (ENs) can be used to develop delivery systems that enhance oral bioavailability by increasing nutraceutical equilibrium in foods and the GIT, enhancing nutraceutical dissolution in intestinal fluids, allowing nutraceutical absorption by the GIT, and lowering first-pass metabolism in the gut and liver (Mingfei, 2015). Several ENs have been developed and tested for use as delivery systems with the goal of enhancing the health benefits of nutraceuticals by encapsulation, safety, and/or controlled release (Yao et al., 2015; McClements, 2013; McClements and Xiao, 2014). A possible method for increasing the effectiveness of nutraceuticals in people is to increase their oral bioavailability. Significant progress has recently been made in the design and research of ENs to improve the oral absorptivity of nutraceuticals. A nutraceuticals passes through the upper GIT, where it is subjected to major transformations in the environment's composition, structure, and flow behavior. The physical state and chemistry of the nutraceutical may change as a result of its circumstances, lowering its bioaccessibility. ENs were created to safeguard nutraceuticals against harmful GI conditions. For instance, the pH of small intestine fluids makes epigallocatechin gallate (EGCG), a polyphenol present in green tea, unstable. According to Zou et al. (2014), encapsulating EGCG in nanoliposomes made of Tween 80, cholesterol and phospholipids significantly slowed down its breakdown in simulated intestinal fluids. Additionally, nutraceuticals may be enclosed in lipid NPs or biopolymer NPs that are intended to prevent early degradation and increase the stability of the nutraceuticals in the GIT (Xu et al., 2013; Harde et al., 2011).

A nutraceutical must be dissolved inside the GIT in order to be bioaccessible for enterocyte uptake. Lipophilic nutraceuticals like carotenoids and curcumins having reduced dissolution in aqueous GI fluids have low bioaccessibility. It has been common practice to employ lipid-based ENs to increase the bioabsorptivity of lipophilic nutraceuticals. In the GIT, lipases hydrolyze digestible carrier oils in ENs to create monoacylglycerols and free fatty acids. These lipid digestion by-products along with phospholipids and bile salts in the small intestinal lumen create "mixed micelles" with intricate topologies. When nutrients contained in ENs are digested, they are transported to the mixed micelles, considerably increasing the bioaccessibility of the nutrients (Porter and Charman, 2001; Sun et al. 2015; Salvia-Trujillo et al., 2013).

Most nutraceuticals are absorbed in the small intestine after consumption (Oehlke et al., 2014). Lipid-based ENs have been typically used to entrap lipophilic functional components such as curcumin, β-carotene, vitamin E, and Co-Q10 in order to improve their intestinal absorption (Qian et al., 2012; Yang et al., 2013; Gong et al., 2012; Cho et al., 2014; Salvia-Trujillo et al., 2013). Lipophilic nutraceuticals are transported through the aqueous mucus layer by mixed micelles that are produced following the digestion of NEs and are then accessible for absorption in enterocytes. Lipophilic supplements are packed into chylomicrons inside enterocytes because of their high lipophilicity (Grolier et al., 1995; Pouton et al., 2008). The enterocytes create the chylomicrons, which are lipid particles made of free fatty acids, monoacylglycerols, and cholesterol that are supplied by mixed micelles (Yanez et al., 2011). Chylomicron production in enterocytes stimulated by mixed nanomicelles made of ethylenediaminetetraacetic acid (EDTA) (which opens intracellular secure junctions), chitosan (CS) (leads to the dissociation of restricted junction components), surfactants (disturbs plasma membrane integrity), and free fatty acids (increases plasma membrane permeability) was linked to an increase in absorption (Yao et al., 2014). To improve the assimilation of nutraceuticals, these chemicals can be added to delivery methods. Encapsulated nutrients for digestible ENs may be liberated and solubilized in intestinal fluids before being taken in by enterocytes by passive absorption or active transport (Hu et al., 2008).

18.4.2 Nanocapsules and Nanocarriers

According to Esfanjani et al. (2018), nanocapsules manufactured from lipid formulations with greater surface areas than micro-sized carriers can successfully be used in functional meals and more efficiently increase the bioavailability, solubility, and regulated release of nanoencapsulated phenolic chemicals. Even though these fields cover a sizable portion of the particle/solution interface and the rate of release is dependent on the solid domain properties, the breakdown of encapsulated bioactive compounds via solid unbreakable domains across the particle/solution interface is only hindered when the dimension of the domain is substantially smaller than the size of NPs. This was found while using Monte Carlo models to analyze the effects of solid domain features on the rate of chemical release from lipid carriers containing nanostructured domains (Dan, 2016). CS-infused solid lipid nanocarriers embedding this nutraceutical after oral administration also demonstrated increased bioavailability of encapsulated curcumin when contrasted with that of curcumin suspensions and extended physical stability at room and refrigerator temperatures (Ramalingam et al., 2016).

By acting as a nanocoating, polysaccharides with various enzymatic susceptibilities may ensure targeted breakdown in the intestinal track, thereby postponing the imprecise diffusion of bioactive substances that have been encapsulated until the coating is exposed to the environment where the release is planned. Such encased nanocarriers may also be directed to various GIT organs, where they will be taken up by enterocytes and increase oral bioavailability (Sampathkumar & Loo, 2018). Vitamin D3 was enclosed in high amylose corn and potato starch nanocarriers, with encapsulating efficiencies ranging up to 94.8%. These nanocarriers were granular in form and varied in size to 99.2 nm. The vitality of a probiotic strain (Lactobacillus rhamnosus ATCC 9595) was increased by their nanoencapsulation in lecithin and cellulose nanocrystals to alginate microbeads throughout stomach transit and storage, as well as at normal room temperatures and cool storage conditions (Khan et al., 2018; Huq et al., 2017). Folic acid (FA), added by post-diffusion to food grade alginate or CS nanolaminates created using the layer-over-layer method, was found to be more stable during ultraviolet (UV) light exposure than free FA, according to estimates. According to Acevedo-Fani et al. (2018), the greater level of FA released from nanolaminates at neutral pH compared to acidic pH showed that these materials can be employed in culinary applications. The photostability and bioaccessibility of curcumin were significantly improved by protein–polysaccharide surfactant complex particles made by co-precipitation in anti-solvent employing propylene glycol alginate, zein and either rhamnolipid or lecithin, indicating that they could be used as carriers of lipophilic nutraceuticals for use in food and pharmaceutical products (Dai et al., 2018).

In order to perfect the encapsulation, preservation, and dissolution of bioactive substances, Fathi et al. (2018) outlined a novel protein nanoencapsulation technology. Ramos et al. (2017) presented a review paper outlining the most recent research on the nanolevel problems of whey protein degradation and amalgamation, which may help in developing a variety of protein nanostructures with novel or enhanced characteristics for facilitating the inclusion and controlled release of nutraceuticals in food frameworks. Parthasarathi and Anandharamakrishnan (2016) proposed a spray/freeze-drying-derived microencapsulation approach as a potential alternative to increase the oral biosorptibility of slightly hydrophobic bioactive compounds.

At stomach digestion circumstances, zein NPs carrying lutein (ZLNPs) of size 75 nm were found to significantly aggregate. In absence of salt, the aggregation of the ZLNPs which were not completely digested by stomach enzymes was reduced and digestion was sped up. Protein–lipid hybrid NPs with a three-layered structure—a layer of barley protein, a layer of tocopherol, and a layer of phospholipid—as well as an interior compartment made of water for storing the hydrophilic vitamin B12 nutraceutical—displayed regulated release behavior in simulated GI medium. In a real-world experiment, vitamin B12-loaded NPs significantly reduced the amount of methylmalonic acid and increased serum concentrations of vitamin B12 in rats after oral administration. These NPs may be used to enhance oral vitamin B12 absorption, claim Liu et al. (2018). According to Lin et al. (2016), vitamin D3 nanocomplexes made of maize protein hydrolysate with spherical shapes and diameters of 102–121 nm exhibited increased physico-chemical endurance and in vitro bioaccessibility. Potato protein may be employed as a safe delivery system for hydrophobic nutraceuticals suitable for supplementing clear liquids as well as other food or drink items having beneficial effects on human health. The nanoassociation in vitamin D-potato protein co-assemblies offered notable protection and reduced vitamin D losses during processing and preservation (David and Livney, 2016). Dehydrated and reconstituted reassembled casein micelles (r-CMs) were found to have a significant protective effect against the gastric breakdown of vitamin D and to boost the in vitro metabolism of the vitamin in a Caco-2 cell line when compared to free vitamin D (Cohen et al., 2017).

Layered double hydroxides (LDHs) and composites made from silica or aluminosilicate are examples of inorganic porous materials that have emerged as promising candidates for the delivery of a variety of drugs and offer some benefits in designing. Because they have a nice design, have an ample surface area, and are sustainable in biosystems, they are used to achieve high loading capacity, gradual release, and increased targeting (Trofimov et al., 2018; Sayed et al., 2018; Mishra et al., 2018).

18.4.3 Nanoliposomes and Nanoemulsions

Nanoliposomes, or nanometric bilayer phospholipid vessels, have a very promising future for the nutraceutical industry since they can concurrently encapsulate lipophilic and hydrophilic substances, ensuring an additive effect, and because they may preserve highly reactive bioactive compounds, improve their adsorption, ensure sustained release, and aid in prolonging shelf life. Due to their unique properties, nanoliposomes are excellent candidates for use in Drug Information Service (DISs) for effective health promotion and prevention (Khorasani et al., 2018). The creation of novel functional foods and beverages may use one of the most contemporary lipid-based nanocarriers, the nanophytosome, which permits the distribution of botanical-based nutraceuticals (Ghanbarzadeh et al., 2016).

The maximum physico-chemical stability (during a month of storage) was discovered to be provided by nanophytosome–phosphatidylcholine (PC)—rutin complexes with an encapsulation efficiency (EE) of 99%. The EE of cobalamin was 56%, alpha-tocopherol was 76%, and ergocalciferol was 57% in NEs made with various bioactive chemicals. Due to the lipid composition utilized, these nanovesicles and their contents remained undamaged for more than 10 days when incubated under circumstances that mimicked an extracellular environment (Bochicchio et al., 2016). Both kinds of liposomes may be employed as curcumin biocarriers in dietary supplements and functional foods because curcumin liposomes demonstrated a lower delivery rate and reduced overall release percentage for the compound, improved acid base and thermal stability, and noticeably enhanced digestion in simulated GIT (Li et al., 2018).

Utilizing smart nanodelivery system for nutraceuticals with both medicinal and nutritional potential is necessary for the development of novel functional meals. Dey et al. (2018) created an omega-3 PUFA-enriched NE using sesame protein isolate (SPI) for an organic surfactant. The hydrodynamic droplet dimension successfully boosted the shelf-life durability of NEs. About 90% of the fatty acids in the NE droplets were released during the course of the 120-minute replicated two-step experimental digestion. Even at 40°C, long-chain triglyceride-based NEs retained vitamin E well, and the retention was enhanced by storage in the dark. Temperatures over 25°C were too high for short-chain triglyceride-based NEs containing vitamin E to tolerate (Hategekimana et al., 2015). A saponin-coated NE (diameter 277 nm) and vitamin E encapsulation was demonstrated to be more resistant to droplet coalescence than a conventional emulsion under heat processing (30°C–90°C), extended storage, and mechanical abuse. Cholecalciferol (vitamin D3) minitablets and a specially made bile salt/lipase alginate–glycerine film were combined to create a bioactive association platform (BAP) capsule, which delivered the main nutraceutical component from its production framework and improved cholecalciferol's performance (Parthasarathi et al., 2016). Figure 18.3 shows the different surface properties that can be modified to formulate a NE.

18.4.4 Nanocomposites

Due to their improved capabilities in the food packaging sector and for the transportation of nutraceutical goods, biopolymer nanocomposites are a growing subject in

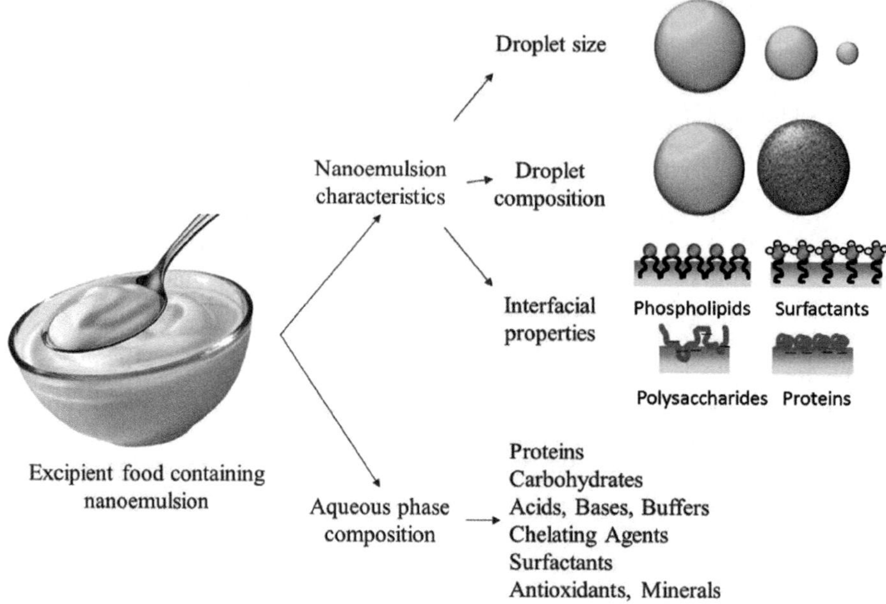

FIGURE 18.3 Schematic representation of a NE and its characteristics. (Salvia-Trujillo et al., 2016)

the study area of food preservation. In addition, the biopolymer and nanocomposite come from natural sources that are cheap, biodegradable, plentiful in nature, and environmentally beneficial. The primary building element of plants, cellulose, is also found in many marine-dwelling organisms and aquatic microflora. They are highly hygroscopic materials that are soluble in dilute acids and solvents but insoluble in water, where they swell. For the creation of lightweight, inexpensive products with great mechanical strength, cellulose nanoreinforcements are appealing materials. To reduce water vapor permeability, various levels of cellulose nanofiber were combined with mango pulp, while the nanofiller cellulose boosts the elongation and tensile strength of the nanofilm (de Azeredo et al. 2001). Chitin is a polymer that resembles cellulose and is widely distributed in shrimp, crabs, and other marine crustaceans and sponges. It has a repeating structure of (1,4)-b-N-acetyl glycosaminoglycan. Acid hydrolysis is used to create chitin whiskers, which are also employed as nanofillers since they are inexpensive, tasteless and odorless, and have high biocompatibility and biodegradability. When used as a reinforcing agent, a mixture of gelatin and chitin whiskers improved the mechanical performance and gelling ability (Wan and Tai, 2013; Ge et al., 2018). It is widely employed in multiple industries, including medicines, food, agriculture, and food engineering since it is a complex cationic polymer with positive charges on its amino group that is also harmless and biocompatible.

The creation of bio-nanocomposites is best suited for protein polymers. The inclusion of amino acid residues with the polypeptide chain determines the chemical and physical properties of the protein. Protein and polymer blends, such as keratin–CS, gluten–methylcellulose, and keratin–polypropylene, increase the strength, flexibility, and water vapor permeability of films. Protein-based films serve as carriers for taste, antioxidants, and bacteriostats, which enhance food quality and provide end consumers with health advantages. In addition to carbs and lipids, sources of protein that were used in the edible film included soybean, corn, milk, peanut, sunflower seeds, and corn. To preserve the quality of food goods, several films such as gelatin, milk protein, silk protein, and maize zein film have been developed (Gupta and Nayak, 2014).

The physico-chemical characteristics, concentration, and viscosity of the biomaterial are all taken into account during the manufacturing of biopolymer nanocomposites in order to create various composites, such as fibers, aerogels, and patterned microstructures. Today, however, a variety of wet chemical techniques are employed to create polymer nanocomposites, including 3D printing, freeze-drying, cast drying, ink-jet printing, electrospinning, masking micropatterns, and layer-by-layer assembly.

In actuality, encapsulating nutritional compounds in nanostructured composite materials might provide certain benefits like (i) shielding the nutritional supplement from environmental agents that could lead to quality deterioration during processing or storage; (ii) covering up unpleasant tastes; (iii) increasing its solubility and dispersibility, which would make it easier to process; (iv) regulating and/or extending its release; and (v) increasing its oral bioavailability (Penalva et al., 2014).

18.5 NANOMATERIAL WITH DIFFERENT FUNCTIONALITIES

Nanomaterials are not only viable carriers but also they are themselves functionally rich and versatile due to their structural and surface properties. These properties make them excellent candidates for incorporation in dietary supplements and medical purpose food. The following sections highlight a few of its crucial functional properties which have made the NPs the most sought-after and researched material to be exploited for the development of newer genre of functional foods and nutraceuticals.

18.5.1 Antioxidant Effects

One of the most exciting areas of study in the hunt for better antioxidants is nanomaterials. Some nanomaterials, such as those based on metals (such as gold and platinum) or organic (such as melanin and lignin) or metal oxides (such as cerium oxide), display inherent redox activity that is frequently linked to radical trapping, as well as superoxide dismutase (SOD)- and catalase (CAT)-like activities. By attaching low molecular weight reductants to redox inactive nanomaterials, antioxidants can be created (Valgimigli et al., 2018).

The oxidative breakdown of organic materials, such as biological components like lipids and proteins, is caused by a radical chain process in which alkyl radicals transform into peroxyl radicals (ROO•) by atmospheric oxygen. These radicals then spread the oxidative chain. Because it happens under benign conditions and for no discernible reason, this reaction is often referred to as "autoxidation" or a "peroxidation", as the primary first-formed products are hydroperoxides (alkyl hydroperoxide and hydrogen peroxide) (Ingold and Pratt, 2014). Since hydroperoxides can cleave homolytically, hydroxyl (HO•) or alkoxyl (RO•) radicals can be produced.

These radicals are very reactive and can target even generally stable compounds like DNA bases (Cadet and Wagner, 2014). The oxidative damage is exacerbated by the creation of reactive carbonyl species (such as 4-hydroxynonenal) as a consequence of alkyl hydroperoxide cleavage (Zhang and Forman, 2017). Oxidative stress is the accumulation of irreparable damage to DNA, proteins, and lipids that causes cell death and mutations. Reactive oxygen species (ROS) are produced in an unbalanced ratio to the cell's ability to mount an antioxidant defence (Morry et al., 2017). Similar to every radical chain reaction, autoxidation has three stages: initiation, propagation, and termination.

A substance (molecule or nanomaterial) known as an antioxidant inhibits or delays the oxidation of oxidizable molecules when it is added in very small doses to those molecules (Ingold and Pratt, 2014). Antioxidants typically come in two varieties: chain-breaking and preventive. Antioxidants that serve as preventives lower the start rate (Amorati and Valgimigli, 2015). This group of substances, which includes sunscreens, metal chelators, hydroperoxide-decomposing enzymes and their analogues, is diverse (Polefka et al., 2012, Perron and Brumaghim, 2009, Lu and Holmgren, 2014, Brand et al., 2004). The Fenton reaction involving hydrogen peroxide or organic hydroperoxides (ROOH) and transition metal ions in their reduced form, such as Fe^{2+}, is one of the primary sources of initiation. Effective preventive antioxidants include molecules like CAT, glutathione (GSH) peroxidase (GPX), and tiny compounds with chalcogen atoms (mostly Se and Te) that react with hydroperoxides without producing free radicals. Chain-breaking antioxidants, also known as radical-trapping antioxidants, compete with the propagation processes to slow down (or prevent) the autoxidation; as a result, peroxyl radicals engage with them faster than the substrate. A hydroperoxide and the antioxidant's radical (A•), which entraps a second ROO• and produces non-radical end products, are the usual results of the interaction between the antioxidant (AH) and a peroxyl radical (ROO•) (Valgimigli et al., 2018).

Nanoantioxidants are described as nanomaterials that have the ability to reduce the number of initiation events or trap chain-carrying radicals in order to lower the overall rate of autoxidation. These nanoantioxidants provide a special possibility since they can be made to target certain areas, have longer stability compared to small molecules, and delay metabolic clearance. Generally speaking, nanomaterials can substitute as passive carriers for the delivery of small-molecule antioxidants, or they can naturally have antioxidant capabilities (Morry et al., 2017). In vitro chemical experiments to gauge the antioxidant activity of new nanoantioxidants are crucial for directing the development of these compounds.

Many different kinds of nanomaterials have inherent antioxidant effects that arise from the surface characteristics of the material rather than from their functionalization with antioxidants.

CAT-mimicking action: By breaking down hydrogen peroxide to produce water and oxygen, CAT simulates work, such as metal (platinum, palladium, silver, and gold) and metal oxide NPs that exhibit CAT–mimic activity (Valgimigli et al., 2018). However, this action only takes place at neutral or alkaline pH, whereas pro-oxidant effects resembling those of peroxidase enzymes are seen at acidic pH levels.

GPX-mimicking action: GPX activity has only been identified in the case of vanadium pentoxide or vanadium oxide and manganese oxides, in contrast to CAT activity, which is typical for many metals or metal oxide materials. Under physiological settings, vanadium oxide nanowires can facilitate the reduction of hydrogen peroxide to water at the expense of GSH. This is possible because vanadium oxide has the unusual capacity to produce polar peroxido species rather than HO• radicals (Vernekar et al., 2014; Ragg et al., 2016)

SOD-mimicking action: Antioxidants that entrap superoxide radicals must be considered individually because, despite the fact that superoxide is a component of the peroxyl radical family, its exclusive chemistry sets it apart from alkylperoxyl radicals. Since the predominant form of superoxide at physiological pH is deprotonated oxygen, the conjugated acid of superoxide (HOO•) has a pKa value of 4.5. Superoxide exhibits a dual behavior when protonated (i.e. neutral and HOO•), since it may either extract a hydrogen atom to generate HOOH or give the hydrogen atom to form oxygen (Cedrowski et al., 2016). Deprotonated oxygen, concurrently, functions as a reducing species (Hayyan et al., 2016). While in organic solvents and at low pH, the interaction between two protonated species becomes significant, the self-degradation of superoxide is caused by the interaction between the two species (protonated and deprotonated). In reality, SOD-like activity has been shown for nanomaterials with extremely varied surface arrangement, including melanin, noble metals (palladium, platinum, and gold), metal oxides (cobalt, cerium, and manganese oxides), carbon clusters, carbon nanotubes (CNTs) and fullerenes (Valgimigli et al., 2018).

Intriguingly, a "multi-nanozyme" based on MnO_2 NPs placed on vanadium oxide nanowires by polydopamine was able to simultaneously produce GPX- and SOD-like activity (Huang et al., 2016).

Chain breaking: An antioxidant must neutralize alkylperoxyl radicals by turning them into hydroperoxides in order to perform its chain-breaking function (Valgimigli et al., 2018). Alkylperoxyl radicals must be quenched using an electron and a proton, which can be delivered either jointly by an antioxidant that donates hydrogen atoms or separately by an antioxidant that donates electrons and a protic solvent. Antioxidants of this kind are active to varying degrees in all mediums, from water to apolar solvents (Amorati et al., 2016). Similar behavior is seen in NPs with cleavable a hydroxy or hydroxyl group on their surface, such as those found in lignin. Lignin NPs have antioxidant action in methanol and apolar polymers like natural rubber (Barana et al., 2016; Tian et al., 2017).

Hydroperoxyl radical quenching: Initiating radicals and sources of damage to macromolecules like DNA and proteins frequently include the HO• radical. Its great reactivity toward all organic substrates, however, makes it unlikely that an antioxidant will catch it before it damages the substrate in the majority of systems.

Singlet oxygen: Singlet oxygen is a potent oxidant that is created when energy is transferred from a higher photosensitizer state to triplet oxygen, which is in its ground state. It causes many biological components, especially unsaturated lipids, to undergo non-radical oxidation (Akazawa-Ogawa et al., 2015). By exposing photo-sensitive natural dyes (excitation at 560 nm) or NPs like ZnO (excitation at 340 nm), singlet oxygen may be produced in a test tube (Wen et al., 2015).

18.5.2 Anticarcinogenic Properties

Malignancy or cancer can cause a variety of pathological alterations in cellular settings. It develops by a variety of signaling systems, including metastasis, angiogenesis, and cell proliferation (Jason et al., 2004; Seigneuric et al., 2010). Aerobic glycolysis, changes in respiratory tracts, mitochondrial DNA degeneration, and genetic expressions are all atypical metabolic processes in cancer cells. At certain stages, the effectiveness of physical and chemical cancer therapies is restricted. However, presently existing treatments have a negative impact and interfere with normal cell activity while exposing patients to high doses of medication and radiation therapy (Rothwell et al., 2010; Wu et al., 2011). AgNPs' remarkable potential as combination partners is further shown by recent reports that they control Pgp function and hence improve the chemotherapeutic efficiency against resistant or mutagenic cancer cells (Igaz et al., 2016). AgNPs were created by Saratale et al. (2018) using the popular medicinal herb dandelion, *Taraxacum officinale*, and they had a strong cytotoxic impact on HepG2 liver cancer cells. With reference to *Commelina nudiflora* L. aqueous extract-treated HCT-116 colon cancer cells, AgNPs developed by Kuppusamy and colleagues (2016) demonstrated lower cell viability and increased cytotoxicity. Four distinct cancer cell models were used to create biofunctionalized silver NPs using a variety of guava and clove plant extracts (Raghunandan et al., 2011). The biological effects of several metal NPs were investigated using simulated tumour stroma, metastasis models, and p53-deficient tumour cells (Melaiye et al., 2004). The silver NPs with a diameter of 5 nm had a greater cytotoxicity than those with a bigger diameter. Additionally, it was determined that in the absence of the tumour suppressor p53, silver NPs might cause apoptosis-dependent programmed cell death. In p53-deficient cancer cells, conventional cancer treatment frequently fails to induce cell death. Such developed AgNPs' exceptional chemotherapeutic potential was established.

Furthermore, it was shown that targeting mitochondrial structure and function was the main mechanism by which NPs (5–35 nm) caused cell death. The cytotoxic action mechanism of Ag NPs of 5 and 35 nm was equivalent (Melaiye et al., 2005), despite the fact that smaller Ag NPs are more lethal. It is interesting to note that the cytotoxic properties of silver and silver hybrid NPs vary depending on the cell type. In this field, cancer cells were found to be more cytotoxic than non-cancerous fibroblasts. In conclusion, a conventional treatment approach involves stimulating tumour-associated fibroblast cells with metal NPs.

According to Geetha et al. (2013), gold NPs made with aqueous *C. guianensis* flower extract have anticancer properties. It is plausible to assume that the anticancer activity of freshly generated gold NPs is provided by the pharmacological characteristics of *C. guianensis*. It is interesting to note that the functionalization of gold NPs as anticancer nanomaterial was accomplished without the doping of molecules.

Antibacterial and anticancer applications have made advantage of ZnONPs' photo-triggered ROS production and the phototoxicity that results in cells. To improve the photocatalytic effectiveness and ROS production capacity of ZnONPs, further chemical modifications, such as doping with metal NPs, modification with polymers, metal hybridization and sensitization by organic photosensitizers, have been developed. Modified ZnONPs' increased ROS production efficiency therefore boosts their antibacterial and anticancer properties (Sivakumar et al., 2018).

Another effective method is photothermal treatment, which uses NPs like CNTs or gold NPs to transform near-infrared (NIR) light into vibrational energy, which then produces heat powerful enough to kill cancer cells. The suspension of polyvinylpyrrolidone-coated graphene sheets subjected to NIR light (808 nm, 2 W/cm^2) produced more heat than DNA or sodium dodecylbenzene sulfonate-solubilized single-wall CNT under identical circumstances, in spite of having a lower NIR-absorbing capability. As a result, graphene NPs greatly outperformed CNT in causing the in vitro photothermal degradation of U251 human glioma cells. The greater dispersity of graphene sheets, due to the shape as well as the thermodynamic and optical features of the two types of carbon NPs, might be substantially responsible for their higher photothermal sensitivity. According to the processes, oxidative stress and membrane depolarization in mitochondria led to mixed cell death, which are, respectively, distinguished by caspase activation/DNA fragmentation and cell membrane damage.

Notably, research shows that metal NPs are a viable future possibility for cancer treatment since their anticancer effectiveness is superior to that of its macro-structure sister due to improved dispersivity/smaller particle size. These NPs are attractive prospects for the treatment of cancer due to their high surface area, minimal toxicity, and incredibly low cost.

18.5.3 Increased Micronutrient Bioavailability, Absorptions and Stability

Through their encapsulating property, food grade NPs can help to increase the effectiveness, stability, and utilization of micronutrients (Hildeliza et al., 2010). The bioavailability of a NP is determined by its bioaccessibility, absorption during oral consumption and transformation in the digestive system (Figure 18.4). During this process, the characteristics of bioactive components may change due to interactions between them or changes in the environment in which they are found. Vitamin C and vitamin D are nutrient enhancers that can increase iron and calcium absorption in human body. For instance, according to Teucher et al. (2004), vitamin C can enhance iron absorption by twofold to threefold. Concurrently, inhibitors prevent the absorption of nutrients by either binding them to other substances or reducing their absorption by making them insoluble. The bioavailability of micronutrients is reduced or hampered by phytic acid, a typical antinutritional factor that is embedded in many vegetarian/vegan diets and has a considerable binding potential for minerals like zinc, calcium, and iron (Zhou et al., 2010). In this situation, using nanotechnology to block these inhibitors of bioactive particles can be a viable strategy.

Curcumin mixed with colloidal NPs has greater absorption effectiveness than natural curcumin, according to Sasaki et al. (2011). A research found that the addition of

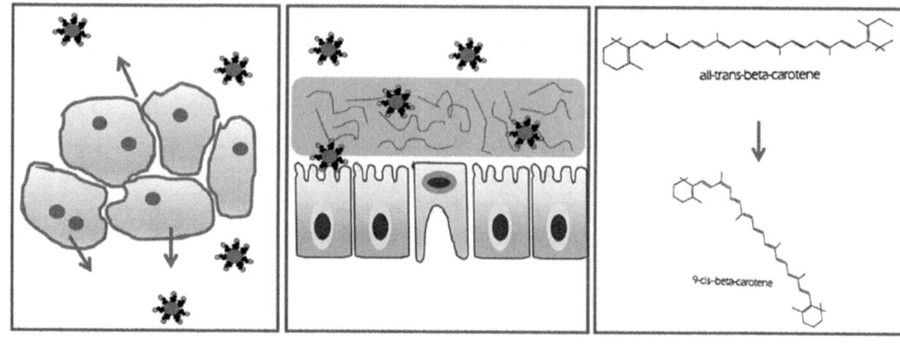

FIGURE 18.4 Biosorption of food grade NP. (Salvia-Trujillo et al., 2016.)

a chemical inhibitor significantly slowed chromogenic deterioration rate of beta-carotene in NEs because of its desire to chelate transition elements (such as Fe^{2+}) that typically favor oxidation. Additionally, when given with a (piperine) absorption enhancer, curcumin's oral bioavailability may increase by nine times (Shaikh et al., 2009; Qian et al., 2012; Haq et al., 2020).

A micronutrient's breakdown depends greatly on its physical, chemical, and intracellular characteristics, as well as the proximate composition of food and its storage circumstances. Within a food product, essential nutrients may be susceptible to enzymatic, physico-chemical instability. Chemical variability comprises adjustments to the molecular structure, which can result in significant fluctuation in the bioactive component's physical characteristics and nutritional qualities. The common processes that lead to the chemical breakdown of micronutrients include hydrolysis, oxidation, isomerization, and reduction. The enzymes found in dietary items can carry out these processes (McClements et al., 2009; McClements, 2015). Physical variability is defined as a change in the location of micronutrients caused by processes such as gravitational separation, aggregation, phase alterations and melting, while it is crucial to understand the main processes of degradation and important variables (such as pH, temperature, and water activity) for a certain micronutrient (Joye et al., 2014; Manzoor et al., 2019).

Materials that prevent the diffusion of multiple reactants into the particles may be placed on top of NPs. According to Matalanis et al. (2011), trapping the fat molecules inside a microgel enwrapped by protein miscellas can reduce the degree of autooxidation in oil-based emulsions (Matalanis et al., 2011; Zhang et al., 2013). For instance, when fish oil droplets are contained within microgels of casein pectin complex, the onset and rate of oxidation are decreased (Zhang et al., 2013). By acting as an antioxidant, chelating transition metals, and preventing reactant spread, these microgels may suppress oxidation (McClements, 2015).

Nanotechnology applications can offer fresh perspectives in the disciplines of biochemistry, nutrition, food science, and medicine (Pérez-Esteve et al., 2016). Wholesome applications of nanofortificants, however, still have a long way to go to be established worldwide (Gallocchio et al., 2015). Because there are still a lot of unknowns regarding the toxicities of NPs, it is imperative that the safety issues surrounding nanomaterials are addressed. However, it is essential to study the food–NP interaction and their fate after ingestion.

18.5.4 Nanoparticles with Other Functional Properties

Improved sensory properties: NPs can be used to improve the texture, color, flavor, and appearance of food products. For example, titanium dioxide NPs can be used to make food products appear whiter and brighter.

Enhanced delivery: NPs can be used to target specific cells or tissues in the body, thereby improving the delivery of active ingredients. For example, gold NPs can be employed to deliver drugs targeted to cancer cells.

Controlled release: NPs can be designed to release active ingredients slowly over time, improving their efficacy and reducing side effects. For example, silver NPs can be used to deliver antibiotics to infected tissues, reducing the need for frequent dosing.

Improved stability: NPs can protect active ingredients from degradation and oxidation, improving their shelf life and efficacy. For example, vitamin E NPs can protect the antioxidant from oxidation, ensuring that it remains effective for longer periods.

Reduced toxicity: NPs can reduce the toxicity of active ingredients by reducing their dosage and minimizing their exposure to non-target tissues. For example, zinc oxide NPs can be used to deliver zinc, which is toxic in high doses, without causing harm to the body.

18.6 POTENTIAL FATE OF NANOPARTICLES AFTER INGESTION

NPs are widely used in food to improve sensory properties such as color, flavor, and texture, increase stability, and expand shelf life. Well-planned application of NPs fortifies food, enhances functionality and bioavailability, and improves nutritional properties. Moreover, NPs are efficiently used to perceive the slightest chemical, physical, and biological changes that arise during food preparation, processing, storage and transport, which is greatly enhanced by nanosensors. These sensors are also used in smart packaging to assist in the detection of food poisons, microbial toxins, hazardous chemicals, and food pathogens. As NP applications become increasingly popular across the food industry, they have become integral parts of three major areas, such as food processing, preservation, safety, packaging and storage of food (Mohammad et al., 2022; Singh et al., 2017). Regarding the safety of human health, the biggest concern with NPs is their exposure and eventual fate in living systems including the GIT, respiratory tract, and renal tract. Nanomaterials have large active surface area and are small in size, but they have the potential to be incredibly chemically active within the body, being able to participate easily in biological reactions,

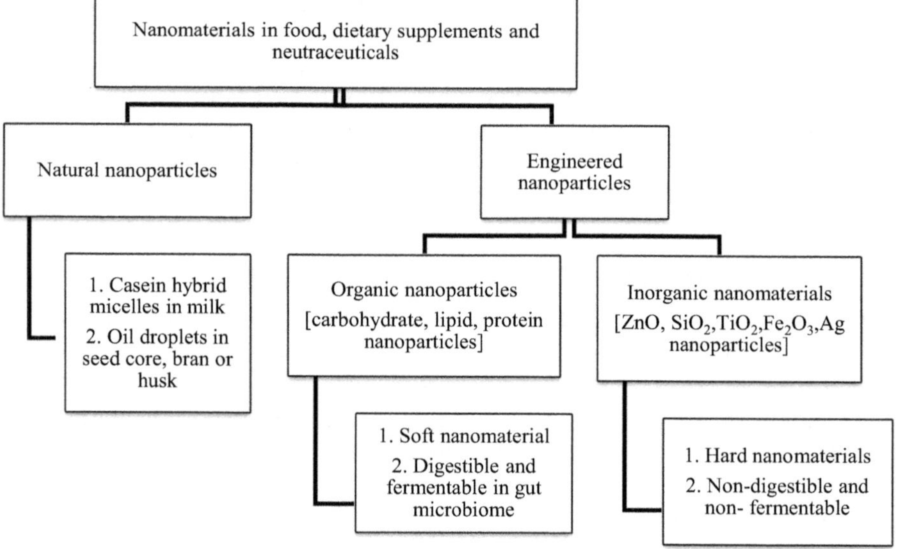

FIGURE 18.5 Nanomaterials in food, dietary supplements and nutraceuticals. (Adopted from McClements and Xiao, 2017; Zhou & McClements, 2022.)

and being able to enter the circulation with ease after rapid absorption, which implies that their fate and possible toxicity must be carefully reevaluated (McClements and Xiao, 2017).

Natural NPs are universally present in common commodities such as oil droplets in seed core, bran or husk, and casein hybrid micelles in milk (Figure 18.5). Different nanomaterials applied in food, dietary supplements and nutraceuticals are commonly known as ENs (Figure 18.5). This can be further classified into organic nanomaterials and inorganic nanomaterials (McClements and Xiao, 2017).

Orally ingested NPs interact with different gastrointestinal juices, pH, and hydrolytic enzymes that affect their physico-chemical properties, particle behavior, bioavailability and fate in living body. These can lead to altered functional performance, bioavailability, and toxicity (Zhou & McClements, 2022). NPs can have a variety of characteristics that are innate (intrinsic) to them or linked to how they behave in exposed environment (extrinsic). A number of intrinsic and extrinsic properties of NPs are responsible for altering the gastrointestinal tract fate. The intrinsic properties of the particle include its size, shape, surface area, morphology, molecular mass, core composition, density, and surface area. The extrinsic properties include zeta potential, aggregation state, oxidative state, stability, dissolution, mobility within the system, and interfacial properties such as polarity and chemical reactivity, all of which take into account changing fates and behaviors (Casals et al., 2017).

Particle dimension solely influences functional properties of particles, digestibility and optical clarity. Smaller particle size of digestible NP increases the pace of digestion and epithelial absorption due to the interaction with digestive hydrolytic enzymes and acids with a larger exposed surface area. The smaller size of

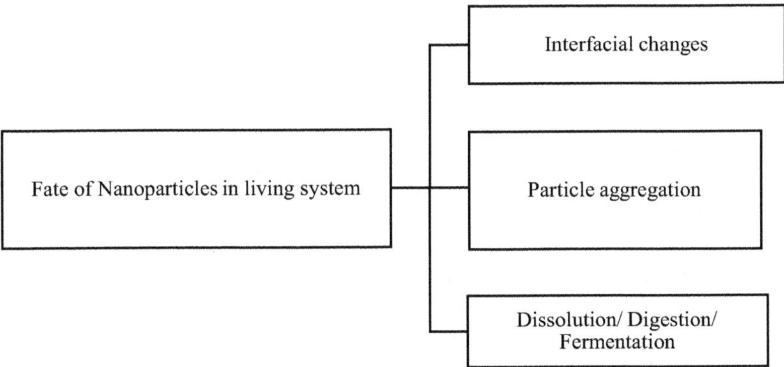

FIGURE 18.6 Potential fate of NPs after ingestion. (Adopted from Zhou & McClements, 2022.)

indigestible NPs facilitates absorption through the GIT mucus layer (Figure 18.6). The influence of particle shape on digestion and absorption is that spherical particles absorb faster than nanofiber or nanocube. A high length-to-width ratio of NPs increases chyme viscosity, causing abdominal distension and delaying GI transit time which improves nutrient feedback signaling (Zhou & McClements, 2022, Tucker & Mattes, 2013).

NPs can boost the availability of bioactive constituents in the body in two ways: On the one hand, the bioactive substance is incorporated within the NPs in the delivery system approach. On the other hand, excipient systems combine an excipient food containing bioactive NPs prepared for oral consumption. In both instances, designed systems are specially intended to boost the bioavailability of the active substances in the GIT by enhancing bioaccessibility or absorption. High amounts of NPs may slow or prevent carbohydrate, fat or protein digestion in the GIT. This effect is most noticeable in inorganic NPs, although it may also be present in certain indigestible organic NPs. Interfacial characteristics of NPs, such as charge, polarity, thickness and chemical reactivity, impact NP interaction with food systems and other GIT components. However, surface properties of NPs can be modified in ENs during designing by the use of food grade organic coating materials (McClements et al., 2017, Powell et al., 2010). The composition of the NP serves as a crucial aspect that impacts the behavior of NPs in the body and its many system components, as well as GI fate. Inorganic NPs are seldom absorbed or fermented in the GIT. There are certain exceptions, such as ZnO and Fe_2O_3 particles dissolved in stomach acid. Organic NPs consisting of mineral oil, resistant starch, flavor or essential oils, however, are indigestible (Feliu et al., 2016).

Consumption of organic NP*s and their fate:* NPs with a characteristic size of less than 100 nm that are generated from carbohydrates, lipids, fractional protein, and other organic components are frequently employed in the wellness food sector as texture modifiers, taste enhancers, stability enhancers, and shelf-life extenders. These organic nanomaterials are frequently employed to improve the bioavailability of important nutrients or bioactive compounds, boost nutritional value, and facilitate the administration of highly sensitive bioactive components and medications with controlled release qualities. Tailored organic composite NPs made up of combination of any carbohydrate, protein, fat and microbial polysaccharides have potential future in health and nutrition industry (Maisel et al., 2015). Carbohydrate-based NPs such as alginate, pectin, agar, CS, starch, carrageenan, and others are not digested by the GI juices because they are resistant polysaccharides. These components are with no trouble fermented by colonic microflora and offer gut health benefits. Protein NPs (zein-, gliadin-, casein-, and soy protein-based NPs) are normally digested inside the GIT unless modified with inorganic coating materials or charged biopolymers. Proteolytic digestive enzymes like as pepsin, trypsin, and chymotrypsin are involved in the breakdown of protein NPs. Different digestive lipases in the stomach and intestine break down phospholipid, triglyceride, and cholesterol-based NPs. Lipid NPs are digested at a faster pace than other organic NPs because they have a larger surface area to interact with. Emulsifier coating on tailored lipid NPs can impair digestion by interfering with bile salt interaction, despite the fact that mineral oil or essential oil-based NPs are indigestible (Zhang et al., 2019).

Consumption of inorganic NPs and their fate: The use of inorganic NPs in different areas of food production, including the direct insertion as nanoadditives, is fast developing in the nanotechnology field in order to improve desirable attributes in food production, application, and storage. The most often used inorganic NPs in commercial food, beverages, vitamin supplements, and food additives include titanium dioxide (TiO_2), iron oxide (Fe_2O_3), zinc oxide (ZnO), silicon dioxide (SiO_2), gold (Au), and silver (Ag). Metal oxide NPs are commonly employed in dairy, processed foods, beverages, and some medications. ZnO and Fe_2O_3 improve nutritional value and system stability while delivering highly sensitive active substances with a regulated release pattern. These NPs dissolve quickly in stomach acid. SiO_2 and TiO_2 are two efficient delivery agents. SiO_2 (food additive E551) is extensively used as anticaking agent in icing sugar, instant food mix, milk powders and other products, while TiO_2 (food additive E171) is used as a whitening agent in chewing gum, candy and milk powder (Byrne et al, 2010). Many mineral-based NPs, including but not limited to titanium dioxide, gold, silicon dioxide, iron dioxide, silver, and zinc oxide, have the ability to influence the gut microbiome and induce pathological conditions such as colitis, and immunological dysfunction. Several studies, however, have demonstrated that inorganic NPs, which are listed above, have a dynamic relationship with gut microbiome and contribute to positive GI microbial habitat. Non-absorbed fractional mineral NPs build up in the intestinal lumen as a result of regular consumption and interact directly with the intestinal bacteria that colonies the lumen and mucosal layers of the epithelial surface. Monitoring the influence of food-derived NPs on colonic microbes and the GIT tract epithelial environment is critical to the secure and efficient implementation of nanotechnology in the health and nutrition sector.

18.7 SAFETY CONCERNS AND POTENTIAL LONG-TERM EFFECT

Over the past few decades, NPs have been widely applied in the food industry for a myriad of different applications ranging from food processing and packaging to food storage and preservation. The key concern with NPs in terms of health security is their human exposure. There are several entrance points for NPs, including ingestion, inhalation, and skin absorption. It is worth noting that nanomaterials possess special properties, such as their large surface area-to-volume ratio, that contribute to making them more chemically active in the human body than bulk materials, so they could become involved in most biological reactions that could even harm human health in the future. Upon absorption, NPs can effortlessly reach circulation, where they may settle in various regions like the brain, liver and kidney or cause immunological reactions. So, it may be worthwhile to assess their fate and potential toxicity. A nanomaterial dissipates more quickly and improves bioavailability compared to a similar substance not manufactured as a nanomaterial. In addition to allowing active ingredients to be targeted directly to specific sites, nanomaterials can also be targets of the complement system and mononuclear phagocytes. Several hydrophilic nanomaterials are excreted by the kidneys. The active targeting of tumours typically requires the attachment of specific molecules to the surface of nanomaterials that are recognized by cancer cells' receptors based on their size or charge (Guo et al., 2021).

The physico-chemical and fundamental characteristics of the NPs in food products define how they behave in the GIT and whether they are harmful. Due to their smaller size, NPs can boost the availability of bioactive constituents in the body which can lead to potential toxicity. However, the probable toxicity mechanisms of NPs are fully dosage-dependent. Organic NPs are digested by hydrolytic enzymes, fermented by gut bacteria or dissolved in stomach acid before being absorbed by the GI epithelium. Inorganic metal NPs, however, bypass digestion and fermentation processes and enter directly through the epithelial layer to interact with the target tissue or organ. A high dosage of metallic NPs in the GI system for an extended length of time might cause massive ROS production in the cytoplasm. These damage intracellular organelles, cell membrane and intracellular enzymes leading to cellular dysfunction via down-regulating Na+/K+ ATPase activity. Hence, before applying NPs to food, it is necessary to check for cellular safety and toxicity potential (Peng et al., 2022).

Despite its antibacterial capabilities, ZnO and Fe_2O_3 produce ROS in biological systems. Overuse over an extended length of time may induce oxidative damage. Nevertheless, no damage or accumulation in functioning tissue or organ was identified at doses ranging from 250 to 1,000 mg/kg body weight. A high amount of powder SiO_2 can induce cytotoxicity and genotoxicity. Nevertheless, no accumulating data were discovered in the rat-feeding experiment. TiO_2 found to be banned in France for promoting cellular toxicity, altering gut microbiota (Proquin et al., 2017). However, it possesses low toxicity and accumulation rate in case of prolonged use. Gold and silver NPs are usually applied as delivery agents or packaging materials that leak into the body circulation. They had a decreased accumulation rate and were largely eliminated via urine and faeces. Yet, if taken in significant quantities over an extended period of time, such NPs can cause long-term chronic toxicity.

Since the Food and Drug Administration (FDA) approved gold NPs for use in many biomedical applications, there have been more uses in fields including cancer treatment, medication delivery, and other biological applications (Hu et al., 2023). Food-derived extracellular vesicles present in dietary supplements such as exosomes of bovine milk, grapes and ginger can alleviate inflammatory reactions (Peng et al., 2022).

Nanocomposite as active component delivery agent may possess toxicity by interacting with other chemical components of the body or nutrients circulating in the body as summarized in Table 18.1. CNTs and graphene nanoplates are frequently employed in the medical field. Along with arsenic, graphite oxide restricts the metabolism of carbohydrates and fatty acids and disrupts urea cycle but promotes the metabolism of amino acids and secondary compounds. Together with enhanced arsenic cellular absorption, graphite oxide also causes electrolyte leakage and intracellular structural damage. AgNPs interact with free chloride ions (Cl^-) in the circulation. This nano-bio-interaction leads to high Cl/Ag ratios, which contribute advanced toxic effects (Honarvar et al., 2016; He et al., 2019; Sarikhani et al., 2022).

An increase in the absorption of organic NPs synthesized from polysaccharides, peptides, and lipids could be linked to allergic responses. Even consumed NPs that are not absorbed may have harmful consequences if they cause changes in the usual gut microbiota. Besides that, a pre-existing disturbed microbiota may influence NP absorption, possibly through NP adhesion to lipopolysaccharides (LPS) (Ranjan et al., 2019; Bergin & Witzmann, 2013). Inorganic NPs, however, may have extensive implications, such as tissue deposition and chronic CVD (Tarhan, 2020).

TABLE 18.1
Toxicity and Potential Long- Term Effect Possesses by Inorganic Nanoparticles

Nanoparticle	Toxicity Type	Toxic Effect	Reference
ZnO	Hepatotoxic	Interrupt zinc homeostasis, prompt oxidative stress in hepatocytes	Youn and Choi, (2022); Pei et al. (2023)
TiO_2	Cytotoxic	DNA damage, cellular senescence	Sarikhani et al. (2022)
Ag NP	Biosynthesized Ag NPs: immune modulator (at high doses) Chemically synthesized Ag NPs: ROS generator	Bio-Ag NPs are nontoxic up to 2,000 mg/kg body weight in mice compared to the chemically synthesized Ag NPs	Shanker et al. (2017); Rajan et al. (2022)
Au NP	ROS-induced cytotoxic	Oxidative damage of liver, spleen and kidney	Sani et al. (2021)
SiO_2	ROS-induced cytotoxic (dose-dependent)	Lipid peroxidation and cellular membrane damage	Zarafshar et al. (2015)
Fe_2O_3	ROS-induced cytotoxic (dose- and time-dependent)	Particles bigger than 100 nm are bio-accumulated in intercellular space	Sadeghi and Espanani (2015)

The effects of SiO_2, Fe_2O_3, ZnO, and TiO_2 NPs on RKO and Caco-2 cell were studied using whole human genomic oligonucleotide microarrays. Only ZnO NP (which disintegrated extensively) was particularly cytotoxic, involving the upregulation of genes associated with protein folding and stress responses. Exposure to TiO_2 NPs amplified respiratory inflammation and intracellular damage via inhalation and penetration through the lungs and skin. Intracellular stress response is triggered by Ag NP exposure. Copper NPs have demonstrated antibacterial effectiveness in vitro and have been recommended as antibiotic substitutes in public health and agriculture. Cu–CS complex NPs reduce harmful bacteria in the cecum such as *Salmonella* sp., *Escherichia coli*, and *Clostridium* sp., increase good bacteria (e.g. *Lactobacilli*) and may promote nutritional absorption by enhanced digestive enzyme production (Ranjan et al, 2019; Bergin & Witzmann, 2013). The photocatalytic activity and phototoxicity of TiO_2 NPs were significantly influenced by humic acid coating. Sulphur-doped TiO_2 caused DNA damage in zebrafish embryos. Nitrogen–fluorine-codoped TiO_2 NPs hasten the generation of ROS (He et al., 2019). Additional drug delivery vehicles incorporate quantum dots and CNTs. Carbon NPs have also been linked to pulmonary inflammation and cardiovascular illness. Possible dangers and toxicity issues associated with the swallowing and inhalation of those tiny NPs should be addressed and minimized. Many nanomaterials, particularly inorganic compounds, have the potential to accumulate in tissues. Excessive exposure can cause damage to tissue and organs, which can lead to a variety of health problems. Manufacturers and suppliers must meet the terms of the risk assessment analysis defined by international bodies (Tarhan, 2020).

18.8 CURRENT REGULATIONS OF NANOPRODUCTS

Any product claiming to use nanoscale materials should take into account if the material exhibits dimension-dependent phenomena having functional effects within 1–100 nm at any single dimension. These occurrences are thought to promote many positive benefits to the end products, but they also result in higher bioavailability, which leads to toxicity. U.S. Food and Drug Administration (FDA) guidelines assess the efficacy, safety, and public health consequences, of nanotechnology-based products and provide product-specific guidance to deal with problems related to the above. FDA has published elaborate guideline for products that contain nanomaterials along with special emphasis on drugs and biological products for industries. Although FDA (2017) has not established a definition of nanomaterials, the guideline has instruction to consider nanomaterial as materials and end product materials with at least one dimension in the size of 1–100 nm range that exhibit dimension-dependent properties. The Food and Drug Administration (2014) defines drug product and biological product as any human drug at its final form of administration and drug containing biologically active substances, respectively. Before commercializing, these medications must go through premarket testing and product certification. Non-prescription-based over-the-counter medications, however, do not necessitate the same. It is the obligation of the maker to assure security while avoiding dangers. There should be a common technical document (CTD) on the nanomaterials in the drug product as well as the attributes of the nanomaterials themselves, such as size, surface charge, morphology, and composition, in a level appropriate to the stage of the product development in which the study is being conducted. The CTD must contain attributes such as chemical composition, morphology, particle average size and distribution, stability and aggregation characters, surface properties, hydrophobicity and distribution of the active components within the particle and system. In order to effectively assess the quality of the drug substance, a detailed description of its physical and chemical attributes must be provided, as critical quality attributes. An applicant should utilize risk assessments and examine them during the development of the product, as well as during its formulation in the market.

To provide regulatory oversight responsibility for nanotechnology regulation, the Environment Protection Agency (EPA), the Occupational Health and Safety Administration (OSHA), and the Consumer Product Safety Commissioner (CPSC) were part of the decentralized approach toward those nanotechnology regulations. Moreover, the USFDA mandates premarket review, for product approval applied to food additives, food contact compounds in packaging material, additives, and nutritional supplements. Post-market tracking is another method used to monitor and document nano-based food items in circulation. This method is additionally utilized for market surveillance if there is no premarket evaluation. The possible health concerns of nanomaterials are demonstrated by a number of investigations that include their detrimental consequences in bulk form. Moreover, they examine acute toxicity using markers that indicate carcinogenicity, neurotoxicity, respiratory and cardiovascular risks. The EPA has created a systematic technique called NanoRiskCat to analyze the exposure and impact level of NP-containing goods. The evaluation procedure contains five color-coded categories, three exposure categories represent handlers, consumers, and the ecosystem, and two risk concerns represent humans and environmental hazards. Based on the use of nanomaterials, the four possible exposure levels are nominated including high, medium, low, and unknown. The Japanese government makes regulatory decisions jointly through the Ministry of Education, Culture, Sports, Science, and Technology (MEXT); the Ministry of Economic, Trade and Industries (METI); the Ministry of Health, Labor, and Welfare (MHLW); and the Ministry of the Environment (MOE). China has set up national nanotechnology standards through the National Center for Nanoscience and Technology (NCNST), which was established in March 2003. Several protocols have been developed for the characterization of nanomaterials and the development of safety requirements for manufacturing. Food Standards Australia New Zealand (FSANZ) ensures that hazardous risks associated with nanomaterials and nanocomponents in food or packaging are assessed and managed. With the support of other Australian regulatory agencies, the Application Handbook is designed to provide practical guidance for the application process. To ascertain the safe application of food nanomaterials, FSANZ has also established a Scientific Nanotechnology Advisory Group (SNAG), which consists of experts in nanotechnology, nanotoxicology, and nanosafety. The purpose of this group is to advise on the safe application of food nanomaterials. In India, the Food Safety and Standards Authority of India (FSSAI) has launched the NanoMission, a mission-mode program operated as part of the Department of

Science and Technology (DST), with the Nano Mission Council (NMC) in charge, which raised concerns about the potential health and environmental risks associated with nanotechnology (Tarhan, 2020; He et al, 2019; Park & Yeo, 2016).

The above guidance relies on a risk-based framework that was tested in vitro human body system. This framework for evaluation comprises the nanomaterial's characterization, an understanding of its clearly intended application, and how the properties of the nanomaterial influence the quality of end product, general safety, and therapeutic efficacy. Asia Nano Forum, NanoForum, World Nano Conference, and International Conference on Advanced Nanotechnology are concerning bodies participating constantly to generate more and more specific guide on nanomaterial safety. Further regulatory guidelines on labeling and waste management and disposal are required. Collaboration is required to direct research toward a more thorough safety evaluation of nanomaterials and to aid regulatory authorities in their policymaking (Ranjan et al, 2019; He et al., 2019; Jain et al., 2018).

18.9 FUTURE PERSPECTIVE

A number of applications of nanotechnology have been successfully utilized to enhance the quality and safety of food products by detecting pathogens or toxins, fortifying food with minerals, antioxidants, vitamins, and essential oils, enhancing sensory quality with flavor and color enhancement, extending shelf life, and packaging that is antimicrobial. The market for nano-based products in the food sector has reached close to $1 billion USD. The majority of this is generated by the area of nanocoatings in packaging, and crucial component in wellness items. The top companies in the global food business are substantially investing in development and incorporation of nanotechnology into various kinds of food items. In the food production practice, nanotechnology and nanomaterials can be brought into use in several phases, including the processing stage, packaging and labeling stage, transportation phase, and post-production quality control phase. With the recent advances in nanosciences, it is possible to develop innovative approaches to the growth of functional foods, when it comes to the inclusion of bioactive components in order to increase the uptake of certain ingredients without affecting the sensory perception of the consumer. As a result, nutrients such as minerals, vitamins, bioactive ingredients, antioxidants, and phytochemicals can be packaged into biocompatible and biodegradable NPs so as to improve their bioavailability and delivery (Patel et al, 2018).

The majority of the in vivo data produced in accordance with standards is still used in the regulatory safety evaluation of NPs. Establishing specific parameters for this research is widely questioned. In addition to the extensive lists of factors necessary for proper material characterization, considerations for biological consequences relevant to nanomaterials must be considered. There are many unanswered questions underlying the various opinions that the FDA and European Food Safety Authority (EFSA) have issued on the suitability of the risk evaluation approach and standards for the industry with regard to the safety evaluation of NPs. This is primarily because there are no reliable data on the characterization of the nanomaterial in the commodity, and the toxicological studies. It has long been understood that regular analytical procedures must be developed, put into action, and validated in order to illustrate possible health effect concerned with the NP application. In addition, it was necessary to create experimental methods for evaluating the different health and environmental risks posed by NPs (Bouwmeester et al., 2014; Chau et al., 2007).

In the approaching years, consumables generated from nanotechnology are projected to broaden the possibilities for manufacturing, marketing and utilization of functional foods. Once rules and restrictions specific to nanotechnology are put in place to address the many safety hazards involved with this technology, it might completely transform the food processing industry. Nanotechnology is predicted to become the most advanced technology within a bounded development rate by the year 2050, solving the bulk of industrial and social obstacles through its capacity for finding creative solutions at both the micro- and macro-levels (Ramkumar et al., 2019; Sahoo et al., 2021).

18.10 CONCLUSIONS

Dietary supplements and medical purpose foods are categorised as special medical items under the law. Globally, these special medical items are governed, for instance, by regulatory authorities like the European Food Safety Authority, the U.S. Food and Drug Administration, and a number of national rules, the majority of which are typically issued by the Ministry of Public Health/Ministry of Agriculture of certain nations. They are a rich supply of antioxidants, PUFA, vitamins, minerals, and other substances with a nutritional or medicinal impact that are present in food or feed and are meant to be consumed directly in moderation. Nanotechnology is widely used for designing new generation of drug formulations, in the food industries and in production of nutritional supplements, as it gives many current materials "a new dimension" along with novel properties. There is no denying the significance of a balanced diet that contains essential nutrients, such as vitamins or antioxidants, in the proper quantities for both human and animal health.

Additionally, doctors now recognize the importance of consuming food products with specific, efficient ingredients to help those with certain diseases (such as cancer, diabetes, hyperlipidaemia, bone health, mental disorders and stunned nutrient absorption) avoid getting sick and to improve their health. When sustainability of the active component in the formulation could be assured till expiration date, the enrichment of food items with dietary supplements may be employed in practice with ease. For these uses, biodegradable natural or semi-synthetic nanocarriers such as polymer matrices, liposomes, NEs, nanomicelles, solid lipid NPs, nanostructured lipid carriers or inorganic/metal matrices are particularly advantageous, ensuring not only improved durability but also controlled release of nutrients. Based on prior rigorous research, it is certain that the most practical nanoformulation may be chosen and utilized for adding particular beneficial nutrients to bakery, dairy, fermented food products or beverages. Contrary to nutraceuticals that are sold in pharmacies and may be misused by certain unwary customers, leading to potential negative side effects, excessive use of these substances is not permitted when food items are fortified with dietary supplements or nutraceuticals. Despite the fact that nanoformulations improve the bioabsorption and stability of certain active ingredients, each and every nanoscale materials used in the food processing should only be used after thorough cytotoxicity testing (e.g. surface reactivity of NPs), which could have unspecified effects in humans or other animals as well. The toxicity of NPs is dependent on a number of variables, including size, shape, surface chemistry, and dosage. As a result, it is critical to carefully assess the harmful effects of NPs before incorporating them into foods and medications. International regulatory organizations are striving to create policies and rules for the secure consumption of NPs in food and supplements.

REFERENCES

Acevedo-Fani, A., Soliva-Fortuny, R. and Martín-Belloso, O., 2018. Photo-protection and controlled release of folic acid using edible alginate/chitosan nanolaminates. *J. Food Eng.*, 229, 72–82.

Akazawa-Ogawa, Y., Shichiri, M., Nishio, K., Yoshida, Y., Niki, E. and Hagihara, Y., 2015. Singlet-oxygen-derived products from linoleate activate Nrf2 signaling in skin cells. *Free Radical Biol. Med.*, 79, 164–175.

Akihisa, T., Tokuda, H., Ogata, M., Ukiya, M., Lizuka, M., Suzuki, T., Metori, K., Shimizu, N. and Nishino, H. 2004. Cancer chemopreventive effects of polyunsaturated fatty acids. *Cancer Lett.*, 205, 9–13.

Amorati, R. and Valgimigli, L., 2015. Advantages and limitations of common testing methods for antioxidants. Free Radic. Res., 49, 633–649.

Amorati, R., Baschieri, A., Morroni, G., Gambino, R. and Valgimigli, L., 2016. Peroxyl radical reactions in water solution: A gym for proton-coupled electron-transfer theories. *Chem. Eur. J.*, 22, 7924–7934.

Anderson, G. J., Connor, W.E. and Corliss, J.D., 1990. Docosahexaenoic acid is the preferred dietary n-3 fatty acid for the development of the brain and retina. *Pediatr. Res.*, 27, 89–97.

Arora, D. and Jaglan, S., 2016. Nanocarriers based delivery of nutraceuticals for cancer prevention and treatment: A review of recent research developments. *Trends Food Sci. Technol.*, 54, 114–126.

Arshad, R., Gulshad, L., Haq, I.U., Farooq, M.A., Al-Farga, A., Siddique, R., Manzoor, M.F. and Karrar, E., 2021. Nanotechnology: A novel tool to enhance the bioavailability of micronutrients. *Food Sci. Nutr.*, 9, 3354–3361.

Avella, M., Bruno, G., Errico, M., Gentile, G., Piciocchi, N., Sorrentino, A. and Volpe, M., 2007. Innovative packaging for minimally processed fruits. *Packag. Technol. Sci.: Int. J.*, 20(5), 325–335.

Babcock, T., Helton, W.S. and Espat, N.J., 2000. Eicosapentaenoic acid (EPA): An anti-inflammatory ω-3 fat with potential clinical applications. *Nutrition,* 16, 1116–1118.

Barana, D., Danish Ali, S., Salanti, A., Orlandi, M., Castellani, L., Hanel, T. and Zoia, L., 2016. Influence of lignin features on thermal stability and mechanical properties of natural rubber compounds. *ACS Sustain. Chem. Eng.*, 4, 5258−5267.

Bergin, I.L. and Witzmann, F.A., 2013. Nanoparticle toxicity by the gastrointestinal route: Evidence and knowledge gaps. *Int. J. Biomed. Nanosci. Nanotechnol.*, 3(1–2), 163–210.

Bochicchio, S., Barba, A.A., Grassi, G. and Lamberti, G., 2016. Vitamin delivery: Carriers based on nanoliposomes produced via ultrasonic irradiation. *LWT Food Sci. Technol.*, 69, 9–16.

Bouwmeester, H., Brandhoff, P., Marvin, H.J., Weigel, S. and Peters, R.J., 2014. State of the safety assessment and current use of nanomaterials in food and food production. *Trends Food Sci. Technol.*, 40(2), 200–210.

Bouwmeester, H., Dekkers, S., Noordam, M.Y., Hagens, W.I., Bulder, A.S., De Heer, C., Ten Voorde, S.E., Wijnhoven, S.W., Marvin, H.J. and Sips, A.J., 2009. Review of health safety aspects of nanotechnologies in food production. *Reg. Toxicol. Pharmacol.*, 53, 52–62.

Brand, M.D., Affourtit, C., Esteves, T.C., Green, K., Lambert, A.J., Miwa, S., Pakay, J.L. and Parker, N., 2004. Mitochondrial superoxide: Production, biological effects, and activation of uncoupling proteins. *Free Radic. Biol. Med.*, 37, 755–767.

Byrne, H.J., Lynch, I., De Jong, W.H., Kreyling, W.G., Loft, S., Park, M.V.D.Z., Riediker, M. and Warheit, D., 2010. *Protocols for Assessment of Biological Hazards of Engineered Nanomaterials*. NanoImpactNet Reports.

Cadet, J. and Wagner, J.R., 2014. Oxidatively generated base damage to cellular DNA by hydroxyl radical and one-electron oxidants: Similarities and differences. *Arch. Biochem. Biophys.*, 557, 47–54.

Casals, E., Gusta, M. F., Piella, J., Casals, G., Jiménez, W. and Puntes, V., 2017. Intrinsic and extrinsic properties affecting innate immune responses to nanoparticles: The case of cerium oxide. *Front. Immunol.*, 8, 970.

Cedrowski, J., Litwinienko, G., Baschieri, A. and Amorati, R., 2016. Hydroperoxyl radicals (HOO.): Vitamin E regeneration and H-bond effects on the hydrogen atom transfer. *Chem. Eur. J.*, 22, 16441–16445.

Chai, J., Jiang, P., Wang, P., Jiang, Y., Li, D., Bao, W., Liu, B., Liu, B., Zhao, L., Norde, W. and Yuan, Q., 2018. The intelligent delivery systems for bioactive compounds in foods: Physicochemical and physiological conditions, absorption mechanisms, obstacles and responsive strategies. *Trends Food Sci. Technol.*, 78, 144–154.

Chau, C.F., Wu, S.H. and Yen, G.C., 2007. The development of regulations for food nanotechnology. *Trends Food Sci. Technol.*, 18(5), 269–280.

Cheng, Q., Li, C., Pavlinek, V., Saha, P. and Wang, H., 2006. Surface-modified antibacterial TiO2/Ag+ nanoparticles: Preparation and properties. *Appl. Surface Sci.*, 252, 4154–4160.

Cho, H.Y., Lee, T., Yoon, J., Han, Z., Rabie, H., Lee, K.B., Su, W.W., and Choi, J.W., 2018. Magnetic oleosome as a functional lipophilic drug carrier for cancer therapy. *ACS applied materials & interfaces*, 10(11), 9301–9.

Cohen, Y., Levi, M., Lesmes, U., Margier, M., Reboul, E. and Livney, Y.D., 2017. Re-assembled casein micelles improve in vitro bioavailability of vitamin D in a Caco-2 cell model. *Food Funct.*, 8, 2133–2141.

Dai, T., Chen, J., McClements, D.J., Hu, P., Ye, X., Liu, C., and Li, T., 2019. Protein–polyphenol interactions enhance the antioxidant capacity of phenolics: Analysis of rice glutelin–procyanidin dimer interactions. *Food & Function*, 10(2), 765–74.

Damián, M.R., Cortes-Perez, N.G., Quintana, E.T., Ortiz-Moreno, A., Garfias Noguez, C., Cruceño-Casarrubias, C.E., Sánchez Pardo, M.E. and Bermúdez-Humarán, L.G., 2022. Functional foods, nutraceuticals and probiotics: A focus on human health. *Microorganisms*, 10(5), 1065.

Dan, N., 2016. Compound release from nanostructured lipid carriers (NLCs). *J. Food Eng.*, 171, 37–43.

David, S. and Livney, Y.D., 2016. Potato protein based nanovehicles for health promoting hydrophobic bioactives in clear beverages. *Food Hydrocoll.*, 57, 229–235.

deAzeredo, H.C., Mattoso, L.C. and McHugh, T.H., 2001. Nanocomposites in food packaging—a review. In Boreddy Reddy (ed.) *Advances in Diverse Industrial Applications of Nanocomposites*, pp. 57–78. InTech, Rijeka, Croatia.

Dey, T.K., Banerjee, P., Chatterjee, R. and Dhar, P., 2018. Designing of ω-3 PUFA enriched biocompatible nanoemulsion with sesame protein isolate as a natural surfactant: Focus on enhanced shelf-life stability and biocompatibility. *Colloids Surf. A Physicochem. Eng. Asp.*, 538, 36–44.

Esfanjani, A.F., Assadpour, E. and Jafari, S.M., 2018. Improving the bioavailability of phenolic compounds by loading them within lipid-based nanocarriers. *Trends Food Sci. Technol.*, 76, 56–66.

Ezhilarasi, P., Karthik, P., Chhanwal, N. and Anandharamakrishnan, C., 2013. Nanoencapsulation techniques for food bioactive components: A review. *Food Bioprocess Technol.*, 6(3), 628–647.

Fathi, M., Donsi, F. and McClements, D.J., 2018. Protein-based delivery systems for the nano-encapsulation of food ingredients. *Compr. Rev. Food Sci.*, 17, 920–936.

FDA, 2017. Drug Products, Including Biological Products, that Contain Nanomaterials - Guidance for Industry, https://www.federalregister.gov/documents/2017/12/18/2017-27133/drug-products-including-biological-products-that-contain-nanomaterials-draft-guidance-for-industry

Feliu, N., Docter, D., Heine, M., Del Pino, P., Ashraf, S., Kolosnjaj-Tabi, J., Macchiarini, P., Nielsen, P., Alloyeau, D., Gazeau, F. and Stauber, R.H., 2016. In vivo degeneration and the fate of inorganic nanoparticles. *Chem. Soc. Rev.*, 45(9), 2440–2457.

Filippini, T., Naska, A., Kasdagli, M.I., Torres, D., Lopes, C., Carvalho, C., Moreira, P., Malavolti, M., Orsini, N., Whelton, P.K. and Vinceti, M., 2020. Potassium intake and blood pressure: A dose-response meta-analysis of randomized controlled trials. *J. Am. Heart Assoc.*, 9, e015719.

Foodand Drug Administration, 2014. *Guidance for Industry Considering Whether an FDA-Regulated Product Involves the Application of Nanotechnology.* U.S. Department of Health and Human Services, Office of the Commissioner, Food and Drug Administration.

Gallocchio, F., Belluco, S. and Ricci, A., 2015. Nanotechnology and food: Brief overview of the current scenario. *Procedia Food Sci.*, 5, 85–88.

Gálvez, A., Abriouel, H., López, R.L. and Omar, N.B., 2007. Bacteriocin-based strategies for food biopreservation. *Int. J. Food Microbiol.*, 120, 51–70.

Gangadoo, S., Nguyen, H., Rajapaksha, P., Zreiqat, H., Latham, K., Cozzolino, D., Chapman, J. and Truong, V.K., 2021. Inorganic nanoparticles as food additives and their influence on the human gut microbiota. *Environ. Sci.: Nano*, 8(6), 1500–1518.

Ge, S., Liu, Q., Li, M., Liu, J., Lu, H., Li, F., Zhang, S., Sun, Q. and Xiong, L., 2018. Enhanced mechanical properties and gelling ability of gelatin hydrogels reinforced with chitin whiskers. *Food Hydrocoll.,* 75, 1–12.

Geetha, R., Ashokkumar, T., Tamilselvan, S., Govindaraju, K., Sadiq, M. and Singaravelu, G., 2013. Green synthesis of gold nanoparticles and their anticancer activity. *Cancer Nanotechnol.*, 4, 91–98.

Ghanbarzadeh, B., Babazadeh, A. and Hamishehkar, H., 2016. Nano-phytosome as a potential food-grade delivery system. *Food Biosci.*, 15, 126–135.

Goncalves, R.F.S., Martins, J.T., Duarte, C.M.M., Vicente, A.A. and Pinheiro, A.C., 2018. Advances in nutraceutical delivery systems: From formulation design for bioavailability enhancement to efficacy and safety evaluation. *Trends Food Sci. Technol.*, 78, 270–291.

Gong, G., Xu, Y., Zhou, Y., Meng, Z., Ren, G., Zhao, Y., Zhang, X., Wu, J., and Hu, Y., 2012. Molecular switch for the assembly of lipophilic drug incorporated plasma protein nanoparticles and in vivo image. *Biomacromolecules*, 13(1), 23–8.

Grolier, P., Agoudavi, S., Azais-Braesco, V., 1995, Comparative bioavailability of diet-, oil- and emulsion-based preparations of vitamin A and β-carotene in rat. *Nutrition Research*, 15(10), 1507–16.

Guo, S., Liang, Y., Liu, L., Yin, M., Wang, A., Sun, K., Li, Y. and Shi, Y., 2021. Research on the fate of polymeric nanoparticles in the process of the intestinal absorption based on model nanoparticles with various characteristics: Size, surface charge and pro-hydrophobics. *J. Nanobiotechnol.*, 19(1), 1–21.

Gupta, P. and Nayak, K.K., 2014. Characteristics of protein-based biopolymer and its application. *Polym. Eng. Sci.,* 55(3), 485–498.

Haq, I.U., Imran, M., Nadeem, M., Tufail, T., Tanweer, A.G. and Mubarak, M.S., 2020. Piperine: A review of its biological effects. *Phytother. Res.*, 35(2), 680–700.

Harde, H., Das, M. and Jain, S., 2011. Solid lipid nanoparticles: An oral bioavailability enhancer vehicle. *Expert Opin. Drug. Deliv.*, 8, 1407–1424.

Hategekimana, J., Chamba, M.V.M., Shoemaker, C.F., Majeed, H. and Zhong, F., 2015. Vitamin E nanoemulsions by emulsion phase inversion: Effect of environmental stress and long-term storage on stability and degradation in different carrier oil types. *Colloids Surf. A Physicochem. Eng. Asp.*, 483, 70–80.

Hayyan, M., Hashim, M.A. and AlNashef, I.M., 2016. Superoxide ion: Generation and chemical implications. *Chem. Rev.*, 116, 3029–3085.

He, X., Deng, H., Aker, W.G. and Hwang, H.M., 2019. Regulation and safety of nanotechnology in the food and agriculture industry. In Gustavo Molina, Inamuddin, Franciele Maria Pelissari, and Abdullah Mohamed Asiri (eds.) *Food Applications of Nanotechnology*, pp. 525–536. CRC Press. Boca Raton.

Helmke, B.P. and Minerick, A.R., 2006. Designing a nano-interface in a microfluidic chip to probe living cells: Challenges and perspectives. *Proc. Nat. Acad. Sci. U.S.A.*, 103, 6419–6424.

Henderson, L., Gregory, J. and Swan G., 2003. Vitamin and mineral intake and urinary analytes. In Beverley Bates, Alison Lennox, Chris Bates, and Gillian Swan (eds.) *The National Diet and Nutrition Survey: Adults Aged 19 to 64 Years*, p. 3. Department of Health and the Food Standards Agency, UK, London.

Hildeliza, Q.B., Chanona-pe, J., Jose, L.S.M., Gutie, G.F. and Jimene, A., 2010. Nano-encapsulation: A new trend in food engineering processing. *Food Eng. Rev.*, 2, 39–50.

Honarvar, Z., Hadian, Z. and Mashayekh, M., 2016. Nanocomposites in food packaging applications and their risk assessment for health. *Electron. Physician*, 8(6), 2531–2538.

Howe, P.R.C., 1997. Dietary fats and hypertension: Focus on fish oil. *Ann. NY Acad. Sci.*, 827, 339–352.

Howell, B.R., Day, O.J., Ellis, T. and Baynes, S.M., 1998. Early life stages of farmed fish. In Black, K.D. and Pickering, A.D. eds., *Biology of Farmed Fish*, pp. 27–66. Sheffield Academic Press Ltd., Sheffield, UK.

Hu, W., Wang, C., Gao, D. and Liang, Q., 2023. Toxicity of transition metal nanoparticles: A review of different experimental models in the gastrointestinal tract. *J. Appl. Toxicol.*, 43(1), 32–46.

Huang, Y., Liu, C., Pu, F., Liu, Z., Ren, J. and Qu, X., 2017. GO–Se nanocomposite as an antioxidant nanozyme for cytoprotection. *Chem. Commun.*, 53, 3082–3085.

Huang, Y., Liu, Z., Liu, C., Ju, E., Zhang, Y., Ren, J., and Qu, X., 2016. Self-assembly of multinanozymes to mimic an intracellular antioxidant defense system. *Angewandte Chemie*, 128(23), 6758–62.

Huq, T., Fraschini, C., Khan, A., Riedl, B., Bouchard, J. and Lacroix, M., 2017. Alginate based nanocomposite for microencapsulation of probiotic: Effect of cellulose nanocrystal (CNC) and lecithin. *Carbohydr. Polym.*, 168, 61–69.

Igaz, N., Kovács, D., Rázga, Z., Kónya, Z., Boros, I.M., and Kiricsi, M., 2016. Modulating chromatin structure and DNA accessibility by deacetylase inhibition enhances the anticancer activity of silver nanoparticles. *Colloids and Surfaces B: Biointerfaces*, 146, 670–7.

Ilkay, J., 2010. Nanoceuticals — Does their potential outweigh their risk? *Today's Dietitian*, 12(10), 28.

Ingold, K.U. and Pratt, D.A., 2014. Advances in radical-trapping antioxidant chemistry in the 21st century: A kinetics and mechanisms perspective. *Chem. Rev.*, 114, 9022–9046.

Jain, A., Ranjan, S., Dasgupta, N. and Ramalingam, C., 2018. Nanomaterials in food and agriculture: An overview on their safety concerns and regulatory issues. *Crit. Rev. Food Sci. Nutr.*, 58(2), 297–317.

Jason, T.L., Koropatnick, J., and Berg, R.W., 2004. Toxicology of antisense therapeutics. *Toxicology and applied Pharmacology*, 201(1), 66–83.

Joye, I.J., Davidov-Pardo, G. and McClements, D.J., 2014. Nanotechnology for increased micronutrient bioavailability. *Trends Food Sci. Technol.*, 40(2), 168–182.

Karimi, S., Javadi, M. and Jafarzadeh, F., 2012. Economic burden and costs of chronic diseases in Iran and the world. *Health Inf. Manag.*, 8(7), 984–996.

Katouzian, I. and Jafari S.M., 2016. Nano-encapsulation as a promising approach for targeted delivery and controlled release of vitamins. *Trends Food Sci. Technol.*, 53, 34–48.

Kelly, D.S., 2001. Modulation of human immune and inflammatory responses by dietary fatty acids. *Nutrition* 17, 669–673.

Khan, A., Wen, Y.B., Huq, T. and Ni, Y.H., 2018. Cellulosic nanomaterials in food and nutraceutical applications: A review. *J. Agric. Food Chem.*, 66, 8–19.

Khorasani, S., Danaei, M. and Mozafari, M.R., 2018. Nanoliposome technology for the food and nutraceutical industries. *Trends Food Sci. Technol.*, 79, 106–115.

Kimoto, H., Endo, Y. and Fujimoto, K., 1994. Influence of interesterification on the oxidative stability of marine oil triacylglycerols. *J. Am. Oil Chem. Soc.*, 71, 469–473.

Kinsella, J.E., 1986. Food components with potential therapeutic benefits: The n-3 polyunsaturated fatty acids of fish oils. *Food Technol.*, 40, 89–97.

Koo, O.M., Rubinstein, I. and Onyuksel, H., 2005. Role of nanotechnology in targeted drug delivery and imaging: A concise review. *Nanomed. Nanotechnol. Biol. Med.*, 1, 193–212.

Krause, M.V., 1979. *Food, Nutrition and Diet Therapy*, p. 963. Saunders, UNFAO, Michigan.

KrishnaMohan, I. and Das, U.N., 2001. Prevention of chemically induced diabetes mellitus in experimental animals by polyunsaturated fatty acids. *Nutrition*, 17, 126–151.

Kunwar, A. and Priyadarsini, K.I., 2011. Free radicals, oxidative stress and importance of antioxidants in human health. *J. Med. Allied. Sci.*, 1, 53–60.

Kuppusamy, P., Ichwan, S.J., Al-Zikri, P.N.H., Suriyah, W.H., Soundharrajan, I., Govindan, N., Maniam, G.P. and Yusoff, M.M., 2016. In vitro anticancer activity of Au, Ag nanoparticles synthesized using *Commelina nudiflora* L. aqueous extract against HCT-116 colon cancer cells. *Biol. Trace Elem. Res.,* 173(2), 297–305.

Lamprecht, A., Saumet, J.L., Roux, J. and Benoit, J.P., 2004. Lipid nanocarriers as drug delivery system for ibuprofen in pain treatment. *Int. J. Pharma.*, 278, 407–414.

Li, K., Liu, C., Kuang, X., Deng, Q., Zhao, F. and Li, D., 2018. Effects of multivitamin and multimineral supplementation on blood pressure: A meta-analysis of 12 randomized controlled trials. *Nutrients*, 10, 1018.

Li, Z.L., Peng, S.F., Chen, X., Zhu, Y.Q., Zou, L.Q., Liu, W. and Liu, C.M., 2018. Pluronics modified liposomes for curcumin encapsulation: Sustained release, stability and bioaccessibility. *Food Res. Int.*, 108, 246–253.

Lin, Y., Wang, Y.H., Yang, X.Q., Guo, J. and Wang, J.M., 2016. Corn protein hydrolysate as a novel nano-vehicle: Enhanced physicochemical stability and in vitro bioaccessibility of vitamin D3. *LWT Food Sci. Technol.*, 72, 510–517.

Liu, G., Huang, W., Babii, O., Gong, X., Tian, Z., Yang, J., Wang, Y., Jacobs, R.L., Donna, V., Lavasanifar, A. and Chen, L., 2018. Novel protein-lipid composite nanoparticles with an inner aqueous compartment as delivery systems of hydrophilic nutraceutical compounds. *Nanoscale*, 10, 10629–10640.

Lu, J. and Holmgren, A., 2014. The thioredoxin antioxidant system. *Free Radic. Biol. Med.*, 66, 75–87.

Maisel, K., Ensign, L., Reddy, M., Cone, R. and Hanes, J., 2015. Effect of surface chemistry on nanoparticle interaction with gastrointestinal mucus and distribution in the gastrointestinal tract following oral and rectal administration in the mouse. *J. Control. Release.*, 197, 48–57.

Mann, J.R. and DuBois, R.N., 2004. Cancer chemoprevention: Myth or reality? *Drug Discov. Today Ther. Strateg.*, 1(4), 403–410.

Manzoor, M.F., Ahmad, N., Ahmed, Z., Siddique, R., Zeng, X.-A., Rahaman, A., Muhammad Aadil, R. and Wahab, A., 2019. Novel extraction techniques and pharmaceutical activities of luteolin and its derivatives. *J. Food Biochem.*, 43(9), e12974.

Markovic, Z.M., Harhaji-Trajkovic, L.M., Todorovic-Markovic, B.M., Kepić, D.P., Arsikin, K.M., Jovanović, S.P., Pantovic, A.C., Dramićanin, M.D. and Trajkovic, V.S., 2011, In vitro comparison of the photothermal anticancer activity of graphene nanoparticles and carbon nanotubes, *Biomaterials*, 32(4), 1121–1129.

Martin, A.A., Davidson, T.L., and McCrory, M.A., 2018. Deficits in episodic memory are related to uncontrolled eating in a sample of healthy adults. *Appetite*, 124, 33–42. doi: 10.1016/j.appet.2017.05.011

Matalanis, A., Jones, O.G. and McClements, D.J., 2011. Structured biopolymer-based delivery systems for encapsulation, protection, and release of lipophilic compounds. *Food Hydrocoll.*, 25, 1865–1880.

Mathers, C., 2008. *The Global Burden of Disease: 2004* Update. World Health Organization, Geneva.

McClements, D.J., 2015. Nanoscale nutrient delivery systems for food applications: Improving bioactive dispersibility, stability, and bioavailability. *J. Food Sci.*, 80(7), N1602–N1611.

McClements, D.J. and Xiao, H., 2014. Excipient foods: Designing food matrices that improve the oral bioavailability of pharmaceuticals and nutraceuticals. *Food Funct.*, 5, 1320–1333.

McClements, D.J. and Xiao, H., 2017. Is nano safe in foods? Establishing the factors impacting the gastrointestinal fate and toxicity of organic and inorganic food-grade nanoparticles. *npj Science of Food*, 1(1), 6.

McClements, D.J., 2013. Utilizing food effects to overcome challenges in delivery of lipophilic bioactives: Structural design of medical and functional foods. *Expert Opin. Drug Discov.*, 10, 1621–1632.

McClements, D.J., Decker, E.A., Park, Y. and Weiss, J., 2009. Structural design principles for delivery of bioactive components in nutraceuticals and functional foods. *Crit. Rev. Food Sci. Nutr.*, 49(6), 577–606.

Melaiye, A., Simons, R.S., Milsted, A., Pingitore, F., Wesdemiotis, C., Tessier, C.A. and Youngs, W.J., 2004. Formation of water-soluble pincer silver(I)-carbene complexes: A novel antimicrobial agent. *J. Med. Chem.*, 47(4), 973–977.

Melaiye, A., Sun, Z., Hindi, K., Milsted, A., Ely, D., Reneker, D.H., Tessier, C.A. and Youngs, W.J., 2005. Silver(I)-imidazole cyclophane gem-diol complexes encapsulated by electrospun tecophilic nanofibers: Formation of nanosilver particles and antimicrobial activity. *J. Am Chem. Soc.*, 127(7), 2285–2291.

Mishra, V., Bansal, K.K., Verma, A., Yadav, N., Thakur, S., Sudhakar, K., and Rosenholm, J.M., 2018. Solid lipid nanoparticles: Emerging colloidal nano drug delivery systems. *Pharmaceutics*, 10(4), 191.

Mohammad, Z.H., Ahmad, F., Ibrahim, S.A. and Zaidi, S., 2022. Application of nanotechnology in different aspects of the food industry. *Discover Food*, 2(1), 12.

Morry, J., Ngamcherdtrakul, W. and Yantasee, W., 2017. Oxidative stress in cancer and fibrosis: Opportunity for therapeutic intervention with antioxidant compounds, enzymes, and nanoparticles. *Redox Biol.*, 11, 240–253.

Nakagawa, K., 2014. Nano- and micro-encapsulation of flavor in food systems. In H.-S. Kwak, ed., *Nano- and Microencapsulation for Foods*, pp. 249–272. John Wiley & Sons, Oxford.

Oehlke, K., Adamiuk, M., Behsnilian, D., Gräf, V., Mayer-Miebach, E., Walz, E., and Greiner, R., 2014. Potential bioavailability enhancement of bioactive compounds using food-grade engineered nanomaterials: a review of the existing evidence. *Food & Function*, 5(7), 1341–59.

Park, H.G. and Yeo, M.K., 2016. Nanomaterial regulatory policy for human health and environment. *Mol. Cell. Toxicol.*, 12, 223–236.

Parthasarathi, S. and Anandharamakrishnan, C., 2016. Enhancement of oral bioavailability of vitamin E by spray-freeze drying of whey protein microcapsules. *Food Bioprod. Process.*, 100, 469–476.

Parthasarathi, S., Muthukumar, S.P. and Anandharamakrishnan, C., 2016. The influence of droplet size on the stability, in vivo digestion, and oral bioavailability of vitamin E emulsions. *Food Funct.*, 7, 2294–2302.

Patel, A., Patra, F., Shah, N. and Khedkar, C., 2018. Application of nanotechnology in the food industry: Present status and future prospects. In Alexandru Mihai Grumezescu and Alina Maria Holban (eds.) *Impact of Nanoscience in the Food Industry*, pp. 1–27. Academic Press, San Diego.

Paul, S.D. and Dewangan, D., 2016. Nanotechnology and neutraceuticals. *Int. J. Nanomater. Nanotechnol. Nanomed.,* 2(1), 009–012.

Pei, X., Jiang, H., Li, C., Li, D. and Tang, S., 2023. Oxidative stress-related canonical pyroptosis pathway, as a target of liver toxicity triggered by zinc oxide nanoparticles. *J. Hazard. Mater.*, 442, 130039.

Penalva, R., Esparza, I., Agüeros, M., Gonzalez-Navarro, C.J., Gonzalez-Ferrero, C. and Irache, J.M., 2014. Casein nanoparticles as carriers for the oral delivery of folic acid. *Food Hydrocoll.*, 44, 399–406.

Peng, C., Lu, W. and Fang, Y., 2022. An insight into the effect of food nanoparticles on the metabolism of intestinal cells. *Curr. Opin. Food Sci.*, 43, 174–182.

Pérez-Esteve, É., Ruiz-Rico, M., de la Torre, C., Villaescusa, L.A., Sancenón, F., Marcos, M.D., Amorós, P., Martínez-Máñez, R. and Barat, J.M., 2016. Encapsulation of folic acid in different silica porous supports: A comparative study. *Food Chem.*, 196, 66–75.

Perron, N.R. and Brumaghim, J.L., 2009. A review of the antioxidant mechanisms of polyphenol compounds related to iron binding. *Cell. Biochem. Biophys.*, 53, 75–100.

Pinto, R.J.B., Daina, S., Sadocco, P., Neto, C.P. and Trindade, T., 2013. Antibacterial activity of nanocomposites of copper and cellulose. *BioMed Res. Int.*, 6, 280512.

Polefka, T.G., Meyer, T.A., Agin, P.P. and Bianchini, R.J., 2012. Effects of solar radiation on the skin. *J. Cosmet. Dermatol.,* 11, 134–143.

Poorolajal, J., Zeraati, F., Soltanian, A.R., Sheikh, V., Hooshmand, E. and Maleki, A., 2017. Oral potassium supplementation for management of essential hypertension: A meta-analysis of randomized controlled trials. *PLoS One*, 12, e0174967

Porter, C.J. and Charman, W.N., 2001. In vitro assessment of oral lipid based formulations. *Adv. Drug Deliv. Rev.*, 50(Suppl 1), S127–147.

Pouton, C.W., and Porter, C.J., 2008. Formulation of lipid-based delivery systems for oral administration: materials, methods and strategies. *Advanced drug delivery reviews*, 60(6), 625–37.

Powell, J.J., Faria, N., Thomas-McKay, E. and Pele, L.C., 2010. Origin and fate of dietary nanoparticles and microparticles in the gastrointestinal tract. *J. Autoimmun.*, 34(3), J226–J233.

Powell, M. and Colin, M., 2008. Nanotechnology and food safety: Potential benefits, possible risks. CAB reviews: Perspectives in agriculture, veterinary science. *Nutr. Nat. Res.,* 3, 123–142.

Proquin, H., Rodríguez-Ibarra, C., Moonen, C.G., Urrutia Ortega, I.M., Briedé, J.J., de Kok, T.M., van Loveren, H. and Chirino, Y.I., 2017. Titanium dioxide food additive (E171) induces ROS formation and genotoxicity: Contribution of micro and nano-sized fractions. *Mutagenesis*, 32(1), 139–149.

Qian, C., Decker, E. A., Xiao, H. and McClements, D.J., 2012. Inhibition of beta-carotene degradation in oil-in-water nanoemulsions: Influence of oil-soluble and water-soluble antioxidants. *Food Chem.*, 135(3), 1036–1043.

Radimer, K., Bindewald, B., Hughes, J., Ervin, B., Swanson, C. and Picciano, M.F., 2004. Dietary supplement use by US adults: Data from the National Health and Nutrition Examination Survey, 1999–2000. *Am J. Epidemiol.*, 160(4), 339–349.

Ragg, R., Tahir, M.N. and Tremel, W., 2016. Solids go bio: Inorganic nanoparticles as enzyme mimics. *Eur. J. Inorg. Chem.*, 13, 1906–1915.

Raghunandan, D., Ravishankar, B., Sharanbasava, G., Mahesh, D.B., Harsoor, V., Yalagatti, M.S., Bhagawanraju, M. and Venkataraman, A., 2011. Anti-cancer studies of noble metal nanoparticles synthesized using different plant extracts. *Cancer Nanotechnol.*, 2(1–6), 57–65.

Rajan, R., Huo, P., Chandran, K., Dakshinamoorthi, B.M., Yun, S.I. and Liu, B., 2022. A review on the toxicity of silver nanoparticles against different biosystems. *Chemosphere*, 292, 133397.

Ramalingam, P., Yoo, S.W. and Ko, Y.T., 2016. Nanodelivery systems based on mucoadhesive polymer coated solid lipid nanoparticles to improve the oral intake of food curcumin. *Food Res. Int.*, 84, 113–119.

Ramkumar, C., Vishwanatha, A. and Saini, R., 2019. Regulatory aspects of nanotechnology for food industry. In Lohith Kumar Dasarahally-Huligowda, Megh R. Goyal, and Hafiz Ansar Rasul Suleria (eds.) *Nanotechnology Applications in Dairy Science*, pp. 169–184. Apple Academic Press, New York.

Ramos, O.L., Pereira, R.N., Martins, A., Rodrigues, R., Fucinos, C., Teixeira, J.A., Pastrana, L., Malcata, F.X. and Vicente, A.A., 2017. Design of whey protein nanostructures for incorporation and release of nutraceutical compounds in food. *Crit. Rev. Food Sci. Nutr.*, 57, 1377–1393.

Ranjan, S., Dasgupta, N., Singh, S. and Gandhi, M., 2019. Toxicity and regulations of food nanomaterials. *Environ. Chem. Lett.*, 17, 929–944.

Rautiainen, S., Wang, L., Lee, I.-M., Manson, J.E., Gaziano, J.M., Buring, J.E. and Sesso, H.D., 2016. Multivitamin use and the risk of hypertension in a prospective cohort study of women. *J. Hypertens.*, 34, 1513–1519.

Renton, A., 2006. Welcome to the World of Nano Foods.

Ronis, M.J., Pedersen, K.B. and Watt, J., 2018. Adverse effects of nutraceuticals and dietary supplements. *Annu. Rev. Pharmacol. Toxicol.*, 58, 583–601.

Rose, D.P. and Connolly, J.M., 1999. Omega-3 fatty acids as cancer chemopreventive agents. *Pharmcol. Ther.*, 83, 217–244.

Rothwell, P.M., Wilson, M., Elwin, C.E., Norrving, B., Algra, A., Warlow, C.P. and Meade, T.W., 2010. Long-term effect of aspirin on colorectal cancer incidence and mortality: 20-year follow-up of five randomised trials. *Lancet*, 376(9754), 1741–1750.

Sadeghi, L. and Espanani, H.R., 2015. Toxic effects of the Fe2O3 nanoparticles on the liver and lung tissue. *Bratislavske lekarske listy*, 116(6), 373–378.

Sahoo, M., Vishwakarma, S., Panigrahi, C. and Kumar, J., 2021. Nanotechnology: Current applications and future scope in food. *Food Front.*, 2(1), 3–22.

Salvia-Trujillo, L., Martín-Belloso, O. and McClements, D.J., 2016. Excipient nanoemulsions for improving oral bioavailability of bioactives. *Nanomaterials*, 6, 1–17.

Salvia-Trujillo, L., Qian, C., Martín-Belloso, O. and McClements, D.J., 2013. Influence of particle size on lipid digestion and beta-carotene bioaccessibility in emulsions and nano-emulsions. *Food Chem.*, 141, 1472–1489.

Sampathkumar, K. and Loo, S.C.J., 2018. Targeted gastrointestinal delivery of nutraceuticals with polysaccharide-based coatings. *Macromol. Biosci.*, 18, 1700363.

Sani, A., Cao, C. and Cui, D., 2021. Toxicity of gold nanoparticles (AuNPs): A review. *Biochem. Biophys. Rep.*, 26, 100991.

Saratale, R.G., Benelli, G., Kumar, G., Kim, D.S. and Saratale, G.D., 2018. Biofabrication of silver nanoparticles using the leaf extract of an ancient herbal medicine, dandelion (*Taraxacum officinale*), evaluation of their antioxidant, anticancer potential, and antimicrobial activity against phytopathogens. *Environ. Sci. Pollut. Res. Int.*, 25, 10392–10406.

Sarikhani, M., Vaghefi Moghaddam, S., Firouzamandi, M., Hejazy, M., Rahimi, B., Moeini, H. and Alizadeh, E., 2022. Harnessing rat derived model cells to assess the toxicity of TiO2 nanoparticles. *J. Mater. Sci. Mater. Med.*, 33(5), 41.

Sasaki, H., Sunagawa, Y., Takahashi, K., Imaizumi, A., Fukudu, H., Hashimoto, T., Wada, H., Katanasaka, Y., Kakeya, H., Fujita, M., Hasegawa, K. and Morimoto, T., 2011. Innovative preparation of curcumin for improved oral bioavailability. *Biol. Pharm. Bull.*, 34(5), 660–665.

Sayed, D., Monroe, F., Orr, W.N., Phadnis, M., Khan, T.W., Braun, E., Manion, S., and Nicol, A., 2018. Retrospective analysis of intrathecal drug delivery: outcomes, efficacy, and risk for cancer-related pain at a high volume academic medical center. *Neuromodulation: Technology at the Neural Interface*, 21(7), 660–4.

Schirmer, B.C., Heiberg, R., Eie, T., Møretrø, T., Maugesten, T. and Carlehøg, M., 2009. A novel packaging method with a dissolving CO2 headspace combined with organic acids prolongs the shelf life of fresh salmon. *Int. J. Food Microbiol.* 133, 154–160.

Schmidt, E.B., Skou, H.A., Christensen, J.H. and Dyerberg, J., 2000. n-3 Fatty acids from fish and coronary artery disease: Implications for public health. *Pub. Health Nutr.*, 3, 91–98.

Seigneuric, R., Markey, L., SA Nuyten, D., Dubernet, C., TA Evelo, C., Finot, E. and Garrido, C., 2010. From nanotechnology to nanomedicine: Applications to cancer research. *Curr. Mol. Med.*, 10(7), 640–652.

Shahidi, F., 2008. Omega-3 oils: Sources, applications, and health effects. In Barrow, C. and Shahidi, F. eds., *Marine Nutraceuticals and Functional Foods*, pp. 23–61. CRC Press. Boca Raton, FL.

Shahidi, F., 2012. Nutraceuticals, functional foods and dietary supplements in health and disease. *J. Food Drug Anal.*, 20(1), 78.

Shaikh, J., Ankola, D., Beniwal, V., Singh, D. and Kumar, M.R., 2009. Nanoparticle encapsulation improves oral bioavailability of curcumin by at least 9-fold when compared to curcumin administered with piperine as absorption enhancer. *Eur. J. Pharm. Sci.*, 37(3–4), 223–230.

Shanker, K., Mohan, G.K., Hussain, M.A., Jayarambabu, N. and Pravallika, P.L., 2017. Green biosynthesis, characterization, in vitro antidiabetic activity, and investigational acute toxicity studies of some herbal-mediated silver nanoparticles on animal models. *Pharmacogn. Mag.*, 13(49), 188.

Singh, A., Kumari, K., and Kundu, P.P., 2017. Extrusion and evaluation of chitosan assisted AgNPs immobilized film derived from waste polyethylene terephthalate for food packaging applications. *Journal of Packaging Technology and Research*, 1, 165–80.

Sivakumar, P., Lee, M., Kim, Y.S. and Shim, M.S., 2018. Photo-triggered antibacterial and anticancer activities of zinc oxide nanoparticles. *J. Mater. Chem. B*, 6, 4852–4871.

Stickel, F., Kessebohm, K., Weimann, R. and Seitz, H.K., 2011.Review of liver injury associated with dietary supplements. *Liver Int.*, 31(5), 595–605.

Sun, Y., Xia, Z., Zheng, J., Qiu, P., Zhang, L., McClements, D.J. and Xiao, H., 2015. Nanoemulsion-based delivery systems for nutraceuticals: Influence of carrier oil type on bioavailability of pterostilbene. *J. Funct. Foods*, 13, 61–70.

Tarhan, Ö., 2020. Safety and regulatory issues of nanomaterials in foods. In Seid Mahdi Jafari (ed.) *Handbook of Food Nanotechnology*, pp. 655–703. Elsevier, Oxford.

Tarver, T., 2006. Food nanotechnology. *Food Technol.*, 60(11), 22–26.

Teucher, B., Olivares, M. and Cori, H., 2004. Enhancers of iron absorption: Ascorbic acid and other organic acids. *Int. J. Vitamin Nutr. Res.*, 74(6), 403–419.

Tian, D., Hu, J., Bao, J., Chandra, R.P., Saddler, J.N. and Lu, C., 2017. Lignin valorization: Lignin nanoparticles as high-value bio-additive for multifunctional nanocomposites. *Biotechnol. Biofuels*, 10, 192–202.

Trofimov, A.D., Ivanova, A.A., Zyuzin, M.V., and Timin, A.S., 2018. Porous inorganic carriers based on silica, calcium carbonate and calcium phosphate for controlled/modulated drug delivery: Fresh outlook and future perspectives. *Pharmaceutics*, 10(4), 167.

Tucker, R.M. and Mattes, R.D., 2013. Satiation, satiety: The puzzle of solids and liquids. In John E. Blundell and France Bellisle (eds.) *Satiation, Satiety and the Control of Food Intake*, pp. 182–201. Woodhead Publishing, Cambridge.

Ubbink, J. and Kruger, J., 2006. Physical approaches for the delivery of active ingredients in foods. *Trends Food Sci. Technol.*, 17, 244–254.

Valgimigli, L., Baschieri, A. and Amorati, R., 2018. Antioxidant activity of nanomaterials. *J. Mater. Chem. B.*, 6(14), 2036–2051.

Vernekar, A.A., Sinha, D., Srivastava, S., Paramasivam, P.U., D'Silva, P. and Mugesh, G., 2014. An antioxidant nanozyme that uncovers the cytoprotective potential of vanadia nanowires. *Nat. Commun.*, 5, 5301.

Wan, A.C. and Tai, B.C., 2013. Chitin - a promising biomaterial for tissue engineering and stem cell technologies. *Biotechnol. Adv.,* 31(8), 1776–1785.

Wang, C., Li, Y., Zhu, K., Dong, Y.-M. and Sun, C.-H., 2009. Effects of supplementation with multivitamin and mineral on blood pressure and C-reactive protein in obese Chinese women with increased cardiovascular disease risk. *Asia Pac. J. Clin. Nutr.*, 18, 121–130.

Wang, X., Jiang, Y., Wang, Y.W., Huang, M.T., Ho, C.T. and Huang, Q., 2008. Enhancing anti-inflammation activity of curcumin through O/W nanoemulsions. *J. Food Chem.*, 108(2), 419–424.

Weiss, J., Takhistov, P., and McClements, J., 2006. Functional materials in food nanotechnology. *J. Food Sci.*, 71, R107–R116.

Wen, T., He, W., Chong, Y., Liu, Y., Yin, J.-J. and Wu, X., 2015. Exploring environment-dependent effects of Pd nanostructures on reactive oxygen species (ROS) using electron spin resonance (ESR) technique: Implications for biomedical applications. *Phys. Chem. Chem. Phys.*, 17, 24937–24943.

WorldHealth Organisation, n.d. Available from: https://www.who.int/health-topics/noncommunicable-diseases#tab=tab_1.

Wu, X., Patterson, S. and Hawk, E., 2011. Chemoprevention--history and general principles. *Best Pract. Res. Clin. Gastroenterol.,* 25(4–5), 445–459.

Xu, J., Zhao, W., Ning, Y., Bashari, M., Wu, F., Chen, H., Yang, N., Jin, Z., Xu, B., Zhang, L. and Xu, X., 2013. Improved stability and controlled release of ω3/ω6 polyunsaturated fatty acids by spring dextrin encapsulation. *Carbohydr. Polym.*, 92(2), 1633–1640.

Yan, S.S. and Gilbert, J.M., 2004. Antimicrobial drug delivery in food animals and microbial food safety concerns: An overview of in vitro and in vivo factors potentially affecting the animal gut microflora. *Adv. Drug Deliv. Rev.*, 56, 1497–1521.

Yáñez, J.A., Wang, S.W., Knemeyer, I.W., Wirth, M.A., and Alton, K.B., 2011. Intestinal lymphatic transport for drug delivery. *Advanced Drug Delivery Reviews*, 63(10–11), 923–42.

Yang, Y., Bai, L., Li, X., Xiong, J., Xu, P., Guo, C., and Xue, M., 2014. Transport of active flavonoids, based on cytotoxicity and lipophilicity: An evaluation using the blood–brain barrier cell and Caco-2 cell model. *Toxicology in Vitro*, 28(3), 388–96.

Yao, M., McClements, D.J. and Xiao, H., 2015. Improving oral bioavailability of nutraceuticals by engineered nanoparticle-based delivery systems, *Curr. Opin. Food Sci.*, 2, 14–19.

Yao, M.F., Xiao, H. and McClements, D.J., 2014. Delivery of lipophilic bioactives: Assembly, disassembly, and reassembly of lipid nanoparticles. *Annu. Rev. Food Sci. Technol.*, 5, 53–81.

Youn, S.M. and Choi, S.J., 2022. Food additive zinc oxide nanoparticles: Dissolution, interaction, fate, cytotoxicity, and oral toxicity. *Int. J. Mol. Sci.*, 23(11), 6074.

Hu, Y., Smith, D.E., Ma, K., Jappar, D., Thomas, W., and Hillgren, K.M. 2008. Targeted Disruption of Peptide Transporter Pept1 Gene in Mice Significantly Reduces Dipeptide Absorption in Intestine. *Molecular Pharmaceutics*, 5(6), 1122–1130, doi: 10.1021/mp8001655

Zarafshar, M., Akbarinia, M., Askari, H., Hosseini, S. M., Rahaie, M. and Struve, D., 2015. Toxicity assessment of SiO_2 nanoparticles to pear seedlings. *Int. J. Nanosci. Nanotechnol.*, 11(1), 3–22.

Zhang, H. and Forman, H.J., 2017. 4-hydroxynonenal-mediated signaling and aging. *Free Radic. Biol. Med.*, 111, 219–225.

Zhang, T., Lv, C., Chen, L., Bai, G., Zhao, G. and Xu, C., 2014. Encapsulation of anthocyanin molecules within a ferritin nanocage increases their stability and cell uptake efficiency. *Food Res. Int.* 62, 183–192.

Zhang, X.P., Le, Y., Wang, J.X., Zhao, H. and Chen, J.F., 2013. Resveratrol nanodispersion with high stability and dissolution rate. *Lwt-Food Sci. Technol.*, 50, 622–628.

Zhang, Z., Zhang, R., Xiao, H., Bhattacharya, K., Bitounis, D., Demokritou, P. and McClements, D.J., 2019. Development of a standardized food model for studying the impact of food matrix effects on the gastrointestinal fate and toxicity of ingested nanomaterials. *NanoImpact*, 13, 13–25.

Zhou, H. and McClements, D.J., 2022. Recent advances in the gastrointestinal fate of organic and inorganic nanoparticles in foods. *Nanomaterials*, 12(7), 1099.

Zhou, H., Yue, Y., Liu, G., Li, Y., Zhang, J., Gong, Q., Yan, Z. and Duan, M., 2010. Preparation and characterization of a lecithin nanoemulsion as a topical delivery system. *Nanoscale Res. Lett.*, 5(1), 224–230.

Zou, L.Q., Peng, S.F., Liu, W., Gan, L., Liu, W.L., Liang, R.H., Liu, C.M., Niu, J., Cao, Y.L., Liu, Z. and Chen, X., 2014. Improved in vitro digestion stability of (−)-epigallocatechin gallate 337 through nanoliposome encapsulation. *Food Res. Int.*, 64, 492–499.

19 Application of Polymeric Nanomaterials and Liposomes in the Food Industry

Prerona Saha, Varnit Jain, Jaideep Adhikari, and Manojit Ghosh

19.1 INTRODUCTION

Food habits, cultivation, and diversity have had a direct impact on the evolution of human civilization. A society is defined by its food culture and the variety of nourishment it provides to its species. Globalization has brought a socio-economic paradigm shift to the development of the food industry. The food industry is constantly expanding in all aspects ranging from nutritional values to exhibition and palate. Advancements in food engineering have always focused on compacting and improving the efficiency of the nutrients in edible supplements. Nanomaterials have exhibited lucrative opportunities for this purpose. Polymeric nanomaterials are being extensively deployed in the selective distribution of nutrients or bioactive molecules at targeted sites (Faridi Esfanjani and Jafari, 2016; Rehman et al., 2019). Protein-based nanoparticles have made their way into edible items because protein solubility aids in the assembly of certain proteins with specific functionality in food (Xu et al., 2018).

An important aspect of the food industry is the packaging of the final processed product. Ever since globalization, the food customs of different cultures have been entangled, modified, and spread widely across the world. This prospect has only been possible because of the efficient packaging of edible materials. Polymeric nanomaterials have been in use for packaging for quite some time now, but recent advancements in sensor-based nanotechnology have led to the development of smart packaging methods (Madhusudan et al., 2018). These encasing methods are now able to keep tabs on the quality and safety of food products. They can provide a barrier against external contamination (Jordan et al., 2005). Stiffness and strength are other important properties that these packings are able to handle. Novel nanomaterial-based polymeric packaging can also further enhance the economic and environmental standards of the food industry.

The shift in consumer trends and habits in the food industry has led to the emergence of customizable food products. One way of customization is the addition of functional compounds. These compounds act as flavour enhancers and preservatives

 DOI: 10.1201/9781003432661-19

and help improve the colour and texture of the product (Garti and McClements, 2012). Food engineers have constantly been developing and working on methods to integrate functional compounds with edible products. Liposomes provide a lucrative encapsulation structure for the delivery of these compounds at specific sites. They have been used in the transportation of enzymes, vitamins, and hormones into the body (Wu and Guy, 2009).

The objective of this chapter is to thoroughly discuss polymeric nanomaterials and liposomes, their implementation, and their future scope in the food industry. These liposomes and polymeric nanomaterials are of varied types, ranging from metallic nanoparticles and nano-encapsulates to polysaccharide matrices and protein-based carriers. The study involves the understanding of these materials, their types, and their applications.

19.2 WHAT ARE DIETARY SUPPLEMENTS AND MEDICAL-PURPOSE FOOD?

Dietary supplements and medical-purpose foods are often referred to together as nutraceuticals. These are food products that consist of any functional food or functional component that can enhance the performance of any fundamental nutritional value of that particular food product. Depending on the enhancement, they can be classified as dietary supplements or medical-purpose foods. Dietary supplements are generally preferred to improve the overall performance of an individual's body, whereas medical-purpose foods manipulate the actions of specific bodily functions. These special dietary intakes should always be accompanied by a prescription from a medically qualified authority and monitored under medical supervision. In comparison to drugs, the concentration of active compounds or active substances in these products is quite low. The main objective of all these products is to revamp the nutritional values of conventional foods and to decrease the risk of diseases (Paolino et al., 2021).

19.3 TYPES AND APPLICATIONS OF NANOMATERIALS USED IN DIETARY SUPPLEMENTS

Food varieties used for nourishment and medicinal needs are known as nutraceuticals. Nanotechnology, when paired with nutraceuticals, has the power of enhancement due to the presence of nanostructured frameworks. Nanoliposomes, nano emulsions, lipid nanocarriers, micelles, and polylactide co-glycolide nanoparticles are known for their biocompatibility.

19.3.1 Nano-Vesicular Carriers and Nanoscale Emulsion

A nanoliposome can be defined as a submicron phospholipid vesicle that is bilayer and has been found to be in great use in nanotechnology for the delivery of bioactive agents. A schematic diagram of a nanoliposome is shown in Figure 19.1. The uses of nanoliposomes can also be seen in encapsulation, especially for lipophilic and

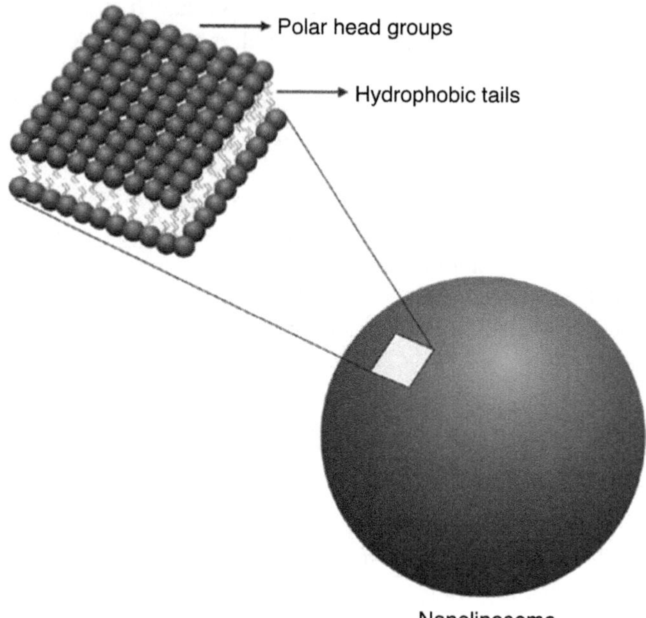

FIGURE 19.1 A nanoliposome is enlarged and its phospholipid bilayer is observed. (Reproduced from Mozafari (2010), with permission from Springer Nature, Copyright 2010.)

hydrophilic materials. Due to their biodegradable, biocompatible nature with nano size, nanoliposomes have potential usage in various fields, including nano therapy, food technology, cosmetics, and agriculture (Mozafari, 2010). They can also enhance the overall operation of bioactive agents. They also help improve the bioavailability, solubility, and storage stability (especially in vivo and in vitro) and prevent interaction with other molecules. They are helpful for the sustained release of a drug and can also be helpful for the promotion of health (Jampilek et al., 2019).

Liposomes are microscopic vesicles that are artificial. They are formed from phospholipids and attain the characteristic of being amphiphilic in nature. They are found naturally in foods like breast milk (Subramani and Ganapathyswamy, 2020). Liposomes are mainly classified into four different categories. They are dependent on their composition and type of delivery, mainly intracellular like conventional liposomes, cationic liposomes, immunoliposomes, and long-circulating liposomes. The composition of liposomes mainly comprises synthetic phospholipids. Bilayers of liposomes may also have a different composition, such as water and cholesterol and hydrophilic polymer conjugated lipids. Cholesterol mainly helps in improving the fluidity of the membrane and stability of the bilayer liposome and also decreases the water-soluble molecules from being permeable (Laouini et al., 2012). Lipid composition in liposomes determines by the chemical properties of liposomes (Kothalawala et al., 2018). Liposomes are used in the drug delivery system due to their ability to lag the duration of clearance and also enhance the blood circulation of the intravascular system, leading to the alteration of bio-distribution. Digestion of liposomes by

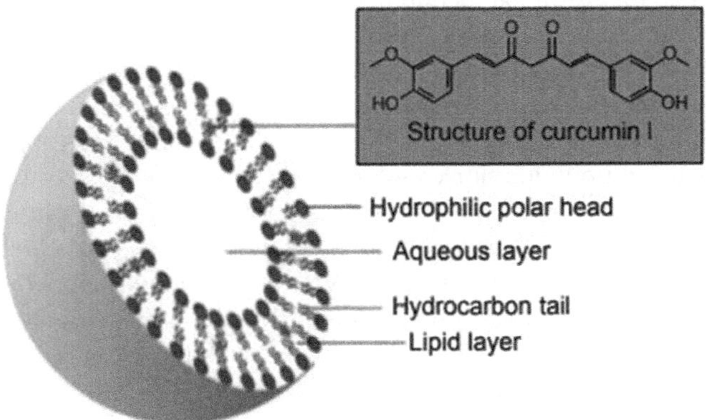

FIGURE 19.2 A CUR liposome. (Reproduced from Feng et al. (2017), http://creativecommons.org/licenses/by/4.0/.)

macrophages of the reticuloendothelial system can be reduced if liposomes are varied with polyethylene glycol (PEG) and these liposomes are meant to be PEGylated (Dutta et al., 2018).

Figure 19.2 shows the labelled diagram of a CUR liposome, a yellow-coloured compound obtained from the turmeric plant, a rhizome. *Curcuma longa* is known as curcumin (CUR) and is also known to be a lipophilic molecule that can test the permeability of the cell membrane. If CUR liposomes are modified with PEGylated liposomes, then they provide better stability (Feng et al., 2017).

A new type of formulation with better absorption and bioavailability than many other plant extracts is phytosomes which are mainly herbal extracts. To produce the above, phospholipid and phyto-active compounds and non-polar solvents are required. They are compatible with lipophilic compounds (Ghanbarzadeh et al., 2016). Nano-phytosomes are defined as nanocarriers which are mainly formed of lipids that help the delivery of botanical nutraceuticals. These can be used potentially in food products (Jampilek et al., 2019).

When non-ionic surfactants cover an aqueous core of microscopic vesicles, they form a bilayer with a wrapped structure. This forms niosomes, which are amphiphilic in nature. Niosomes, which are not formed spontaneously, require energy to be input. Cholesterol and diacetyl phosphate are non-ionic surfactants which, when hydrated, form the niosomes. In order to improve the stability of niosomes dispersion and to prevent the aggregation of niosomes, diacetyl phosphate can be incorporated into the formulation of niosomes. Cholesterol addition to the dispersion can also increase the membrane stability of non-ionic surfactant vesicles (niosomes). Niosomes are cheaper, require no condition for storage, and scaling is easier when compared to liposomes.

Then, there are transferosomes which are known to surround a non-ionic edge activator and phosphatidyl choline. The edge activators possess both types of characteristics—hydrophobicity and hydrophilicity. The properties of transferosomes are dependent on factors like lipid-surfactant ratio, surfactant-lipid concentration, type of solvent used and its concentration, the hydration medium, and bioactive concentration. Transferosomes exhibit both the properties of liposomes and niosomes (Dehnad et al., 2022).

Emulsifiers are active substances that work only on the surface and play two critical roles in creating emulsions. They have a dual purpose—promoting emulsion stability and helping to increase emulsion formation. They find a great application in the food industry as natural alternatives to synthetic surfactants. Natural protein-based emulsifiers like whey proteins and caseins are obtained from bovine milk. There are more plant sources like peas, lupin, and soy proteins. There are examples of surface-active polysaccharides, like gum Arabic and pectin. Saponins from a tree bark *Quillaja saponaria* are available commercially (Ozturk and McClements, 2016). Each type of natural emulsifier has different types of interfacial structures, and the difference can be observed in Figure 19.3.

Nano emulsions (NEs) can increase the bioavailability of the substances that fail to get miscible with water or hydrophobic substances. These nano emulsions can be

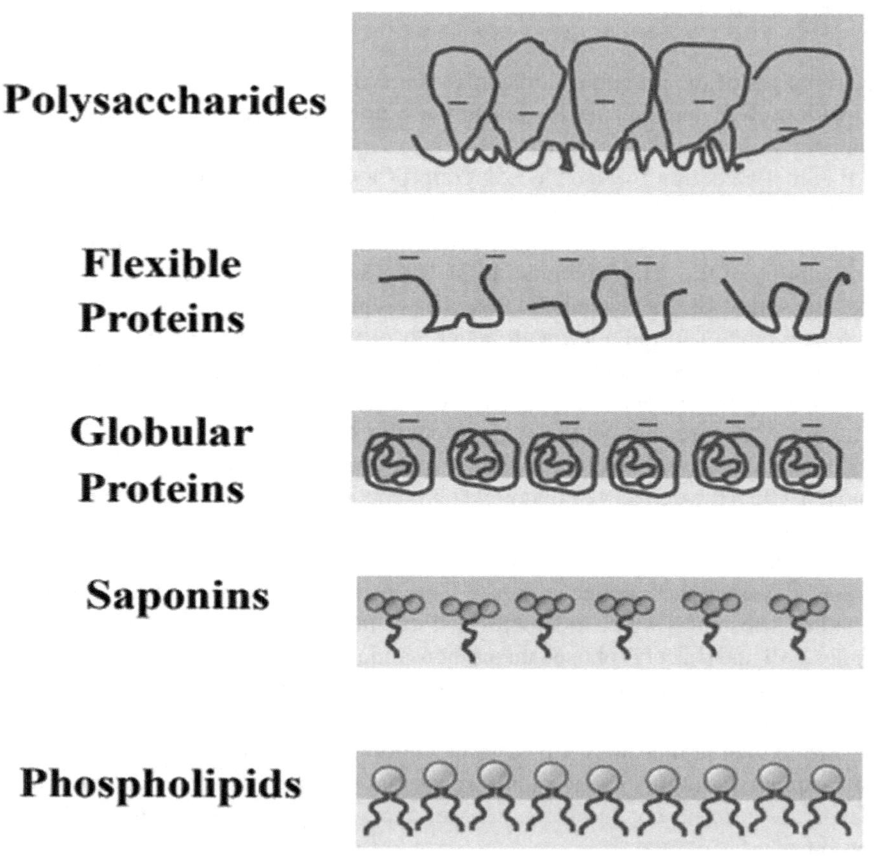

FIGURE 19.3 The interfacial structures of the natural emulsifiers—polysaccharides, proteins, saponins, and phospholipids. (Reproduced from Ozturk and McClements (2016) with permission from Elsevier, Copyright 2016.)

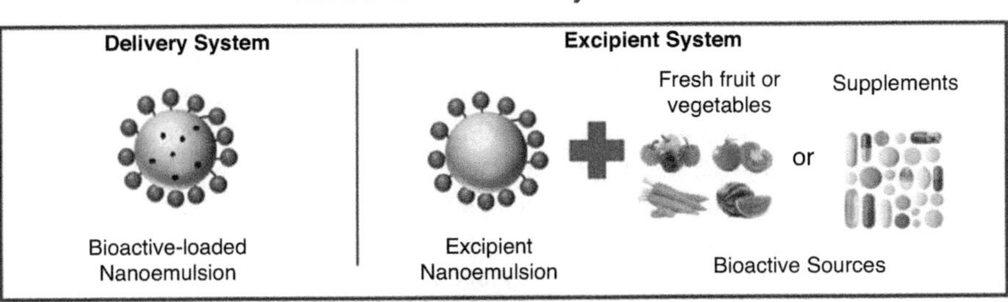

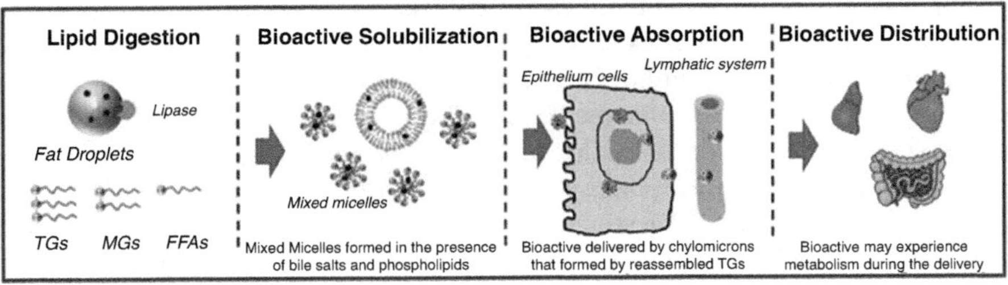

FIGURE 19.4 The gastrointestinal fate of delivery systems of nano emulsion-based foods which are bioactive. (Reproduced from Zhang et al. (2020) with permission from Elsevier, Copyright 2020.)

used as both fluids and solids. Powdered forms can be used in capsules or tablets. The hydrophobic substances include nutraceuticals (foods derived from healthy sources that have an additional benefit for human physiology), pharmaceuticals (used for medicinal purposes), and nutrients. The constituents of these edible substances and their respective structures can be easily controlled. It is due to this reason that they are flexible for bioavailability uses (Zhang et al., 2020). Figure 19.4 below represents the delivery systems of nano emulsion-based foods.

Glycerolipids are of different types depending on the number of bonds formed by the esters with the fatty acids and glycerol, which form the backbone of the compound. These compounds are mainly found in prokaryotes (in their cell membranes) and eukaryotes. They are generally regarded as reservoirs that store energy (Park et al., 2021).

19.3.2 Polysaccharide Matrices

Polysaccharides are known to have ideal bioactivities and properties related to physiochemical activities. There are mixed polysaccharide dietary supplements. Ambrotose® complex is a mixed polysaccharide dietary supplement containing rice starch, *Aloe vera* gel extract, and gums like ghatti and tragacanth. Ingesting this substance orally can help the human body fight diseases (Marzorati et al., 2010).

Some soluble polysaccharides can reduce the increased risk of coronary disease as they happen to decrease the total concentration of plasma cholesterol. Different kinds of foods can be classified as thickeners and stabilizers. *Cyanopsis tetragonoloba L.* is the scientific name of the Indian cluster bean, and guar gum is produced and extracted from the endosperm of this cluster bean. This gum can be categorized as a galactomannan. Xanthate gum is an edible gum extracted and produced by the bacterium *Xanthomonas campestris*. This xanthate gum contains glucose, mannose, and glucuronic acid (Castro et al., n.d.). Polysaccharides are believed to have excellent characteristics in biological activities such as promoting growth, preventing tumours due to their antioxidant properties, and promoting immunomodulation. The root of Astragalus helps produce Astragalus polysaccharides, mainly used in stock forming as sedative drugs and immunostimulants. Major bioactive components are *Lycium barbarum* polysaccharides, which are mainly helpful in liver repair, kidney strengthening, and improvement in eyesight (Serhan et al., 2019).

Starch nanoparticles are mainly used for packaging food exhibiting appropriate mechanical properties for packaging applications. Also, starch nanoparticles help treat the diseases causing cardiovascular diseases and are also helpful in drug delivery (Qin et al., 2016). The monomer of starch is glucose, and the amylase enzyme breaks starch into smaller molecules for absorption in the human body. However, like starch, the monomer of cellulose is glucose; it still cannot be digested due to the unavailability of cellulose-digesting enzymes (cellulase) in the human body. Starch is composed of α-glucose subunits, whereas cellulose is composed of β-glucose subunits. Cellulosic nanomaterials can be used as an emulsifier to stabilize emulsions and immobilize cells and enzymes. The grafting of functional groups on cellulose nanomaterials helps in improving colloidal stability (Khan et al., 2018).

19.3.3 Protein-Based Carriers

Nano-encapsulation regarding protein-based carrier approaches requires modification of the protein. It is considered to see an improvement in retention, protection, and encapsulation compared to their functionality in non-carrier systems. This nano-encapsulation also releases bioactive agents (Jampilek et al., 2019). An egg has several nutrients that are essential to our life. Water and proteins are the primary nutrients of an egg. Macronutrients of the egg consist of proteins, fat, carbohydrates, and inorganic elements like phosphorous and sulphur in trace amounts. Triglycerides and phospholipids are the most dominant components which are part of the fatty acid composition in the egg (Cherian, n.d.).

Mammalian milk secretes calcium-binding phosphoproteins, which are insoluble. These proteins are collectively known as casein. Denaturation of casein proteins leads to low sensitivity. These proteins are unfolded and flexible due to the absence of α-helices and β-sheets. Milk has caseins in definite but various proportions, even from various breeds of cows. A casein micelle is a stable form of an agglomerate form of casein peptides and is porous in its internal structure. The cross-section of the casein-micelle particle is shown in Figure 19.5. Caseins are believed to have an affinity for intermolecular bonds with phosphorous, calcium, and sequences rich in glutamine and proline. Casein is generally secreted by the epithelial cells of mammals and, therefore, is an essential part of evolution (Głąb and Boratyński, 2017).

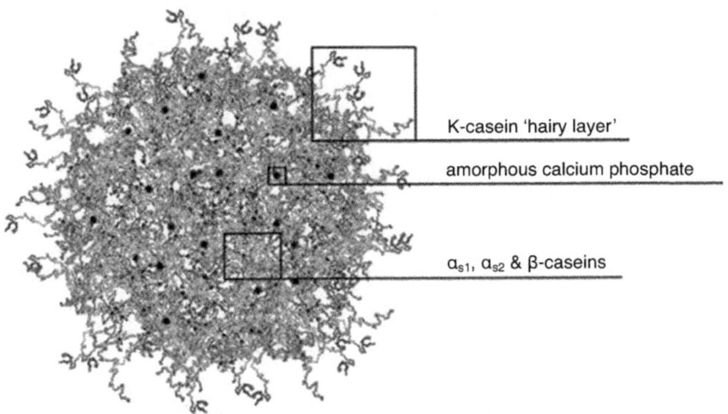

FIGURE 19.5 Cross-section of the casein-micelle particle. Reproduced from Głąb and Boratyński (2017), http://creativecommons.org/licenses/by/4.0/.) It is to be noted that the graphical representation adapted by Głąb and Boratyński (2017) was based on the model proposed by Kruff and Holt (2003).

In food processing, whey proteins are used in a wide variety and have high yields. Non-polar bioactive molecules are lutein, astaxanthin, quercetin, and curcumin. Protein-based nano complexes can assemble to form and deliver the molecules mentioned above. Studies show that the nano complexes of proteins (for example, carrageenan and chitosan), when coated with polysaccharides, depict improvement in stability and functional properties. They are sensitive when there is an addition of salt and pH (Wang et al., 2021). Amino acids are the backbone or the main building components of proteins. These are synthesized in organisms with the help of intermediate metabolites, which are a significant part of the metabolism of lipids and carbohydrates. There are free amino acids that are mainly seen in the cellular cytoplasm. They also help in protein synthesis, acting as a stock. Food products and their quality can be affected by amino acids and their chemical reactions since side products will form. The decomposition of proteins is enhanced due to thermal processing. It happens when the native proteins are denatured (Ribarova, 2018).

Spirulina is a high protein source and contains vitamin B12 and minerals, mainly iron, and it is also known to contain phenolic compounds (these are known to be antioxidants). A protein source can be included in our diet to increase nutritional efficiency (Santos et al., 2016). There are also legume proteins (LPs) which are carriers that can encapsulate the ingredients which are highly reactive and unstable. LPs are used as the devices for delivery, but they are mainly needed for controlled release. The structure of the LPs can be altered, and the functionality could be enhanced to enfold the bioactive core materials. The processes are pressure pre-heat treatments, homogenization, and the enzymatic cross-linking of LPs. In order to encase probiotics and nutraceuticals, the most common LPs are isolates of proteins and concentrates of soy and peas (Gharibzahedi and Smith, 2021). Milk-based supplements can be produced by fortification of readily available food sources (Milne et al., 2009).

Glutenin polymers are built up with high and low molecular weight subunits, which are known to remain attached with the help of disulphide bonds. These polymers make hydrogen bonds and noncovalent hydrophobic interactions with the gliadins. Bread and making of dough are related to gluten proteins.

Zein protein is classified under the group of prolamins, which has biocompatibility and biodegradability and is also less toxic. These nanoparticles also help in protecting antioxidant compounds. Polysaccharides can interact with zein protein through electrostatic interactions and hydrogen bonds (Tapia-Hernández et al., 2018).

19.3.4 Inorganic Matrices

CRM stands for certified reference materials. The availability of food matrix CRMs has become quite limited (Wise and Phillips, 2019). The use of CRMs is now demanding as it has many advantages, like validating material in many operations and estimating unpredictability. CRMs also test the stability of a material. This test also helps to get the shelf life of the CRM. Some factors that promote the instability of CRMs are temperature, moisture, oxidation, and properties of the container used for storage, as well as exposure to UV light. Each CRM has protocols that differ from the others and varied statistical calculations (Olivares et al., 2018).

Selenium can be used as a dietary supplement. Heavy metals such as cadmium and lead are responsible for intoxication, and selenium protects the human body against these. Selenium is also known to possess anticarcinogenic properties. This inorganic element is also helpful in treating neoplastic diseases. Selenium dietary supplements are generally found in the form of tablets (Zembrzuska et al., 2014). The consumption of multivitamins is increasing for the safety of public health. Several factors are responsible for the safety of multivitamins or dietary supplements. They are the conditions for growing and extracting raw materials and their manufacturing processes. These dietary supplements can contain higher amounts of elements like lead and arsenic, concerning their safety. Therefore, the determination of the composition of these dietary supplements is required. Some elements, such as chromium, copper, zinc, and manganese, are considered essential parts yet will be toxic if the dose changes (Avula et al., 2011). The most abundant element in our body is calcium, the cation found in the most quantity in our human body and almost 99% of the total body calcium is found in teeth and bones. Calcium is stored in the matrix of the bone in the form of hydroxyapatite crystals. These are responsible for the strength and rigidity of the bone. Homeostasis of calcium in the body is mainly taken care of by Vitamin D3 in different ways like absorption of calcium in the intestine, bone turnover modulation and growth of the cartilaginous plate and its mineralization. Calcium salts-based dietary supplements are mainly used for improving bone health. It is found in combination with cholecalciferol. These calcium salts also have a problem with intoxicating elements like lead (Santos et al., 2022).

Some particles are designed mainly for the controlled delivery of bioactive molecules. Mesoporous silica particle (MSP) is one such particle of increased interest nowadays. Figure 19.6a depicts the synthesis of mesoporous particles, and Figure 19.6b reveals their microstructures under Field Emission Scanning Electron Microscope (FESEM) and Transmission Electron Microscope (TEM). After these

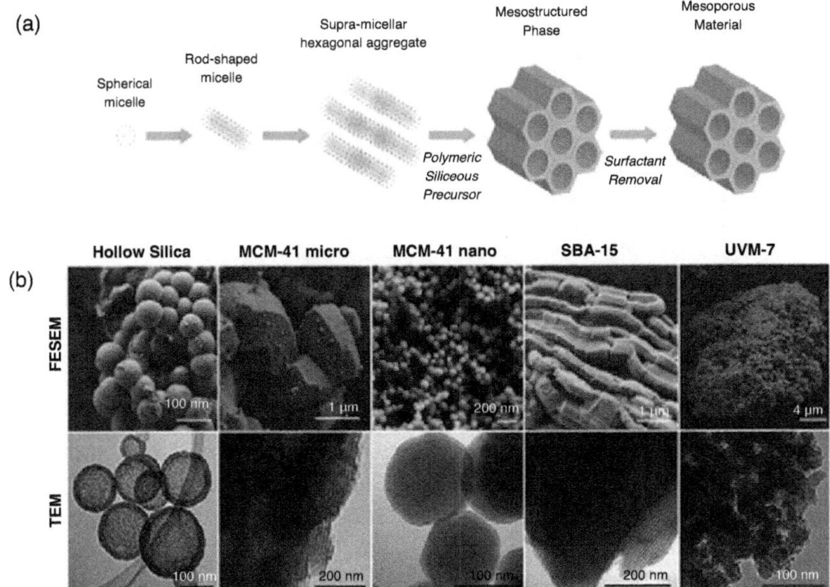

FIGURE 19.6 (a) Synthesis of mesoporous silica particles. (Reproduced from Pérez-Esteve et al. (2015) with permission from John Wiley and Sons, Copyright 2015). (b) Observation of the microstructures of mesoporous silica particles (MSPs). (Reproduced from Pérez-Esteve et al. (2015) with permission from John Wiley and Sons, Copyright 2015.)

MSPs are encapsulated with the bioactive molecules, there is a need to increase biological stability and improve the bioaccessibility of the molecules in the digestive or gastrointestinal tract (Pérez-Esteve et al., 2015).

19.4 USES AND IMPLEMENTATION OF NANOMATERIALS IN MEDICAL-PURPOSE FOOD

Since ancient times, people have been interested in medical-purpose food. The advancement of nanomaterials and their application in the food business has enabled researchers and food engineers to create enhanced food items with distinct characteristics. This section has explored various nanomaterials that can have a significant influence on the development of improved medical-purpose foods.

19.4.1 Metal Nanoparticles

Food technology uses metallic nanoparticles (MNPs) to protect and preserve the shelf life of food. MNPs help to improve the packaging characteristics by introducing antibacterial properties and being permeable to water vapour, allowing retainment of freshness of foods. MNPs have potential applications in nano sensors and new food analysis techniques (Couto and Almeida, 2022). The materials used for food packaging should possess toughness, flexibility, easy fabrication, lightness, and prevention of water vapour. The two polymeric packaging materials widely used in food

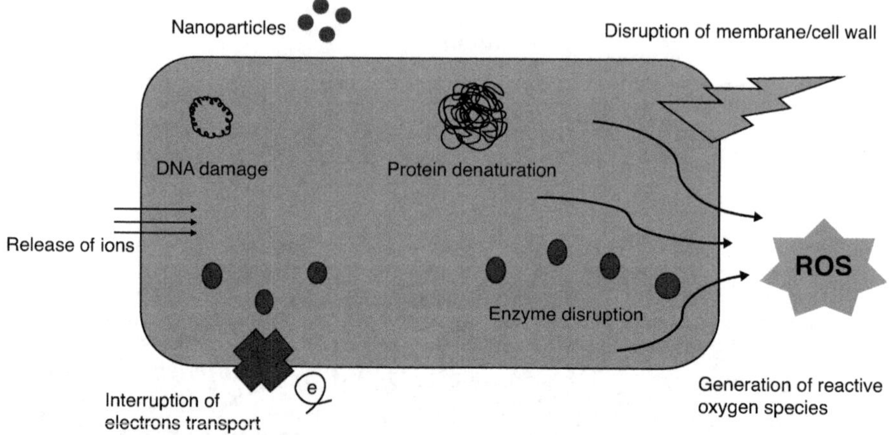

FIGURE 19.7 Mechanisms shown by the metal nanoparticles (MNPs). (Reproduced from Jafarzadeh et al. (2020) with permission from Elsevier, Copyright 2020.)

packaging are polyethylene (PE) and polypropylene (PP). MNPs can be of great help in preventing contamination through microbial contact. The mechanism of action for antimicrobial action is shown in the schematic diagram in Figure 19.7. Antimicrobial activity exerted by metal nanoparticles is the culmination of several factors, including generating reactive oxygen species (ROS) to induce oxidative stress, the release of metal ions, or non-oxidative mechanisms. The positively charged nanoparticles get attached to the bacterial membrane through electrostatic attractions. Additionally, van Der Waals forces, hydrophobic interaction or receptor-ligand mechanism facilitate attachment. After penetration, the membrane shape and structure get altered as the nanoparticles hinder the metallic pathways. Further, enzyme inhibition, protein and DNA impairment, and gene expression alteration lead to cellular metabolism disruption. Also, ROS generation causes leakage of cellular materials. These multifaceted attacks effectively kill bacteria. The categories of MNPs are divided into nanofibres, nanolayers, and nanoparticles. Nanoparticles have applications in active and intelligent packaging, bioplastics, surface biocides, and nanocomposites. They can be a barrier against microbes, bacteria, or water or oxide formation. (Jafarzadeh et al., 2020).

Platinum is used to diagnose diseases like cancer, HIV, and Parkinson's disease. Silver nanoparticles (AgNPs) are essential in biomedical applications such as antimicrobial and anti-cancerous agents. Gold nanoparticles (AuNPs) are used effectively as carriers of drugs. These nanoparticles are also known to have cytotoxic effects (Rai et al., 2016). AuNPs find their application in surface-enhanced Raman scattering sensors (SERS) where bisphenol or milk is used as film, analyte, or food. AuNPs are applied in optical sensors when the food is poultry meat. POC biosensors are used for food allergens. Honey is used in immunochromatographic sensors. AgNPs find their application as edible coatings in fresh-cut melon. These AgNPs are mixed with gamma irradiation, and the food used is fresh button mushrooms. Strawberries are packaged in active nanocomposite film. These films can assist in detecting food spoilage in fresh milk. Copper nanoparticles (CuNPs) are also used for the packaging of meat and soft drinks. These CuNPs act as electrochemical sensors for vegetable extracts. Zinc

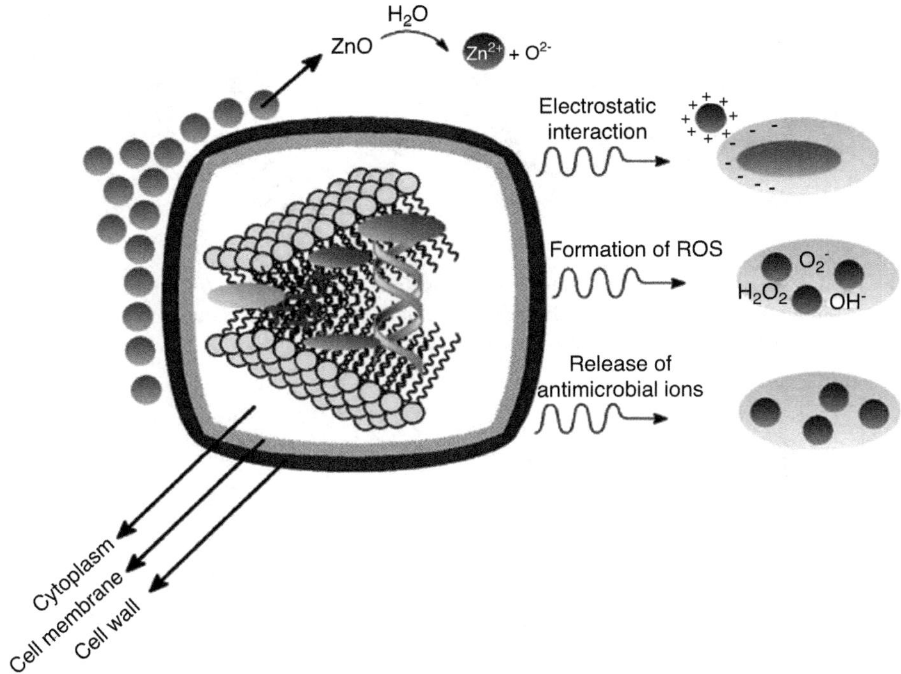

FIGURE 19.8 This shows the microbial activities and the mechanisms which are exhibited by ZnO nanoparticles. (Reproduced from Jafarzadeh et al. (2020) with permission from Elsevier, Copyright 2020.)

nanoparticles (ZnNPs) are used in biodegradable films for apple peels and meat from fresh poultry. ZnNPs are also used for the packaging of cheese. Figure 19.8 shows the mechanism exhibited by ZnONPs. Ultraviolet rays, as used in fish oil, can also be used for minced meat and skimmed milk acid-coagulated cheese packaging. Other MNPs are also used in active food packaging (Rai et al., 2016).

19.4.2 Nano-Encapsulates

Nano-encapsulation is one of the promising new nanotechnologies that keeps and protects components that are usually bioactive and can be delivered to the targeted systems in the body of a living organism. Nano-encapsulation enables the dispersibility of hydrophobic components like omega-3 fish oil, which is soluble through a micelle-based system. Nano-encapsulation increases the surface area of the ingredient, and it is also observed that there is an enhancement in the flavour of foods (Tahir et al., 2021). Lipid-based nano-encapsulation is known to be the most developed among the recent nanotechnologies and can trap materials irrespective of their different solubilities. These act as a shield to the encapsulated ingredients from the metal ions and enzymes and any free radicals resulting in the degradation of ingredients. Lipid-based nano-encapsulation can give stability, allowing targeted delivery to

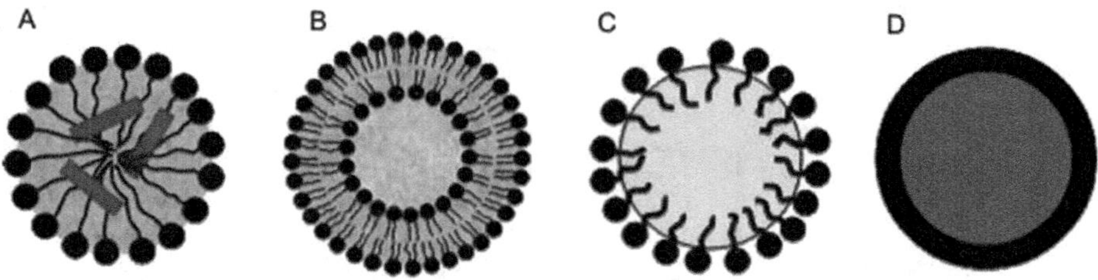

FIGURE 19.9 Liquid-liquid systems of encapsulated nanoparticles; (a) Microemulsion; (b) Liposome; (c) Nano emulsion; (d) Biopolymeric nanoparticle. (Reproduced from Khare and Vasisht (2014) with permission from Elsevier, Copyright 2014.)

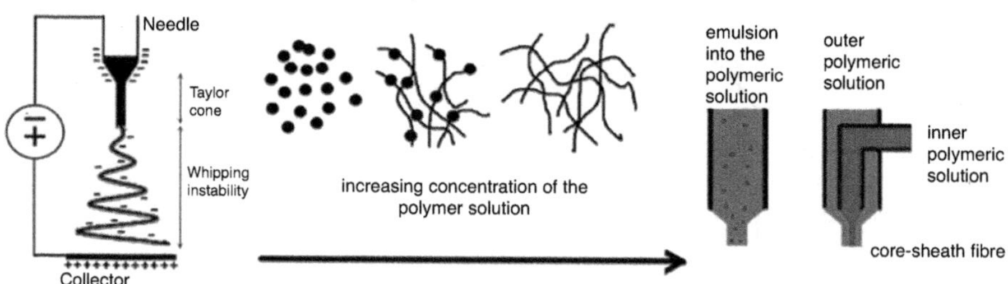

FIGURE 19.10 Setup for electrospinning. (Reproduced from Munteanu and Vasile (2021) https://creativecommons.org/licenses/by/4.0/.)

the specified areas. Mainly, this is used for the protection of foods and nutraceuticals (Mozafari et al., 2006).

In the food industry, nano-encapsulates have limited usage due to their cost and complexity. Figure 19.9 shows the different types of nano-encapsulates. The active ingredient encapsulated is the molecule in the nanoscale. Nano emulsions like oils have droplets of size less than 100 nm. These are optically transparent (Khare and Vasisht, 2014). Nano-encapsulation can be classified into "top-down" and "bottom-up." Particle size is one of the crucial factors that can be considered during encapsulation. In the "top-down" approach, with the help of tools, particle size is reduced during encapsulation. While in the latter "bottom-up" technique, the size of the particle is increased. There are some cases where both types of techniques can be combined. Emulsification is considered a top-down technique, whereas nanoprecipitation is a bottom-up technique (Pateiro et al., 2021).

Electrospinning, as shown in Figure 19.10, is another method of encapsulation. It is used to encapsulate bioactive compounds. This method does not require any severe temperature conditions or too much pressure. This method has increased the efficiency of encapsulation and has also increased the stability. It also improves the bioavailability of bioactive compounds. As the process does not require heat, the efficiency of encapsulation increases while preserving the structure of the compounds (Wen et al., 2017). The fibres that undergo electrospinning show thermal stability and they are more reliable for food packaging (Munteanu and Vasile, 2021).

19.4.3 Nanoscale Nutraceuticals

Nutraceuticals mainly comprise dietary supplements, plant-origin products, and foods that will be genetically engineered. However, limited solubility in an aqueous state leads to a low profile for bioavailability (Ali et al., 2019).

There is a classification of nutraceuticals as shown in Figure 19.11 – first, traditional nutraceuticals and second, non-traditional nutraceuticals. Traditional nutraceuticals can be divided into nutraceutical enzymes and probiotic enzymes. Non-traditional nutraceuticals can be divided into fortified and recombinant nutraceuticals. There are common bioactive agents which act as nutraceuticals. Carotenoids in citrus foods and tomatoes, act as antioxidants and help prevent heart diseases. Omega-3 fatty acids help in lowering the risk of heart disease. Onion, apple skin, and red grapes are sources of flavanols that help as antioxidants and lower blood lipids. Turmeric is a source of curcuminoids that protects against chronic diseases and acts as an antioxidant and anti-cancerous. Ubiquinone can be derived from meat or seafood and is an antioxidant (Ali et al., 2019). Nutraceuticals can be used as a substitute for contemporary medicine and enhance human life quality. They also act as immune boosters or even as antioxidants. They are helpful in processing nutrients like an aroma encapsulation and protect the food from degradation by

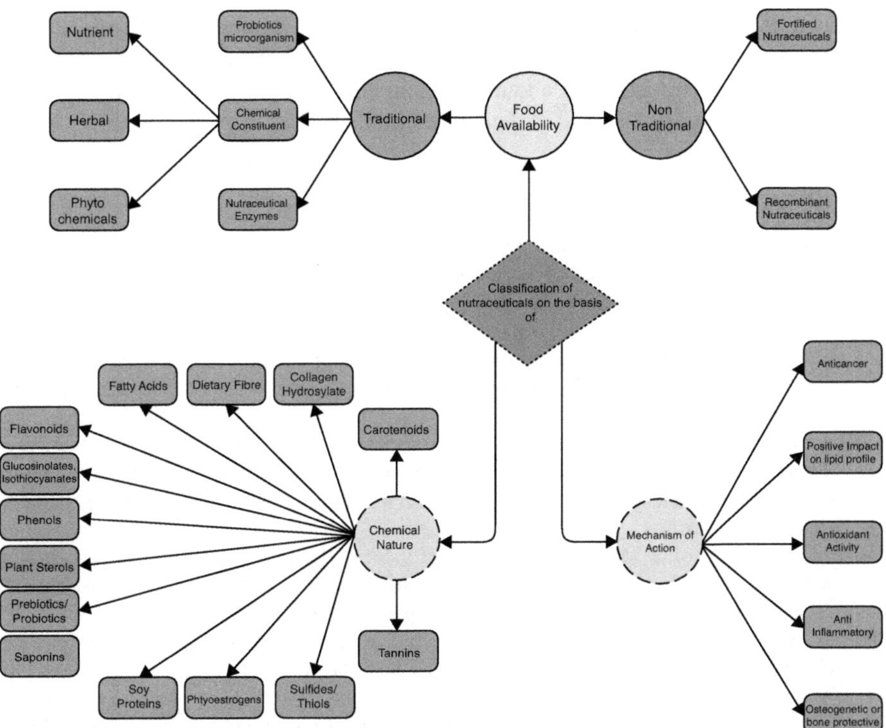

FIGURE 19.11 Classification of nutraceuticals. (Reproduced from Ali et al. (2019) with permission from Elsevier, Copyright 2019.)

UV rays (Singh et al., 2022). Nutraceuticals possess the good property of cytocompatibility. Nanotechnologies are involved in improving the solubility and bioavailability of nutraceuticals. Curcumin quercetin and flavone are regarded as bioactive nutraceuticals and act as anti-cancer (in-vitro) and antioxidants (Bansode et al., 2019). Stimuli-responsive nanoparticles have been observed to interact with charged components and hydrophobic components. These substances are mainly produced when proteins or polysaccharides undergo thermal treatment. As a result, these substances get a size that is tuneable and have physicochemical properties. These thermal-treated NPs are responsible for the pH and salt content. They also can act as nanocarriers of nutraceuticals (Papagiannopoulos and Vlassi, 2019).

19.5 CONCLUSIONS

A variety of nanomaterials and liposomes can be utilized to tailor food products. These changes cause variations in the features of edible items, such as colour, taste, texture, and nutritional or dietary qualities. They boost these qualities in vivo and serve as performance boosters for dietary supplements and medical-purpose foods. These nanomaterials include polysaccharide matrices, protein-based transporters, and nanoscale nutraceuticals. The food chemical sector has many complex applications, including oxidative stress management. Although these materials enhance the attributes of food products, their effects on the environment should also be considered. As a result, there should be specific and unambiguous guidelines for understanding pertinent information about nanomaterials used in the product, which can lead to safer consumer disposal and consumption.

REFERENCES

Ali, A., Ahmad, U., Akhtar, J., Khan, M.M., 2019. Engineered nano scale formulation strategies to augment efficiency of nutraceuticals. *J Funct Foods*. https://doi.org/10.1016/j.jff.2019.103554

Avula, B., Wang, Y.H., Duzgoren-Aydin, N.S., Khan, I.A., 2011. Inorganic elemental compositions of commercial multivitamin/mineral dietary supplements: Application of collision/reaction cell inductively coupled-mass spectroscopy. *Food Chem* 127, 54–62. https://doi.org/10.1016/j.foodchem.2010.12.083

Bansode, P.A., Patil, P. V., Birajdar, A.R., Somasundaram, I., Bachute, M.T., Rashinkar, G.S., 2019. Anticancer, antioxidant and antiangiogenic activities of nanoparticles of bioactive dietary nutraceuticals. *ChemistrySelect* 4, 13792–13796. https://doi.org/10.1002/slct.201903946

Castro, I.A., Tirapegui, J., Márcia, M., Benedicto, L., 2003. Effects of diet supplementation with three soluble polysaccharides on serum lipid levels of hypercholesterolemic rats. *Food Chemistry* 80(3), 23–330. https://doi.org/10.1016/S0308-8146(02)00267-4

Cherian, G., 2009. Eggs and health: Nutrient sources and supplement carriers. In: *Complementary and Alternative Therapies and the Aging Population* (pp. 333–346). Academic Press.

Couto, C., Almeida, A., 2022. Metallic nanoparticles in the food sector: A mini-review. *Foods*. https://doi.org/10.3390/foods11030402

De Kruif, C.G. and Holt, C., 2003. Casein micelle structure, functions and interactions. In Advanced dairy chemistry—1 proteins: part a/part b (pp. 233–276). Boston, MA: Springer US.

Dehnad, D., Emadzadeh, B., Ghorani, B., Rajabzadeh, G., Kharazmi, M.S., Jafari, S.M., 2022. Nano-vesicular carriers for bioactive compounds and their applications in food formulations. *Crit Rev Food Sci Nutr*. https://doi.org/10.1080/10408398.2022.2156474

Dutta, S., Moses, J.A., Anandharamakrishnan, C., 2018. Encapsulation of nutraceutical ingredients in liposomes and their potential for cancer treatment. *Nutr Cancer*. https://doi.org/10.1080/01635581.2018.1557212

Faridi Esfanjani, A., Jafari, S.M., 2016. Biopolymer nano-particles and natural nano-carriers for nano-encapsulation of phenolic compounds. *Colloids Surf B Biointerfaces* 146, 532–543. https://doi.org/https://doi.org/10.1016/j.colsurfb.2016.06.053

Feng, T., Wei, Y., Lee, R.J., Zhao, L., 2017. Liposomal curcumin and its application in cancer. *Int J Nanomed*. https://doi.org/10.2147/IJN.S132434

Garti, N., McClements, D.J., 2012. *Encapsulation Technologies and Delivery Systems for Food Ingredients and Nutraceuticals*. Elsevier, Cambridge.

Ghanbarzadeh, B., Babazadeh, A., Hamishehkar, H., 2016. Nano-phytosome as a potential food-grade delivery system. *Food Biosci*. https://doi.org/10.1016/j.fbio.2016.07.006

Gharibzahedi, S.M.T., Smith, B., 2021. Legume proteins are smart carriers to encapsulate hydrophilic and hydrophobic bioactive compounds and probiotic bacteria: A review. *Compr Rev Food Sci Food Saf*. https://doi.org/10.1111/1541-4337.12699

Głąb, T.K., Boratyński, J., 2017. Potential of casein as a carrier for biologically active agents. *Top Curr Chem*. https://doi.org/10.1007/s41061-017-0158-z

Jafarzadeh, S., Salehabadi, A., Jafari, S.M., 2020. Metal nanoparticles as antimicrobial agents in food packaging, In: *Handbook of Food Nanotechnology: Applications and Approaches*. Elsevier, pp. 379–414. https://doi.org/10.1016/B978-0-12-815866-1.00010-8

Jampilek, J., Kos, J., Kralova, K., 2019. Potential of nanomaterial applications in dietary supplements and foods for special medical purposes. *Nanomaterials*. https://doi.org/10.3390/nano9020296

Jordan, J., Jacob, K.I., Tannenbaum, R., Sharaf, M.A., Jasiuk, I., 2005. Experimental trends in polymer nanocomposites—a review. *Mater Sci Eng A* 393, 1–11. https://doi.org/https://doi.org/10.1016/j.msea.2004.09.044

Khan, A., Wen, Y., Huq, T., Ni, Y., 2018. Cellulosic nanomaterials in food and nutraceutical applications: A review. *J Agric Food Chem*. https://doi.org/10.1021/acs.jafc.7b04204

Khare, A.R., Vasisht, N., 2014. Nanoencapsulation in the food industry: Technology of the future, In: *Microencapsulation in the Food Industry: A Practical Implementation Guide*. Elsevier, pp. 151–155. https://doi.org/10.1016/B978-0-12-404568-2.00014-5

Kothalawala, N., Mudalige, T.K., Sisco, P., Linder, S.W., 2018. Novel analytical methods to assess the chemical and physical properties of liposomes. *J Chromatogr B Analyt Technol Biomed Life Sci* 1091, 14–20. https://doi.org/10.1016/j.jchromb.2018.05.028

Laouini, A., Jaafar-Maalej, C., Limayem-Blouza, I., Sfar, S., Charcosset, C., Fessi, H., 2012. Preparation, characterization and applications of liposomes: State of the art. *J Colloid Sci Biotechnol* 1, 147–168. https://doi.org/10.1166/jcsb.2012.1020

Madhusudan, P., Chellukuri, N., Shivakumar, N., 2018. Smart packaging of food for the 21st century – A review with futuristic trends, their feasibility and economics. *Mater Today Proc* 5, 21018–21022. https://doi.org/https://doi.org/10.1016/j.matpr.2018.06.494

Marzorati, M., Verhelst, A., Luta, G., Sinnott, R., Verstraete, W., de Wiele, T. v., Possemiers, S., 2010. In vitro modulation of the human gastrointestinal microbial community by plant-derived polysaccharide-rich dietary supplements. *Int J Food Microbiol* 139, 168–176. https://doi.org/10.1016/j.ijfoodmicro.2010.02.030

Milne, A.C., Potter, J., Vivanti, A., Avenell, A., 2009. Protein and energy supplementation in elderly people at risk from malnutrition. *Cochrane Database Syst Rev*. https://doi.org/10.1002/14651858.CD003288.pub3

Mozafari, M.R., 2010. Nanoliposomes: preparation and analysis. *Methods Mol Biol* 605, 29–50. https://doi.org/10.1007/978-1-60327-360-2_2

Mozafari, M.R., Flanagan, J., Matia-Merino, L., Awati, A., Omri, A., Suntres, Z.E., Singh, H., 2006. Recent trends in the lipid-based nanoencapsulation of antioxidants and their role in foods. *J Sci Food Agric.* https://doi.org/10.1002/jsfa.2576

Munteanu, B.S., Vasile, C., 2021. Encapsulation of natural bioactive compounds by electrospinning—applications in food storage and safety. *Polymers.* https://doi.org/10.3390/polym13213771

Olivares, I.R.B., Souza, G.B., Nogueira, A.R.A., Toledo, G.T.K., Marcki, D.C., 2018. Trends in developments of certified reference materials for chemical analysis - Focus on food, water, soil, and sediment matrices. *Trends Analyt Chem.* https://doi.org/10.1016/j.trac.2017.12.013

Ozturk, B., McClements, D.J., 2016. Progress in natural emulsifiers for utilization in food emulsions. *Curr Opin Food Sci.* https://doi.org/10.1016/j.cofs.2015.07.008

Paolino, D., Mancuso, A., Cristiano, M.C., Froiio, F., Lammari, N., Celia, C., Fresta, M., 2021. Nanonutraceuticals: The new frontier of supplementary food. *Nanomaterials* 11. https://doi.org/10.3390/nano11030792

Papagiannopoulos, A., Vlassi, E., 2019. Stimuli-responsive nanoparticles by thermal treatment of bovine serum albumin inside its complexes with chondroitin sulfate. *Food Hydrocoll* 87, 602–610. https://doi.org/10.1016/j.foodhyd.2018.08.054

Park, J., Choi, J., Kim, D.D., Lee, S., Lee, B., Lee, Y., Kim, S., Kwon, S., Noh, M., Lee, M.O., Le, Q.V., Oh, Y.K., 2021. Bioactive lipids and their derivatives in biomedical applications. *Biomol Ther.* https://doi.org/10.4062/biomolther.2021.107

Pateiro, M., Gómez, B., Munekata, P.E.S., Barba, F.J., Putnik, P., Kovačević, D.B., Lorenzo, J.M., 2021. Nanoencapsulation of promising bioactive compounds to improve their absorption, stability, functionality and the appearance of the final food products. *Molecules.* https://doi.org/10.3390/molecules26061547

Pérez-Esteve, É., Ruiz-Rico, M., Martínez-Máñez, R., Barat, J.M., 2015. Mesoporous silica-based supports for the controlled and targeted release of bioactive molecules in the gastrointestinal tract. *J Food Sci* 80, E2504–E2516. https://doi.org/10.1111/1750-3841.13095

Qin, Y., Liu, C., Jiang, S., Xiong, L., Sun, Q., 2016. Characterization of starch nanoparticles prepared by nanoprecipitation: Influence of amylose content and starch type. *Ind Crops Prod* 87, 182–190. https://doi.org/10.1016/j.indcrop.2016.04.038

Rai, M., Ingle, A.P., Birla, S., Yadav, A., dos Santos, C.A., 2016a. Strategic role of selected noble metal nanoparticles in medicine. *Crit Rev Microbiol.* https://doi.org/10.3109/1040841X.2015.1018131

Rehman, A., Ahmad, T., Aadil, R.M., Spotti, M.J., Bakry, A.M., Khan, I.M., Zhao, L., Riaz, T., Tong, Q., 2019. Pectin polymers as wall materials for the nano-encapsulation of bioactive compounds. *Trends Food Sci Technol* 90, 35–46. https://doi.org/https://doi.org/10.1016/j.tifs.2019.05.015

Ribarova, F., 2018. Amino acids: Carriers of nutritional and biological value foods, In: *Food Processing for Increased Quality and Consumption.* Elsevier, pp. 287–311. https://doi.org/10.1016/B978-0-12-811447-6.00010-2

Santos, W.M. dos, de Souza, M.L., Nóbrega, F.P., de Sousa, A.L.M.D., de França, E.J., Rolim, L.A., Rolim Neto, P.J., 2022. A review of analytical methods for calcium salts and cholecalciferol in dietary supplements. *Crit Rev Anal Chem.* https://doi.org/10.1080/10408347.2020.1823810

Santos, T.D., de Freitas, B.C.B., Moreira, J.B., Zanfonato, K., Costa, J.A.V., 2016. Development of powdered food with the addition of *Spirulina* for food supplementation of the elderly population. *Innov Food Sci Emerg Technol* 37, 216–220. https://doi.org/10.1016/j.ifset.2016.07.016

Serhan, M., Sprowls, M., Jackemeyer, D., Long, M., Perez, I.D., Maret, W., Tao, N., Forzani, E., 2019. Total iron measurement in human serum with a smartphone, In: *AIChE Annual Meeting, Conference Proceedings. American Institute of Chemical Engineers.*

Singh, A.R., Desu, P.K., Nakkala, R.K., Kondi, V., Devi, S., Alam, M.S., Hamid, H., Athawale, R.B., Kesharwani, P., 2022. Nanotechnology-based approaches applied to nutraceuticals. *Drug Deliv Transl Res*. https://doi.org/10.1007/s13346-021-00960-3

Subramani, T., Ganapathyswamy, H., 2020. An overview of liposomal nano-encapsulation techniques and its applications in food and nutraceutical. *J Food Sci Technol*. https://doi.org/10.1007/s13197-020-04360-2

Tahir, A., Shabir Ahmad, R., Imran, M., Ahmad, M.H., Kamran Khan, M., Muhammad, N., Nisa, M.U., Tahir Nadeem, M., Yasmin, A., Tahir, H.S., Zulifqar, A., Javed, M., 2021. Recent approaches for utilization of food components as nano-encapsulation: A review. *Int J Food Prop*. https://doi.org/10.1080/10942912.2021.1953067

Tapia-Hernández, J.A., Rodríguez-Felix, F., Juárez-Onofre, J.E., Ruiz-Cruz, S., Robles-García, M.A., Borboa-Flores, J., Wong-Corral, F.J., Cinco-Moroyoqui, F.J., Castro-Enríquez, D.D., Del-Toro-Sánchez, C.L., 2018. Zein-polysaccharide nanoparticles as matrices for antioxidant compounds: A strategy for prevention of chronic degenerative diseases. *Food Res Int*. https://doi.org/10.1016/j.foodres.2018.05.036

Wang, C., Ren, J., Song, H., Chen, X., Qi, H., 2021. Characterization of whey protein-based nanocomplex to load fucoxanthin and the mechanism of action on glial cells PC12. *LWT* 151. https://doi.org/10.1016/j.lwt.2021.112208

Wen, P., Zong, M.H., Linhardt, R.J., Feng, K., Wu, H., 2017. Electrospinning: A novel nano-encapsulation approach for bioactive compounds. *Trends Food Sci Technol*. https://doi.org/10.1016/j.tifs.2017.10.009

Wise, S.A., Phillips, M.M., 2019. Evolution of reference materials for the determination of organic nutrients in food and dietary supplements—a critical review. *Anal Bioanal Chem*. https://doi.org/10.1007/s00216-018-1473-0

Wu, X., Guy, R.H., 2009. Applications of nanoparticles in topical drug delivery and in cosmetics. *J Drug Deliv Sci Technol* 19, 371–384. https://doi.org/https://doi.org/10.1016/S1773-2247(09)50080-9

Xu, W., Wang, X., Sandler, N., Willför, S., Xu, C., 2018. Three-dimensional printing of wood-derived biopolymers: A review focused on biomedical applications. *ACS Sustain Chem Eng* 6, 5663–5680. https://doi.org/10.1021/acssuschemeng.7b03924

Zembrzuska, J., Matusiewicz, H., Polkowska-Motrenko, H., Chajduk, E., 2014. Simultaneous quantitation and identification of organic and inorganic selenium in diet supplements by liquid chromatography with tandem mass spectrometry. *Food Chem* 142, 178–187. https://doi.org/10.1016/j.foodchem.2013.05.004

Zhang, R., Zhang, Z., McClements, D.J., 2020. Nanoemulsions: An emerging platform for increasing the efficacy of nutraceuticals in foods. *Colloids Surf B Biointerfaces* 194. https://doi.org/10.1016/j.colsurfb.2020.111202

20 Nanotechnology and its Application in the Science of Beauty

Nano Formulation for Cosmetics and Beauty Creams

Suhasini Mallick and Rina Rani Ray

20.1 INTRODUCTION

Cosmeceuticals draw an alliance between pharmaceuticals and over-the-counter personal care products. They have created a space for themselves in people's daily lives or routines and framed a personal relationship with their customers. It is perceived as a personal affair since studies have testified that it unveils a complex relationship with a person's individuality and offers an overall confidence boost (Evangelista et al., 2022). The US Society of Cosmetic Chemists used the term "cosmetics" for the first time in 1961. It is defined as the personal care items that enhance the appearance and promote beautiful skin with intensive cleansing of the skin (Gautam et al., 2011). Similarly, there have been different definitions of cosmetics over time and in specific countries; one such example would be that of the US Food and Drug Administration (US-FDA), designating cosmetics as "particles intended to be applied onto human bodies or any part thereof for cleansing, beautifying, promoting attractiveness, or altering the appearance' (Center for Food Safety and Applied Nutrition, 2023). Considering its prevalence for ages, there have been alterations and innovations adhering to the concept of beauty. One such modification would be the use of nanotechnology by the Greeks, Romans, and Egyptians as early as 4,000 BC in preparing hair dyes (Bangale et al., 2012). Nanotechnology upholds demand in the science of beauty as it delivers innovation in its designs, delivery, production, and application. The basis of the innovation arises from a wide scheme of inherent properties that allow the nanomaterials to be different from their higher-scaled states. They range across a nanometer to 100 nanometers in scale and are crucial, as this dictates the fate of a given cosmetic product. For the manufacturers, nanoscale ingredients are a holistic component settling quality measures of deeper dermal seepage, better color and UV protection, higher product

 DOI: 10.1201/9781003432661-20

quality and long-standing effects, etc. (Raj et al., 2012). Since nanotechnology is associated with unique rearrangement of their structure owing to their nanodimension, they exhibit greater surface area, allowing their interaction with the biological systems differently compared to the micro/millidimension associates (Oberdörster et al., 2005). The nanomaterials are lucrative for point-of-care industries, as they achieve a cumulative value by having products that exceed in solubility, reactivity, transparency, and color (Aziz et al., 2019). Nanoformulation creates a unique delivery system of uplifting and restorative compounds without affecting the integrity of the purpose and broadens the scope of interaction with the biological tissues. The point-of-care dictates the type of formulation most suitable for nanocosmetology. They are commonly used to achieve the right chemical at the right site in the right concentration at the right time. One such example would be that of skin aging. It is a natural process but is speeded upon exposure to UV radiation; this can be subsided with the help of protective layering of nanoblockers that absorb the UV radiation, delaying skin aging. Additionally, lifestyle sits at the very core of health and beauty; any compromises in terms of extended stress, insufficient sleep, addictions, malnutrition, or environmental issues can reflect upon health and beauty. Since all the factors cannot be tackled altogether, the go-to quick fix is usually topical treatments containing nanoformulations. Such formulations are often accompanied by the aspects of enhanced permeation across the skin owing to their ability to conduct site-specific delivery, better hydration, and occlusive properties (Kaul et al., 2018). Upon considering these value-added benefits to a cosmetic product, nanotechnology also fulfills a wide range of layouts required for the ever-expanding global beauty market. The blueprint of which remains the paradigm of design, storage, and delivery of the desired beautification. This delicate framework is assisted primarily by nanoformulations that intensify and magnify the benefits to be drawn from a cosmeceutical product. The chapter gives a summative overview of the most likely nanoformulations used across a wide spectrum of cosmetics and does not list an exhaustive list of all the potentially available nanoformulations.

20.2 TYPES OF NANOFORMULATIONS

The formulation decides the prospect of bioavailability of the bioactive agent and destines the therapeutic concentration that will reach the target. (Salehi et al., 2019). This bioavailability depends heavily on the form of dosage rather than the inherent properties of the bioactive compounds, as they might not reach the therapeutic levels by themselves and will therefore require a framework to have an astute conveyance (Bhadoriya et al., 2011). The physical states of cosmetic applications can be presented in various forms, such as solids, liquids, or semi-solids. Semi-solid formulations are most sought after since they offer the advantage of leaching and dispersing within the dermis. Since skin hones at refraining xenobiotics; permeation within the skin via topical administration becomes an ineffective layout for bringing about any cosmetic reformations; hence, the application must be encased within a system that brings forth a desirable change with no drawbacks (Dokhani et al., 2017).

20.2.1 Emulsions

Nanoemulsions are a metastable system of the dispersion of nanoscale droplets within another liquid. They are capable of being curated by altering the method of preparation as per the requirement of the cosmetic application (Elavia, 2018). The emulsification helps in stretching the lifespan of the product. When the surfactants acquire an optimal concentration of surfactants, they reach the critical micellization concentration. This allows for the formation of tiny oil droplets with one segment facing toward the hydrophilic medium while the surfactant entraps it with a hydrophobic segment (Lee et al., 1970). The selection of the surfactant is predominantly based on its emulsification ability. Mostly nonionic surfactants are used in cosmetics due to higher biocompatibility compared to ionic surfactants (Azeem et al., 2009). The choice of nonionic surfactants is mostly based on the hydrophilic-lipophilic balance value, especially when used in oil-water (OW) nanoemulsions (Komaiko & McClements, 2015). Among the different forms of nanoemulsions, OW nanoemulsions are more frequently used in cosmetic formulations. Nanoemulsion-based cosmeceuticals tend to possess elevated kinetic and thermal stability due to greater surface charge arising from the nanodimension of the micelles that assist them in taming sedimentation, flocculation, and the Ostwald ripening phenomenon (Sadurní et al., 2005). Another aspect is that they are watery and transparent compared to their traditional formats, which are mostly creamy and semi-solid in texture (Khosa et al., 2018.). Further, these also put forth the advantage of reduced transdermal water loss, thereby retaining hydrated skin that permits a better influx of any active compounds (Bernardi et al., 2011).

20.2.2 Gels

Gels have a higher aqueous content, enabling them to dissolve a higher ratio of hydrophilic substances, helping in homogeneous spreading on the skin and assisting in transporting nanocosmetic systems incompatible with emulsions. Owing to their hydrophilic nature, they are readily used in the production of skin cleansers as they wash off easily. The limiting factor of gels is their inability to deliver active hydrophobic ingredients. Emulgels can overcome this disadvantage, as they consist of an emulsion dispersed across a gel base (Leon-Méndez et al., 2018).

20.2.3 Nanosomes

20.2.3.1 Liposomes

Concentric lipid bilayer vesicles are composed of generally regarded as safe (GRAS) phospholipids that enclose the active components and are termed liposomes. Moreover, the phospholipid bilayers can either be natural or synthetic and can fuse with the bilayers of cell membranes to stimulate the delivery of their cosmetic contents. Liposomes comprise a phosphatidylcholine-enriched phospholipid bilayer in the shape of a sphere and are excellent carriers of active ingredients and protein antigens in cosmetics. Cosmetic liposomes can be classified into Marinosomes,

Novasomes, Transferosomes, and Ultrasomes depending on their composition (Effiong et al., 2020; Hamid et al., 2016; Kaul et al., 2018; Moraes & Vieira, 2020). Regardless of their progress in synthesis, certain limitations loom over the aspect of liposomal applications due to inferior effective penetration, poor physical and chemical stability, and obstacles in attaining large-scale production (Van Tran et al., 2019).

20.2.3.2 Niosomes

Analogous to liposomes, niosomes are also self-assembled bilayer structures with hydrated nonionic surfactants arranged in the lamellar phase that meliorate the skin penetration by reducing interactions with the horny layer of the skin. They are associated with the delivery of antioxidants like resveratrol, ellagic acid, and ascorbic acid (Nasir et al., 2012). Additionally, they offer superior benefits over liposomes, as they are more cost-effective and can assure long-term stability to the cosmetic ingredients (Shegokar, 2016).

20.2.3.3 Polymersomes

The cosmetic industry uses polymersomes to enhance the rejuvenation and elasticity of skin cells. Polymersomes are vesicle-based, self-assembled block copolymers (Dhadwal et al., 2020). They are proficient in trapping and protecting sensitive active substances like proteins, drugs, enzymes, peptides, DNA, and RNA fragments. (Discher & Eisenberg, 2002).

20.2.3.4 Cubosomes

Cubosomes are particles of cubic liquid crystalline-phased nanostructures arranged in a self-assembled cubic and cavernous fashion with a size of 10–500 nm in diameter. They contain surfactants with relative water content and are often used in OW emulsions as stabilizers and render absorbability of pollutants (Raj et al., 2012). Another advantage of cubosomes is transporting both hydrophobic and hydrophilic compounds, creating a desirable mould for credible drug delivery (Barriga et al., 2019).

20.2.4 Lipid Carriers

Biocompatible nanomaterials are the most sought after to ensure ruling out any side effects or toxicities. On that note, lipid nanoemulsions occupy an elevated status due to their biocompatibility and the diversity of compositions, namely, nanostructured lipid carriers or solid lipid nanoparticles (NPs). Additionally, since it forms a lipid layer over the dermis, it has moisture-locking features that improve skin hydration. (Souto et al., 2020a). The solid lipid nanocarriers (SLNs) and nanostructured lipid nanocarriers (NLCs) are non-vesicular heterogeneous systems comprising a dispersion of immiscible phases and are stabilized with the help of surfactants (Salvioni et al., 2021).

20.2.4.1 Solid Lipid Nanocarriers

SLNs are composed of solid fat of approximately 0.1–30 (% w/w) and dispersed within an aqueous phase, followed by surfactants attached to it to enhance the stability of the system. The SLNs often contain fatty acids, glycerides, triglycerides, steroids, and waxes (Zielińska & Nowak 2016). The system enables the lipidic constituents to retain as solids at both body and ambient temperatures. (Lima et al., 2013). An advantage of SLNs is that they have greater entrapment efficiency than liposomes and can carry both hydrophilic and hydrophobic drugs (Joshi & Müller 2009).

20.2.4.2 Nanostructured Lipid Nanocarriers

NLCs are the second generation carriers propagated to overcome the restrictions of SLN usage. It is used across the products of hair serums and conditioners (Patel & Joshi, 2012). The structure organizes itself by creating voids to increase the accommodation of the active compounds, making it superior in occlusive and skin-adherence properties. This adherence helps gain superiority over the SLNs as it develops a thin film on the particles, enhancing skin hydration and stability (Pardeike et al., 2009). In a similar context, NLCs are a blend of solid and liquid lipids, providing an elevated loading capacity for lipophilic active agents over storage compared to SLNs (Souto et al., 2020a). They are addressed as nanobeads or nanopearls when used for different cosmetic applications.

20.2.5 Dendrimer

Dendrimers are vigorously branched globular and unimolecular micellar and multivalent nanostructures that can stretch into successive series of branches from their core. They often distribute themselves in a spherical pattern with three-dimensional morphology with sizes ranging from 2 to 20 nm in diameter (Fruchon & Poupot, 2017). Dendrimers allow for the proficient controlled release of vital components with high precision and selectivity due to the branched nature of the structure (Yapar & Inal, 2012). Interestingly, the dendrimers offer monodispersity, stability, polyvalence, and easy functionalization as delivery vehicles (Souto et al., 2020c).

20.2.6 Nanotubes

Nanotubes (NTs) are tubular structures that are used to entrap dyes and pigments. Among them, carbon nanotubes (CNTs) have been used extensively to color eyebrows, eyelashes, and hair. The nanotubes can alter shapes when coated with biopolymers like peptides and proteins. This occurs due to the presence of covalent bonding, which increases the affinity toward hair in peptide-based CNTs. This works by incorporating hair-binding peptides into the surface of the CNTs. Moreover, due to their abundance in nature, lower toxicity, and costs, NTs occupy a large share of hair care products (Panchal et al., 2018).

20.2.7 Nanospheres

Nanospheres can either be biodegradable like gelatine nanospheres or non-biodegradable like polylactic acid nanospheres and are typically core-shell structures, this commissions them to deliver the active constituent efficiently with precision (Kaul et al., 2018). They are made up of a polymeric matrix that entraps the active agents or adsorbs them, thereby carrying a higher load and spreading it due to their high surface area (Santos et al., 2019; Severino et al., 2016). The size of the nanospheres ranges between 10 to 200 nm in diameter and can either be crystalline or amorphous. Due to the encapsulation, dissolution, and attachment of the drug, the nanospheres protect it from chemical and enzymatic degradation (Singh et al., 2010).

20.2.7.1 Nanocrystals

Nanocrystals are drug particles that are stabilized by a surfactant or a polymer. The stabilizer plays a crucial role in nanocrystal-based formulations and is of different types based on the requirement of the cosmetic application as ionic, nonionic, and polymeric (Cardoza et al., 2022). Poor delivery of the soluble ingredients is overcome by nanocrystalline aggregates possessing acrystalline clusters of numerous atoms in 10–400 nm size. They tend to exhibit physiochemical properties like those of bulk-like and molecular solids (Petersen, 2008). Rutin, an antioxidant, was used as a nanosuspension, where 5% of it was in nanocrystal form. This formulation resulted in a whopping 500 times greater bioactivity than that of a water-soluble rutin glycoside derivative, demonstrating the ease of spreading in the skin to provide better photoprotection (Petersen, 2008). Further, the nanocrystals aid in increasing the substance's solubility, especially in the case of dispersing lipophilic active agents (Shegokar, 2016.).

20.2.7.2 Nanocapsules

The nanocapsule is a shell-based vesicular system that encompasses a liquid core of either water/oil in which the active drug is infused and wrapped within a polymeric membrane (Qorri et al., 2021). The major advantage of these nanocapsules is their ability to degrade into carbon dioxide and water, making them environmentally friendly (Yadwade et al., 2021). Research has also shown the development of fullerene nanocapsules containing vitamin E and ascorbic acid helps in combating premature aging of the skin (Goodarzi et al., 2017).

20.2.7.3 Nanopigments

Nanopigments engage in a safe, harmless, and colorful display of pigments often utilized as lipsticks and lip tints. This benefit is due to the nanodimension of the components since they exhibit and transform light differently. For example, inorganic nanoformulations mainly comprised of silver and gold exhibit yellow and red colors, respectively, in nanometer size (Garg et al., 2007). Studies have also demonstrated that the use of nanopigments in the form of metallic NPs can facilitate the reduction of the number of chemicals influencing the functionalization of nail polish (Lau et al., 2017). Thereby reducing the use of several other chemicals to achieve a preferred color effect.

20.3 APPLICATIONS OF NANOCARE IN BEAUTY

The sole purpose of cosmetics is to supplement, embroider, and boost the appearance and beauty of an individual (Gautam et al., 2011). Based on the purpose and coverage, they can be segregated into three broad categories-restorative, regenerative, and protective cosmetology. They showcase the areas of beauty and wellness that are most popular among the masses. Extending to that notion, it is important to realize that the categories display a wide spectrum of cosmeceuticals, offering multiple benefits and are not exclusive of the other categories.

20.3.1 Restorative Cosmetology

Restorative cosmetology revolves around bringing back the existing state to its former health and glory. Such beauty products entail the aspects of hydration, color correction, reversing the effects of aging, reviving cells, and reduction of scars. Alongside, it also aims to prevent further damage to the region by restoring it to its native form. Such strategies often turn toward casting barriers, promoting regrowth, and reviving the skin/scalp. Hair care products comprise several different nanomaterials like gold NPs, nanoemulsions, poly lactic-co-glycolic acid (PLGA) nanospheres, niosomes, liposomes, etc. that create a desirable effect on the scalp and hair follicles by shielding with a preventive film over them (Rosen et al., 2015). These barriers also ensure the prevention of excess water loss. Moisturizing cream containing nanoformulation also showcases a well-sustained barrier function for the skin even after 5 hours of single usage; demonstrating enhanced dispersion and fabrication of the proactive constituent (Barreto et al., 2017).

Due to diet, lack of nourishment and care, hyperpigmentation, discoloration, or tanning of the skin is seen. Consumers look for products with easy application modules. Since nanocomponents are dispersed in various forms, their topical administration is not an obstacle for the consumer. Additionally, they also bring forth better results in color correction. For instance, arbutin inhibits the melanin synthesis by inhibiting tyrosinase, the preliminary coordinator of melanin production (Chawla et al., 2008). Upon utilizing this strategy, Ayumi et al. (2019) stated that the α- and β-arbutin chitosan NPs offer an extended absorption rate by steadily releasing the active agent over 52 hours (Ayumi et al., 2019). Acne was seen to cause depression, low self-esteem, and suicidal thoughts among individuals (Golchai et al., 2010). Thus, it suggests that mental ailments can be rinsed out if treatments can be forged against their prevalence. Acne treatment is a very delicate arena since the incorrect evaluation of the acne and irritants can cause it to plummet into a downward spiral. Utilizing a biocompatible erythromycin-containing cubosomal formulation leads to a non-invasive passage to get rid of acne effectively (Khan et al., 2018). Another important obstacle of maintaining beauty is delaying the effect of aging. Similarly, liposome-based lip volumizers rule out wrinkles by filling them in the lip contours, giving them a well-endowed outline (Kaul et al., 2018).

Body dissatisfaction, poor mental health, and lower self-esteem have a psychological correlation to obesity (Weinberger et al., 2016). Nanotechnology-based obesity-reversing strategies include converting the white adipose tissues (WATs) into brown adipose tissues (BATs), inhibiting the angiogenesis of the WATs, and using photothermal lipolysis of the WATs. These, in comparison to conventional therapies, have much better targetability with high tolerability and efficiency, along with reduced side effects (Sibuyi et al., 2019). A polycation-based nanomedicine, polyamidoamine generation-3, when delivered intraperitoneally, uses a selective system to target the visceral fat due to its greater charge density. Moreover, it was observed that the treatment inhibited the visceral adiposity in obese mice by increasing energy expenditure, thereby alleviating the associated metabolic dysfunctions. The mechanism behind it is the uncoupling of adipocyte lipid synthesis and retarding the hypertrophic growth in the adipocyte development by modulating the associated nutrient-sensing signaling pathways by nanomedicine (Wan et al., 2022).

A white and bright smile can make or break the way for an individual. Tooth whitening is in demand now since people want to look and feel their best, especially due to the peer pressure of social media. It can help in making a good impression or cover bad oral hygiene. Shang et al. (2022) studied the impact of toothpaste containing hydroxyapatite NPs on teeth whitening by application and then by testing it to mechanical stress. The investigation revealed that the whitening effect was sustained after the stress in a concentration-dependent manner (Shang et al., 2022).

20.3.2 Regenerative Cosmetology

Active molecules drive across the dermal layers via passive diffusion, guided by a gradient concentration of extracellular and intrinsic pathways. The bulkier ones get cast out as they cannot penetrate the skin, thereby failing to satisfy the cosmetic requests (Bolzinger et al., 2012). Therefore, nanocosmetology can pave the way to deal with several fine-scale factors of the skin and scalp to regenerate and replenish the given area. Counteractive measures help cater to reversing the photodamage to the skin; for instance, spherical CeO_2 NPs ranging between 3 and 5 nm demonstrated that they could mitigate the photodamage caused by UV-A light and favored the survival and proliferation of the skin cells (Ribeiro et al., 2020). Healing of wounds can leave unfavoring scars. To eradicate them, a study suggests nanofibers such as PLGA can contain the carboxylic acid groups in the wound and exhibit enhanced fibroblast cell adhesion and proliferation, facilitating the avoidance of scar formation (Mulholland, 2020.). Further, numerous medical conditions offshooting from diabetes, physical aberrations, cancer treatments, biopsies, etc. can diminish the scale of the beauty of an individual. Hence, nanotechnology can furnish solutions to such needs that not only dwell on healing but also on providing scar-free, compatible, speedy modules that match beauty standards. (Mallick et al., 2022).

Minoxidil is a drug used to treat baldness and is approved by Health Canada and the US FDA (Gupta & Foley, 2014). A study led by Pravalika et al. (2020) demonstrated the incorporation of minoxidil within ethosomal vesicles and used it as a gel formulation to treat hair loss. The gel had improved penetration compared to other marketed formulations. In addition, it delivered good ex vivo permeability and hair growth (Pravalika et al., 2020). Researchers have found that on using chitosan and surface-deacetylated chitin nanofibers, there was a boost of proliferation in the follicular dermal papilla cells alongside an increased synthesis of fibroblast growth factor-7 in these cells within 3 days of its application, inducing growth of normal hair follicles (Azuma et al., 2019). Thus, delivering targeted therapies that ensure regenerative aspects with rapid action.

Beauty is determined by an individual's and society's perspective. "Deemed beauty" is the concept of beauty that helps achieve the basic beauty standards, especially in medically challenged skin conditions. These beautifications involve the remediation of worn-out skin, burnt skin from radiotherapy, melasma, psoriasis, or vitiligo of the skin. These deformities can compromise the perspective of beauty; therefore, nanocosmetics can become a viable and versatile agent in reforming the medically challenged skin. For instance, among the patients that receive radiotherapy, approximately 95% of them tend to develop radiation-induced dermatitis. This leads to a decreased quality of life and treatment outcomes (Iacovelli et al., 2020). Copper nanoarchitectures when dispersed in cosmetic cream, aided in recovering radiation-damaged skin. It delivered significant dermal healing on in vivo models and reduced the inflammation at the site by slashing the expression of cytokines. Additionally, the biocompatible nature of the nanoarchitecture displayed no signs of toxicity and therefore is a competent treatment for radiation dermatitis and skin burns (Ermini et al., 2023).

The spikes in melanin levels can prompt inconvenient color disorders in the skin, like melasma. The topical delivery of α-arbutin by functionalized chitosan NPs in gel formulation had a sustained release of the arbutin over 24 hours. The NPs showcased high stability and entrapment efficiency, especially in ex vivo studies. Additionally, there were no interactions between the carrier and the drug, hence maintaining the chemical stability of the active ingredient. Further, the α-arbutin-loaded NP hydrogel delivered better modifications to the melasma-affected region compared to the drug-free hydrogen (Hatem et al., 2022). Another depigmentation disorder in the skin is the occurrence of vitiligo. A study formulated ultradeformable liposomes (UDL) loaded with psoralen and resveratrol to treat vitiligo. Psoralen, in combination with UV-A, can stimulate melanin production and tyrosinase activity in melanocytes. On the other hand, resveratrol is seen to reduce oxidative stress, which in turn favors the reduction of vitiligo. Liposomes ensure that these active agents reach the target sites at therapeutical levels. The entrapment efficiency of psoralen and resveratrol was 74.09% and 76.91%, respectively. Thus, multiple agents loaded in the liposome helped significantly reduce the triggers of vitiligo, thereby reducing the depigmentation itself (Doppalapudi et al., 2017).

Psoriasis is an immune-mediated skin disorder. It can convert into multiple phenotypes in the same individual. Among them, Psoriasis vulgaris is the most common occurrence (Sarac et al., 2016). A nanoemulsion that combines clobetasol propionate (CP) and calcipotriol (CT) and incorporates it within a Carbopol® hydrogel was used on an induced psoriasis murine model. The treatment showed a larger reduction in erythema, inflammation, skin thickness, and scaling compared to treatment with free CP-CT gel and betamethasone dipropionate 0.05% gel. The superiority of the loaded gel is due to its prolonged drug release, as seen from high-performance liquid chromatography analysis. It showed that in comparison to the free drug, the nanoformulation had a sixfold increase in the duration of drug release (Kaur et al., 2017).

Thus, nanoformulations can combat several types of skin issues and assist in the regeneration, reformation, and beautification of extrinsic or intrinsic skin conditions.

20.3.3 Protective Cosmetology

Protective cosmetology deals with the areas that are frequently exposed to external irritants that devour the integrity of the region and destroy its natural state. Such irritants are mostly reactive oxygen species (ROS), environmental ambience, pollution, UV radiation, microbial entities, etc. UV radiation affects the skin by generating photo-oxidative stress on skin cells. UV-A is specifically responsible for promoting the collagen and elastin-degrading matrix metalloproteinases causing loss of skin elasticity (Battie et al., 2014). The driving force behind any protective agent is to provide a flourishing ambience without compromising on its state due to external influences and to constrict itself from creating any hindrance to the status quo. Such cases can be witnessed from ZnO and TiO_2 NPs that are used in large-scale UV-filtering products without harmful cutaneous health effects (Morganti, 2010).

To protect the hair, keratin treatments are a popular choice as they maintain the luster and texture of the hair. The proposal of loading natural halloysite clay nanotubes with free keratin produces a micrometer-thick protective coating on hair. This nanocomposite had a hair surface coverage of 50–60% with only 1wt % suspension application. Hair samples with the coating could inhibit the cysteine oxidation of the product upon irradiation with UV for up to 72 hours. Thus, showcasing minimal nanomaterials can offer maximized physical and chemical protection to the hair. (Cavallaro et al., 2020). Further zinc and chitin nanofibril complexes are also studied to assist in curbing hair flakes and sebum both *in vitro* and *in vivo* trials (Morganti et al., 2012).

Metallic nanoformulations have a spectrum of antimicrobial applications largely required in the domain of beauty. For instance, upon treating acne vulgaris with silver NP gel with clindamycin antibiotic gel, it demonstrated that the former showcased enhanced tolerability and satisfaction scores (Jurairattanaporn et al., 2017). The metal and metal oxide NPs also play a role in warding off toenail infections, thereby also rendering antimicrobial properties that ensure beauty enhancements stay undisturbed (Pereira et al., 2014).

To maintain cellular integrity and immune mechanisms, the body indulges in a series of chemical reactions that produce ROS, capable of rapidly transforming the fundamental requirements of maintaining cutaneous homeostasis (Pelle et al., 2005). Antioxidants are substances that prevent oxidative damage to cells and tissues by neutralizing the ROS generated from systematic natural processes (Sindhi et al., 2013). Naringenin, nordihydroguaiaretic acid (NDGA), and kaempferol are three natural agents that were encapsulated into NLCs aimed at delivering a potent formulation with antioxidant properties. There was a prolonged release of the bioactive compounds in *in vitro* studies with an encapsulation efficiency of over 90% and stability for 30 days. Further upon investigating the NLC's antioxidant effects against oxidative stress caused by tert-butyl hydroperoxide (t-BHP), the loaded NLC had an effective protective effect. Owing to the NLCs, the biodelivery and bioavailability of the compounds increased, enabling the tackling of the oxidative agents (Gonçalves et al., 2021).

A diverse overview of a few nanoformulations with their applications is shown in Table 20.1, and the range of nanocosmetic products is represented in Figure 20.1.

TABLE 20.1
Different Cosmetic Applications of Nanoformulations

Point-of-Care	Nanoformulation	Application	Reference
Skin	Hydroquinone-cellulose nanocrystal complex	Hyperpigmentation	Taheri and Mohammadi (2015)
	Cubosome formulation containing erythromycin	Anti-acne	Khan et al. (2018)
	SLNs containing coenzyme Q10 incorporated into a semisolid emulsion	Anti-wrinkles	Farboud et al. (2011)
	Nanoemulsion using pomegranate seed oil	Growth	Dhawan and Nanda (2019)
	Nano-hyaluronic acid formulations	Hydration	Jegasothy et al. (2014)
	Buckminster fullerene	Anti-oxidative	Bakry et al. (2007)
	Zinc oxide and titanium oxide NP	UV block	Schneider and Lim (2019)
	Carbon black	Face mask	Fytianos et al. (2020)
	Ethosomes incorporating phenylethyl resorcinol	Lightening	Yang and Kim (2018)
	Micellar NPs of polysaccharide-enriched fraction isolated from the byproduct of *A. sisalana*	Moisturizing	Barreto et al. (2017)
Hair	Pluronic lecithin organogel with roxithromycin-loaded NPs	Hair loss	Główka et al. (2014)
	Combination of minoxidil and caffeine in transfersomes	Regeneration	Ramezani et al. (2018)
	Seracin, derived from silkworms, incorporated into the conditioning agents as cationic nanoparticles	Conditioning	Pereda et al. (2012)
	p-phenylenediamine incorporated NPs using hyaluronic acid	Color	Lee et al. (2013)
	Fullerene nanomaterials	Volumizer	Zhou et al. (2009)
Nails	Metallic NPs	polish	Lau et al. (2017)
	Rosa indica L-mediated biogenic ZnO NP	anti-fungal	Tiwari et al. (2017)
Body	Poly-L-lactic acid (PLLA) nanocapsules	Fragrance	Yadwade et al. (2021)
	Biogenic silver NPs	Soap	Bansod et al. (2015)
Teeth	Carbamide peroxide polymeric NP bleaching gel	Whitening	Favoreto et al. (2021)
	Zinc-carbonate hydroxyapatite nanocrystals	Mouthwash	Almutairi and Asmari (2019)
	Nano-gold and nano-silver	Antimicrobial toothpaste	Junevičius et al. (2015)
Lip	Rice bran oil liposome	Antioxidant	Amnuaikit et al. (2008)

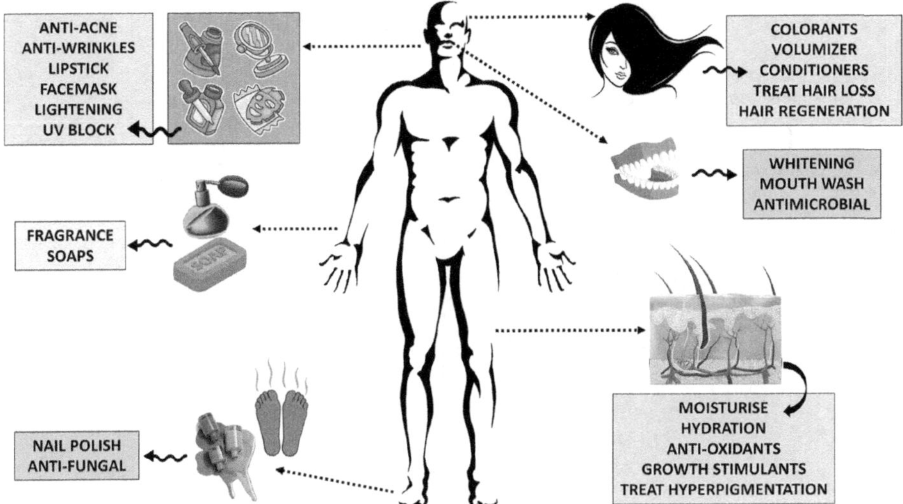

FIGURE 20.1 Cosmetic commercial products of nanoformulations.

20.4 DRAWBACKS OF NANOCOSMETOLOGY

The Environmental Working Group states that, on average, women use 12 products a day that contain a diverse range of 168 chemicals (*Exposures Add Up – Survey Results*, 2004). Thus, providing insight into the daily uptake of cosmeceuticals around the globe. Among the numerous advantages lurks the cunning downside of nanocosmeceuticals that may have gender-specific impacts, owing to the patterns of consumption. These deliberately require active invigilation in terms of clinical trials, sustainable and regulatory limits, and permits to ensure the safety of the consumers (Souto et al., 2020b). Given the nanodimension of the substances, their inherent physiochemical properties differ tremendously from the larger particles. At the nanolevel, the higher surface-area-to-volume ratios furnish greater chemical reactivity and biological activity to the particles. Such reactivity ensures the vigorous production of ROS, including free radicals detrimental to the biological system (Brown et al., 2002) (Figure 20.2). NPs used in powders, perfumes, setting sprays, etc. can enter the respiratory tract upon exposure. Studies on animals, prove that the inhaled NPs that enter the pulmonary tract may travel through the nasal nerves to the brain and can gain access to other organs via blood (Tsuji et al., 2006). Likewise, nanocosmetics may irritate the skin, which may also go overlooked during trials or assessments (Jeswani et al., 2019).

The use of nanoformulations is frequently admonished since it can trigger the formation of ROS, yielding toxic consequences like oxidative stress, inflammatory response, DNA damage, etc., in the biological setup (Doktorovova et al., 2011; Doktorovová et al., 2014). Carbon-based nanomaterials demonstrate severe cytotoxic effects in human beings and other mammals. This is due to its accumulation in different organs, such as lungs and kidney tissues, which destabilizes the organs' functioning upon reaching a threshold concentration (Wang et al., 2011). Medical conditions like psoriasis make the skin vulnerable, allowing deeper penetration of

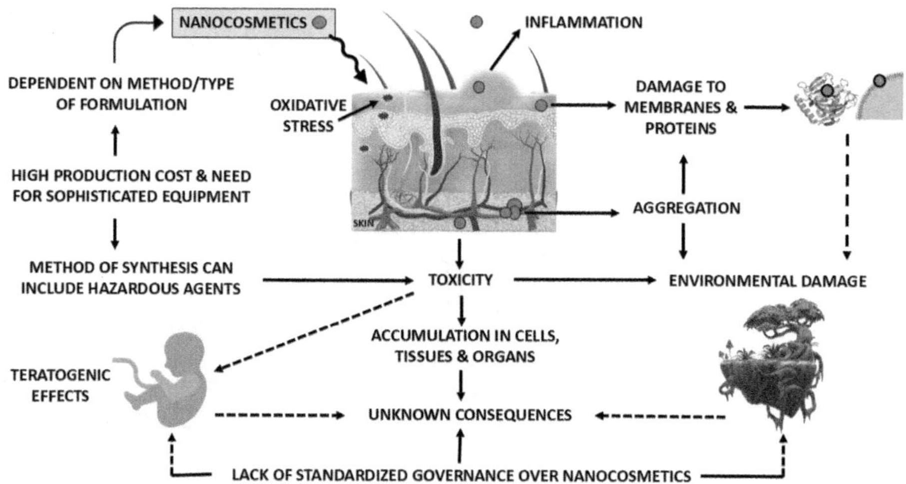

FIGURE 20.2 Disadvantages of nanocosmetic formulations.

the NPs than unaffected skin (Prow et al., 2011). On the other hand, fullerenes of molecular weight 500–600 Da not only penetrate easily into the skin but can also create radicals without oxygen, posing as a pro-oxidant. This is another common obstacle for an antioxidant to switch as a pro-oxidant under specific biological circumstances (Mousavi et al., 2017).

The multiple factors that can contribute to toxicity are the size, shape, and concentration of the nanomaterials. The most studied reports are on the ill effects of metallic NPs, giving them a dazed reputation. For example, upon ingesting gold NPs of size 13.5 nm, there was a significant reduction in red blood cells, body weight, and the spleen index of mice. Similarly, there was a sharp reduction in the size of neuronal cells along with irregularities among rats exposed to silver NPs. This consequently also hampered cell viability and mitochondrial functions (Zhang et al., 2010). Another crucial aspect of NPs is concentration. A study led by Wu et al. (2010) led to the investigation of the neurotoxicity of ZnO NPs ranging between 10–200 nm on cultures of mouse neural stem cells. The cell viability tests demonstrated that after 24 hours, NPs inflicted dose-dependent but not size-dependent toxic effects on cells (Wu et al., 2010).

The US Government Accountability Office (GAO) investigated the nanomaterials present in sunscreens and stated that they could gain access through damaged skin, offshooting serious side effects (Ostiguy et al., 2010). The existence of contradictory studies makes it erroneous to side with either the helpful or the harmful nature of nanocosmetics. For instance, a study on subcutaneous application of TiO_2 NPs in pregnant mice reveals that it was transferred to offspring, resulting in brain damage and diminished sperm production among the male offspring (Posada et al., 2015). On the same note, titanium dioxide NPs of 500 nm size can instigate breakage of the DNA strand, while those of 20 nm can destroy the super-coiled DNA, even at low doses (Donaldson et al., 1996). This indicates that the downfalls and safety of nanocosmetics are heavily based upon their usage and dynamics with the biological system.

Chemical and physical processes of synthesizing nanocarriers can procure high developmental costs, poor solubility, reduced shelf life, and jeopardize drug stacking owing to leaching and hydrolysis. Similarly, green synthesized nanocarriers can fall prey to reduced stability of the nanosystem. Such scenarios can lead to biased effects or burst release of the loaded drug molecules. (Chauhan & Chauhan, 2021). The physicochemical properties of the selected nanoingredients will have to be scrupulously verified for their biocompatibility, polarity, and the possible routes of toxicity, especially with concerning genotoxic and immunogenic side effects that might occur. These non-negotiables play a pivotal role in the benefit and safety of nanocosmetics.

The NPs have also been studied for their plausibility of binding to contaminants such as petrochemicals and cadmium that heighten the immanence in the environment. This prolongs the longevity and range of permeating transport of contaminants via groundwater (Wong et al., 2008). Another quandary is that the NPs have an affinity to bond with pollutants like cadmium and petrochemicals that already reside in the environment, providing a prolonged and unwavering magnitude to their toxicity (Marzuki et al., 2019). Nano-titanium dioxide prevalent in personal care products can reduce the biological roles of bacteria within less than an hour of exposure. This is suggestive of the conclusion that such particles reaching the municipal sewage treatment plants could obliterate microbes crucial to the ecosystems and that are involved in treating wastewater (Cimitile, 2009).

One of the measures to constrict the unethical usage of nanocosmetics is to govern them with competent bodies that adhere to maintaining standard products with low complicacies to health and the environment. The governance related to nanomaterial applications is well addressed across different literary sources. Two supervising international bodies, namely, the World Health Organization and Cosmetics Harmonization and International Cooperation, watch over the safety and efficacy of cosmeceuticals around the globe. Likewise, additional information on the marketed nanocosmetics can be accessed from two additional resources (Kuenen et al., 2020): the "Global Nanotechnology Database", launched by StatNano in 2014, and the "Nanotechnology Consumer Products Inventory", created in 2005 (Vance et al., 2015).

20.5 FUTURE PROSPECT

Futuristic cosmetology involves looking for products and compounds that integrate personal care without heavily indulging in pharmacology. Moreover, since nanocosmeceutical formulations align with the requirements of non-invasive, effective, and precision skin care, they certainly have greater potential to advance in the future. Fortunately, it can also be tuned to have non-surgical reforms and healing of the skin, thereby furthering the science behind attaining beauty (Chauhan & Chauhan, 2021). Better alternatives must be developed to avoid the complications that may arise from the current usage of nanocosmetics. Nanobiotechnology can help formulate biomimetic particles that can induce the desired benefits at the target of interest.

Such formulations can also enable diverse transcutaneous penetration through the epidermal and dermal layers effectively (Nafisi & Maibach, 2018; Santini et al., 2015).

On that note, the governance over nanocosmetics is not standardized across the globe and sets irregular control over the extent of integration of nanotechnology among the cosmeceuticals. Such diversities in regulation are being checked by advancing the country's policies to match the rest of the world. Like, as of 2021, the Canadian government has commenced screening the priority products that utilize nanoforms of TiO_2 and ZnO to quantize commercial consumptions and collect information on the potential exposure toward humans and the environment (Health Canada, 2022). Finally, the integration of artificial intelligence in the frontiers of cosmetology can help develop predictive models of an individual's state of skin, hair, and overall beauty to predict the treatments or cosmetic applications that would be customized as per requirements. This would eliminate the non-judicious usage of nanomaterials in the science of beauty.

20.6 CONCLUSION

Nanoformulations have established markets across sectors of pharmaceutics, wellness, dermatology, and cosmetics. They enable the reinforcement of a prolonged effect alongside preoperative status by managing a uniform and controlled release of the compounds. So far, nanocosmetology has proved to ameliorate the performance of cosmetics by escalating the entrapment efficiency and dermal penetration, manipulating the release of active compounds, and enhancing the moisturizing capacity and physical stability. Apart from that, the focus is shifting to the green synthesis and propagation of nanomaterials to make them more appropriate for applications in biological systems. Green technology is a plausible solution for biocompatible and energy-efficient consumption, alongside restricting ecological destruction by limiting the usage of harsh chemicals in their synthesis.

The real peril arises from the inconsistent standardized regulations over nanocosmetics across the global market. The lack of an inconclusive status on the consumption and regulation of most nanocosmetics creates a distorted perspective on the bewildered safety of nanocosmetics. There must be punctilious scrutiny of the nanomaterials used in the composition of cosmetics, irrespective of the type of care they provide. Moreover, nanomaterials are diverse in shape, size, form, and function; it is essential to overcome this problem. Complexing the problem is that the biological and environmental hindrances arising from these nanomaterials can be case-specific and irrational to investigate. Hence, the manufacturers, the stakeholders, and the respective authorities must come up with inclusive solutions to tackle the problem of nanomaterial toxicity and spillage. Additionally, the consumer's awareness and education can compel the maintenance of regulations. Such advances to keep a check on nanocosmetics can prevent unprecedented fallouts of nanomaterials in natural systems. They must be treated as pseudo-pharmaceutical products, irrespective of mostly being over-the-counter products. The overall goal for any cosmetic must be to not jeopardize health in the drive to attain beauty.

REFERENCES

Amnuaikit, T., Pinsuwan, S., Ingkatawornwong, S., & Worachotekamjorn, K. (2008) 'Development of lipsticks containing rice bran oil liposome'. *Planta Medica, 74*, p. PD14.

Almutairi, A.S., & Asmari, D.A. (2019) 'Clinical evaluation of zinc-carbonate hydroxyapatite nanocrystals mouthwash in controlling plaque induced gingivitis: A randomized clinical trial', *IP International Journal of Periodontology and Implantology, 4*(3), pp. 98–102. https://doi.org/10.18231/j.ijpi.2019.021

Ayumi, N. S., Sahudin, S., Hussain, Z., Hussain, M., & Samah, N. H. A. (2019) 'Polymeric nanoparticles for topical delivery of alpha and beta arbutin: Preparation and characterization'. *Drug Delivery and Translational Research, 9*(2), pp. 482–496. https://doi.org/10.1007/s13346-018-0508-6

Aziz, Z. A. A., Mohd-Nasir, H., Ahmad, A., Mohd. Setapar, S. H., Peng, W. L., Chuo, S. C., Khatoon, A., Umar, K., Yaqoob, A. A., & Mohamad Ibrahim, M. N. (2019) 'Role of nanotechnology for design and development of Cosmeceutical: Application in makeup and skin care', *Frontiers, 7*. https://doi.org/10.3389/fchem.2019.00739

Azeem, A., Rizwan, M., Ahmad, F. J., Iqbal, Z., Khar, R. K., Aqil, M., & Talegaonkar, S. (2009) 'Nanoemulsion components screening and selection: A technical note', *AAPS PharmSciTech, 10*(1), pp. 69–76. https://doi.org/10.1208/s12249-008-9178-x

Azuma, K., Koizumi, R., Izawa, H., Morimoto, M., Saimoto, H., Osaki, T., Ito, N., Yamashita, M., Tsuka, T., Imagawa, T., Okamoto, Y., Inoue, T., & Ifuku, S. (2019) 'Hair growth-promoting activities of chitosan and surface-deacetylated chitin nanofibers', *International Journal of Biological Macromolecules, 126*, pp. 11–17. https://doi.org/10.1016/j.ijbiomac.2018.12.135

Bakry, R., Vallant, R. M., Najam-ul-Haq, M., Rainer, M., Szabo, Z., Huck, C. W., & Bonn, G. K. (2007) 'Medicinal applications of fullerenes', *International Journal of Nanomedicine, 2*(4), pp. 639–649.

Bangale, M. S., Mitkare, S. S., Gattani, S. G., & Sakarkar, D. M. (2012) 'Recent nanotechnological aspects in cosmetics and dermatological preparations', *International Journal of Pharmacy and Pharmaceutical Sciences, 4*(2), pp. 88–97.

Bansod, S. D., Bawaskar, M. S., Gade, A. K., & Rai, M. K. (2015) 'Development of shampoo, soap and ointment formulated by green synthesised silver nanoparticles functionalised with antimicrobial plants oils in veterinary dermatology: Treatment and prevention strategies', *IET Nanobiotechnology, 9*(4), pp. 165–171. https://doi.org/10.1049/iet-nbt.2014.0042

Barreto, S. M. A. G., Maia, M. S., Benicá, A. M., de Assis, H. R. B. S., Leite-Silva, V. R., da Rocha-Filho, P. A., de Negreiros, M. M. F., de Oliveira Rocha, H. A., Ostrosky, E. A., Lopes, P. S., de Farias Sales, V. S., Giordani, R. B., & Ferrari, M. (2017) 'Evaluation of in vitro and in vivo safety of the by-product of *Agave sisalana* as a new cosmetic raw material: Development and clinical evaluation of a nanoemulsion to improve skin moisturizing', *Industrial Crops and Products, 108*, pp. 470–479. https://doi.org/10.1016/j.indcrop.2017.06.064

Barriga, H. M. G., Holme, M. N., & Stevens, M. M. (2019) 'Cubosomes: The next generation of smart lipid nanoparticles?', *Angewandte Chemie (International ed. in English), 58*(10), pp. 2958–2978. https://doi.org/10.1002/anie.201804067

Battie, C., Jitsukawa, S., Bernerd, F., Del Bino, S., Marionnet, C., & Verschoore, M. (2014) 'New insights in photoageing, UVA induced damage and skin types', *Experimental Dermatology, 23*(Suppl 1), pp. 7–12. https://doi.org/10.1111/exd.12388

Bernardi, D. S., Pereira, T.A., Maciel, N. R., Bortoloto, J., Viera, G. S., Oliveira, G. C., & Rocha-Filho, P. A. (2011) 'Formation and stability of oil-in-water nanoemulsions containing rice bran oil: *In vitro* and *in vivo* assessments', *Journal of Nanobiotechnology, 9*, p. 44. https://doi.org/10.1186/1477-3155-9-44

Bhadoriya, S. S., Mangal, A., Madoriya, N., & Dixit, P. (2011) 'Bioavailability and bioactivity enhancement of herbal drugs by "Nanotechnology": A review', *Journal of Current Pharmaceutical Research*, *8*, pp. 1–7.

Dhadwal, A., Sharma, D., Pandit, V., Ashawat, M., & Kumar, P. (2020) 'Cubosomes: A novel carrier for transdermal drug delivery', *Journal of Drug Delivery and Therapeutics*, *10*(1), pp. 123–130. doi: 10.22270/jddt.v10i1.3814.

Bolzinger, M., Briançon, S., Pelletier, J., & Chevalier, Y. (2012) 'Penetration of drugs through skin, a complex rate-controlling membrane', *Current Opinion in Colloid & Interface Science*, *17*(3), pp. 156–165. https://doi.org/10.1016/j.cocis.2012.02.001

Brown, J. S., Zeman, K. L., & Bennett, W. D. (2002) 'Ultrafine particle deposition and clearance in the healthy and obstructed lung', *American Journal of Respiratory and Critical Care Medicine*, *166*(9), pp. 1240–1247. https://doi.org/10.1164/rccm.200205-399OC

Cardoza, C., Nagtode, V., Pratap, A., & Mali, S. N. (2022) 'Emerging applications of nanotechnology in cosmeceutical health science: Latest updates', *Health Sciences Review*, *4*, p. 100051. https://doi.org/10.1016/j.hsr.2022.100051

Cavallaro, G., Milioto, S., Konnova, S., Fakhrullina, G., Akhatova, F., Lazzara, G., Fakhrullin, R., & Lvov, Y. (2020) 'Halloysite/keratin nanocomposite for human hair photoprotection coating', *ACS Applied Materials & Interfaces*, *12*(21), pp. 24348–24362. https://doi.org/10.1021/acsami.0c05252

Center for Food Safety and Applied Nutrition. 'Is it a cosmetic, a drug, or both? (or is it soap?)', *U.S. Food and Drug Administration*. https://www.fda.gov/cosmetics/cosmetics-laws-regulations/it-cosmetic-drug-or-both-or-it-soap (Accessed: 29 January 2023).

Chauhan, A., & Chauhan, C. (2021), 'Emerging trends of nanotechnology in beauty solutions: A review', *Materials Today: Proceedings*. https://doi.org/10.1016/j.matpr.2021.04.378

Chawla, S., deLong, M. A., Visscher, M. O., Wickett, R. R., Manga, P., & Boissy, R. E. (2008) 'Mechanism of tyrosinase inhibition by deoxyArbutin and its second-generation derivatives', *The British Journal of Dermatology*, *159*(6), pp. 1267–1274. https://doi.org/10.1111/j.1365-2133.2008.08864.x

Cimitile, M. (2009) 'Nanoparticles in sunscreen damage microbes', *Scientific American*. https://www.scientificamerican.com/article/nanoparticles-in-sunscreen/

Dhawan, S., & Nanda, S. (2019) 'In vitro estimation of photo-protective potential of pomegranate seed oil and development of a nanoformulation', *Current Nutrition & Food Science*, *15*(1), pp. 87–102. https://doi.org/10.2174/1573401314666180223134235.

Discher, D. E., & Eisenberg, A. (2002). Polymer vesicles. *Science*, *297*(5583), pp. 967–973. https://doi.org/10.1126/science.1074972

Dokhani, A., Amini, J., Gortzi, O., Danaei, M., Mozafari, M. R., & Maherani, B. (2017) 'Enhanced efficacy and bioavailability of skin-care ingredients using liposome and nano-liposome technology', *Modern Applications of Bioequivalence & Bioavailability*, *2*(2). https://doi.org/10.19080/MABB.2017.02.555584.

Doktorovova, S., Shegokar, R., Rakovsky, E., Gonzalez-Mira, E., Lopes, C. M., Silva, A. M., Martins-Lopes, P., Muller, R. H., & Souto, E. B. (2011) 'Cationic solid lipid nanoparticles (cSLN): Structure, stability and DNA binding capacity correlation studies', *International Journal of Pharmaceutics*, *420*(2), pp. 341–349. https://doi.org/10.1016/j.ijpharm.2011.08.042

Doktorovová, S., Santos, D. L., Costa, I., Andreani, T., Souto, E. B., & Silva, A. M. (2014) 'Cationic solid lipid nanoparticles interfere with the activity of antioxidant enzymes in hepatocellular carcinoma cells', *International Journal of Pharmaceutics*, *471*(1–2), pp. 18–27. https://doi.org/10.1016/j.ijpharm.2014.05.011

Donaldson, K., Beswick, P. H., & Gilmour, P. S. (1996) 'Free radical activity associated with the surface of particles: A unifying factor in determining biological activity?', *Toxicology Letters*, *88*(1–3), pp. 293–298. https://doi.org/10.1016/0378-4274(96)03752-6

Doppalapudi, S., Mahira, S., & Khan, W. (2017) 'Development and in vitro assessment of psoralen and resveratrol co-loaded ultradeformable liposomes for the treatment of vitiligo', *Journal of Photochemistry and Photobiology. B, Biology*, *174*, pp. 44–57. https://doi.org/10.1016/j.jphotobiol.2017.07.007

Effiong, D., Uwah, T., Jumbo, E., & Akpabio, A. (2020) 'Nanotechnology in cosmetics: Basics, current trends and safety concerns—A review', *Advances in Nanoparticles*, *9*, pp. 1–22. https://doi.org/10.4236/anp.2020.91001.

Elavia, P. (2018) 'A review on applications of nanotechnology in cosmetics', *International Research Journal of Pharmacy, 9*(4). https://doi.org/10.7897/2230–8407.09452

Ermini, M. L., Summa, M., Zamborlin, A., Frusca, V., Mapanao, A. K., Mugnaioli, E., Bertorelli, R., & Voliani, V. (2023) 'Copper nano-architecture topical cream for the accelerated recovery of burnt skin', *Nanoscale Advances*, *5*(4), pp. 1212–1219. https://doi.org/10.1039/d2na00786j

Evangelista, M., Mota, S., Almeida, I. F., & Pereira, M. G. (2022) 'Usage patterns and self-esteem of female consumers of antiageing cosmetic products', *Cosmetics*, *9*(3), p. 49. https://doi.org/10.3390/cosmetics9030049

Exposures Add Up – Survey Results. (2004). https://www.ewg.org/news-insights/news/2004/12/exposures-add-survey-results (Accessed: 3 February 2023).

Farboud, E., Nasrollahi, S.A., & Tabakhi, Z. (2011) 'Novel formulation and evaluation of a Q10-loaded solid lipid nanoparticle cream: In vitro and in vivo studies', *International Journal of Nanomedicine*, *6*, pp. 611–617. https://doi.org/10.2147/IJN.S16815

Favoreto, M. W., Madureira, M. P., Hass, V., Maran, B. M., Parreiras, S. O., Borges, C. P. F., Reis, A., & Loguercio, A. D. (2021) 'A novel carbamide peroxide polymeric nanoparticle bleaching gel: Color change and hydrogen peroxide penetration inside the pulp cavity', *Journal of Esthetic and Restorative Dentistry*, *33*(2), pp. 277–283. https://doi.org/10.1111/jerd.12652

Fruchon, S., & Poupot, R. (2017) 'Pro-inflammatory versus anti-inflammatory effects of dendrimers: The two faces of immuno-modulatory nanoparticles', *Nanomaterials*, *7*(9), p. 251. https://doi.org/10.3390/nano7090251

Fytianos, G., Rahdar, A., & Kyzas, G. Z. (2020) 'Nanomaterials in cosmetics: Recent updates', *Nanomaterials*, *10*(5), p. 979. https://doi.org/10.3390/nano10050979

Garg, G., Saraf, S., & Saraf, S. (2007) 'Cubosomes: An overview', *Biological & Pharmaceutical Bulletin*, *30*(2), pp. 350–353. https://doi.org/10.1248/bpb.30.350

Gautam, A., Singh, D., & Vijayaraghavan, R. (2011) 'Dermal exposure of nanoparticles: An understanding', *Journal of Cell and Tissue Research*, *11*, pp. 2703–2708.

Główka, E., Wosicka-Frąckowiak, H., Hyla, K., Stefanowska, J., Jastrzębska, K., Klapiszewski, Ł., Jesionowski, T., & Cal, K. (2014) 'Polymeric nanoparticles-embedded organogel for roxithromycin delivery to hair follicles', *European Journal of Pharmaceutics and Biopharmaceutics: Official Journal of Arbeitsgemeinschaft fur Pharmazeutische Verfahrenstechnik e.V*, *88*(1), pp. 75–84.

Golchai, J., Khani, S. H., Heidarzadeh, A., Eshkevari, S. S., Alizade, N., & Eftekhari, H. (2010) 'Comparison of anxiety and depression in patients with acne vulgaris and healthy individuals', *Indian Journal of Dermatology*, *55*(4), pp. 352–354. https://doi.org/10.4103/0019-5154.74539

Gonçalves, C., Ramalho, M. J., Silva, R., Silva, V., Marques-Oliveira, R., Silva, A. C., Pereira, M. C., et al. (2021) 'Lipid nanoparticles containing mixtures of antioxidants to improve skin care and cancer prevention', *Pharmaceutics*, *13*(12), p. 2042. https://doi.org/10.3390/pharmaceutics13122042

Goodarzi, S., Da Ros, T., Conde, J., Sefat, F., & Mozafari, M. (2017). Fullerene: Biomedical engineers get to revisit an old friend. *Materials Today*, *20*(8), pp. 460–480. https://doi.org/10.1016/j.mattod.2017.03.017

Gupta, A. K., & Foley, K. A. (2014) '5% Minoxidil: Treatment for female pattern hair loss', *Skin Therapy Letter*, *19*(6), pp. 5–7.

Hamid Reza Ahmadi Ashtiani, P. B., Bishe, P., Lashgari, N. A., Nilforoushzadeh, M. A., & Zare, S. (2016) 'Liposomes in cosmetics', *Journal of Skin and Stem Cell*, *3*(3), p. e65815. https://doi.org/10.5812/jssc.65815

Hatem, S., Elkheshen, S. A., Kamel, A. O., Nasr, M., Moftah, N. H., Ragai, M. H., Elezaby, R. S., & El Hoffy, N. M. (2022) 'Functionalized chitosan nanoparticles for cutaneous delivery of a skin whitening agent: An approach to clinically augment the therapeutic efficacy for melasma treatment', *Drug Delivery*, *29*(1), pp. 1212–1231. https://doi.org/10.1080/10717544.2022.2058652

Health Canada (2022) 'Nanomaterials', *Government of Canada*. Canada.ca. https://www.canada.ca/en/health-canada/services/chemical-substances/nanomaterials.html (Accessed: 10 January 2023).

Iacovelli, N. A., Torrente, Y., Ciuffreda, A., Guardamagna, V. A., Gentili, M., Giacomelli, L., & Sacerdote, P. (2020) 'Topical treatment of radiation-induced dermatitis: Current issues and potential solutions', *Drugs in Context*, *9*, p. 2020-4-7. https://doi.org/10.7573/dic.2020-4-7

Jegasothy, S. M., Zabolotniaia, V., & Bielfeldt, S. (2014) 'Efficacy of a new topical nano-hyaluronic acid in humans', *The Journal of Clinical and Aesthetic Dermatology*, *7*(3), pp. 27–29.

Jeswani, G., Das Paul, S., Chablani, L., & Ajazuddin (2019) 'Safety and toxicity counts of nanocosmetics', in: Cornier, J., Keck, C., & Van de Voorde, M. (eds), *Nanocosmetics*, pp. 299–335. https://doi.org/10.1007/978-3-030-16573-4_14

Joshi, M. D., & Müller, R. H. (2009) 'Lipid nanoparticles for parenteral delivery of actives', *European Journal of Pharmaceutics and Biopharmaceutics: Official Journal of Arbeitsgemeinschaft fur Pharmazeutische Verfahrenstechnik e.V*, *71*(2), pp. 161–172. https://doi.org/10.1016/j.ejpb.2008.09.003

Junevičius, J., Žilinskas, J., Česaitis, K., Česaitienė, G., Gleiznys, D., & Maželienė, Ž. (2015) 'Antimicrobial activity of silver and gold in toothpastes: A comparative analysis', *Stomatologija*, *17*(1), pp. 9–12.

Jurairattanaporn, N., Chalermchai, T., Ophaswongse, S., & Udompataikul, M. (2017) 'Comparative trial of silver nanoparticle gel and 1% clindamycin gel when use in combination with 2.5% benzoyl peroxide in patients with moderate acne vulgaris', *Journal of the Medical Association of Thailand = Chotmaihet thangphaet*, *100*(1), pp. 78–85.

Kaul, S., Gulati, N., Verma, D., Mukherjee, S., & Nagaich, U. (2018) 'Role of nanotechnology in cosmeceuticals: A review of recent advances', *Journal of Pharmaceutics*, 2018, p. 3420204. https://doi.org/10.1155/2018/3420204

Kaur, A., Katiyar, S. S., Kushwah, V., & Jain, S. (2017) 'Nanoemulsion loaded gel for topical co-delivery of clobitasol propionate and calcipotriol in psoriasis', *Nanomedicine: Nanotechnology, Biology, and Medicine*, *13*(4), pp. 1473–1482. https://doi.org/10.1016/j.nano.2017.02.009

Khan, S., Jain, P., Jain, S., Jain, R., Bhargava, S., & Jain, A. (2018) 'Topical delivery of erythromycin through cubosomes for acne', *Pharmaceutical Nanotechnology*, *6*(1), pp. 38–47. https://doi.org/10.2174/2211738506666180209100222

Khosa, A., Reddi, S., & Saha, R. N. (2018) 'Nanostructured lipid carriers for site-specific drug delivery', *Biomedicine & Pharmacotherapy = Biomedecine & pharmacotherapie*, *103*, pp. 598–613. https://doi.org/10.1016/j.biopha.2018.04.055

Komaiko, J., & McClements, D. J. (2015) 'Low-energy formation of edible nanoemulsions by spontaneous emulsification: Factors influencing particle size', *Journal of Food Engineering*, *146*, pp. 122–128. https://doi.org/10.1016/j.jfoodeng.2014.09.003

Kuenen, J., Pomar-Portillo, V., Vilchez, A., Visschedijk, A., Gon, H. D. van der, Vázquez-Campos, S., Nowack, B., & Adam, V. (2020) 'Inventory of country-specific emissions of engineered nanomaterials throughout the life cycle', *Environmental Science: Nano*, *7*, pp. 3824–3839.

Lau, M., Waag, F., & Barcikowski, S. (2017) 'Direct integration of laser-generated nanoparticles into transparent nail polish: The plasmonic 'Goldfinger'', *Industrial & Engineering Chemistry Research*, *56*(12), pp. 3291–3296. https://doi.org/10.1021/acs.iecr.7b00039

Lee, B.K. (1970) The effect of anionic and nonionic detergents on soil microfungi, *Canadian Journal of Botany*, *48*(3), pp. 583–9.

Lee, H. Y., Jeong, Y. I., Kim, D. H., & Choi, K. C. (2013) 'Permanent hair dye-incorporated hyaluronic acid nanoparticles', *Journal of Microencapsulation*, *30*(2), pp. 189–197. https://doi.org/10.3109/02652048.2012.714412

Leon-Méndez, G., Osorio-Fortich, M., Ortega-Toro, R., Pajaro-Castro, N., Torrenegra-Alarcón, M., & Herrera-Barros, A. (2018) 'Design of an emulgel-type cosmetic with antioxidant activity using active essential oil microcapsules of thyme (*Thymus vulgaris L.*), cinnamon (*Cinnamomum verum J.*), and clove (*Eugenia caryophyllata T.*)', *International Journal of Polymer Science*, *8*, p. 287439.

Lima, A. M., Pizzol, C. D., Monteiro, F. B., Creczynski-Pasa, T. B., Andrade, G. P., Ribeiro, A. O., & Perussi, J. R. (2013) 'Hypericin encapsulated in solid lipid nanoparticles: Phototoxicity and photodynamic efficiency', *Journal of Photochemistry and Photobiology. B, Biology*, *125*, pp. 146–154. https://doi.org/10.1016/j.jphotobiol.2013.05.010

Mallick, S., Nag, M., Lahiri, D., Pandit, S., Sarkar, T., Pati, S., Nirmal, N. P., Edinur, H. A., Kari, Z. A., Ahmad Mohd Zain, M. R., & Ray, R. R. (2022) 'Engineered nanotechnology: An effective therapeutic platform for the chronic cutaneous wound', *Nanomaterials*, *12*(5), pp. 1–34. https://doi.org/10.3390/nano12050778.

Marzuki, N.H.C., Wahab, R.A., & Hamid, M.A. (2019) 'An overview of nanoemulsion: Concepts of development and cosmeceutical applications', *Biotechnology & Biotechnological Equipment*, *33*, pp. 779–797. https://doi.org/10.1080/13102818.2019.1620124

Moraes, C. A. P., & Vieira, A. R. (2020) 'Nanomaterials for lip and nail cares applications', in *Nanocosmetics*, pp. 375–389. https://doi.org/10.1016/B978-0-12-822286-7.00029-2

Morganti, P., Fabrizi, G., Palombo, P., Palombo, M., Guarneri, F., Cardillo, A., Morganti, G. (2012) New chitin complexes and their anti-aging activity from inside out. *The Journal of Nutrition, Health and Aging*, *16*(3), pp. 242–5.

Morganti, P. (2010) 'Use and potential of nanotechnology in cosmetic dermatology', *Clinical, Cosmetic and Investigational Dermatology*, *3*, pp. 5–13. https://doi.org/10.2147/ccid.s4506

Mousavi, S. Z., Nafisi, S., & Maibach, H. I. (2017) 'Fullerene nanoparticle in dermatological and cosmetic applications', *Nanomedicine: Nanotechnology, Biology, and Medicine*, *13*(3), pp. 1071–1087. https://doi.org/10.1016/j.nano.2016.10.002

Mulholland, E. J. (2020) 'Electrospun biomaterials in the treatment and prevention of scars in skin wound healing', *Frontiers in Bioengineering and Biotechnology*, *8*, p. 481. https://doi.org/10.3389/fbioe.2020.00481

Nafisi, S., & Maibach, H. I. (2018) 'Skin penetration of nanoparticles', in *Emerging Nanotechnologies in Immunology*, pp. 47–88. https://doi.org/10.1016/B978-0-323-40016-9.00003-8

Nasir, A., Harikumar, S., & Amanpreet, K. (2012) 'Niosomes: An excellent tool for drug delivery', *International Journal of Research in Pharmacy and Chemistry*, *2*(2), pp. 479–487.

Oberdörster, G., Oberdörster, E., & Oberdörster, J. (2005) 'Nanotoxicology: An emerging discipline evolving from studies of ultrafine particles', *Environmental Health Perspectives*, *113*(7), pp. 823–839. https://doi.org/10.1289/ehp.7339

Ostiguy, C., Roberge, B., Woods, C., & Soucy, B. (2010) 'Engineered nanoparticles: Current knowledge about OHS risks and prevention measures', *Robert-Sauvé Research Institute for Occupational Health and Safety, Studies and Research Projects*, 2nd Edition. Institut de recherche Robert-Sauvé en santé et en sécurité du travail, Montréal (Québec). https://www.irsst.qc.ca/media/documents/PubIRSST/R-656.pdf

Panchal, A., Fakhrullina, G., Fakhrullin, R., & Lvov, Y. (2018) 'Self-assembly of clay nanotubes on hair surface for medical and cosmetic formulations', *Nanoscale, 10*(38), pp. 18205–18216. https://doi.org/10.1039/c8nr05949g

Pardeike, J., Hommoss, A., & Müller, R. H. (2009) 'Lipid nanoparticles (SLN, NLC) in cosmetic and pharmaceutical dermal products', *International Journal of Pharmaceutics, 366*(1–2), pp. 170–184. https://doi.org/10.1016/j.ijpharm.2008.10.003

Patel, R. P., & Joshi, J. R. (2012) 'An overview on nanoemulsion: A novel approach', *International Journal of Pharmaceutical Sciences and Research, 3*(12), pp. 4640–4650. https://doi.org/10.13040/IJPSR.0975-8232.3(12).4640-50

Pelle, E., Mammone, T., Maes, D., & Frenkel, K. (2005) 'Keratinocytes act as a source of reactive oxygen species by transferring hydrogen peroxide to melanocytes', *The Journal of Investigative Dermatology, 124*(4), pp. 793–797. https://doi.org/10.1111/j.0022-202X.2005.23661.x

Pereda, M.D.C.V., Polezel, M.A., de Campos Dieamant, G., Nogueira, C., Marcelino, A.G., Rossan, M.R., & Santana, M.H.A. (2012) *Sericin Cationic Nanoparticles for Application in Products for Hair and Dyed Hair*, United States Patent and Trademark Office. Patent US20120164196 A1, 28 June 2012. https://patents.google.com/patent/US20120164196A1/en (Accessed: 12 January, 2023).

Pereira, L., Dias, N., Carvalho, J., Fernandes, S., Santos, C., & Lima, N. (2014) 'Synthesis, characterization and antifungal activity of chemically and fungal-produced silver nanoparticles against *Trichophyton rubrum*', *Journal of Applied Microbiology, 117*(6), pp. 1601–1613. https://doi.org/10.1111/jam.12652

Petersen, R. (2008). *Nanocrystals for Use in Topical Cosmetic Formulations and Method of Production Thereof.* U.S. Patent and Trademark Office. US Patent 60/866233. https://patents.google.com/patent/US9114077B2/en (Accessed: 12 January, 2023).

Posada, O. M., Tate, R. J., & Grant, M. H. (2015) 'Toxicity of cobalt-chromium nanoparticles released from a resurfacing hip implant and cobalt ions on primary human lymphocytes in vitro', *Journal of Applied Toxicology, 35*(6), pp. 614–622. https://doi.org/10.1002/jat.3100

Pravalika, G., Chandhana, P., Chiranjitha, I., & Dhurke, R. (2020) 'Minoxidil ethosomes for treatment of alopecia', *International Journal of Recent Scientific Research, 11*, pp. 37112–37117.

Prow, T. W., Grice, J. E., Lin, L. L., Faye, R., Butler, M., Becker, W., Wurm, E. M., Yoong, C., Robertson, T. A., Soyer, H. P., & Roberts, M. S. (2011) 'Nanoparticles and microparticles for skin drug delivery', *Advanced Drug Delivery Reviews, 63*(6), pp. 470–491. https://doi.org/10.1016/j.addr.2011.01.012

Qorri, B., DeCarlo, A., Mellon, M., & Szewczuk, M. R. (2021) 'Drug delivery systems in cancer therapy', in *Drug Delivery Devices and Therapeutic Systems*, pp. 423–454. https://doi.org/10.1016/B978-0-12-819838-4.00016-X

Ramezani, V., Honarvar, M., Seyedabadi, M., Karimollah, A., Ranjbar, A.M., & Hashemi, M. (2018) 'Formulation and optimization of transfersome containing minoxidil and caffeine', *Journal of Drug Delivery Science and Technology, 44*, pp. 129–135. https://doi.org/10.1016/j.jddst.2017.12.003

Ribeiro, F. M., de Oliveira, M. M., Singh, S., Sakthivel, T. S., Neal, C. J., Seal, S., Ueda-Nakamura, T., Lautenschlager, S. O. S., & Nakamura, C. V. (2020) 'Ceria nanoparticles decrease UVA-induced fibroblast death through cell redox regulation leading to cell survival, migration and proliferation', *Frontiers in Bioengineering and Biotechnology, 8*, p. 577557. https://doi.org/10.3389/fbioe.2020.577557

Rosen, J., Landriscina, A., & Friedman, A. (2015) 'Nanotechnology-based cosmetics for hair care', *Cosmetics*, *2*(3), pp. 211–224. https://doi.org/10.3390/cosmetics2030211

Sadurní, N., Solans, C., Azemar, N., and García-Celma, M. J. (2005) 'Studies on the formation of O/Wnano-emulsions, by low-energy emulsification methods, suitable for pharmaceutical applications', *European Journal of Pharmaceutical Sciences*, *26*, pp. 438–445. https://doi.org/10.1016/j.ejps.2005.08.001

Salehi, B., Venditti, A., Sharifi-Rad, M., Kręgiel, D., Sharifi-Rad, J., Durazzo, A., Lucarini, M., Santini, A., Souto, E. B., Novellino, E., Antolak, H., Azzini, E., Setzer, W. N., & Martins, N. (2019) 'The therapeutic potential of apigenin', *International Journal Molecular Sciences*, *20*(6), p. 1305. https://doi.org/10.3390/ijms20061305

Salvioni, L., Morelli, L., Ochoa, E., Labra, M., Fiandra, L., Palugan, L., Prosperi, D., & Colombo, M. (2021) 'The emerging role of nanotechnology in skincare', *Advances in Colloid and Interface Science*, *293*, p. 102437. https://doi.org/10.1016/j.cis.2021.102437

Santini, B., Zanoni, I., Marzi, R., Cigni, C., Bedoni, M., Gramatica, F., Palugan, L., Corsi, F., Granucci, F., & Colombo, M. (2015) 'Cream formulation impact on topical administration of engineered colloidal nanoparticles', *PLoS One*, *10*(5), p. e0126366. https://doi.org/10.1371/journal.pone.0126366

Santos, A. C., Morais, F., Simões, A., Pereira, I., Sequeira, J. A. D., Pereira-Silva, M., Veiga, F. & Ribeiro, A. (2019) 'Nanotechnology for the development of new cosmetic formulations', *Expert Opinion on Drug Delivery*, *16*(4), pp. 313–330. https://doi.org/10.1080/17425247.2019.1585426

Sarac, G., Koca, T. T., & Baglan, T. (2016) 'A brief summary of clinical types of psoriasis', *Northern Clinics of Istanbul*, *3*(1), pp. 79–82. https://doi.org/10.14744/nci.2016.16023

Schneider, S. L., & Lim, H. W. (2019) 'A review of inorganic UV filters zinc oxide and titanium dioxide', *Photodermatology, Photoimmunology & Photomedicine*, *35*(6), pp. 442–446. https://doi.org/10.1111/phpp.12439

Severino, P., Fangueiro, J. F., Chaud, M. V., Cordeiro, J., Silva, A. M., & Souto, E. B. (2016) 'Advances in nanobiomaterials for topical administrations: New galenic and cosmetic formulations', in: Grumezescu, A. M. (ed), *Nanobiomaterials in Galenic Formulations and Cosmetics*, Vol. 10, pp. 1–23. https://doi.org/10.1016/B978-0-323-42868-2.00001-2

Shang, R., Kaisarly, D., & Kunzelmann, K. H. (2022) 'Tooth whitening with an experimental toothpaste containing hydroxyapatite nanoparticles', *BMC Oral Health*, *22*(1), p. 331. https://doi.org/10.1186/s12903-022-02266-3

Shegokar, R. (2016) 'What nanocrystals can offer to cosmetic and dermal formulations', in *Nanobiomaterials in Galenic Formulations and Cosmetics*, pp. 69–91. https://doi.org/10.1016/B978-0-323-42868-2.00004-8

Sindhi, V., Gupta, V., Sharma, K., Bhatnagar, S., Kumari, R, & Dhaka, N. (2013) 'Potential applications of antioxidants – A review', *Journal of Pharmacy Research*, *7*(9), pp. 828–835. https://doi.org/10.1016/j.jopr.2013.10.001

Sibuyi, N. R. S., Moabelo, K. L., Meyer, M., Onani, M. O., Dube, A., & Madiehe, A. M. (2019) 'Nanotechnology advances towards development of targeted-treatment for obesity', *Journal of nanobiotechnology*, *17*(1), p. 122. https://doi.org/10.1186/s12951-019-0554-3

Singh, A., Garg, G., & Sharma, P. K. (2010) 'Nanospheres: A novel approach for targeted drug delivery system', *International Journal of Pharmaceutical Sciences Review and Research*, *5*(3), p. 105.

Souto, E. B., Baldim, I., Oliveira, W. P., Rao, R., Yadav, N., Gama, F. M., & Mahant, S. (2020a) 'SLN and NLC for topical, dermal, and transdermal drug delivery', *Expert Opinion on Drug Delivery*, *17*(3), pp. 357–377. https://doi.org/10.1080/17425247.2020.1727883

Souto, E. B., Dias-Ferreira, J., Shegokar, R., Durazzo, A., & Santini, A. (2020b) 'Ethical issues in research and development of nanoparticles', *Drug Delivery Aspects*, pp. 157–168. https://doi.org/10.1016/B978-0-12-821222-6.00007-5

Souto, E. B., Fernandes, A. R., Martins-Gomes, C., Coutinho, T. E., Durazzo, A., Lucarini, M., Souto, S. B., Silva, A. M., & Santini, A. (2020c) 'Nanomaterials for skin delivery of cosmeceuticals and pharmaceuticals', *Applied Sciences*, *10*(5), p. 1594. https://doi.org/10.3390/app10051594

Taheri, A., & Mohammadi, M. (2015) 'The use of cellulose nanocrystals for potential application in topical delivery of hydroquinone', *Chemical Biology & Drug Design*, *86*(1), pp. 102–106. https://doi.org/10.1111/cbdd.12466

Tiwari, N., Pandit, R., Gaikwad, S., Gade, A., & Rai, M. (2017) 'Biosynthesis of zinc oxide nanoparticles by petals extract of *Rosa indica* L., its formulation as nail paint and evaluation of antifungal activity against fungi causing onychomycosis', *IET Nanobiotechnology*, *11*(2), pp. 205–211. https://doi.org/10.1049/iet-nbt.2016.0003

Tsuji, J. S., Maynard, A. D., Howard, P. C., James, J. T., Lam, C. W., Warheit, D. B., & Santamaria, A. B. (2006) 'Research strategies for safety evaluation of nanomaterials, part IV: Risk assessment of nanoparticles', *Toxicological Sciences: An Official Journal of the Society of Toxicology*, *89*(1), pp. 42–50. https://doi.org/10.1093/toxsci/kfi339

Raj, S., Jose, S., Sumod, U. S., & Sabitha, M. (2012) 'Nanotechnology in cosmetics: Opportunities and challenges', *Journal of Pharmacy & Bioallied Sciences*, *4*(3), pp. 186–193. https://doi.org/10.4103/0975-7406.99016

Wan, Q., Huang, B., Li, T., Xiao, Y., He, Y., Du, W., Wang, B. Z., Dakin, G. F., Rosenbaum, M., Goncalves, M. D., Chen, S., Leong, K. W., & Qiang, L. (2022) 'Selective targeting of visceral adiposity by polycation nanomedicine', *Nature Nanotechnology*, *17*(12), pp. 1311–1321. https://doi.org/10.1038/s41565-022-01249-3

Wang, K., Ruan, J., Song, H., Zhang, J., Wo, Y., Guo, S., & Cui, D. (2011) 'Biocompatibility of Graphene Oxide', *Nanoscale Research Letters*, *6*(1), p. 8. https://doi.org/10.1007/s11671-010-9751-6

Weinberger, N. A., Kersting, A., Riedel-Heller, S. G., & Luck-Sikorski, C. (2016) 'Body dissatisfaction in individuals with obesity compared to normal-weight individuals: A systematic review and meta-analysis', *Obesity Facts*, *9*(6), pp. 424–441. https://doi.org/10.1159/000454837

Wong, M. S., Alverez, P. J. J., Akcin, N., Nutt, M. O., Miller, J. T., & Heck, K. N. (2008) 'Cleaner water using bimetallic nanoparticle catalysts', *Journal of Chemical Technology and Biotechnology*, *84*(2), pp. 158–166. https://doi.org/10.1002/jctb.2002

Wu, W., Samet, J. M., Peden, D. B., & Bromberg, P. A. (2010) 'Phosphorylation of p65 is required for zinc oxide nanoparticle-induced interleukin 8 expression in human bronchial epithelial cells', *Environmental Health Perspectives*, *118*(7), pp. 982–987. https://doi.org/10.1289/ehp.0901635

Van Tran, V., Moon, J., & Lee, Y. (2019) 'Liposomes for delivery of antioxidants in cosmeceuticals: Challenges and development strategies', *Journal of Controlled Release*, *300*, pp. 114–140. https://doi.org/10.1016/j.jconrel.2019.03.003

Vance, M. E., Kuiken, T., Vejerano, E. P., McGinnis, S. P., Hochella, M. F., Jr., Rejeski, D., & Hull, M. S. (2015) 'Nanotechnology in the real world: Redeveloping the nanomaterial consumer products inventory', *Beilstein Journal of Nanotechnology*, 6, pp. 1769–1780. https://doi.org/10.3762/bjnano.6.181

Yadwade, R., Gharpure, S., & Ankamwar, B. (2021) 'Nanotechnology in cosmetics pros and cons', *Nano Express,* 2(2), p. 022003. https://doi.org/10.1088/2632-959X/abf46b

Yang, J., & Kim, B. (2018) 'Synthesis and characterization of ethosomal carriers containing cosmetic ingredients for enhanced transdermal delivery of cosmetic ingredients', *Korean Journal of Chemical Engineering*, *35*, pp. 792–797. https://doi.org/10.1007/s11814-017-0344-2

Yapar, E. A., & Inal, O. (2012) 'Nanomaterials and cosmetics', *Journal of Pharmacy of Istanbul University*, *42*(1), pp. 43–70.

Zhang, X. D., Wu, H. Y., Wu, D., Wang, Y. Y., Chang, J. H., Zhai, Z. B., Meng, A. M., Liu, P. X., Zhang, L. A., & Fan, F. Y. (2010) 'Toxicologic effects of gold nanoparticles in vivo by different administration routes', *International Journal of Nanomedicine*, *5*, pp. 771–781. https://doi.org/10.2147/IJN.S8428

Zhou, Z., Lenk, R., Dellinger, A., MacFarland, D., Kumar, K., Wilson, S. R., & Kepley, C. L. (2009) 'Fullerene nanomaterials potentiate hair growth', *Nanomedicine: Nanotechnology, Biology, and Medicine*, *5*(2), pp. 202–207. https://doi.org/10.1016/j.nano.2008.09.005

Zielińska, A., & Nowak, I. (2016) 'Solid lipid nanoparticles and nanostructured lipid carriers as novel carriers for cosmetic ingredients', in *Nanobiomaterials in Galenic Formulations and Cosmetics*, pp. 231–255. https://doi.org/10.1016/B978-0-323-42868-2.00010-3

21 Stimuli-Responsive DNA Device for Biomedical Applications

Garima Tripathi, Sagnik Nag, Pratik Gravit, Shrestha Dutta, Purvesh Kadam, Soumyadeep Basu, and Shubhrima Ghosh

21.1 INTRODUCTION

One of the most progressive areas of DNA nanotechnology is the emergence and advancement of stimuli-dependent nanodevices, which function on the programmability of the dynamic structure and motifs of DNA. The dynamic DNA nanostructures (DDNs) are smart nanograde molecules, which are responsive to different kinds of external stimuli like pH, heat, temperature, metal ions, light, etc. and endogenous stimuli of biomolecules like ATP, GSH, ROS, etc. (Chen and Shi, 2022). Due to their dynamic nature and superior stimuli-responsive characteristics, they are now being widely used in biomedical applications like sensing, bioimaging, and detection of different molecules (Figure 21.1). The most important challenge to overcome while handling nanodevices is the management of the self-assembly of nucleotides. Assembly of these DDNs can be improved under the conjugation of nanoparticles, which are further modified and responsive to different stimuli subjected to them. This makes them biocompatible and suitable for different kinds of therapeutic applications. The DNA origami technology has facilitated the formulation of different types of nanodevices, which have a spatial design, accurate geometries, and dynamic nanograde reactivity (Loretan et al., 2020). Different kinds of functional molecules, like peptides, fluorescent probes, nanoparticles, and proteins, can be easily incorporated in the DDNs, with nanoscale precision. These structures, according to the stimuli responses, can change their respective conformations, making them fit for different types of biomedical applications. The combination of biomolecular logic gates with nanostructures has paved a new path in the medical diagnostics of diseases. It has made the Boolean logic computation utilized for biorecognition, biocatalysis, and bioinformation. Due to the specificity and reduced side effects, stimuli-responsive DNA nanodevices can be used as intelligent carriers for drug delivery in diseases such as cancer and neurodegenerative disorders. The engineered framework of DDNs, associated with different endogenous and exogenous stimuli, helps initiate a sorted arrangement of reactions that simultaneously have paved paths for targeted drug delivery using DNA nanodevices. These devices, in conjugation with the nanoparticles, facilitate controlled and

DOI: 10.1201/9781003432661-21

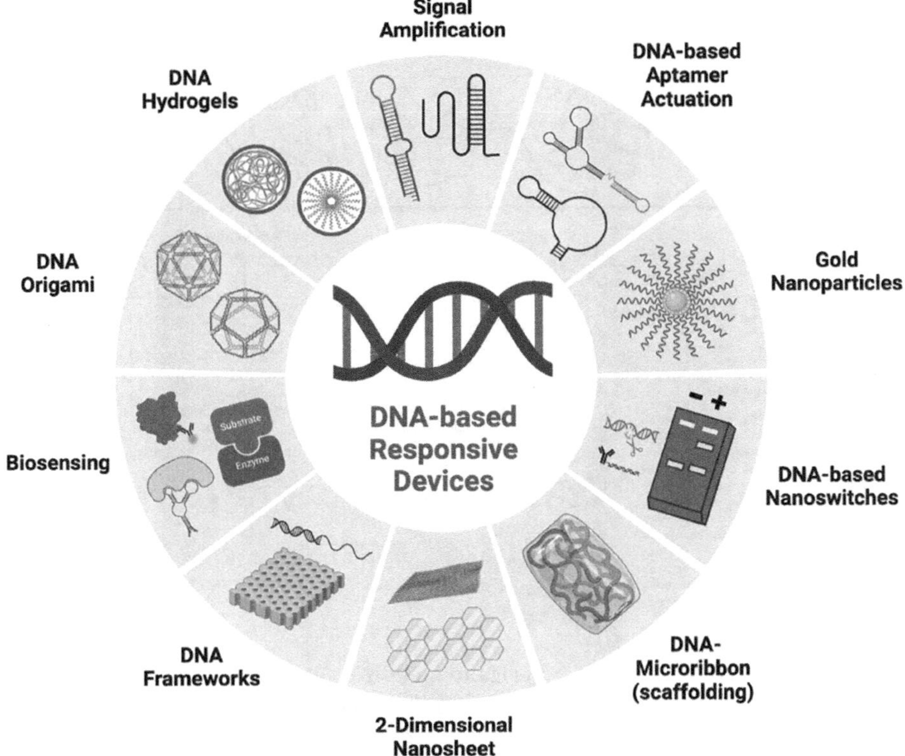

FIGURE 21.1 Multimodal applications of DNA responsive devices. Diagrammatic representation of the various implementation areas of DNA based responsive systems.

sustained release of the drug, which further attributes to the regulation of cellular behavior and enhances regenerative therapeutics.

Switchable DNA hydrogels are a very recent mode of diagnosis that has been exclusively constructed from the DNA molecule (Motoi et al., 2019). DNA molecules are used in cross-linking the hydrogels, increasing their specificity and making them stimuli-responsive. The different kinds of stimuli that the DNA nanodevices are sensitive to are - pH, light, temperature, metal ions, molecular modifications, enzymes, and others. These stimuli make these devices suitable for a specific and sensitive detection of the molecule under consideration. The consequent implications of these works are noticed in different biomedical applications like biosensors, drug delivery, biocompatibility, detection, and diagnosis of diseases.

21.2 DNA-BASED SYSTEMS AND DESIGN CONSIDERATIONS

DNA has been conceived as an important and intelligent tool for building functional nanomaterials, and this has not only been highlighted in its biocompatible, easily programmable, and manipulative attributes but also in its implementation in the form of varied systems and designs for biomedical applications (Figure 21.2). DNA-template

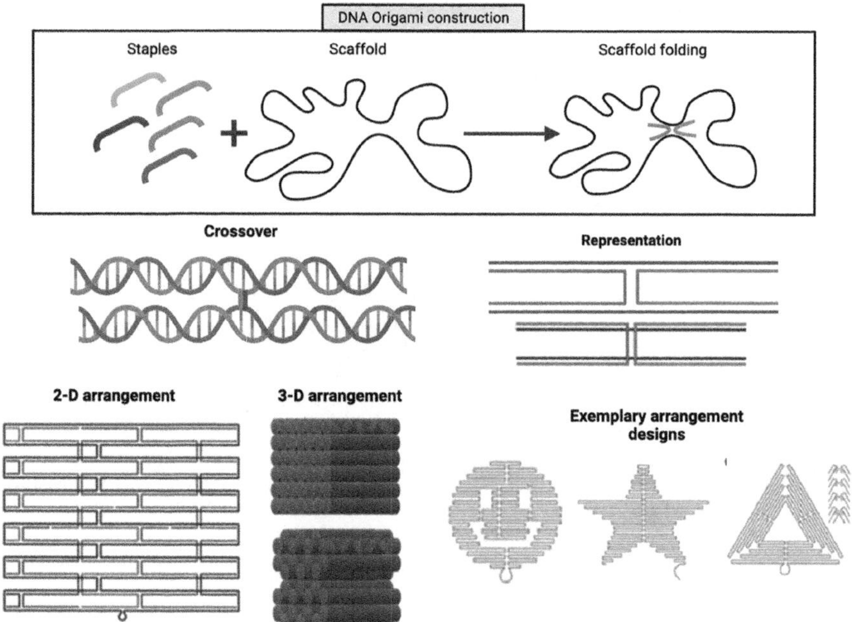

FIGURE 21.2 Overall DNA based origami and different shapes. Diagrammatic representation of how DNA origami is constructed by the process of scaffold folding, he different structural arrangement formations (2-dimensional and 3-dimensional) along with exemplary design configurations.

systems and their unique designs have been applied in various sectors such as nanoelectronics, biosensing, bioimaging, and so on. Single-stranded DNA or RNA moieties, which exhibit increased specificity termed as aptamers, upon conjugation with the nanoparticle surface bind exclusively to the overexpressed receptor molecules on the tumor cells, thereby undergoing receptor-mediated endocytosis for enhanced cellular uptake. In recent studies, the catalytic performance of DNA-aptamer-Cu nanocatalyst was analyzed, wherein the nanocatalyst showcased improved levels of fluorescence, which remained constant in its absence otherwise (You et al., 2022).

Past years have seen a surging attention on the dynamism that DNA nanodevices have shown. The controlled transitional states, directional, and rotational migration when induced by specific DNA sequences or external stimuli such as pH changes, irradiation, electromagnetic spectral induction, etc., have raised its bar in uniqueness. Hybridized arrangement and displacement reactivity within the strands of DNA aid in the manipulation of complicated migration and attaining time-dependent behavioral patterns. DNA-based molecular tweezer structure was created whereby, toward the two ends, fluorescent-labeled donor and acceptor reporters were tagged to monitor the closing and opening effects of the tweezer using the fluorescence resonance energy transfer (FRET) technique (Liu et al., 2019). Versatile and biocompatible cross-linkers amalgamated with synthetic polymers along with functional short, sequenced DNA grafts help in building customized DNA-based hydrogels that exhibit remarkable biospecificity. Um et al. (2006) beautifully demonstrated the flexibility and three-dimensional adaptability of DNA. Since then, several effective processes have been utilized to formulate DNA-based hydrogels. DNA-based hydrogels have also displayed hierarchical architectonics, becoming catalytically active by the administration of the streptavidin-modified horseradish peroxidase when the biotinylated bottlebrush primers, which serve as interesting platforms for sheathing specific guest molecules without losing out on any portion of protein functionality, get amplified. Moreover, DNA-based hydrogels that are bound with polymer scaffolds imparting enhanced hydrophilicity result in optimized functionality due to their chemical versatility, stable nature, and availability toward hydrophilic polymers (Jian et al., 2021). Targeting the RNA configurations and reconfiguring the DNA nanoswitches from a linear "switch off" condition to a looped "switch on" condition. Specific microRNAs, ribosomal RNAs, transfer RNAs, and messenger RNAs that are isolated from complicated mixture solutions, show specific binding affinity toward the nanoswitches, and then the RNA-bound nanoswitches are effectively quantified to separate the pure RNA of a single sequence.

21.3 TYPES OF STIMULI-RESPONSIVE DNA DEVICES

Apart from being a hereditary molecule, double-stranded helical deoxyribonucleic acid (DNA) can be incorporated for the development of various nanodevices and nanostructures. The complementary base-pairing property of DNA, where G pairs with C by triple bond and A pairs with T by double bond, allows easy self-assembly of DNA structures. These DNA structures are easy to modify with the addition of some functional groups like biotin, fluorescent markers, and various enzymes like restriction endonucleases, exonucleases, and DNA ligases. They may be either single or double-stranded and respond to various stimuli like heat, light, pH, and metal ions, making them smart materials, which are easy to program for biomedical applications.

21.3.1 Thermal and Light-Responsive Systems

DNA itself is not light-responsive; hence, light-responsive material is incorporated in DNA structures to make them photoresponsive. Light as a stimulus directly interacts with molecules or bonds, which results in either bond formation or bond breakage, which indirectly affects the conformation of the molecule. Also, it is easy to control light irradiation with spatial and temporal resolution. Various mechanisms are used to control dehybridization and hybridization of DNA structures, including photocleavage, photoisomerization, photo-dimerization, photothermal and photo-rearrangement, or photo cross-linking by using light of different wavelengths such as ultraviolet (UV) 200–400 nm, visible light (vis) 400–700 nm, and near infrared light (NIR) 700–1,000 nm. Till date, various photoresponsive molecules or chromophores have been studied, such as azobenzene and its derivatives, spiropyran, and nitrobenzyl. Out of which azobenzene is widely used as switching moieties to regulate DNA hybridization. They either exist as *cis* or *trans* form, and when incorporated in helices, it either causes or inhibits DNA hybridization, where light irradiation wavelength plays a crucial role, resulting in *cis-trans* interconversion. On the other hand, spiropyrans (SP) belongs to a family of molecular photo-switches, which results in changes in chemical configuration upon light irradiation. Irradiation of UV light causes heterocyclic cleavage, forming *trans*-merocyanine form (MC), which can be reversibly brought to SP state with heat or irradiation with visible light. Škugor et al. reported a light-responsive non-autonomous DNA walker that can travel in both directions on a one-dimensional path. Two azobenzene derivatives were incorporated to facilitate *cis-trans* conformation change (Škugor et al., 2019).

In another study, Liu et al. reported a photoresponsive DNA nanotweezer, which upon UV irradiation, switched from close to open state. This conformation is brought about by the degradation of 6 nitropiperonyloxymethyl (NPOM) caging groups of the poly T (thymidine) trigger strand, which are inhibiting hybridization between the hairpin loop. UV light exposure causes cleavage of these NPOM groups, allowing the trigger strand to be open for hybridization, causing conformation change. This photocaged tweezer assembly has potential application in the efficient cargo delivery in cellular compartments (Liu et al., 2018).

DNA hybrid systems are now the topic of research because of their potential applications in sensing, drug delivery, etc. One such newly developed system is the DNA hydrogel, which can be prepared by chemical bonding (either ionic or covalent) or physical interaction with DNA strands with biocompatible polymers either natural or synthetic. Both mechanical and swelling characteristics of the gel are significantly influenced by the cross-linker, which also determines the transition from the gel to fluid state. They come in two varieties: pure (made solely of DNA and constructed by enzymatic ligation and hybridization) and hybrid (made by linking DNA strands to polymers like polyacrylamide to enable complementary base pairing). Peng et al. have engineered photo switchable light-driven hybrid DNA cross-linked hydrogel using acrylamide and azobenzene. UV and vis light were used to cause conformational change from *cis* to *trans* state (Peng et al. 2012).

Other than DNA, there are some thermo-responsive materials, which are generally incorporated in stimuli-responsive devices, such as thermo-responsive polymers like poly(N-isopropylacrylamide, PNIPAAm) and poly (propylene oxide, PPO). Out of which PNIPAAm is extensively studied as a smart material. These smart temperature-responsive polymers are usually classified into two types depending upon how they respond to changes in temperature (i) polymers having a lower critical solution temperature (LCST) and (ii) polymers having an upper critical solution temperature (UCST). PNIPAAm has been reported to have LCST behavior with LCST temperature ranging from 30°C–35°C. Nagahara et al. have reported the first water-soluble DNA hydrogel using water-soluble copolymer poly (N, N, - dimethylacrylamide co-N-acryloyloxysuccinimide)s in which oligodeoxyribonucleotides (ODNs) were incorporated in the side chains of the polymer using complementary base pairing (Nagahara & Matsuda, 1996). In another study, Xu et al. prepared a 3D assembled graphene/DNA composite hydrogel having higher mechanical strength and self-healing properties (Xu et al., 2010).

21.3.2 Enzymatic-Responsive Systems

Enzymes are also one of the widely used stimuli incorporated in nanodevices. The majority of the metabolic pathways in the living system are regulated by various classes of enzymes. These molecular machineries catalyze broad range of biochemical reactions, which are highly substrate-specific and have a greater turnover rate in terms of product formation. Moreover, these enzymes play a significant role in the clinical state, exhibiting altered expression and serving as a disease biomarker in a wide range of diseases, including cancer and numerous metabolic disorders, for example, in terms of cancer, these enzymes facilitate tumor progression and metastasis, which includes several proteases and phospholipases. Hence, enzymes are one of the promising candidates to be used in DNA nanotechnology.

Several DNA-specific enzymes that employ DNA as a substrate, such as nucleases, ligases, and polymerases, cause modifications to DNA structure. Del Grosso et al. have constructed DNA nanodevices incorporating various classes of proton-generating enzymes, which brought pH change in the systems regulating nanoswitching dynamics. First, a detoxifying enzyme called glutathione (GSH) transferase was added along with its substrate, which causes the production of a strong acid called HCl and the formation of triplex, which closes the nanoswitching. By varying the concentration of GSH, the dynamics of the nanoswitch can be precisely controlled. This closed nanoswitched structure was further opened by the addition of urease, a hydrolase that forms ammonia and CO_2, when urea is introduced. Triplex structure destabilization caused by ammonia generation causes the nano switch to open, and it may be precisely controlled by changing the substrate's concentration. Under acidic conditions (HCl production), the system favors formation of a stable DNA triplex, which acts as padlock which restricts strand, displacement whereas the basic condition (ammonia production) causes strand displacement as a result of the unstable triplex. These DNA nanoswitches belong to the family of DNA nanodevices, which further includes tweezers, molecular motors, walkers, and nanomachines. Acetylcholinesterase (AchE), a type of hydrolase, was incorporated to further analyze its use in drug/ligand unloading. When its substrate, acetylcholine, is present, AchE produces acetic acid along with thiocholine, which causes cytosines in the helix to behave as bases and accept proton from the acetic acid that was produced as a result of hydrolysis of acetylcholine (Del Grosso et al., 2015). These enzyme-responsive DNA-based nanomachines can be a useful substitute for controlled drug or ligand release at a defined target region.

The sensitivity, time assay, and efficiency of DNA walkers depend on various factors such as orientation, steric effects, binding affinity, charges, DNA structure, and most importantly, driving force, which can be either strand displacement, enzymatic reactions (protein or DNAzyme), photoinitiated reactions, or environmental or chemical stimulus-driven reactions. A self-assembling track is used by Yin et al. to create an autonomous unidirectional DNA walker that moves as a result of ATP hydrolysis. The three evenly spaced double-stranded anchorages on the walker track were strategically placed to allow for walker binding. In order to move forward, walker gets ligated to a subsequent anchor and chopped off from one that is behind by a restriction endonuclease. This cleavage constraint stops the walker from moving backward, enabling unidirectional mobility. Forward movement of the walker is based on alternate cleavage and ligation of anchorages. These anchorages have complementary sticky ends, making them hybridize with each other, which are further ligated by ligase, and this step consumes energy, which is obtained as a result of ATP hydrolysis. The restriction enzyme PflM I recognizes this newly created strand as its target and proceed to cleave the hybridized strand in order to produce sticky ends that are complementary to successive anchorages, and so on. DNA walker mobility is favored by this cyclical process (Yin et al., 2004). These walker devices can be promising candidates for therapeutic drug delivery and biosensor applications.

21.3.3 pH-Responsive Systems

Homeostasis is a state of body at which all the systems in the body are balanced, well functioned, and self-regulated in terms of temperature, blood pressure, and pH. The physiological pH of the human body ranges from 7.35 to 7.45, with an average of 7.40 and is necessary for multiple biochemical activities in the various metabolic pathways, including protein folding, oxygen transport, cell and enzyme function, and protein synthesis. Alteration of physiological pH is usually associated with diseased state causing either acidemia (decreased pH) or alkalemia (increased pH). Hence pH serves as an important external stimulus to be incorporated in DNA nanodevices necessary for diagnosis, targeted drug delivery, and other therapeutic applications. pH-responsive DNA machinery primarily works in response to pH variability between the target (or diseased) cell/tissue and normal cells. For example, tumor cells exhibit relatively higher cellular pH and lower extracellular pH (as a result of accumulated acidic metabolites) than the normal cells, which makes them suitable targets for pH-dependant DNA devices.

These pH-sensitive DNA systems are categorized into five types: (i) i-motif, (ii) triplex structure, (iii) organic molecule either protonated or deprotonated, (iv) $A^{+}{\cdot}C$ wobble pair, and (v) coordinate bonds. Out of which i-motif structures have attracted researchers' interest because of their unique hemi-protonated structure. These intercalated motifs (i-motifs) occur when two antiparallel cytosine-rich DNA sequences are joined at cytosine bases where one of the cytosines is protonated, forming a hemi-protonated quadruplex structure. It was discovered in the late 1900s by Maurice Guéron. These i-motifs are pH-sensitive and can change their configuration in acidic pH. D. Liu and Balasubramanian have reported pH-responsive DNA-based nanomachines having i-motif structure. The fundamental working principle of the machine is pH-dependent complementary base pairing of oligonucleotides. The i-motif structure is composed of two strands of ssDNA, one having four stretches of cytosine (CCC) (21nts) and the later one having only 17nts and are complementary to each other. Cytosine-rich strands being protonated in nature pair with unprotonated strands at acidic pH (pH5.0), forming a closed quadruplex i-motif structure, which further opens when the pH of the system is elevated to the basic range (pH 8.0), forming an extended duplex structure (Liu & Balasubramanian, 2003). In another study, Surana et al. have demonstrated *in vivo* application of i-motif-containing pH-sensitive DNA device for spatiotemporal mapping inside multicellular living organisms. The DNA device consists of three oligonucleotides, which upon hybridization form a four-strand structure (i-motif) referred to as i-switch, which shows open and closed configurations in response to pH ranging from 5.3 to 6.6. To analyze the *in vivo* activity of DNA i-switch scavenger cells of *C. elegans* were chosen (Surana et al., 2011).

21.3.4 Molecular Responsive Systems

NA identification plays a major role in forensic and medical studies, as simple as the structural change from linear DNA strand to loop-formed structure shows off and on signals in the absence and presence of NAs. In detail, two detector oligonucleotides can be added to the ends of one strand of DNA. This detector sequence must have a complementary sequence to the target sequence, upon which addition or presence of that the strand will get bound with the detector in the adjacent space along with the target joining that detector and proceeding to form a loop on the second strand. This oligonucleotide-induced loop DNA structure easily gets detected by normal gel electrophoresis and leads to quantification of the molecular targets (Chandrashekhar et al., 2017).

For active medication delivery at the malignant site, oligonucleotides like siRNA and microRNA have been utilized as active agents. Using nanoparticles, oligonucleotides are delivered to cancerous areas. The nanocarriers can be rearranged and released via strand displacement. The double-stranded DNA is rehybridized and dehybridized using a single-stranded oligonucleotide that is complementary to the area of the double-stranded DNA (Sabir et al., 2021). Cellular pathways in cancerous cells are very tough to be targeted with normal drugs. But therapeutic oligonucleotides (TOs) treat this cellular damage by modulating their pathways in a very precise manner. TOs, which are short DNA or RNA oligomers, are a new class of medications that can either interact with disease-related genes through complementary Watson-Crick base pairing or also recognize target proteins by forming three-dimensional secondary structures in a sequence-specific way (Wu et al., 2022). To stop the transmission of genetic information at all levels, TOs may easily be designed. TOs are frequently utilized for selective identification and binding to corresponding target molecules with high affinities to block their activities because of their structure. Several methods have been created by creating adaptable nanoparticles that can load and transport TOs to the desired target in a programmed manner in order to overcome delivery challenges. With the application of stimuli-responsive TOs, one can achieve targeted drug release in severe conditions and protect normal tissues, which otherwise get harmed by the toxicity effects.

As a quick response to regulate normal physiological processes in the body, nanofingers were invented with the help of DNA origami technology. These nanofingers are mainly made of three tweezers supported with aptamers at the end, which facilitates specific binding to the respective proteins. This binding is facilitated by reducing the distance of two aptamers upon activation by tweezer aptamer binding. A signal would cause the device to release thrombin and catch an anti-coagulation agent, such as hirudin, in the event that a person is harmed and needs temporary increased blood coagulation (Wu et al., 2016). In order to release an anti-coagulation factor and lower the level of thrombin to bring the coagulation potential back to normal, the device's structure would need to be reversed after the damage was fixed. This would assist the body to reestablish homeostasis. Nanofingers were found to detect accurate blood glucose levels, coagulation, and several metabolic processes.

21.3.5 Metal Ion-Responsive Systems

The phenomenon of sequence-specific DNA hybridization through complementary base pairing is critical to many biological processes and has also emerged as an important factor in the development of DNA-based materials.This stability enhancement can be leveraged for applications such as the metal-responsive conversion of DNA structures and the allosteric regulation of DNAzymes (Kanai et al., 2016). The potential applications of metal-mediated artificial base pairs in various fields are still being actively explored. Studies have demonstrated that metal cations can create either an ion-bridging complex or a stable intramolecular structure with the DNA backbone. Multiple metal-mediated base pairs can be incorporated within the DNA duplex, leading to the formation of specific metal assemblies that can accommodate a certain number of base pairs. These assemblies can consist of two, four, or five base pairs, depending on the nature of the metal cation involved.

DNAzymes are synthetic DNA molecules that can catalyze chemical reactions, and the activity of these molecules can be controlled by metal ions through metal-mediated base pairing. Labile metal ions, which are useful for various biochemical processes, led to numerous complications in cellular behavior in their high concentration beyond required measures. The quantification of DNAzymes produced signal can be calculated by FRET (Hwang et al., 2019). FRET is majorly used to calculate the signals from fluorescent-based sensor proteins and NAs. Also, it overcomes the concentration-based sensor and autofluorescence problem.

The scientists developed a new kind of nanocomplex termed DP-PM that is intended for gene therapy and is activated by NIR light. The two parts of DP-PM are the DNA particle (DP) and polydopamine-MnO_2 coating (PM). The DP is a nanostructure created by the synthesis of very long DNA chains with repeating DNAzyme units. The PM is created by a redox reaction between $KMnO_4$ and dopamine and is then constructed on the surface of DP by stacking interactions between DNA bases and polydopamine. NIR light radiation can activate DP-PM when it is administered to the tumor site through the increased permeability and retention effect (Zhao et al., 2021). The polydopamine in PM has the ability to transform light energy into heat, raising the temperature near the tumor. Heat stress may result from the temperature rise brought on by DP-PM, and this might further slow tumor development.

21.4 BIOMEDICAL APPLICATIONS OF STIMULI-RESPONSIVE DNA DEVICES

21.4.1 Drug Delivery

DNA molecules, due to their predictability and programmability, illustrate their capability for drug delivery. Several stimuli-responsive DNA drug delivery systems have evolved because of the ongoing advancement of DNA nanotechnology. To selectively deliver cargo to selected spaces and activate the release of loads in response to stimuli, DDNs are used as delivery systems for drugs (Wang et al., 2022).

Under an acidic pH, DNA sequences rich in cytosine tend to fold into i-motifs, which are four-stranded intercalated DNA structures. Significant advances in recent studies have shown how chemists can regulate these structures for medicines and nanobiotechnology. DNA delivery techniques now frequently use double-stranded or free structures folded into triplex and quadruplexed pH-responsive dynamic DNA (Debnath et al., 2019). The advancement and progression of different diseases are closely correlated with pH disturbances. For instance, tumor tissues showing anaerobic metabolism result in the production of numerous acidic metabolites, and acidic substances are not easily excreted because the density of blood vessels in tumor tissues is low, leading to an imbalance in the pH of the tumor tissue, which promotes the endurance and growth of cancer cells as well as transfer conditions (Alfarouk et al., 2020).

Functional NAs have been used extensively to design stimuli-responsive medication delivery in the tumor microenvironment because of their capability to target cancer cells. The main constraints on the formation of DNA-based drug delivery nanocarriers currently are their high cost, poor biostability, and difficult fabrication procedure. Rolling circle amplification (RCA) is utilized to design doxorubicin (Dox)-delivering nanoparticles for tumor-targeting chemotherapy. RCA enables the efficient collection of many functional DNAs. Additionally, the extremely long sequence of a RCA product can be suitably condensed by a magnesium ion (is a significant electrolyte in the human body), with great biocompatibility. The resulting DNA nanoparticle has a high level of biostability, which makes it a safe and suitable nanomaterial for *in vivo* application (Zhao et al., 2018).

According to recent research, double-stranded DNA forms a DNA tetrahedron (nasTET) that is used to deliver nuclear localization signal (NLS) peptide and disulfide bond-conjugated ASOs (silencing the proto-oncogene c-raf) and releases ASOs in response to reduction and the environment around the nucleus. Thus, the levels of mRNA and protein expression are significantly decreased (Yang et al., 2018). Moreover, the transport of molecular payloads has been regarded as a crucial trigger for the creation of novel molecular therapeutics. This difference provides ATP with a great amount of scope for use in the formation of responsive drug delivery systems. In order to deliver molecular payloads to living cells in response to varied stimuli, framework NA (FNA) nanocarriers controlled by a DNA-computation circuit are developed for mRNA imaging. With the use of a square pyramid (TSP) cage and a duplex cargo, scientists created an FNA, which has an embedded i-motif that can respond to pH and an ATP aptamer (ABA27) that can respond to ATP. The reaction consists of an FNA device controlled by a DNA circuit that can help in payload stimulus-response release, followed by mRNA imaging by introducing the reaction chain of target mRNA. To trigger the toehold-mediated strand displacement (TMSD) reaction, ATP and pH are used as trigger units and trigger footholds in turn (Wang et al., 2020).

21.4.2 Point-of-Care (POC) Devices

Point-of-care testing is a type of test where medical tests for diagnosis are performed near the patient. In contrast to the conventional strategy, which involves conducting tests primarily in central laboratories and requires hours or days to conclude the results, POC provides a faster diagnostic option. For POCT, biosensors are frequently employed. When biological recognition structures are amalgamated with physical transducers, a biosensor can distinguish target analytes by translating the biological reaction into a quantifiable signal (Su et al., 2017).

Lateral flow tests are frequently used in medical diagnosis because they are quick, affordable, and typically yield results in 5–20 minutes. Not only for proteins and small molecules, but lateral flow tests can also be applied to identify various analytes such as lysophospholipids, pathogens, and NAs (Tominaga, 2019). A novel class of Cas-nucleases has been recently used to produce CRISPR/Cas-based NA detection methods for COVID-19 detection, which showed significant benefits like sensitivity, specificity, speed, and simplicity for detection. The CRISPR Cas13- and Cas12-based tests have been designed to detect SARS-CoV-2 using extracted NAs as input. When Cas12 binds to its target sequence as an RNA-guided DNase, it can indiscriminately break ssDNA. Researchers developed a CRISPR-Cas12-based lateral flow test to rapidly identify betacoronavirus severe acute respiratory syndrome (SARS-CoV-2) from extracted patient sample RNA in 40 minutes (Broughton et al., 2020).

Nanomaterials can be used to enhance and automate the purification of samples, which also makes sample pre-processing easier for users and boosts specificity in the POCT technique. Researchers created an easy NA purification method that utilizes magnetic nanoparticles that are introduced into the NA extraction process and is carried out in a plastic Pasteur pipette. Contrary to conventional methods, the system could extract NA in 15 minutes from a wide range of objects, including swabs, serum, milk, and pork, and the extracted material had a low detection limit for amplification after that. This technology provides an innovative concept for integrated detection in POCT devices (Kang et al., 2021).

21.4.3 Diagnosis and Therapeutics

DNA nanodevices are being actively used for the detection and sensing of biomolecules in the recent developing course of theranostics. They use nanoprobes and chips, which make it highly sensitive and durable. This helps easy detection and processing of the molecule under consideration (Yang et al., 2019). In the case of disease analysis or treatment, it helps in the quantification of the detrimental particle or biomolecule under study. DNA nanoswitches play an important role as the quantitative platform of single-molecule analysis and help in the amplification and detection of the same. Thus, DNA-mediated detection plays a critical role in clinical and medical diagnosis and testing. However, the low copy number of the DNA obtained from the sample provided makes it difficult for the biosensor to provide accurate results. Hence, hybridization chain reaction (HCR) is taken up into practice, which helps in DNA amplification in an ideal isothermal process, without the aid of any enzymes. Hence, maintaining the purity and integrity of the DNA strand under consideration (Bi et al., 2017). DNA-based nanosensors work on the principle of strand displacement. Studies show that researchers developed a system that helps in the development of a pH-responsive, and full reversible HCR system for imaging induced by pH changes (Jiang et al., 2020). They help in the evaluation of cell surface and molecular grade detection, which can be modulated by the stimuli reprimanded at the given time and temperature.

DNA plays a significant role in controlling biological processes in living cells. Like proteins such as transcription factors, small drug molecules also adhere to DNA to modulate its function. The development of innovative NA-based biosensors using various types of nanostructures has greatly contributed to the growth in nanotechnology. The characteristic of a nanosensor is found in the similarity of the length scale of the nanostructures to the biological targets to promote superior binding interactions that more closely resemble natural interactions, which may further provide *in vivo* applications. Furthermore, the significant surface area-to-volume ratios that nanostructures offer allow a substantial number of biorecognition components to bind and collect the target analyte, greatly increasing the detection sensitivity. The capability of DNA-based fluorescent probes to identify NA and non-NA targets, as well as simple synthesis in production and chemical modifications, has growing attention (Ebrahimi et al., 2020). DNA-based biosensors have recently shown significant potential as candidates to detect and diagnose diseases like malignancies through specialized techniques such as MRI, PDT, and PTT (Figure 21.3).

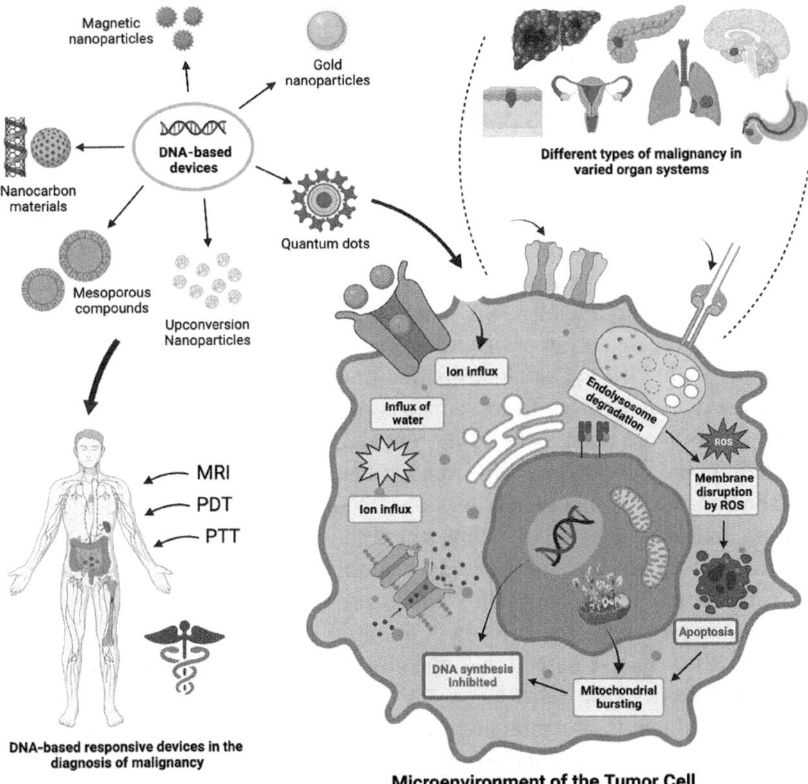

FIGURE 21.3 Mechanism of action of DNA-based devices in Biomedical Diagnostics. Diagrammatic representation of the various mediums of DNA-based responsive systems in targeting and diagnosing diseases like tumor in cancerss and detection of various malignancies in the organ systems of the body through specialized technologies such as MRI (Magnetic Resonance and Imaging), PDT (Photodynamic Therapy) and PTT (Partial Thromboplastin Time).

Silicon dioxide (SiO_2) typically ranges in size from 50 to 200 nm. It has received more attention because of its high drug loading and inert structure, which allow the ingrained pharmaceuticals to be highly stable in cells. However, some scientists have created fluorescent probes based on SiO_2 that can identify tumor-related RNAs in living cells. Wu et al. created nanoplatforms based on Ru-SiO_2@ polydopamine that enable NIR-assisted signal amplification and ratiometric imaging of miRNA in cells (Deng et al., 2021). The probe prevents false-positive signals carried on by DNase I due to its high specificity, stability, and low toxicity, providing a unique method for the specific detection of minute amounts of mRNA. SiO_2's surface has a lot of pores, which creates a suitable surface for drug loading. Hence, by combining detection and drug loading, the SiO_2 probe may utilize the properties of SiO_2.

One of the earliest uses of DNA nanodevices was for the multiplexed detection of antibodies. T switches are a type of DNA nanoswitches based on the pH-triggered triplex duplex transition of DNA strands. This can help in monitoring the pH level changes in living cells (Yan et al., 2013). Recently, studies show that nanoswitches have a great amount of sensitivity to pH changes and responses accordingly. It detects the intracellular changes and was found to be stable in the acidic interference of the endosome. It could then help in the documentation of the development of an endsome by further FRET analysis. A DNA nanomachine was developed that can record the pH changes in the two endocytic pathways and help in the comparative study of the same. G-quadruplex motifs in a particular self-assembled nanostructure can help in the sensitive detection of zinc protoporphyrin IX iridium complex (Yang et al., 2020). This DNA device could readout any fluorescent signal attached to a complex formed by Pb ions and hence could help in the efficient and sensitive detection of lead. An ontriangular-shaped DNA nanotube is a dynamic detection platform that can be used for the detection of different types of target molecules bound to a single system (Dai et al., 2017). The nanotube facilitates the selective recognition with the help of three distinguishable fluorescence signals. In this particular study, three different aptamers were used as building blocks of the DNA nanotube. This can also further help in the generation of different geometries that help further binding events to the sensing device. These features on DNA nanodevices have made diagnosis accessible and available for different scientific endeavors (Liu et al., 2023). Yang et al. recently studied that an antibody-responsive DNA walker was designed that helps in the detection of antibodies and short interfering molecules in the buffer and serum samples of humans (Yang et al., 2021). Majorly pathological detection is attributed to the sensitive detection of the molecules related to the metabolic pathway of the pathogenesis of the disease.

The chemical nature of nanomaterials stimulates cell interaction. The characteristics of nanomaterials such as the size of particles, shape, texture, rigidity, charge, and the presence of functional groups. The cellular uptake and its interaction are stimulated by the hydrophobicity or hydrophilicity of the cellular components. There are many endocytic routes like – phagocytosis, micropinocytosis, Catherine-mediated and Caveolar-mediated endocytosis, and endocytosis mediated without Clathrin and Caveolin that have been described for the internalization of nanoparticles into the cell (Augustine et al., 2020) (Figure 21.4).

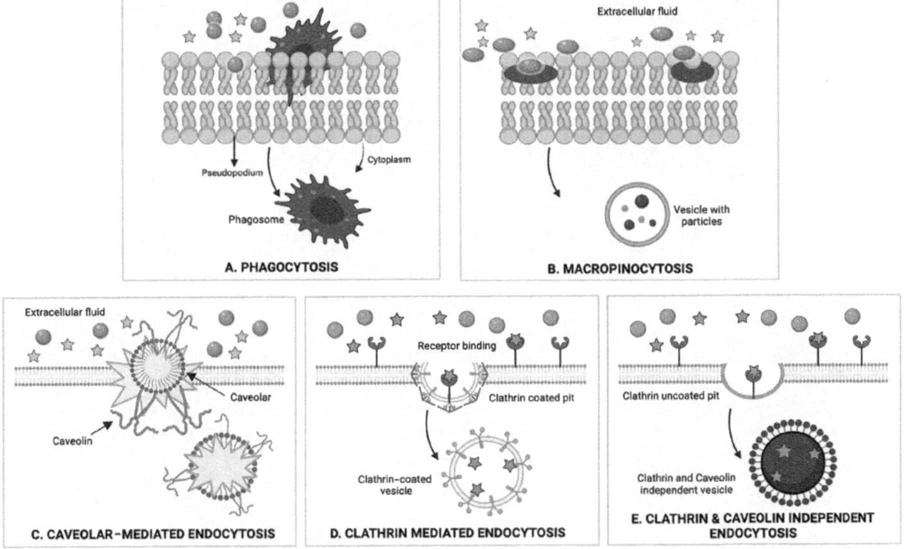

FIGURE 21.4 Mechanistic cascades for internalization DNA-bound nanoparticle hybrid. The various pathways that lead to the internalization of the DNA conjugated nanoparticles are presented as (A) Phagocytosis; (B) Macropinocytosis; (C) Caveolar activated endocytosis pathway; (D) Endocytosis caused through Clathrin and (E) Endocytosis mediated without the action of Clathrin and Caveolin.

Recently, ultrasound energy has also been used to treat cancer effectively. The core of lipospheres is filled with gas molecules that act both as contrast agents for ultrasonic imaging and as delivery systems for drugs such as microbubbles or nanobubbles. Li et al. studied the nanoparticle-assisted drug delivery system and how it can augment the analysis of images and biomedicine. In conjunction with a precision ultrasound imaging system, drug-carrying lipospheres can specifically detect tumor tissue and deliver drugs to tumor cells to augment the capability of nanocomposites for treating cancer (Li et al., 2022) (Figure 21.5).

21.5 FUTURE PROSPECTIVES AND CONCLUSION

DNA nanotechnology is based on DDNs in which the structures and functions of the DNA-based nanoparticles can be predicted, programmed, easily chemically modified, made compatible with other functional NAs, and made non-toxic. The DNA nanodevices can be used as stimuli-responsive materials that have applications in targeted delivery, chemotherapy, biosensing, and immunotherapy. The disadvantages of the stimuli-responsive DNA nanodevice are its response time, which is comparatively slower and takes minutes to hours to finish, the decreased reversibility of the process, the decreased efficiency of the process, and the affected performance of the device due to the accumulation of wastes after a chemically triggered reaction. The DDNs also cannot cross the blood–brain barrier. Thus, sophisticated DNA

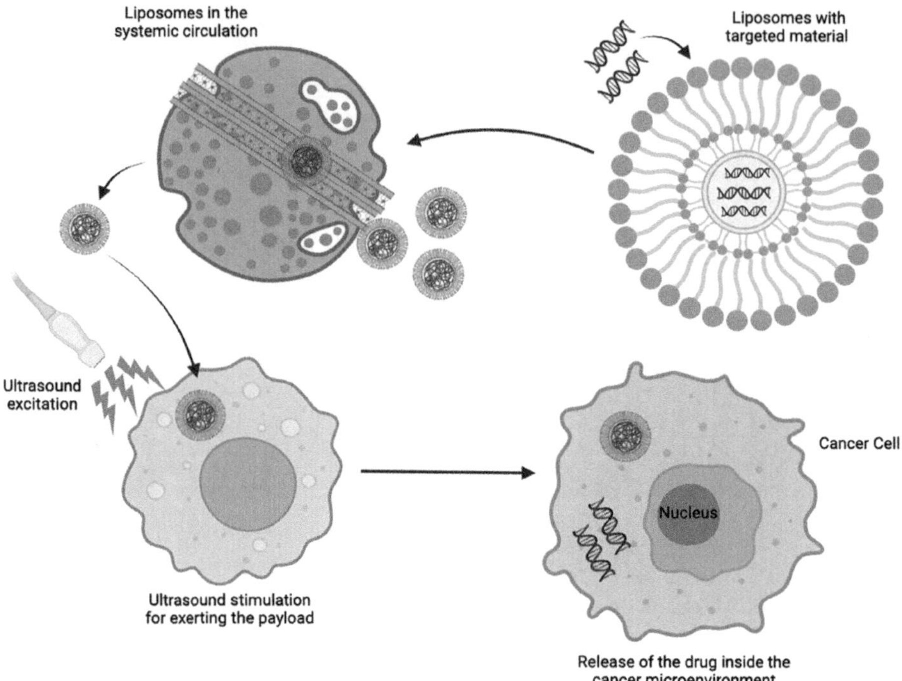

FIGURE 21.5 Ultrasound stimulated Cancer targeting. Schematic portrayal of the administration of ultrasound to excite the liposome-carrier system for targeting cancerous cells and releasing the drug for positive outcome.

nanodevice construction is required to protect against structural disassembly and enzymatic degradation. The DDNs should be designed in a manner that their structural integrity is maintained till reaching the site of action. The non-biological stimuli are cleaner and non-invasive in nature, like the optical, electric, and magnetic stimuli. Among these, the response to the stimulus of light is easier to deal with than the electric response, the NIR being better than the UV light with good depth of penetration and biosafety. The pharmacokinetic studies of the DNA nanocarriers in vivo, like their distribution, circulation, metabolism, and excretion, need to be investigated in their clinical trial stages. The drugs where the use of DDNs has made the system of drug delivery smarter, site-specific, and non-toxic are the chemotherapeutic drugs, NA drugs, and other drugs like vancomycin, melittin, and insulin. The DDNs have also shown promising responses in tissue regeneration where they can promote bone regeneration and angiogenesis in diabetic rats (Jing et al., 2022). The cellular behavior can also be controlled by the DDNs, like the inhibition of in vitro and in vivo migration of cancer cells (Su et al., 2022).

The stimuli-responsive smart DNA-based nanocarriers thus have a wide range of possibilities to be constructed into various sizes and shapes. The application of nanotechnology has made a big impact in the field of nanomedicines, having high specificity and multiple uses in drug delivery, and beneficial roles in cancer diagnosis and treatment. But from this wide spectrum study, only a few have managed to reach the stage of clinical trial and thus need further research work. The delivery of the nanocarriers to humans is also a very challenging aspect. The surface charge, base composition and combination, and the geometry of the structure might play a major role in the pharmacokinetics and the bioavailability of the drug. The maintenance of the stimuli on a large scale is also a potential challenge in the field of DNA-based nanostructures. Thus, the DNA-based stimuli response is a rapidly emerging field with direct biomedical applications like biosensing in COVID-19 and other infectious diseases.

REFERENCES

Alfarouk K, Ahmed SBM, Ahmed A, Elliott RL, Ibrahim ME, Ali HS, Wales CC, Nourwali I, Aljarbou AN, Bashir AHH, Alhoufie STS, Alqahtani SS, Cardone RA, Fais S, Harguindey S, Reshkin SJ. (2020). The interplay of dysregulated ph and electrolyte imbalance in cancer. *Cancers*, 12, 898.

Augustine R, Hasan A, Primavera R, Wilson RJ, Thakor AS, Kevadiya BD. (2020). Cellular uptake and retention of nanoparticles: Insights on particle properties and interaction with cellular components. *Materials Today Communications*, 25, 101692.

Bi S, Yue S, Zhang S. (2017). Hybridization chain reaction: A versatile molecular tool for biosensing, bioimaging, and biomedicine. *Chemical Society Reviews*, 46, 4281–4298.

Broughton JP, Deng X, Yu G, Fasching CL, Servellita V, Singh J, Miao X, Streithorst J, Granados A, Sotomayor-Gonzalez A, et al. (2020). CRISPR–Cas12-based detection of SARS-CoV-2. *Nature Biotechnology*, 38, 870–874.

Chandrashekhar R, Ram B, Bhavani NL, Bakshi V. (2017). Molecular Docking Studies of Hydrazide-Hydrazone Derivatives of Gossypol against Bcl-2 Family Anti-Apoptotic Targets. *Drug Des, An Open Access Journal*, 6(3), 1000155. doi: 10.4172/2169-0138.1000155, ISSN: 2169-0138.

Chen Y, Shi S. (2022). Advances and prospects of dynamic DNA nanostructures in biomedical applications. *RSC advances*, 12(47), 30310–20.

Dai Z, Leung HM, Lo PK. (2017). Stimuli-responsive self-assembled DNA nanomaterials for biomedical applications. *Small*, 13, 1602881.

Debnath M, Fatma K, Dash J. (2019). Chemical regulation of DNA i-motifs for nanobiotechnology and therapeutics. *Angewandte Chemie International Edition*, 58, 2942–2957.

Del Grosso E, Dallaire, AM, Vallée-Bélisle A, Ricci F. (2015). Enzyme-operated DNA-based nanodevices. *Nano Letters*, 15, 8407–8411.

Deng X, Liu X, Wu S, Zang S, Lin X, Zhao Y, et al. (2021). Ratiometric fluorescence imaging of intracellular microRNA with NIR-assisted signal amplification by a Ru-SiO2@ Polydopamine nanoplatform. *ACS Applied Materials and Interfaces*, 13, 45214–45223.

Ebrahimi SB, Samanta D, Mirkin CA. (2020). DNA-based nanostructures for live-cell analysis. *Journal of American Chemical Society*, 142, 11343–11356.

Hwang K, Mou Q, Lake RJ, Xiong M, Holland B, Lu Y. (2019). Metal-dependent DNAzymes for the quantitative detection of metal ions in living cells: recent progress, current challenges, and latest results on FRET ratiometric sensors. *Inorganic Chemistry*, 58(20), 13696–708.

Jian X, Feng X, Luo Y, Li F, Tan J, Yin Y, Liu Y. (2021). Development, preparation, and biomedical applications of DNA-based hydrogels. *Frontiers in Bioengineering and Biotechnology*, 9, 661409.

Jiang X, Lin M, Huang J, Mulan M, Liu H, Jiang Y, Cai X, Leung W, Xu C. (2020). Smart responsive nanoformulation for targeted delivery of active compounds from traditional Chinese medicine. *Frontiers in Chemistry*, 8, 559159.

Jing X, Wang S, Tang H, Li D, Zhou F, Xin L, He Q, Hu S, Zhang T, Chen T, Song J. (2022). Dynamically bioresponsive DNA hydrogel incorporated with dual-functional stem cells from apical papilla-derived exosomes promotes diabetic bone regeneration. *ACS Applied Materials & Interfaces*, 14, 16082–16099.

Kanai M, Tanaka T, Okada Y. (2016). Empirical estimation of genome-wide significance thresholds based on the 1000 Genomes Project data set. *Journal of Human Genetics*, 61(10), 861–6.

Kang J, Li Y, Zhao Y, Wang Y, Ma C, Shi C. (2021). Nucleic acid extraction without electrical equipment via magnetic nanoparticles in Pasteur pipettes for pathogen detection. *Analytical Biochemistry*, 635, 114445.

Li C, Chang, Y., Hsiao M, Chan M-H. (2022). Ultrasound and nanomedicine for cancer-targeted drug delivery: Screening, cellular mechanisms and therapeutic opportunities. *Pharmaceutics*, 14, 1282.

Liu D, Balasubramanian S. (2003). A proton-fuelled DNA nanomachine. *Angewandte Chemie*, 42, 5734–5736.

Liu M, Jiang S, Loza O, Fahmi NE, Šulc P, Stephanopoulos N. (2018). Rapid photoactuation of a DNA nanostructure using an internal photocaged trigger strand. Angewandte Chemie International Edition, 57, 9341–9345.

Liu S, Jiang Q, Wang Y, Ding B. (2019). Biomedical applications of DNA-based molecular devices. *Advanced HealthCare Materials*, 8, 1801658.

Liu X, Cao S, Gao Y, Luo S, Zhu Y, Wang L. (2023). Subcellular localization of DNA nanodevices and their applications. *Chemical Communications*, 59, 3957–3967.

Loretan M, Domljanovic I, Lakatos M, Rüegg C, Acuna GP. (2020). DNA origami as emerging technology for the engineering of fluorescent and plasmonic-based biosensors. *Materials*, 13, 2185.

Motoi Y, Ito Z, Suzuki S, Takami S, Matsuo K, Sato M, Ota Y, Tsuruta M, Kojima M, Noguchi M, Uchiyama K. (2019). FADS2 and ELOVL6 mutation frequencies in Japanese Crohn's disease patients. *Drug Discoveries & Therapeutics*, 13(6), 354–9.

Nagahara S, Matsuda T. (1996). Hydrogel formation via hybridization of oligonucleotides derivatized in water-soluble vinyl polymers. *Polymer Gels and Networks*, 4, 111–127.

Peng L, You M, Yuan Q, Wu C, Han D, Chen Y, Zhong Z, Xue J, Tan W. (2012). Macroscopic volume change of dynamic hydrogels induced by reversible DNA hybridization. *Journal of the American Chemical Society*, 134, 12302–12307.

Sabir F, Zeeshan M, Laraib U, Barani M, Rahdar A, Cucchiarini M, Pandey S. (2021). DNA based and stimuli-responsive smart nanocarrier for diagnosis and treatment of cancer: Applications and challenges. *Cancers*, 13(14), 3396.

Škugor M, Valero J, Murayama K, Centola M, Asanuma H, Famulok M. (2019). Orthogonally photocontrolled non-autonomous DNA walker. *Angewandte Chemie*, 131, 7022–7025.

Su Y, Chen X, Wang H, Sun L, Xu Y, Li D. (2022). Enhancing cell membrane phase separation for inhibiting cancer metastasis with a stimuli-responsive DNA nanodevice. *Chemical Science*, 13, 6303–6308.

Su H, Li S, Jin Y, Xian Z, Yang D, Zhou W, Mangaran F, Leung F, Sithamparanathan G, Kerman K. (2017). Nanomaterial-based biosensors for biological detections. *Archived Journal*, 3, 19–29.

Surana S, Bhat JM, Koushika SP, Krishnan Y. (2011). An autonomous DNA nanomachine maps spatiotemporal pH changes in a multicellular living organism. *Nature Communications*, 2, 340.

Tominaga T. (2019). Rapid detection of coliform bacteria using a lateral flow test strip assay. *Journal of Microbiology and Methods*, 160, 29–35.

Um SH, Lee JB, Park N, Kwon SY, Umbach CC, Luo D. (2006). Enzyme-catalysed assembly of DNA hydrogel. *Nature Materials*, 5, 797–801.

Wang H, Peng P, Wang Q, Du Y, Tian Z, Li T. (2020). Environment recognizing DNA-computation circuits for the intracellular transport of molecular payloads for mRNA imaging. *Angewandte Chemie International Edition*, 59, 6099–6107.

Wang J, Wang C, Wang Q, Zhang Z, Wang H, Wang S, Chi Z, Shang L, Wang W, Shu Y. (2022). Microfluidic preparation of gelatin methacryloyl microgels as local drug delivery vehicles for hearing loss therapy. *ACS Applied Materials & Interfaces*, 14(41), 46212–23.

Wu J, Li Y, He C, Kang J, Ye J, Xiao Z, Zhu J, Chen A, Feng S, Li X, Xiao J. (2016). Novel H2S releasing nanofibrous coating for in vivo dermal wound regeneration. *ACS Applied Materials & Interfaces*, 8(41), 27474–81.

Wu Y, Yi M, Niu M, Mei Q, Wu K. (2022). Myeloid-derived suppressor cells: an emerging target for anticancer immunotherapy. *Molecular Cancer*, 21(1), 184.

Xu Y, Wu Q, Sun Y, Bai H, Shi G. (2010). Three-dimensional self-assembly of graphene oxide and DNA into multifunctional hydrogels. *ACS Nano*, 4, 7358–7362.

Yan Y, Tan J, Lu Y, Yan S, Wong K, Li D, Gu L, Huang Z. (2013). G-Quadruplex conformational change driven by pH variation with potential application as a nanoswitch. *Biochimica et Biophysica Acta (BBA) - General Subjects*, 1830, 4935–4942

Yang H, Zhou Y, Liu J. (2020). G-quadruplex DNA for construction of biosensors. *TrAC Trends in Analytical Chemistry*, 132, 116060

Yang J, Jiang Q, He L, Zhan P, Liu Q, Liu S, Fu M, Liu J, Li C, Ding B. (2018). Self-assembled double-bundle DNA tetrahedron for efficient antisense delivery. *ACS Applied Materials & Interfaces*, 10, 23693–23699.

Yang P, Zhou R, Kong C, Fan L, Dong C, Chen J, Hou X, Li F. (2021). Using nature's "tricks" to rationally tune the binding properties of biomolecular receptors. *ACS Nano*, 15, 16870–16877.

Yang Y, Bang J, Yulin L, Zhaoxiang D. (2019). Stimuli-responsive DNA self-assembly: From principles to applications. *Chemistry*, 25, 9785–9798.

You Y, Deng Q, Wang Y, Sang Y, Li G, Pu F, Ren J, Qu X. (2022). DNA-based platform for efficient and precisely targeted bioorthogonal catalysis in living systems. *Nature Communications*, 13, 1459.

Yin P, Yan H, Daniell X, Turberfield AJ, Reif JH. (2004). A unidirectional DNA walker that moves autonomously along a track. *Angewandte Chemie*, 43, 4906–4911.

Zhao H, Wu L, Yan G, Chen Y, Zhou M, Wu Y, Li Y. (2021). Inflammation and tumor progression: signaling pathways and targeted intervention. *Signal Transduction and Targeted Therapy*, 6(1), 263.

Zhao C, Xiao F, Lin L, Li Y, Tian L. (2018). Magnesium-stabilized multifunctional DNA nanoparticles for tumor-targeted and ph-responsive drug delivery. *ACS Applied Materials & Interfaces*, 10, 15418–15427.

22 Role of Nanostructured Materials towards Futuristic Biomedical Sensing Applications

Souradeep Roy, Anu Bharti, and Ashish Mathur

22.1 INTRODUCTION

Over the past few centuries, gradual advances in materials science research have played a decisive role in shaping the contemporary world. Countless materials have been studied and are implemented in different applications, such as electronics, energy, packaging, biomedical science, pharmacy, defence, wearables, implants, and additive manufacturing/construction to name a few. The choice of selection of suitable materials for a specific application depends on the material properties, such as their geometry/morphology, tensile strength, degree of reflectance/transmittance/absorbance, electronic/thermal conductivity, chemical reactivity, biocompatibility, and magnetic strength/susceptibility to name a few. A plethora of materials exist around us successfully serving in numerous sectors. However, in a bid to break the barrier of conventional technologies and move towards futuristic designs and innovations, most of the available materials can no longer be implemented. For example, in order to increase the processing speed of smartphones and laptops while continuously introducing multiple features/apps, a large number of transistors [beyond very large-scale integration (VLSI)] have to be fabricated on a limited area of integrated chips (ICs), which can no longer be achieved by the conventional silicon-based micromachining. Ensuring accurate and timely treatment for life-threatening diseases, such as cancers/tumours, depends on the diagnosis speed and accuracy. As an example, imaging and identifying a tiny spot of cancer cell in the body requires high-quality contrast agents for magnetic resonance imaging (MRI) and computerized tomography (CT) scans. Such exceptional optical behaviours are beyond the scope of conventional materials being used. Furthermore, implant devices for dental, orthopaedics, cardiac arrythmia (pacemaker) applications demand a high degree of biocompatibility with minimal chemical reactivity with surrounding cells or tissues. Over the past years, technological advancements are being continuously made in various other applications which demand materials with extraordinary properties.

Nanotechnology has been bridging the gap between the development of conventional and emerging/futuristic technologies for a variety of applications over the past few decades. This has been made possible by harnessing the exotic properties of

DOI: 10.1201/9781003432661-22

materials upon scaling them down from the bulk to nanoscale (1–100 nm) (Gajanan and Tijare, 2018, Gao and Xu, 2009, Sharma et al., 2018, Mandal and Ganguly, 2011). Properties at the nanoregime are primarily governed by two features:

i. Surface-to-volume ratio (*S*/*V*) and
ii. Quantum confinement.

The surface-to-volume ratio is an indication of the fraction of atoms or molecules available on the surface of the material as compared to that within its volume. If we consider a sphere of radius R, the surface-to-volume ratio is given by:

$$\frac{S}{V} = \frac{4\pi R^2}{\left(\frac{4}{3}\right)\pi R^3} = \frac{3}{R} \tag{22.1}$$

Considering four spheres of radii 1 m, 1 mm, 1 μm, and 1 nm, the *S*/*V* ratios can be calculated to be 3, 3×10^3, 3×10^6, and 3×10^9, respectively, as shown in Figure 22.1 below.

This indicates a billion times enhancement in the fraction of atoms exposed at the surface as compared to the volume as the sphere radius is scaled down to the nanoregime. A consequence of such a scenario is the presence of huge numbers of dangling bonds – which is highly favourable from surface functionalization viewpoint by introducing various functional groups for biomolecule immobilization. This finds diverse possibilities in the field of biomolecular sensing applications, where electrode surface functionalization is one of the crucial stages for generating optimum response (Wu et al., 2019, Singh et al., 2018, Mathur et al., 2021, Rawat et al., 2023).

Meanwhile, quantum confinement refers to the restriction of degrees of freedom of charge carriers (electrons/holes) within a specific dimension(s) of the material. The various types of dimensional confinement are shown in Figure 22.2.

Electrons/holes in bulk materials obey the free electron gas model where the carriers are free to move in any direction and can thus possess energies within a vast continuum (E_{cont}). However, in the nanoscale, confining the degrees of freedom along specific dimensions results in restricted motion and eventually possessing only

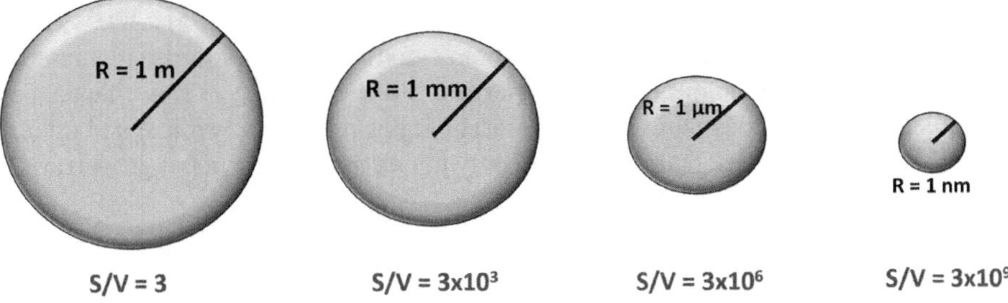

FIGURE 22.1 Variation of surface-to-volume ratios upon scaling the radius of a sphere down from bulk to the nanoscale.

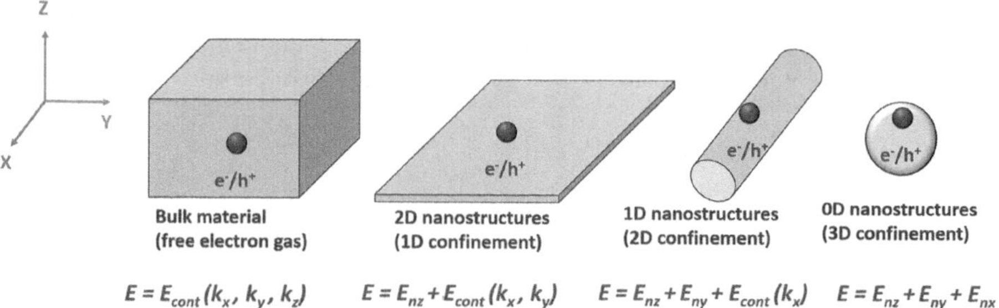

FIGURE 22.2 Dimensional confinement in nanostructures and variation of quantized energy of charge carriers.

certain values of energy. The latter is no longer continuous and hence gets quantized (E_n) (Hanson, 2008). Confining the carriers within a material of the characteristic length scale (de-Broglie wavelength) leads to a drastic decrease in scattering events, thereby resulting in ballistic conduction which enhances electronic properties. The quantization of energy levels also plays a key role in deciding the optical properties of a nanomaterial, which is a characteristic of the material bandgap energy (E_g).

Furthermore, the nanoscale features – namely *S*/*V* ratio and quantum confinement – result in unique interesting properties in the nanostructures of various geometries. The choice of a suitable geometry/morphology of nanomaterials plays a deciding factor in achieving optimum device performance (Roy et al., 2021). The next section will briefly introduce the common nanostructure geometries widely employed, as well as some of their properties with a few examples.

22.2 NANOMATERIAL GEOMETRIES AND THEIR PROPERTIES

Nanostructure geometry plays a very important role in achieving superior and optimum product quality. In the case of biosensors, various geometries exhibit basal and edge-plane-area-specific electrochemical behaviour. A typical nuance in this case is to select a geometry which introduces more edge plane sites which act as regions of high electric field, thereby enhancing heterogeneous electron transfer (Tite et al., 2019, Song and Bazant, 2013, Ji et al., 2006). Similarly, properties, such as surface plasmon resonance (SPR) and fluorescence, which are utilized in calibrating optical biosensors, are also heavily dependent on the nanostructure geometry (Sosa et al., 2003, Wang et al., 2020). This section will discuss the most commonly employed nanomaterial geometries along with some of their properties. Since the scope of this chapter lies in applications of various nanostructure morphologies in electrochemical and optical biosensors, we will restrict our discussion only to electronic and optical properties.

22.2.1 Quantum Dots

Quantum dots (QDs) are 0D nanostructures in which the carriers are confined in all three dimensions, with a high degree of energy quantization. The length scale of QDs is comparable to the Bohr exciton radius (Rani et al., 2022). As a result, the density of states (DOS) profile of such systems is indicated by a series of Dirac delta functions given by:

$$\rho(E) = 2\sum_{n_x n_y n_z} \delta\left(E - E_{n_x n_y n_z}\right) \tag{22.2}$$

where integer 2 represents spin degeneracy. This indicates strong confinement of carriers within the quantum system with a high degree of energy quantization. The electron transport occurs with negligible scattering events in every direction, thereby resulting in ballistic conduction making them suitable for biosensor applications. From the electrochemical perspective, the enhanced curvature of nanoscale dots – especially carbon dots (CDs) and graphene quantum dots (GQDs) results in the exposure of basal and edge plane sites which enable increased space charge capacitance and heterogenous electron transport (Campuzano et al., 2019, Pedrero et al., 2017). Meanwhile, QDs also exhibit fascinating size-dependent fluorescence emission making them suitable for deployment in optical biosensors (Kim and Yoo, 2021). For example, the widely explored and used gold QDs/gold nanoparticles of size 5–6 nm emit longer wavelengths and appear to be of red colour. On the other hand, particles of size 1–3 nm emit shorter wavelengths and hence appear violet or blue in colour. The optical emission in QDs is significantly bright so that they are used as tracers for imaging cancers/tumours as well as probes for colorimetric quantification of biochemicals.

22.2.2 Nanotubes

Nanotubes/wires/fibres are characterized as 1D nanostructures in which the radius/diameter is normally within few tens of nanometre, while the length can range from a few hundreds of nanometre to a few microns. In this case, the carriers are confined to two dimensions while being free to traverse in the other direction. Considering a cylindrical geometry as in Figure 22.2, the electrons/holes can acquire distinct energy values (quantization) along Y and Z axes while being able to achieve energy within a vast continuum. A typical example of such 1D nanostructures is carbon nanotubes. The electronic properties are dependent on the bandgap, which in turn varies on the type of nanotubes, such as single-wall carbon nanotubes (SWCNTs) and multi-wall carbon nanotubes (MWCNTs), which exhibit either metallic or semiconducting behaviour depending on chirality. For example, MWCNT bundles are preferred over SWCNTs as the channels in field effect transistors due to comparatively high electronic conductivity and less contact resistance which enhances device performance (Yang et al., 2021). The TiO_2 nanotubes (TiNTs) have also been widely studied and have advantages over CNTs, such as easy synthesis of free-standing and rigid tubes (Wadhwa et al., 2021, Regonini et al., 2013). However, the wide bandgap of TiO_2 often limits their application in device scenario. Apart from these, the high curvature-induced strain at the nanotube ends exposes the graphene edges which are sites of high electric field. This phenomenon is exploited in the development of electrochemical biosensors by enhancing the interface electron transfer kinetics and overall sensitivity. Furthermore, CNTs also exhibit bright fluorescence in the near-infrared spectrum depending on the tube chirality and dimensions. For example, aqueous SWCNTs fluoresce within the range of 870–2,400 nm without any bleaching (Ackermann et al., 2022). This is suitable primarily for imaging purposes as well as the detection of biochemicals, such as H_2O_2 (Giraldo et al., 2015), riboflavin (Nibler et al., 2021), and neurotransmitters (Kruss et al., 2014) to name a few.

22.2.3 2D Sheet-like Nanostructures

The 2D nanosheets exhibit carrier confinement along the region which defines the material thickness. The latter is typically below 500 nm and is termed as thin film as compared to the thick film counterpart (thickness ~ 10–25 μm). The carriers in nanosheets have quantized energies along the sheet/film thickness while being able to move freely along the surface (length and width). The most commonly used 2D nanomaterials are graphene, transition metal dichalcogenides (TMDs) and graphene-like materials, such as MXenes, borophene, stanene, and phosphorene to name a few. Graphene is a 2D sheet-like framework of sp^2 hybridized carbon atoms arranged in a hexagonal manner. The metal-like (DOS) and quantum confinement in graphene results in a huge electron mobility of $\sim 2 \times 10^5 cm^2/Vs$ (Bernardi et al., 2017). However, the lack of energy bandgap results in leakage currents in transistors which necessitates the gap opening by means of chemical doping. Typical 2D nanostructures in such cases are graphene oxide (GO) and reduced GO. The latter, or any functionalized 2D nanosheets/flakes, are primarily suitable for electroanalysis due to diverse possibilities of surface functionalization and enhanced heterogenous electron transfer as a result of edge plane sites. The 2D nanostructures also exhibit impressive optical properties. For example, the TMDs exhibit light emission which is dependent on the number of atomic layers. Specifically, the group-6 TMDs undergo a transition from indirect to direct bandgap while moving from bilayer to monolayer structures, resulting in brighter emissions in the latter (Splendiani et al., 2010, Mak et al., 2010). With suitable doping strategies, 2D nanostructures can be extensively employed for the detection of various biochemicals using optical transduction.

22.2.4 3D Tetrapodal Nanostructures

The 3D hierarchical materials, such as hollow sea urchins, branched structures, tetrapods, and multipods, exhibiting nanoscale features, have been reported to be equally suitable for diverse applications (Mishra et al., 2014, Zhao and Lei, 2020, Naseri et al., 2018). Over the years, the tetrapodal morphology of ZnO has been of significant research interest for numerous applications. These primarily consist of four interconnected arms having length and thickness/diameter in the microns and nanoscale, respectively. Therefore, the presence of a huge surface area along with the quantum confinement of carriers in each arm makes the tetrapodal geometry highly suitable – especially for biosensing applications. Although ZnO exhibits a wide bandgap of 3.37 eV, the electron transport in its tetrapodal geometry is rather fascinating. Sulciute et al. reported enhanced electron transport in the long ZnO tetrapods as compared to shorter ones, as well as other ZnO morphologies, such as nanowires (NWs) and QDs (Sulciute et al., 2021). Longer tetrapods exhibit a high degree of percolation pathway along with porous features as compared to NWs and QDs. Apart from this, tetrapodal morphology also offers comparatively less inter-particle junctions which drastically reduces electron scattering events, thereby resulting in increased conductivity. The 3D tetrapods are also known to exhibit exotic optical properties suitable for imaging and sensing applications. For example, ZnO tetrapods exhibit UV and green emissions at ~380 and 495 nm, respectively, which occur due to near band-edge and deep level emissions (respectively) (Dai et al., 2002, Fischer et al., 2007).

It can be observed that the electronic and optical properties of nanostructures are highly geometry-specific due to varying surface-to-volume ratios and quantum confinement effects. The nanoscale phenomena have inherent effects on the electronic band structure which governs the transport and optical properties and hence is unique for every nanostructure geometry. In this regard, the choice of a suitable geometry is of utmost importance for ensuring optimum device performance – especially in biosensor development/calibration, considering the huge demand for next-generation biomedical diagnostic devices (connected health). The next section will focus on a brief introduction to biosensors and connected health, and the role of various nanostructure geometries on the electrochemical and optic based detection of bioanalytical species.

22.3 ROLE OF NANOSTRUCTURE GEOMETRY IN BIOSENSING APPLICATIONS

The world of nanostructured materials is extremely fascinating, as it spans a diverse range of fields, from physics and chemistry to medicine, making it a truly exciting area of research. The potential impact of nanomaterials on biology, biotechnology, and medicine is immense, as they can match the size of biological materials, such as enzymes, antibodies, proteins, and nucleotides. As a result, they are well suited for a wide range of medical applications (Anjum et al., 2021). The biomedical field benefits greatly from the versatile applications of nanostructured materials, which can be customized for optical, electrical, and magnetic properties. These materials can take on a variety of forms, including 0D (QDs, nanoparticles), 1D (NWs, nanofibres, or carbon nanotubes), 2D (metallic platelets or graphene sheets), and 3D (nanocubes and tetrapodals), which impact their overall functionality. Ongoing research in this area holds limitless potential for the use of nanostructured materials in biomedical applications, as shown in Figure 22.3.

Nanostructures are a remarkable class of materials with unique physicochemical properties, featuring a large surface-to-volume ratio that makes them ideal for biosensors. Smaller nanomaterials have larger surface areas, resulting in increased sensitivity that can detect even trace amounts of substances. The shape of the nanostructure is crucial in determining its interaction with biological molecules, with different shapes exhibiting varying affinities for specific biomolecules (Gooding, 2006). Researchers can improve the performance of the biosensor by tailoring the surface chemistry of the nanostructure. Surface functionalization with biomolecules or chemical moieties can enhance the biosensor's specificity for a particular target

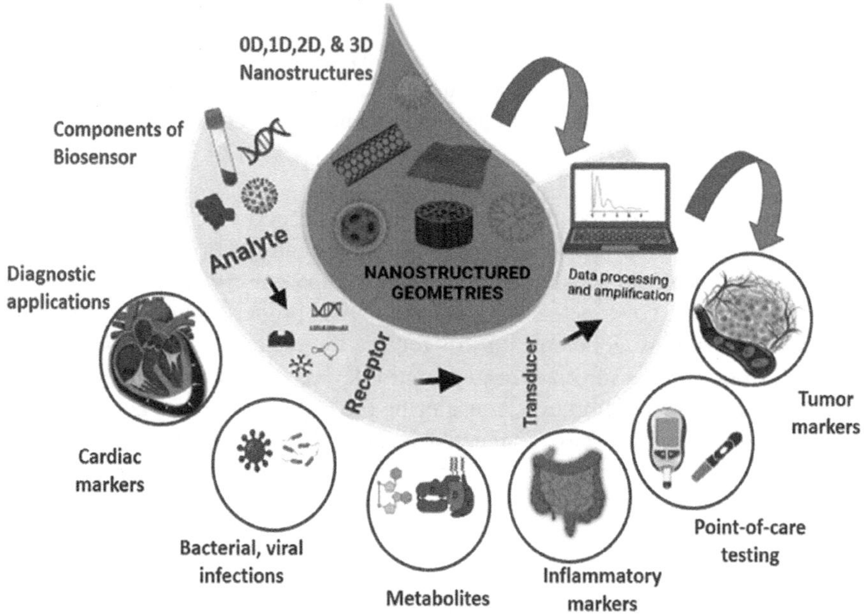

FIGURE 22.3 Applications of nanostructured materials in PoC diagnosis.

analyte while minimizing non-specific binding. Nanostructured materials offer the advantage of real-time monitoring of biological events, enabling early diagnosis and treatment of diseases like cancer, HIV, and infections. In addition to their sensing capabilities, nanostructured materials are also utilized in targeted drug delivery systems and advanced imaging techniques for the diagnosis and treatment of diseases in biomedical science (Sim and Wong, 2021, Harish et al., 2022).

22.3.1 Introduction to Biosensors and Connected Health

A biosensor is an innovative device with the remarkable ability to detect a specific target analyte by binding to its bio-recognition element, which then produces some measurable response picked up by a transducer element. These signals are converted into electrical signals that can be precisely analyzed or quantified. The concept was introduced by Leland C. Clark in 1956, who invented the first biosensor for oxygen detection and was recognized as the "father of biosensors" (Clark and Clark, 1987). Since then, numerous other biosensors have been developed across multiple fields, from nanotechnology and electrochemistry to medical diagnosis. They are widely used in various applications, such as home pregnancy tests, glucose detectors, agriculture, health science, food safety, and environmental monitoring. Biosensors can selectively detect target analytes in the presence of numerous non-specific analytes, making them an essential tool in various diagnostic fields. Their real-time analysis, low cost, and miniaturization have made them an increasingly indispensable technology in medical research, driving growing commercial interest in biosensors (Pirzada and Altintas, 2019). The performance of a biosensor is measured by several parameters that are important in determining their accuracy and effectiveness.

1. **Linearity:** This refers to the maximum linear value of the sensor calibration curve. The linearity of the sensor must be high for the detection of high substrate concentration, which is crucial in many applications.
2. **Sensitivity:** The higher the sensitivity of a biosensor, the more accurate its measurements will be, making it an invaluable tool in various fields of medical diagnosis.
3. **Selectivity:** Selectivity refers to the ability of the device to minimize interference of chemicals and obtain the correct result. The selectivity of a biosensor is vital, as it ensures that the device only detects the targeted biological molecule, avoiding any false readings or misinterpretations of data.
4. **Response time:** A rapid response time is vital in biosensing applications for timely detection of biological molecules which get denatured in long-term storage.
5. **Limit of detection (LOD):** LOD is the smallest amount of a material that may be calculated from its absence (blank signal). It may be calculated using the mean and standard deviation of the blank.

The three main components of a biosensor are the biomarker molecule (sample analyte), bioreceptor (recognition element), and compatible bio-transducer (Bhalla et al., 2016). These components are essential in determining the technical specifications of biosensor design. Biomarkers, which are often expressed abnormally during disease progression, are detected using bioreceptors, such as enzymes, antibodies, cells, DNA, and aptamers, which interact specifically with their targets and generate biochemical signals. Bioreceptors play a critical role in recognizing the analyte of interest to establish a compatible biosensing system. To improve stability and reproducibility, many bioreceptor molecules have been introduced in the biosensing field through advances in technology and synthetic chemistry. After the interaction between the bioreceptor and its target, the appropriate transducer is selected, based on the type of biochemical signal produced. This transducer converts the biological signals into measurable signals, which are usually proportional to the amount of target analyte present. The measured signal is then amplified, and the output is displayed on an easily readable screen (Thévenot et al., 2001). Biosensors can be classified into different categories, such as optical, piezoelectric, calorimetric, and electrochemical biosensors, depending on the transducer system employed. However, discussing the working principle of each type of transducer system is beyond the scope of this chapter. Instead, this chapter focusses on the wide range of capabilities that electrochemical and optical biosensors offer in biomedical diagnosis.

Moreover, the demand for connected health applications is growing rapidly, driven by several factors, including an aging population, rising healthcare costs, and advances in technology. Connected health refers to the use of technology to connect patients, healthcare providers, and other stakeholders in the healthcare system in a way that improves access, quality, and efficiency of care. This includes the use of mobile apps, wearable devices, remote monitoring systems, and other digital tools that enable real-time communication and data sharing between patients and providers. The World Health Organization (WHO) has put forth an exciting challenge for analytical methods: to be affordable, sensitive, specific, user-friendly, rapid, robust, equipment free, and easily deliverable to end-users. These criteria represented by the acronym ASSURED offer a compelling framework for assessing detection devices, particularly in resource-constrained areas or for field applications (Land et al., 2019). The COVID-19 pandemic has also accelerated the adoption of digital health technologies, as more patients and providers seek to reduce the risk of exposure to the virus. The market for connected health applications is a global phenomenon, with strong demand in many countries around the world. While the United States is currently the largest market for connected health applications, other countries are quickly catching up, and many are expected to see significant growth in the coming years. Furthermore, it is also important to note that personalized and affordable healthcare is not just the responsibility of healthcare providers. Individuals also play a critical role in maintaining their own health and wellness. By adopting healthy lifestyles, such as eating a nutritious diet; engaging in regular physical activity; and avoiding harmful behaviours, such as smoking, individuals can reduce their risk of developing chronic diseases and improve their overall health. Personalized and affordable healthcare is an essential component of a modern healthcare system.

22.3.2 Electrochemical Biosensors

The field of clinical diagnostics and monitoring necessitates accurate analyses, which can be challenging due to the high cost of analytical devices and overall measurement expenses. Additionally, the requirement for skilled personnel to conduct clinical analyses emphasizes the need for alternative analytical technologies. Given these challenges, electrochemical sensors offer unique advantages over other strategies. They are easily miniaturized, simple to operate, and have a low-cost detection process, making them a popular diagnostic tool in various medical and pharmaceutical analytical disciplines. Electrochemical biosensors are composed of three electrodes: reference, counter, and working. These biosensors operate on the principle that when a biomolecule is immobilized on an electrode, the subsequent chemical reaction after interaction with the target analyte produces or consumes some electrons or ions. This leads to a measurable change in the electrical signals and this change is employed for the detection process during a redox reaction (Grieshaber et al., 2008). Moreover, selecting the appropriate electrochemical technique is crucial for obtaining accurate measurements and associated parameters. Some commonly used techniques include cyclic voltammetry (CV), differential pulse voltammetry (DPV), impedimetry, and amperometry which are effective in determining analytical signals. Electrochemical biosensors have played a vital role in enabling the timely diagnosis and treatment of diseases by analyzing the biomarkers present in the bloodstream and detecting them using wireless data-collecting systems (Hai et al., 2020). This section provides a detailed exploration of the use of nanostructured geometries to enhance the efficacy of electrochemical diagnosis; some biosensing strategies are also given in Table 22.1.

TABLE 22.1
Some Examples of PoC Electrochemical Diagnostic Approaches Based on Various Nanostructured Geometries

	Nanostructured Material Used	Target Molecule	LOD	References
Electrochemical Biosensors	GQDs	Platelet-derived growth factor (PDGF)	0.82 pg/mL	Zhang et al. (2017)
	GQDs	Heat shock protein 70 (HSP70)	0.05 ng/mL	Sun et al. (2020)
	GQDs	Catechol, epinephrine, and norepinephrine	0.002, 0.065, and 0.035 μM	Erkmen et al. (2021)
	TiO_2 nanotube	L-Tyrosine	0.35 nM	Roy et al. (2019)
	Gold nanowire	miRNA-137	1.7 fM	Azimzadeh et al. (2017)
	ZnO nanofibres	Glucose	1 μM	Ahmad et al. (2010)
	Ribbon conductive nanofibres– MWCNTs	BRCA-1	2.4 pM	Ehzari et al. (2018)
	Manganese (III) oxide (Mn_2O_3) nanofibres	Dengue consensus primer	120 zM	Tripathy et al. (2017)
	SWCNTs	miRNA-25	3.13×10^{-13} M	Asadzadeh-Firouzabadi and Zare (2018)
	Graphene	Zika virus (NS1 antigen)	450 pM	Afsahi et al. (2018)
	GO	miRNA-21 & miRNA-210	0.87 fM	
	Reduced GO	Cancer antigen 15-3 (CA15-3)	0.3 U mL	Amani et al. (2017)
	Reduced GO	H1N1 influenza viruses	0.5 PFU/mL	Singh et al. (2017)
	PdPtCu@black phosphorus bilayer nanosheets	Kidney injury molecule-1 (KIM-1)	32 pg/mL	Yin et al. (2022)
	MXene	miRNA-122	0.0035 aM	Ranjbari et al. (2023)
	Tin disulfide (SnS_2) nanosheets	amyloid-β (42) oligomers (AβOs)	238.9 fg/mL	Tri Murti et al. (2022)
	Boron nitride nanosheet	Cancer antigen 125 (CA-125)	1.18 U/mL	Öndeş et al. (2021)
	MXene	Cytokines [tumour necrosis factor (TNF-α), interferon-γ (IFN-γ)]	0.15 pg/mL 0.12 pg/mL	Noh et al. (2022)
	Nano-PEDOT-graphene aerogel nanocomposite	Prostate-specific antigen (PSA)	0.03 pg/mL	Jia et al. (2018)
	Gold nanocubes	H_2O_2	15×10^{-9} M	Manickam et al. (2019)
	3D PtNi nanocubes	Human epididymis protein 4 (HE4)	0.11 pg/mL	Chen et al. (2022)

22.3.2.1 0D QDs

QDs are popularly utilized in developing various types of sensors due to their exclusive photochemical stability, resistance to photobleaching, and other advantages, such as narrow emission spectrum and size-tunable light emission. Graphene quantum dots (GQDs) have shown in-depth applications in healthcare monitoring through electrochemical biosensing techniques. Because of the quantum-confined properties, GQDs are highly desirable in biosensor design owing to their fast electron transport and excellent conductivity properties (Martynenko et al., 2017). One recent study in this area by Baluta et al. focussed on immobilizing laccase through glutaraldehyde linker on the surface of GQDs-coated glassy carbon electrode (GCE) for the electrochemical detection of epinephrine. The developed laccase-based biosensor displayed a wide detection range of 1–120 μM, and a detection limit of 83 nM was obtained. The biosensor was also successfully used for epinephrine detection in clinical samples, indicating its suitability for various applications (Baluta et al., 2018). Together with other catecholamine neurotransmitters, epinephrine is crucial for the normal functioning of the circulatory system, central nervous system, and a number of metabolic activities. A variety of ailments, such as Parkinson's disease, Alzheimer's disease, and schizophrenia, may be caused by fluctuations in the neurotransmitter concentrations. Moreover, Hepatitis B virus (HBV) is a highly infectious pathogen that can cause liver inflammation in patients. Detection of HBV-deoxyribonucleic acid (DNA) is the most reliable method to determine the degree of infection and replication activity of the virus. Xiang et al. reported a label-free sensing tool for the detection of HBV gene DNA sequence, using a GQD-coated GCE. The -COOH groups present on GQDs were used to immobilize the NH_2-functionalized HBV probe onto the surface of GCE. The biosensor covered with the probe was put through electrochemical tests utilizing CV and DPV procedures in ferro-ferricyanide electrolyte solution to identify the target HBV-DNA. The biosensor showed a linear detection range of 10–500 nM, with a low detection limit of 1 nM. This electrochemical detection strategy exhibits both a remarkable detection sensitivity and ease of application, making it a highly promising tool for future clinical testing (Xiang et al., 2018). Vitamin D, also recognized as the sunshine vitamin, is a crucial lipid-soluble nutrient indispensable for several physiological processes. However, the global prevalence of individuals with insufficient vitamin D is steadily increasing. Considering this, a portable electrochemical aptasensor was developed using a combination of GQD-Au nanoparticles to detect vitamin D3 (Wadhwa et al., 2020). This aptasensor showed a linear detection range from 1 to 500 nM, and an LOD of 0.70 nM with the response time of less than 1 minute. GQDs can be altered with precious metal nanoparticles to enable effective and precise conjugation with various bio-recognition elements. The reported biosensor has a shelf life of more than 35 days, good selectivity for vitamin D3, and over 98% recovery in spiked blood samples. The sensor has also been coupled with controlled electronics resulting in the development of a portable biosensing system.

Numerous other innovations have been developed for biosensing using QDs. Hu et al. conducted a study on an RNA biosensor for the analysis of cancer biomarker miRNA-155 by utilizing GQDs in combination with horseradish peroxidase (HRP)

(Hu et al., 2016). In a study, a bimetallic nanocomposite containing gold-platinum nanoparticles and GQDs was synthesized to simultaneously measure various biomolecule targets – ascorbic acid, uric acid, tryptophan, and dopamine (Yola and Atar, 2016). These QD nanostructures have proven to be efficient nanomaterials for developing various PoC diagnostics in healthcare settings. In addition, fullerenes are also categorized as 0D structures and have been reported to possess favourable characteristics, including great mechanical strength, low cost of production, large surface area, and biological compatibility. Of particular interest to researchers are the electrochemical properties of fullerene-C60, as partially reduced films of this molecule have demonstrated enhanced electrochemical behaviour in aqueous solutions. Consequently, it has been employed for electrode modification purposes (Pilehvar and De Wael, 2015).

22.3.2.2 1D Nanotubes, NWs, and Nanofibres

One-dimensional nanostructures are nanomaterials, which have two dimensions between a scale of 1 and 100 nm and offer significant aspect ratios and better compatibility with a variety of biological systems (Paras et al., 2023). To enhance biosensor sensitivity and molecule accessibility, nanotubes, NWs, and nanofibres are promising materials for electrode modification. These materials exhibit long electron pathway and porous nature and have particularly high potential which help in improving sensing properties. In biosensors and diagnostics, CNTs have been extensively investigated and are considered to be the most exciting 1D nanomaterials. Minor surface perturbations, such as macromolecule binding, can greatly influence the electronic conductance of these nanostructures which corresponds to their large-surface-to volume ratio and faster electron mobility (Murjani et al., 2022). A DNA-based electrochemical aptasensor was constructed by utilizing CNT-loaded poly(3,4-ethylenedi oxythiophene)-poly(styrenesulfonate) (PEDOT) polymer for the testing of MPT64 (responsible for tuberculosis). By exploiting the streptavidin-biotin linkage strategy, the biotin-modified aptamer sequence was effectively coated on the surface of carboxylated CNTs. The aptasensor was subjected to differential pulse voltametric detection of MPT64 in ferri-ferrocyanide redox probe solution showing a detection limit of 0.5 ± 0.2 fg/mL with a response time of 15 minutes and found stable for a remarkable 27-day duration (Thakur et al., 2017).

Nanofibres (NFs) are stranded structures having a high surface area with greater directional versatility and strength. Though they have been researched for quite some time, they only became popular with the advent of nanotechnology in the 1990s. Given their potential and adaptable characteristics, NFs are suitable candidates for biological testing. A mesoporous ZnO nanofibre-based immunosensor was created with excellent sensitivity and efficiency for label-free diagnosis of EGFR-2a (epidermal growth factor receptor) which is a biomarker for breast cancer (Ali et al., 2015). Gupta et al. developed a multiplexed immunosensor for the real-time detection of three biomarkers (i.e. C-reactive protein, cardiac troponin-I, and myoglobin) without the need for any labelling. The immunosensor demonstrated good sensitivity and selectivity for the detection of three specific protein biomarkers present in a complex mixture. Importantly, the immunosensor is free from false positive responses arising from non-specific binding, further validating its accuracy and reliability (Gupta et al., 2016).

NWs are thin structures with high electrical conductivity and show a length-to-diameter ratio of approximately 1000 nm, which is comparatively less than 2D nanotubes. NWs possess great performance in biosensing applications, owing to their large surface area; higher energy; lattice defects; and the inclusion of pores, acute edges, and nanoscale intersections.

Bai and colleagues created an electrochemical detection method using Ni-CuO NWs to provide accurate and enzyme-free glucose sensing (Bai et al., 2017). The electrochemical behaviour of Ni-CuO NWs displayed remarkable characteristics for glucose oxidation showing a low detection limit of 0.07 μM and a wide detection range from 0.2 to 3.0 mM, with high specificity for its target. These outstanding results were attributed to the presence of hierarchical structures and $Ni(OH)_2$ entities within the Ni-CuO NWs. Metal oxide composites designed in this way proved to be an efficient methodology for non-enzymatic sensor development. Liu et al. recently introduced a label-free electrochemical immunosensor utilizing gallium nitride (GaN) NWs. The reported electrochemical method used a combination of GaN-polydopamine (PDA) hybrid with gold nanoparticles for the immobilization of anti-alpha-fetoprotein on the biosensor surface exhibiting a linear range of 0.01 to 100 ng/mL, with an LOD value as low as 0.003 ng/mL (Liu et al., 2019).

22.3.2.3 2D Nanosheets

2D nanomaterials are a class of materials that exhibit two dimensions within the nanoscale range. Prominent examples of these materials include MXenes, graphene sheets, and metal oxide sheets. The carbon allotrope graphene and its various forms possess an exceptional set of optical, electronic, electrochemical, and biomolecular surface adsorption properties that contribute to their PoC biosensing applications (Prattis et al., 2021, Bolotsky et al., 2019). In particular, graphene nanosheets have been utilized for the detection of a cancer biomarker, urokinase plasminogen activator (uPA), by means of FTO electrode-based experimentation. The resulting immunosensor displayed a very low detection limit of about 4.8 fM and a linear detection range of 1 fM to 1 μM (Roberts et al., 2019). GO is gaining attention as a promising matrix material for biosensors due to its 2D framework, robust nature, biological compatibility, and adjustable electrical characteristics. The presence of carboxylic acid and other important oxygen-containing functional groups in GO allows for simple covalent binding of biomolecules without requiring linker molecules. An effective electrochemical aptasensor was developed by using Au-PtBNPs decorated CGO/FTO electrode modified with streptavidin for immobilizing biotinylated aptamers that selectively target the breast cancer biomarker, MUC1. This aptasensor exhibited high specificity for Mucin 1 (MUC1) showing remarkable linear range i.e. 1 fM-100 nM and LOD value of 0.79 fM (Bharti et al., 2020). Recently, an aptamer-based electrochemical sensor for detecting cardiac troponin-I (cTnI) was fabricated using layer-structured MoS_2 nanosheets anchored onto a GCE which is further conjugated with target-specific aptamer sequence (Qiao et al., 2018). When cTnI is present, it forms a defined and rigid tertiary structure that weakens its affinity with MoS_2, causing the release of aptamer-bound cTnI present at the surface of MoS_2 nanosheets and a subsequent decrease in resistance. The aptasensor demonstrated a linear detection range (10 pM–1.0 μM) for cTnI target and a low detection limit of 0.95 pM.

MXenes, a new class of 2D nanomaterials, are gaining attention as potential candidates for electrochemical biosensors due to their high metallic conductivity, hydrophilicity, and biocompatibility. One MXene-based biosensor was designed using 3-aminopropyltriethoxysilane (APTES)-functionalized Ti_3C_2-MXene, achieving a highly sensitive, label-free biosensor for detecting carcinoembryonic antigen (CEA) for cancer detection (Kumar et al., 2018). Another MXene-based biosensor was developed for sensing of a diabetic ketoacidosis biomarker i.e. β-hydroxybutyrate. The biosensor showed a linear detection range of 0.36–17.9 mM, along with a detection limit of 45 μM, making it suitable for analyzing real serum samples (Koyappayil et al., 2020). Wearable biosensor technology has also demonstrated encouraging results with 2D nanomaterial composites. A wearable biosensor was developed by using an epidermal biosensing patch which is a combination of MXene and nanoporous carbon acting as a transducer component (Zahed et al., 2022). The biosensing platform was connected to a miniaturized testing device and demonstrated exceptional sensitivity (100.85 $\mu A/mM/cm^2$) for the physiological concentration of glucose from 0.003 to 1.5 mM. This wearable sensor could accurately monitor glucose levels and electrocardiogram (ECG) signals and was found to be suitable for human use in a variety of settings.

22.3.2.4 3D Nanocubes and Tetrapodal Structures

In biosensing field, complex hierarchical structures and nanocomposites belong to the 3D materials group. Compared to simpler 0D, 1D, and 2D structures, 3D structures have elaborate morphology with biomimetic components that can trap analytes, amplify signals, and enhance biosensor performance. *Helicobacter pylori*, a Gram-negative bacterium responsible for gastric diseases, can be detected using an electrochemical immunosensor utilizing zinc oxide tetrapods (ZnO-T) as a biosensing interface, showing a linear range of 0.2–50 ng/mL and an LOD of 0.2 ng/mL (Chauhan et al., 2018). The resulting sensing interface exhibited good linearity (0.2 to 50 ng/mL) and a low limit of detection (0.2 ng/mL). Recently, Rahmanian et al. employed this method to create a new biosensing approach using 3D nanostructured material for highly sensitive detection of urea. The hierarchical material-based biosensing approach was able to detect urea in a linear range of detection i.e. 5–205 mg/dL and an LOD of 2 mg/dL was calculated (Rahmanian et al., 2017). Fang and colleagues employed a 3D-nanostructure-based synergistic approach for glucose detection by combining the unique properties of gold nanoparticles and the large surface area provided by ZnO. The resulting sensor exhibited reliable performance having an LOD of 0.02 mM and a linear range of detection from 1 to 20 mM (Fang et al., 2015).

Nowadays, researchers are more interested in biosensing applications of metal-organic frameworks (MOFs). These MOFs possess unique properties, including large surface area, high versatility, good porosity, and ease of modification after synthesis. For e.g. nickel and cobalt hydroxides were electrodeposited onto the surface of carbon electrodes, afterwards integrated with an acidic organic solution to create dispersion of MOF flakes. The two metal centres work together synergistically to accelerate the oxidation of glucose by Ni-Co metal organic frameworks (Ezzati et al., 2020). In another study, rim-shaped structures were designed using hierarchical MOF films for sweat sensing. The researchers achieved a macro-meso-micropore like architecture capable of simultaneous lactate and glucose detection showing a linear response for glucose concentrations to 1,592.5 μM and a detection limit of 0.1 μM (Wang et al., 2018). Although 3D nanocomposite assembly can be difficult, it is still a promising approach for developing biosensors. In fact, its assembly can be made simpler to facilitate easier fabrication of biosensors. Therefore, the potential of MOFs in biosensor development is becoming increasingly apparent making them promising material for further exploration.

22.3.3 Optical Biosensors

Optical biosensors offer several superiorities to conventional analytical sensing technology, such as label-free and sensitive biological and chemical substance detection. To develop novel optical biosensors, various advanced multidisciplinary approaches, including nanotechnology and molecular biology, are being employed along with emerging science and technology. Optical detection involves the interplay of the biometric component and electromagnetic radiation. The surface is illuminated by the source of light andthe bio-sensitive layer interact with analytes followedby the recording of the optical signal (luminescence or reflectance). The variation in the optical signal due to the selective recognition of the target species allows the plotting of a dependence of the sensor response on analyte concentration. There are two main variations of optical biosensing: label-free mode and label-based mode. The signals generated as soon as the analytic material comes into contact with the transducer are used for biosensing in the label-free mode. On the other hand, in the label-based mode, the optical signal is produced via suitable tags using techniques like fluorimetry, colorimetry, or luminescence (Damborský et al., 2016). Various nanostructured geometries have been explored in optical biosensing for diagnostic purposes which are summarized below in detail and some are also mentioned in Table 22.2.

22.3.3.1 0D QDs

Semiconductor QDs have been recognized as building blocks that show promise for the development of effective biosensors with enhanced performance, which is attributed to their unique electronic and optical properties. QDs have been extensively used for developing a variety of sensors as well as bioimaging (Ma et al., 2018). Wu et al. reported an immunosensor to detect ovarian cancer by quantifying the presence of the biomarker cancer antigen 125 (CA-125), using chemiluminescence resonance energy transfer to GQDs. The researchers used the photo-Fenton method to synthesize nanodots from Graphene oxide (GO), which were immobilized on glass chips modified with amino groups. The GQDs were further linked covalently to the capture antibody via amide conjugation, which specifically binds to the CA-125 antigen. This approach placed HRP near the GQDs, facilitating the resonant energy transfer and quenching the chemiluminescence. The developed biosensor exhibited a wide linear detection range, ranging from 0.1 U/mL -600 U/mL, along with an LOD of 0.05 U/mL. In another work, Wu et al. developed a label-free electrochemiluminescent immunosensor for quantifying prostate-specific antigen (PSA) levels. This was achieved by immobilizing anti-PSA on the sensor surface and depositing

TABLE 22.2
Nanostructured Geometries Based Optical Biosensing Techniques for Healthcare Applications

	Nanostructured Material Used	Target Molecule	LOD	References
Optical Biosensors	ZnO quantum dots	Cysteine	0.642 μM	Kamaci and Kamaci (2021)
	Silicon quantum dots	Glucose	30 μM	Du et al. (2019)
	QDs	Cardiac troponin	0.04 ng/mL (critical value)	Zhou et al. (2019)
	Carbon nanotubes	Dopamine	18.9 pM	Pathak and Gupta (2019)
	ZnO NWs	α-fetoprotein (AFP) CEA	1 pg/mL 100 fg/mL	Guo et al. (2018)
	GO	25-hydroxyvitamin D3	2.39 fM	Esposito et al. (2021)
	GO	Glucose	1.06 nm/mM	Yang et al. (2020)
	Carbon quantum dots	Cholesterol	1 μM	Li et al. (2022)
	ZnO tetrapods	Apomorphine	1 μM	Picciolini et al. (2015)
	Silver nanocubes	Citrulline	24.5 pM	Walton et al. (2017)
	Lanthanide-functionalized metal organic framework (L-MOF)	Glucose	0.2 μM	Zhang and Yan (2019)

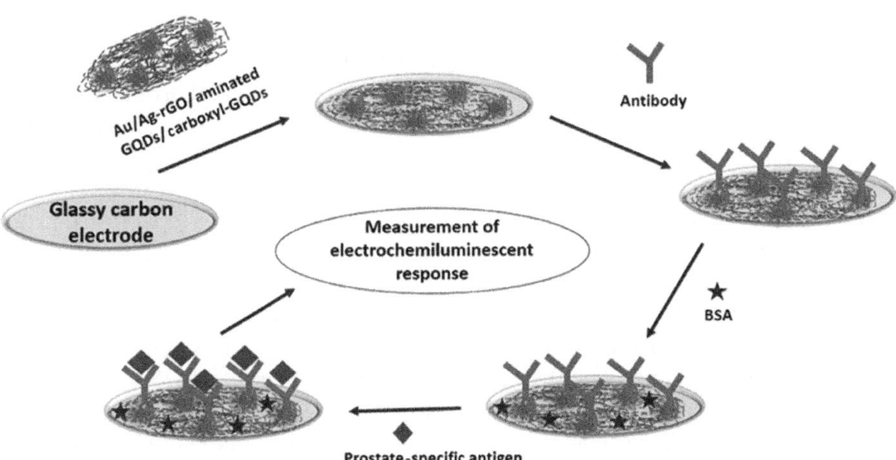

FIGURE 22.4 Schematic representation of electrochemiluminescent immunosensor for PSA detection.

Au/Ag-rGO modified with aminated-GQDs and carboxyl-GQDs onto a GCE, as shown in Figure 22.4. The electrochemiluminescent immunosensor exhibited a detection range from 1 pg/mL to 10 ng/mL and an LOD of 0.29 pg/mL (Wu et al., 2016).

The quantity of Fe^{3+} in living cancer cells can indicate various pathophysiological processes which includes liver damage, anaemia, neurodegenerative disorders, diabetes, and cancer. In order to detect Fe^{3+} levels, a study by Voelcker et al. reported on the development of a fluorescent biosensor based on GQD-functionalized rhodamine B. The authors observed low detection limits of 0.02 μM in pancreatic cancer stem cells by this fluorescent sensor. After the binding process, the bio-nanohybrid displayed orange-reddish emission with a 43% quantum yield, which suggests its potential use as a labelling agent for cancer cells (Guo et al., 2015). Mars et al. developed a biosensor that uses dual electrochemical and fluorescence methods for the detection of apolipoprotein E4 (APOE4) DNA, a marker for Alzheimer's and coronary artery diseases. The sensor consists of an indium tin oxide (ITO) electrode coated with curcumin and GQDs showing an LOD of 0.48 pg/mL for the target DNA (Mars et al., 2018). QDs have also been used as fluorescent tags in cancer diagnostics and their excellent surface-enhanced Raman scattering (SERS) properties can be utilized to develop more sensitive biosensors.

22.3.3.2 1D NWs, Nanotubes, and Nanofibres

Biosensors often use optical transduction mechanisms for their high stability, sensitivity, and possibility of multiplexed detection. One common application of fluorescent sensors and biosensors is the use of CNTs which possess fluorescent properties which depend on their structural features. In a study by Safaee et al., CNTs were integrated with core-shell microfibrous-type textiles to fabricate flexible fluorescent biosensors. To achieve this, single-stranded DNA was bound to SWCNTs via non-covalent interactions followed by dispersing in an aqueous solution. The dispersion was mixed with polycaprolactone and poly-ethylene oxide through electrospinning to produce core-shell microfibres. These nanosensors demonstrated changes in their fluorescent behaviour, allowing the detection of hydrogen peroxide, a type of reactive oxygen species. The core-shell microfibres were subsequently used in wound dressings to track the healing of wounds in real time (Safaee et al., 2021). NWs possess a diameter that is comparable in size to the biological and chemical species that they detect, and they exhibit highly consistent optical characteristics. This makes them an exceptional tool for generating transduction signals that can interface with macroscopic instruments. The optical properties of NWs are also of significant interest, especially with regard to fluorescence-based techniques in bioimaging. When combined with fluorescence microscopy, NWs can improve the performance of biosensing applications, such as the determination of the rate of binding of biomolecules on a surface. Recently, researchers have demonstrated that the light-guiding properties of NWs can be used to boost biosensing based on fluorescent biomolecules. By exploiting the near-field interactions between fluorophores attached to the surface and core of NWs, it is possible to couple light into the nanowire core, similar to an optical fibre (Warren-Smith et al., 2010). Kim et al. conducted a study wherein they created a plasmonic biosensor with high sensitivity using ZnO NWs and gold nanoparticles incorporated in a fibre optic sensor (Kim et al., 2019). Leonardi et al. demonstrated the detection of genomes directly using a label-free and polymerase-chain-reaction-free optical biosensor based on silicon NWs. Their findings indicated that the detection limit for the synthetic genome was two copies/reaction and 20 copies/reaction for the genome extracted from human blood (Leonardi et al., 2018). In addition to NWs, scientists are exploring the potential of nanofibres to detect biologically relevant compounds using optical transducers. Nanofibres have been used to detect dopamine (Ratlam et al., 2020), kanamycin (Abedalwafa et al., 2020), thrombin (Li et al., 2019), and bacteria (Currie et al., 2020) through optical sensing methods.

22.3.3.3 2D Nanosheets

A number of innovative optical biosensors utilizing 2D materials have been recently developed due to their unique optical properties and biocompatibility. Chen et al. reported the development of a label-free ultrasensitive immunosensor employing GO nanosheets and biphasic long-period grating, demonstrating an excellent analytical platform for real-time detection. The study revealed that the refractive index sensitivity of the long-period grating significantly increased by 200% and 155% in the low refractive index and high refractive index regions, respectively, with the deposition of GO (Liu et al., 2017). Cui et al. developed a "turn-on" magnetic fluorescent biosensor utilizing GQDs, Fe_3O_4, and molybdenum disulfide nanosheets for the detection of epithelial cell adhesion molecule (EpCAM) receptors. The biosensor exhibited high sensitivity with a detection limit of 1.19 nM and a linear detection range of 2–64 nM, making it suitable for rapid and efficient detection of circulating tumour cells (Cui et al., 2019). Another notable example is the surface plasmon resonance (SPR) sensor developed by Wang et al. which utilizes AuNPs-modified GO for the detection of miRNA-141. The biosensor demonstrated high sensitivity and selectivity, with a detection limit in the picomolar range and a 1,000-fold higher performance compared to AuNP alone. Additionally, the sensor is easy to operate, low in cost, and non-toxic (Wang et al., 2016). Furthermore, Zhang et al. developed a Cy3-labelled cell surface antigen (CD63) aptamer/Ti_3C_2 MXene nanocomposite utilizing fluorescence resonance energy transfer (FRET) technology for the detection of exosomes (Zhang et al., 2018). This unique biosensor offers a promising tool for detecting exosomes with high sensitivity and selectivity.

22.3.3.4 3D Nanocubes and Tetrapodal Structures

The use of 3D nanostructures, including nanocubes and metallic tetrapods, has become increasingly popular in optical biosensing for biomedical applications. This is due to their unique ability to provide highly enhanced optical signals, owing to their high surface-to-volume ratio. As a result, 3D nanostructures have greatly improved the sensitivity and detection limits of biosensors. For instance, nanocubes have been employed as substrates for SERS, a powerful technique for detecting and identifying biological molecules. Meanwhile, metallic tetrapods have been found to exhibit strong localized surface plasmon resonance (LSPR) signals, which makes them ideal for label-free biosensing applications. With the widespread and devastating impact of COVID-19 on public health and global economies, there has been a significant push to develop biosensors for the rapid and accurate detection of the virus. Leong et al. have developed a handheld COVID-19 biosensor that utilizes SERS to detect specific spectral variations resulting from interactions between respiratory metabolites and multiple molecular receptors on the substrate of silver nanocubes. This biosensor has demonstrated high sensitivity (96.2%) and specificity (99.9%)

in identifying COVID-19-positive individuals within just 5 minutes, with 501 participants successfully tested by blowing on the sensor for 10 seconds. Notably, the biosensor is effective across diverse demographics, including age, gender, smoking habits, and other confounding factors. This technology has the potential to overcome the limitations of traditional gas chromatography–mass spectrometry methods, as it allows for both respiration collection and measurement simultaneously, making it ideal for large-scale testing in a variety of settings (Leong et al., 2022). Recently, Lee et al. have created a biosensor for exosomal miRNAs in breast cancer cells using Au nanopillars. The biosensor is highly sensitive and precise, with uniformly distributed plasmonic Au nanopillars that create dense hot spots, resulting in an enhanced coupling of local plasma fields. It is equipped with LNA (locked nucleic acid) probes that specifically lock onto and hybridize with targeting miRNAs. The biosensor is capable of identifying single base mismatches in miRNA molecules and has a remarkably low detection limit of 1 aM, which is 100 times lower than other SERS methods for detecting micro ribonucleic acid (miRNA). It has a broad dynamic range, ranging from 1 aM to 100 nM, and has the ability to detect multiple targets simultaneously, making it ideal for multiplex sensing (Lee et al., 2019).

22.4 CONCLUSION AND FUTURE PERSPECTIVES

The role of nanostructured materials in futuristic biomedical sensing applications has the potential to revolutionize the healthcare industry and improve patient outcomes. Continued research and development in this field will undoubtedly lead to further advancements and innovations in the years to come. The use of nanostructured materials in biomedical sensing applications has shown promising results in improving the accuracy, speed, and affordability of disease diagnosis and monitoring. The unique properties of nanomaterials, such as high surface-area-to-volume ratio, tunable optical and electrical properties, and biocompatibility, have led to the development of miniaturized sensors for point-of-care (PoC) applications. These sensors have the potential to enhance doctor–patient interaction, improve patient outcomes, and reduce healthcare costs. Various nanostructured materials, such as nanoparticles, nanotubes, NWs, and two-dimensional materials, have been explored in the development of biosensors for the detection of biomolecules, proteins, and cells. The choice of a suitable nanomaterial geometry is vital in determining the biosensor performance and its sensitivity.

Looking towards the future, the use of nanostructured materials in biomedical sensing applications is expected to continue to grow. With advancements in nanofabrication techniques and materials science, it is anticipated that more sophisticated and specialized biosensors will be developed for specific diseases and medical conditions. In addition to the advancements in nanofabrication techniques and materials science, the integration of biosensors with Internet of Things (IoT) technologies and wireless communication networks is expected to significantly impact the healthcare industry. The IoT allows for real-time communication and data exchange between medical devices, healthcare providers, and patients, thereby enabling remote monitoring and management of health conditions. This would be particularly useful in cases where patients require continuous monitoring even in remote areas where access to healthcare facilities is limited. Moreover, personalized medicine is another area that could benefit greatly from the use of nanostructured materials in biomedical sensing applications. Personalized medicine involves tailoring medical treatment to individual patients based on their genetic makeup, lifestyle, and other factors. Biosensors that can detect specific biomarkers or genetic mutations associated with certain diseases can aid in the early diagnosis and treatment of those diseases, improving patient outcomes. However, the development of nanostructured materials for biomedical sensing applications also brings challenges and concerns related to their toxicity and biocompatibility. It is crucial to ensure that the materials used in biosensors are safe for use in human applications and do not cause adverse effects on human health. Therefore, continued research and testing are necessary to ensure the safety and efficacy of nanostructured materials for biomedical sensing applications.

REFERENCES

Abedalwafa, M.A., Tang, Z., Qiao, Y., Mei, Q., Yang, G., Li, Y. & Wang, L. 2020. An aptasensor strip-based colorimetric determination method for kanamycin using cellulose acetate nanofibers decorated DNA–gold nanoparticle bioconjugates. *Microchimica acta,* 187**,** 360.

Ackermann, J., Metternich, J. T., Herbertz, S. & Kruss, S. 2022. Biosensing with fluorescent carbon nanotubes. *Angewandte Chemie International Edition,* 61, e202112372.

Afsahi, S., Lerner, M. B., Goldstein, J. M., Lee, J., Tang, X., Bagarozzi, D. A., Jr., Pan, d., Locascio, L., Walker, A., Barron, F. & Goldsmith, B. R. 2018. Novel graphene-based biosensor for early detection of Zika virus infection. *Biosensors and Bioelectronics,* 100**,** 85–88.

Ahmad, M., Pan, C., Luo, Z. & Zhu, J. 2010. A single ZnO nanofiber-based highly sensitive amperometric glucose biosensor. *The Journal of Physical Chemistry C,* 114**,** 9308–9313.

Ali, M. A., Mondal, K., Singh, C., Malhotra, B. D. & Sharma, A. 2015. Anti-epidermal growth factor receptor conjugated mesoporous zinc oxide nanofibers for breast cancer diagnostics. *Nanoscale,* 7, 7234–7245.

Amani, J., Khoshroo, A. & Rahimi-Nasrabadi, M. 2017. Electrochemical immunosensor for the breast cancer marker CA 15-3 based on the catalytic activity of a CuS/reduced graphene oxide nanocomposite towards the electrooxidation of catechol. *Mikrochim Acta,* 185**,** 79.

Anjum, S., Ishaque, S., Fatima, H., Farooq, W., Hano, C., Abbasi, B. H. & Anjum, I. 2021. Emerging applications of nanotechnology in healthcare systems: Grand challenges and perspectives. *Pharmaceuticals,* 14, 707.

Asadzadeh-Firouzabadi, A. & Zare, H. 2018. Preparation and application of AgNPs/SWCNTs nanohybrid as an electroactive label for sensitive detection of miRNA related to lung cancer. *Sensors and Actuators B: Chemical,* 260, 824–831.

Azimzadeh, M., Nasirizadeh, N., Rahaie, M. & Naderi-Manesh, H. 2017. Early detection of Alzheimer's disease using a biosensor based on electrochemically-reduced graphene oxide and gold nanowires for the quantification of serum microRNA-137. *RSC Advances,* 7**,** 55709–55719.

Bai, X., Chen, W., Song, Y., Zhang, J., Ge, R., Wei, W., Jiao, Z. & Sun, Y. 2017. Nickel-copper oxide nanowires for highly sensitive sensing of glucose. *Applied Surface Science,* 420**,** 927–934.

Baluta, S., Lesiak, A. & Cabaj, J. 2018. Graphene quantum dots-based electrochemical biosensor for catecholamine neurotransmitters detection. *Electroanalysis,* 30, 1781–1790.

Bernardi, M., Ataca, C., Palummo, M. & Grossman, J. C. 2017. Optical and electronic properties of two-dimensional layered materials. *Nanophotonics,* 6**,** 479–493.

Bhalla, N., Jolly, P., Formisano, N. & Estrela, P. 2016. Introduction to biosensors. *Essays in Biochemistry,* 60, 1–8.

Bharti, A., Rana, S., Dahiya, D., Agnihotri, N. & Prabhakar, N. 2020. An electrochemical aptasensor for analysis of MUC1 using gold platinum bimetallic nanoparticles deposited carboxylated graphene oxide. *Analytica Chimica Acta,* 8, 186–195.

Bolotsky, A., Butler, D., Dong, C., Gerace, K., Glavin, N. R., Muratore, C., Robinson, J. A. & Ebrahimi, A. 2019. Two-dimensional materials in biosensing and healthcare: From in vitro diagnostics to optogenetics and beyond. *ACS Nano,* 13, 9781–9810.

Campuzano, S., Yáñez-Sedeño, P. & Pingarrón, J. M. 2019. Carbon dots and graphene quantum dots in electrochemical biosensing. *Nanomaterials,* 9, 634.

Chauhan, N., Gupta, S., Avasthi, D. K., Adelung, R., Mishra, Y. K. & Jain, U. 2018. Zinc oxide tetrapods based biohybrid interface for voltammetric sensing of *Helicobacter Pylori. ACS Applied Materials and Interfaces,* 10, 30631–30639.

Chen, D. N., Jiang, L. Y., Zhang, J. X., Tang, C., Wang, A. J. & Feng, J. J. 2022. Electrochemical label-free immunoassay of HE4 using 3D PtNi nanocubes assemblies as biosensing interfaces. *Mikrochim Acta,* 189, 455.

Clark Jr, L. C. & Clark, E. W. 1987. A personalized history of the Clark oxygen electrode. *International Anesthesiology Clinics,* 25, 1–29.

Cui, F., Ji, J., Sun, J., Wang, J., Wang, H., Zhang, Y., Ding, H., Lu, Y., Xu, D. & Sun, X. 2019. A novel magnetic fluorescent biosensor based on graphene quantum dots for rapid, efficient, and sensitive separation and detection of circulating tumor cells. *Analytical and Bioanalytical Chemistry,* 411, 985–995.

Currie, S., Shariatzadeh, F. J., Singh, H., Logsetty, S. & Liu, S. 2020. Highly sensitive bacteria-responsive membranes consisting of core–shell polyurethane polyvinylpyrrolidone electrospun nanofibers for in situ detection of bacterial infections. *ACS Applied Materials & Interfaces,* 12, 45859–45872.

Dai, Y., Zhang, Y., Li, Q. K. & Nan, C. W. 2002. Synthesis and optical properties of tetrapod-like zinc oxide nanorods. *Chemical Physics Letters,* 358, 83–86.

Damborský, P., Svitel, J. & Katrlík, J. 2016. Optical biosensors. *Essays in Biochemistry,* 60, 91–100.

Du, L., Li, Z., Yao, J., Wen, G., Dong, C. & Li, H.W. 2019. Enzyme free glucose sensing by amino-functionalized silicon quantum dot. *Spectrochimica Acta Part A: Molecular and Biomolecular Spectroscopy,* 216, 303–309.

Ehzari, H., Safari, M. & Shahlaei, M. 2018. A simple and label-free genosensor for BRCA1 related sequence based on electrospinned ribbon conductive nanofibers. *Microchemical Journal,* 143, 118–126.

Erkmen, C., Demir, Y., Kurbanoglu, S. & Uslu, B. 2021. Multi-Purpose electrochemical tyrosinase nanobiosensor based on poly (3,4 ethylenedioxythiophene) nanoparticles decorated graphene quantum dots: Applications to hormone drugs analyses and inhibition studies. *Sensors and Actuators B: Chemical,* 343, 130164.

Esposito, F., Sansone, L., Srivastava, A., Cusano, A. M., Campopiano, S., Giordano, M. & Iadicicco, A. 2021. Label-free detection of vitamin D by optical biosensing based on long period fiber grating. *Sensors and Actuators B: Chemical,* 347, 130637.

Ezzati, M., Shahrokhian, S. & Hosseini, H. 2020. In situ two-step preparation of 3D NiCo-BTC MOFs on a glassy carbon electrode and a graphitic screen printed electrode as non-enzymatic glucose-sensing platforms. *ACS Sustainable Chemistry & Engineering,* 8, 14340–14352.

Fang, L., Liu, B., Liu, L., Li, Y., Huang, K. & Zhang, Q. 2015. Direct electrochemistry of glucose oxidase immobilized on Au nanoparticles-functionalized 3D hierarchically ZnO nanostructures and its application to bioelectrochemical glucose sensor. *Sensors and Actuators B: Chemical,* 222, 1096–1102.

Fischer, A. M., Srinivasan, S., Garcia, R., Ponce, F. A., Guaño, S. E., Di Lello, B. C., Moura, F. J. & Solórzano, I. G. 2007. Optical properties of highly luminescent zinc oxide tetrapod powders. *Applied Physics Letters,* 91, 121905.

Gajanan, K. & Tijare, S. N. 2018. Applications of nanomaterials. *Materials Today: Proceedings,* 5, 1093–1096.

Gao, J. & Xu, B. 2009. Applications of nanomaterials inside cells. *Nano Today,* 4, 37–51.

Giraldo, J. P., Landry, M. P., Kwak, S. Y., Jain, R. M., Wong, M. H., Iverson, N. M., Ben-Naim, M. & Strano, M. S. 2015. A ratiometric sensor using single chirality near-infrared fluorescent carbon nanotubes: Application to in vivo monitoring. *Small,* 11, 3973–84.

Gooding, J. J. 2006. Biosensor technology for detecting biological warfare agents: Recent progress and future trends. *Analytica Chimica Acta,* 559, 137–151.

Grieshaber, D., Mackenzie, R., Vörös, J. & Reimhult, E. 2008. Electrochemical biosensors - sensor principles and architectures. *Sensors,* 8, 1400–1458.

Guo, L., Shi, Y., Liu, X., Han, Z., Zhao, Z., Chen, Y., Xie, W. & Li, X. 2018. Enhanced fluorescence detection of proteins using ZnO nanowires integrated inside microfluidic chips. *Biosensors and Bioelectronics,* 99, 368–374.

Guo, R., Zhou, S., Li, Y., Li, X., Fan, L. & Voelcker, N. H. 2015. Rhodamine-functionalized graphene quantum dots for detection of Fe3+ in cancer stem cells. *ACS Applied Materials & Interfaces,* 7, 23958–23966.

Gupta, R. K., Pandya, R., Sieffert, T., Meyyappan, M. & Koehne, J. E. 2016. Multiplexed electrochemical immunosensor for label-free detection of cardiac markers using a carbon nanofiber array chip. *Journal of Electroanalytical Chemistry,* 773, 53–62.

Hai, X., Li, Y., Zhu, C., Song, W., Cao, J. & Bi, S. 2020. DNA-based label-free electrochemical biosensors: From principles to applications. *TrAC Trends in Analytical Chemistry,* 133, 116098.

Hanson, G. W. 2008. Fundamentals of Nanoelectronics. Pearson/Prentice Hall, Upper Saddle River, NJ.

Harish, V., Tewari, D., Gaur, M., Yadav, A. B., Swaroop, S., Bechelany, M. & Barhoum, A. 2022. Review on nanoparticles and nanostructured materials: Bioimaging, biosensing, drug delivery, tissue engineering, antimicrobial, and agro-food applications. *Nanomaterials*, 12, 457.

Hu, T., Zhang, L., Wen, W., Zhang, X. & Wang, S. 2016. Enzyme catalytic amplification of miRNA-155 detection with graphene quantum dot-based electrochemical biosensor. *Biosensors and Bioelectronics,* 77, 451–456.

Ji, X., Banks, C. E., Crossley, A. & Compton, R. G. 2006. Oxygenated edge plane sites slow the electron transfer of the ferro-/ferricyanide redox couple at graphite electrodes. *Chemphyschem,* 7, 1337–1344.

Jia, H., Xu, J., Lu, L.M., Yu, Y., Zuo, Y., Tian, Q. & Li, P. 2018. Three-dimensional Au nanoparticles/nano-poly(3,4-ethylene dioxythiophene)- graphene aerogel nanocomposite: A high-performance electrochemical immunosensing platform for prostate specific antigen detection. *Sensors and Actuators B: Chemical,* 260, 990–997.

Kamaci, U. D. & Kamaci, M. 2021. Selective and sensitive ZnO quantum dots based fluorescent biosensor for detection of cysteine. *Journal of Fluorescence,* 31, 401–414.

Kim, D. & Yoo, S. 2021. Aptamer-conjugated quantum dot optical biosensors: Strategies and applications. *Chemosensors,* 9, 318.

Kim, H. M., Park, J. H. & Lee, S. K. 2019. Fiber optic sensor based on ZnO nanowires decorated by Au nanoparticles for improved plasmonic biosensor. *Scientific Reports,* 9, 15605.

Koyappayil, A., Chavan, S. G., Mohammadniaei, M., Go, A., Hwang, S. Y. & Lee, M. H. 2020. β-Hydroxybutyrate dehydrogenase decorated MXene nanosheets for the amperometric determination of β-hydroxybutyrate. *Microchimica Acta,* 187, 277.

Kruss, S., Landry, M. P., Vander Ende, E., Lima, B. M. A., Reuel, N. F., Zhang, J., Nelson, J., Mu, B., Hilmer, A. & Strano, M. 2014. Neurotransmitter detection using corona phase molecular recognition on fluorescent single-walled carbon nanotube sensors. *Journal of the American Chemical Society,* 136, 713–724.

Kumar, S., Lei, Y., Alshareef, N. H., Quevedo-Lopez, M. A. & Salama, K. N. 2018. Biofunctionalized two-dimensional Ti**3**C**2** MXenes for ultrasensitive detection of cancer biomarker. *Biosensors and Bioelectronics,* 121, 243–249.

Land, K. J., Boeras, D. I., Chen, X. S., Ramsay, A. R. & Peeling, R. W. 2019. Reassured diagnostics to inform disease control strategies, strengthen health systems and improve patient outcomes. *Nature Microbiology,* 4, 46–54.

Lee, J. U., Kim, W., Lee, H., Park, K. & Sim, S. 2019. Quantitative and specific detection of exosomal miRNAs for accurate diagnosis of breast cancer using a surface-enhanced raman scattering sensor based on plasmonic head-flocked gold nanopillars. *Small,* 15, 1804968.

Leonardi, A. A., Lo Faro, M. J., Petralia, S., Fazio, B., Musumeci, P., Conoci, S., Irrera, A. & Priolo, F. 2018. Ultrasensitive label- and PCR-free genome detection based on cooperative hybridization of silicon nanowires optical biosensors. *ACS Sensors,* 3, 1690–1697.

Leong, S. X., Leong, Y. X., Tan, E. X., Sim, H. Y. F., Koh, C. S. L., Lee, Y. H., Chong, C., Ng, L. S., Chen, J. R. T., Pang, D. W. C., Nguyen, L. B. T., Boong, S. K., Han, X., Kao, Y.-C., Chua, Y. H., Phan-Quang, G. C., Phang, I. Y., Lee, H. K., Abdad, M. Y., Tan, N. S. & Ling, X. Y. 2022. Noninvasive and point-of-care Surface-Enhanced Raman Scattering (SERS)-based breathalyzer for mass screening of coronavirus disease 2019 (COVID-19) under 5 min. *ACS Nano,* 16, 2629–2639.

Li, Q., Ding, L., Zhang, Y. & Wu, T. 2022. A cholesterol optical fiber sensor based on CQDs-COD/CA composite. *IEEE Sensors Journal,* 22, 6247–6255.

Li, X., Wu, Y., Niu, J., Jiang, D., Xiao, D. & Zhou, C. 2019. One-step sensitive thrombin detection based on a nanofibrous sensing platform. *Journal of Materials Chemistry B,* 7, 5161–5169.

Liu, C., Cai, Q., Xu, B., Zhu, W., Zhang, L., Jianlong, Z. & Chen, X. 2017. Graphene oxide functionalized long period grating for ultrasensitive label-free immunosensing. *Biosensors and Bioelectronics,* 94, 200–206.

Liu, Q., Yang, T., Ye, Y., Chen, P., Ren, X., Rao, A., Wan, Y., Wang, B. & Luo, Z. 2019. A highly sensitive label-free electrochemical immunosensor based on an aligned GaN nanowires array/polydopamine heterointerface modified with Au nanoparticles. *Journal of Materials Chemistry B,* 7, 1442–1449.

Ma, F., Li, C.-C. & Zhang, C.-Y. 2018. Development of quantum dot-based biosensors: Principles and applications. *Journal of Materials Chemistry B,* 6, 6173–6190.

Mak, K. F., Lee, C., Hone, J., Shan, J. & Heinz, T. F. 2010. Atomically thin MoS_2: A new direct-gap semiconductor. *Physical Review Letters,* 105, 136805.

Mandal, G. & Ganguly, T. 2011. Applications of nanomaterials in the different fields of photosciences. *Indian Journal of Physics,* 85, 1229–1245.

Manickam, P., Vashist, A., Madhu, S., Sadasivam, M., Sakthivel, A., Kaushik, A. & Nair, M. 2019. Gold nanocubes embedded biocompatible hybrid hydrogels for electrochemical detection of H_2O_2. *Bioelectrochemistry,* 131, 107373.

Mars, A., Hamami, M., Bechnak, L., Patra, D. & Raouafi, N. 2018. Curcumin-graphene quantum dots for dual mode sensing platform: Electrochemical and fluorescence detection of APOe4, responsible of Alzheimer's disease. *Analytica Chimica Acta,* 1036, 141–146.

Martynenko, I. V., Litvin, A. P., Purcell-Milton, F., Baranov, A. V., Fedorov, A. V. & Gun'ko, Y. K. 2017. Application of semiconductor quantum dots in bioimaging and biosensing. *Journal of Materials Chemistry B,* 5, 6701–6727.

Mathur, A., Nayak, H. C., Rajput, S., Roy, S., Nagabooshanam, S., Wadhwa, S. & Kumar, R. 2021. An enzymatic multiplexed impedimetric sensor based on α-MnO_2/GQD nano-composite for the detection of diabetes and diabetic foot ulcer using micro-fluidic platform. *Chemosensors*, 9, 339.

Mishra, Y., Kaps, S., Schuchardt, A., Paulowicz, I., Jin, X., Gedamu, D., Wille, S., Oleg, L. & Adelung, R. 2014. Versatile fabrication of complex shaped metal oxide nano-microstructures and their interconnected networks for multifunctional applications. *Powder and Particle,* 31, 92–110.

Murjani, B. O., Kadu, P. S., Bansod, M., Vaidya, S. S. & Yadav, M. D. 2022. Carbon nanotubes in biomedical applications: Current status, promises, and challenges. *Carbon Letters,* 32, 1207–1226.

Naseri, M., Fotouhi, L. & Ehsani, A. 2018. Recent progress in the development of conducting polymer-based nanocomposites for electrochemical biosensors applications: A mini-review. *Chemical Records,* 18, 599–618.

Nibler, R., Kurth, L., Li, H., Spreinat, A., Kuhlemann, I., Flavel, B. S. & Kruss, S. 2021. Sensing with chirality-pure near-infrared fluorescent carbon nanotubes. *Analytical Chemistry,* 93, 6446–6455.

Noh, S., Lee, H., Kim, J., Jang, H., An, J., Park, C., Lee, M.-H. & Lee, T. 2022. Rapid electrochemical dual-target biosensor composed of an Aptamer/MXene hybrid on Au microgap electrodes for cytokines detection. *Biosensors and Bioelectronics,* 207, 114159.

Öndeş, B., Evli, S., Uygun, M. & Aktaş Uygun, D. 2021. Boron nitride nanosheet modified label-free electrochemical immunosensor for cancer antigen 125 detection. *Biosensors and Bioelectronics,* 191, 113454.

Paras, Yadav, K., Kumar, P., Teja, D. R., Chakraborty, S., Chakraborty, M., Mohapatra, S. S., Sahoo, A., Chou, M. M. C., Liang, C.-T. & Hang, D.-R. 2023. A review on low-dimensional nanomaterials: Nanofabrication, characterization and applications. *Nanomaterials*, 13, 160.

Pathak, A. & Gupta, B. D. 2019. Ultra-selective fiber optic SPR platform for the sensing of dopamine in synthetic cerebrospinal fluid incorporating permselective nafion membrane and surface imprinted MWCNTs-PPy matrix. *Biosensors and Bioelectronics,* 133, 205–214.

Pedrero, M., Campuzano, S. & Pingarrón, J. M. 2017. Electrochemical (bio)sensing of clinical markers using quantum dots. *Electroanalysis,* 29, 24–37.

Picciolini, S., Castagnetti, N., Vanna, R., Mehn, D., Bedoni, M., Gramatica, F., Villani, M., Calestani, D., Pavesi, M., Lazzarini, L., Zappettini, A. & Morasso, C. 2015. Branched gold nanoparticles on ZnO 3D architecture as biomedical SERS sensors. *RSC Advances,* 5, 93644–93651.

Pilehvar, S. & De Wael, K. 2015. Recent advances in electrochemical biosensors based on fullerene-C60 nano-structured platforms. *Biosensors*, 5, 712–735.

Pirzada, M. & Altintas, Z. 2019. Nanomaterials for healthcare biosensing applications. *Sensors*, 19, 5311.

Sharma, V.P., Sharma, U., Chattopadhyay, M. & Shukla, V. N. 2018. Advance applications of nanomaterials: A review. *Materials Today: Proceedings,* 5, 6376–6380.

Prattis, I., Hui, E., Gubeljak, P., Kaminski Schierle, G. S., Lombardo, A. & Occhipinti, L. G. 2021. Graphene for biosensing applications in point-of-care testing. *Trends in Biotechnology,* 39, 1065–1077.

Qiao, X., Li, K., Xu, J., Cheng, N., Sheng, Q., Cao, W., Yue, T. & Zheng, J. 2018. Novel electrochemical sensing platform for ultrasensitive detection of cardiac troponin I based on aptamer-MoS**2** nanoconjugates. *Biosensors and Bioelectronics,* 113, 142–147.

Rahmanian, R., Mozaffari, S. A., Amoli, H. & Abedi, M. 2017. Development of sensitive impedimetric urea biosensor using DC sputtered Nano-ZnO on TiO_2 thin film as a novel hierarchical nanostructure transducer. *Sensors and Actuators B: Chemical,* 256, 760–774.

Rani, P., Dalal, R. & Srivastava, S. 2022. Study of electronic and optical properties of quantum dots. *Applied Nanoscience,* 12, 2127–2138.

Ranjbari, S., Rezayi, M., Arefinia, R., Aghaee-Bakhtiari, S. H., Hatamluyi, B. & Pasdar, A. 2023. A novel electrochemical biosensor based on signal amplification of Au HFGNs/PnBA-MXene nanocomposite for the detection of miRNA-122 as a biomarker of breast cancer. *Talanta,* 255, 124247.

Ratlam, C., Phanichphant, S. & Sriwichai, S. 2020. Development of dopamine biosensor based on polyaniline/carbon quantum dots composite. *Journal of Polymer Research,* 27, 183.

Rawat, R., Singh, S., Roy, S., Kumar, A., Goswami, T. & Mathur, A. 2023. Design and development of an electroanalytical genosensor based on Cu-PTCA/rGO nanocomposites for the detection of cervical cancer. *Materials Chemistry and Physics,* 295, 127050.

Regonini, D., Bowen, C. R., Jaroenworaluck, A. & Stevens, R. 2013. A review of growth mechanism, structure and crystallinity of anodized TiO**2** nanotubes. *Materials Science and Engineering: R: Reports,* 74, 377–406.

Roberts, A., Tripathi, P. P. & Gandhi, S. 2019. Graphene nanosheets as an electric mediator for ultrafast sensing of urokinase plasminogen activator receptor-A biomarker of cancer. *Biosensors and Bioelectronics,* 141, 111398.

Roy, S., John, A., Nagabooshanam, S., Mishra, A., Wadhwa, S., Mathur, A., Narang, J., Singh, J., Dilawar, N. & Davis, J. 2019. Self-aligned TiO2- Photo reduced graphene oxide hybrid surface for smart bandage application. *Applied Surface Science,* 488, 261–268.

Roy, S., Sain, S., Wadhwa, S., Mathur, A., Dubey, S. & Roy, S. 2021. Electrochemical impedimetric analysis of different dimensional (0D-2D) carbon nanomaterials for effective biosensing of L-tyrosine. *Measurement Science and Technology,* 33, 014002.

Safaee, M. M., Gravely, M. & Roxbury, D. 2021. A wearable optical microfibrous biomaterial with encapsulated nanosensors enables wireless monitoring of oxidative stress. *Advanced Functional Materials,* 31, 2006254.

Sim, S. & Wong, N. K. 2021. Nanotechnology and its use in imaging and drug delivery (Review). *Biomedical Reports,* 14, 42.

Singh, C., Ali, M. A., Kumar, V., Ahmad, R. & Sumana, G. 2018. Functionalized MoS_2 nanosheets assembled microfluidic immunosensor for highly sensitive detection of food pathogen. *Sensors and Actuators B: Chemical,* 259, 1090–1098.

Singh, R., Hong, S. & Jang, J. 2017. Label-free detection of Influenza viruses using a reduced graphene oxide-based electrochemical immunosensor integrated with a microfluidic platform. *Scientific Reports,* 7, 42771.

Song, J. & Bazant, M. Z. 2013. Effects of nanoparticle geometry and size distribution on diffusion impedance of battery electrodes. *Journal of the Electrochemical Society,* 160, A15.

Sosa, I. O., Noguez, C. & Barrera, R. G. 2003. Optical properties of metal nanoparticles with arbitrary shapes. *The Journal of Physical Chemistry B,* 107, 6269–6275.

Splendiani, A., Sun, L., Zhang, Y., Li, T., Kim, J., Chim, C.Y., Galli, G. & Wang, F. 2010. Emerging photoluminescence in monolayer MoS2. *Nano Letters,* 10, 1271–1275.

Sulciute, A., Nishimura, K., Gilshtein, E., Cesano, F., Viscardi, G., Nasibulin, A. G., Ohno, Y. & Rackauskas, S. 2021. ZnO nanostructures application in electrochemistry: Influence of morphology. *The Journal of Physical Chemistry C,* 125, 1472–1482.

Sun, B., Wang, Y., Li, D., Li, W., Gou, X., Gou, Y. & Hu, F. 2020. Development of a sensitive electrochemical immunosensor using polyaniline functionalized graphene quantum dots for detecting a depression marker. *Materials Science and Engineering: C,* 111, 110797.

Thakur, H., Kaur, N., Sareen, D. & Prabhakar, N. 2017. Electrochemical determination of M. tuberculosis antigen based on Poly(3,4-ethylenedioxythiophene) and functionalized carbon nanotubes hybrid platform. *Talanta,* 171, 115–123.

Thévenot, D. R., Toth, K., Durst, R. A. & Wilson, G. S. 2001. Electrochemical biosensors: Recommended definitions and classification. *Biosensors and Bioelectronics,* 16, 121–131.

Tite, T., Chiticaru, E., Burns, J. & Ionita, M. 2019. Impact of nano-morphology, lattice defects and conductivity on the performance of graphene based electrochemical biosensors. *Journal of Nanobiotechnology,* 17, 1–22.

Tri Murti, B., Huang, Y. J., Darumas Putri, A., Lee, C. P., Hsieh, C. M., Wei, S. M., Tsai, M. L., Peng, C. W. & Yang, P. K. 2022. Free-standing vertically aligned tin disulfide nanosheets for ultrasensitive aptasensor design toward alzheimer's diagnosis applications. *Chemical Engineering Journal,* 452, 139394.

Tripathy, S., Krishna Vanjari, S. R., Singh, V., Swaminathan, S. & Singh, S. G. 2017. Electrospun manganese (III) oxide nanofiber based electrochemical DNA-nanobiosensor for zeptomolar detection of dengue consensus primer. *Biosensors and Bioelectronics,* 90, 378–387.

Wadhwa, S., John, A., Nagabooshanam, S., Mathur, A. & Narang, J. 2020. Graphene quantum dot-gold hybrid nanoparticles integrated aptasensor for ultra-sensitive detection of vitamin D3 towards point-of-care application. *Applied Surface Science,* 521, 146427.

Wadhwa, S., Roy, S., Mittal, N., John, A., Midha, S., Mohanty, S., Vasanthan, K. & Mathur, A. 2021. Self – aligned mesoporous titania nanotubes – reduced graphene oxide hybrid surface: A potential scaffold for osteogenesis. *International Journal of Materials Research,* 112, 584–590.

Walton, B. M., Jackson, G. W., Deutz, N. & Cote, G. 2017. Surface-enhanced Raman spectroscopy competitive binding biosensor development utilizing surface modification of silver nanocubes and a citrulline aptamer. *Journal of Biomedical Optics,* 22, 75002.

Wang, L., Kafshgari, M. & Meunier, M. 2020. Optical properties and applications of plasmonic-metal nanoparticles. *Advanced Functional Materials,* 30, 2005400.

Wang, Q., Li, Q., Yang, X., Wang, K., Du, S., Zhang, H. & Nie, Y. 2016. Graphene oxide-gold nanoparticles hybrids-based surface plasmon resonance for sensitive detection of microRNA. *Biosensors and Bioelectronics,* 77, 1001–1007.

Wang, Z., Liu, T., Asif, M., Yu, Y., Wang, W., Wang, H., Xiao, F. & Liu, H. 2018. Rimelike structure-inspired approach toward in situ-oriented self-assembly of hierarchical porous MOF films as a sweat biosensor. *ACS Applied Materials & Interfaces,* 10, 27936–27946.

Warren-Smith, S. C., Afshar, S. & Monro, T. M. 2010. Fluorescence-based sensing with optical nanowires: A generalized model and experimental validation. *Optics Express,* 18, 9474–9485.

Wu, D., Liu, Y., Wang, Y., Hu, L., Ma, H., Wang, G. & Wei, Q. 2016. Label-free electrochemiluminescent immunosensor for detection of prostate specific antigen based on aminated graphene quantum dots and carboxyl graphene quantum dots. *Scientific Reports,* 6, 20511.

Wu, L., Yan, H., Wang, J., Liu, G. & Xie, W. 2019. Tyrosinase incorporated with Au-Pt@ SiO_2 nanospheres for electrochemical detection of bisphenol A. *Journal of The Electrochemical Society,* 166, B562–B568.

Xiang, Q., Huang, J., Huang, H., Mao, W. & Ye, Z. 2018. A label-free electrochemical platform for the highly sensitive detection of hepatitis B virus DNA using graphene quantum dots. *RSC Advances,* 8, 1820–1825.

Yang, Q., Ma, L., Xiao, S., Zhang, D., Djoulde, A., Ye, M., Lin, Y., Geng, S., Li, X., Chen, T. & Sun, L. 2021. Electrical conductivity of multiwall carbon nanotube bundles contacting with metal electrodes by nano manipulators inside SEM. *Nanomaterials*, 11, 1290.

Yang, Q., Zhu, G., Singh, L., Wang, Y., Singh, R., Zhang, B., Zhang, X. & Kumar, S. 2020. Highly sensitive and selective sensor probe using glucose oxidase/gold nanoparticles/graphene oxide functionalized tapered optical fiber structure for detection of glucose. *Optik,* 208, 164536.

Yin, Z., Liu, C., Yi, Y., Wu, H., Fu, X. & Yan, Y. 2022. A label-free electrochemical immunosensor based on PdPtCu@BP bilayer nanosheets for point-of-care kidney injury molecule-1 testing. *Journal of Electroanalytical Chemistry,* 917, 116420.

Yola, M. L. & Atar, N. 2016. Functionalized graphene quantum dots with bi-metallic nanoparticles composite: Sensor application for simultaneous determination of ascorbic acid, dopamine, uric acid and tryptophan. *Journal of the Electrochemical Society,* 163, B718.

Zahed, M. A., Sharifuzzaman, M., Yoon, H., Asaduzzaman, M., Kim, D. K., Jeong, S., Pradhan, G. B., Shin, Y. D., Yoon, S. H., Sharma, S., Zhang, S. & Park, J. Y. 2022. A nanoporous carbon-MXene heterostructured nanocomposite-based epidermal patch for real-time biopotentials and sweat glucose monitoring. *Advanced Functional Materials,* 32, 2208344.

Zhang, Q., Wang, F., Zhang, H., Zhang, Y., Liu, M. & Liu, Y. 2018. Universal Ti_3C_2 MXenes based self-standard ratiometric fluorescence resonance energy transfer platform for highly sensitive detection of exosomes. *Analytical Chemistry,* 90, 12737–12744.

Zhang, Y. & Yan, B. 2019. A point-of-care diagnostics logic detector based on glucose oxidase immobilized lanthanide functionalized metal–organic frameworks. *Nanoscale,* 11, 22946–22953.

Zhang, Z., Guo, C., Zhang, S., He, L., Wang, M., Peng, D., Tian, J. & Fang, S. 2017. Carbon-based nanocomposites with aptamer-templated silver nanoclusters for the highly sensitive and selective detection of platelet-derived growth factor. *Biosensors and Bioelectronics,* 89, 735–742.

Zhao, H. & Lei, Y. 2020. 3D Nanostructures for the next generation of high-performance nanodevices for electrochemical energy conversion and storage. *Advanced Energy Materials,* 10, 2001460.

Zhou, P., Liu, H., Gong, L., Tang, B., Shi, Y., Yang, C. & Han, Z. 2019. A faster detection method for high-sensitivity cardiac troponin—POCT quantum dot fluorescence immunoassay. *Journal of Thoracic Disease*, 11, 1506–1513.

23 Therapeutic Nutraceutical Delivery Strategies Using Nanocarrier Systems and their Characterization Methods

Souptik Bhattacharya,
Sayamdipta Das Chowdhury,
and Sayani Debnath

23.1 INTRODUCTION

Nanomaterials are bursting through the realm of science fiction and into our homes; medicines; clothes; cosmetics; and even shockingly into our foods, drinks, and nutritional supplements (Bai et al., 2021). In general, nanotechnology is defined as the engineering and science associated with the design, fabrication, characterization, and utilization of materials and systems having at least one nanoscale aspect (often in the range of 1–100 nm) (Mazumder et al., 2020). At this size, they have special features that alter the pharmacokinetics of the molecules and their resulting outcomes. Products known as nutraceuticals give the body critical nutrients and fight illness. It is a necessity over and above the fundamental nutrients that we receive from our everyday meals. It could include nutritional supplements, items made from plants, nutrients extracted from mixtures, genetically modified food, and processed items like cereals, drinks, and soups. Many traditional nutraceutical merchandizers are already on the market, ranging from straightforward, inexpensive items for everyday use to pricey combinations recommended for specific conditions. In order to stay healthy, individuals are spending more money on purchasing unprocessed food and nutritious foods, which is driving up demand for nutraceuticals globally. However, nutraceuticals have limitations because of their excessive dosage levels; poor regularity and repeatability; issues with structural characterization, solubility; formulation difficulties; issues with longevity for minimum two years; difficulties with wide mass production for high-quality medicines. These challenges limit their proper applicability which needs to be mitigated by sustainable and strategic research and

DOI: 10.1201/9781003432661-23

innovation in the upcoming years (Tundisi et al., 2023). The use of nanomaterials in medicine, food, and nutrition sectors involves creating innovative carrier strategies with improved solubility, durability against heat and light, higher OB, and more profound physiological efficiency. Emulsions and microemulsions, nanoparticles (NPs), or a mixture of both domains can be used as the cores of nanocarrier vehicles [nanostructured lipid carriers (NLCs)]. The aqueous/hydrophobic core of the nano-based materials used to encapsulate hydrophilic/hydrophobic chemicals is separated from the continuous phase by an encapsulating shell. They consist of colloidosomes, liposomes, and nanohydrogels. Either colloidal particles or emulsifying molecules stabilize the nanocarriers in both groups (Pickering emulsions). All of them have been extensively used to deliver hydrophilic/lipophilic drugs effectively. Nanocarriers have demonstrated numerous benefits due to their incredibly small size, including increased aqueous solubility, increased residence time in gastrointestinal (GI) tract regions, improved physicochemical stability in GI tract, increased intestinal permeation, controlled release in GI tract, intracellular delivery, and transcellular delivery (Ali et al., 2019).

Hence, designing blueprints for a better nutraceutical delivery by fusing it with nanotechnology has become crucial. Using nanotechnology would undoubtedly offer superior outcomes than the conventional items already on the market, elevating the role of nutraceuticals. Due to these benefits of nanotechnology, an effort has been made in this chapter to understand how engineered nanosized formulation techniques are facilitating the appropriate management and utilization of nutraceuticals by reducing their drawbacks and increasing their overall effectiveness in the somatic body.

23.2 IMPORTANCE OF ENTRAPMENT OF FOOD BIOACTIVES BY ENCAPSULATING CARRIER MATERIALS

Nutraceuticals, bioactive compounds in food, are influenced by primary composition, texture, flavor profiles, and processing styles (MacDonald and Reitmeier, 2017). Recent advancements in nutrition, science, engineering, and technology have led to minimally processed foods that maintain qualities akin to natural foods, offering extended shelf life, improved nutritional functionality, unique textures, and distinct tastes (Liem and Russell, 2019). The growing market for agro-biological products, such as gummy bears, has promoted innovative formulation methods due to their stability and reduced volatility losses (Čižauskaitė et al., 2019). Encapsulation techniques protect bioactive compounds (e.g., essential oils, aqueous extracts, secondary metabolites) from environmental factors and degradation, enhancing their therapeutic potential. This method ensures the long-term existence of active substances by maintaining environmental factors during storage and preserving the biological integrity of the products (Čižauskaitė et al., 2019). Encapsulation can mitigate the effects of UV light, harsh temperatures, and microbiological agents, which often compromise the integrity and feasibility of these compounds (Bhattacharya et al., 2022b). Consequently, encapsulation strategy might be a solution to these problems as it enables, among other things, the reduction of volatility-related losses, the increment of biological integrity, efficiency enhancement, commercial viability

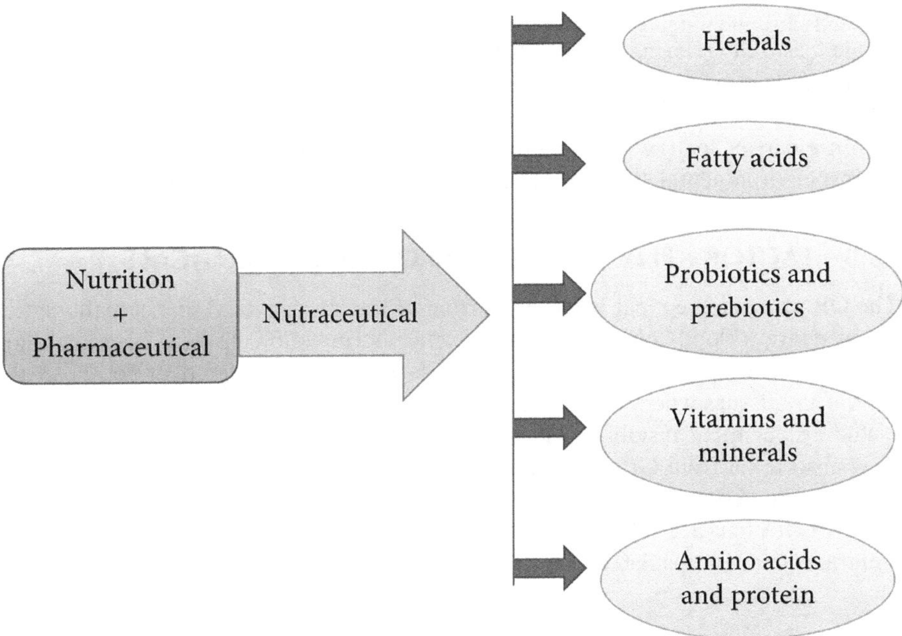

FIGURE 23.1 Classification of nutraceuticals. (Adopted from Khalaf et al. (2021) under the terms and conditions of the Creative Commons Attribution (CC BY) license granting unrestricted reproduction.)

enhancement, and formulation stability enhancement in the agricultural, food, and biopharmaceutical sectors. Figure 23.1 depicts the classification of nutraceuticals (Khalaf et al., 2021).

Encapsulation offers several benefits, including reducing volatility-related losses, enhancing biological integrity, improving efficiency, increasing commercial viability, and stabilizing formulations in agriculture, food, and biopharmaceutical sectors. Various polymers, such as chitosan, gums (Arabic, xanthan, acacia, and shellac), maltodextrin, zein, starch, and sodium alginate, are employed to safeguard the core bioactive chemicals and prolong their release under specific physicochemical conditions (Bhattacharya et al., 2019; Riseh et al., 2022). Encapsulation involves creating a protective zone around a core material (liquid, solid, or gas) within a membrane, which shields the core from chemical and environmental interactions, thereby reducing the deterioration of bioactive components (Levi et al., 2011). Both natural and artificial polymers, including those derived from petroleum, renewable resources, and natural sources, are used in encapsulation (Bhattacharya et al., 2021; Riseh et al., 2022).

Microencapsulation, which forms microcapsules or microspheres, significantly impacts feed and powder qualities based on the process and coating materials. Microspheres, dense matrix structures with a reservoir system, are utilized in the food, chemical, and medicinal industries. The morphologies of microparticles are influenced by core bioactive chemicals, coating materials, and encapsulation methods. Emulsion methods, particularly Pickering emulsions, are prevalent in the food and biopharmaceutical industries due to their resilience against coalescence and economic feasibility (Harman et al., 2019). Encapsulation confines bioactive components like natural antibacterial compounds, antifungals, phenolics, flavonoids, carotenoids, color pigments, fatty acids, phytosterols, probiotics, vitamins, and bioactive peptides within a carrier matrix. This approach enhances the stability of these compounds against environmental changes and controls their release rate (Zabot et al., 2022).

23.3 FACTOR AFFECTING THE OB OF NUTRACEUTICALS

The OB of a nutraceutical is the proportion of the nutraceutical that actually enters the systemic (blood) circulation in an active form following oral administration (Vinarov et al., 2021). Nutraceuticals needs bodily access for distribution in the organs and tissues where they can have a positive impact on health. A few obstacles, including chemical instability during digestion, poor solubility in GI tract fluids, slow absorption from GI tract, reflux by p-glycoprotein, and first-pass metabolism, prohibit ingested nutraceuticals from reaching the systemic circulation in an active state (Bhattacharya, 2020). The following equation can be used to evaluate the OB of a nutraceutical encapsulated (EN) within a carrier matrix (Yao et al., 2015).

$$OB = OB_B \times OB_A \times OB_M \tag{23.1}$$

In this case, OB_B refers to the portion of a consumed nutraceutical that makes it through the upper GI tract and released from the food matrix into the GI tract fluids, becoming bioaccessible for enterocyte absorption. OB_A is the portion of the bioavailable supplement that is actually absorbed by the enterocytes and delivered to the portal blood or lymph (and into the body's circulation). After first-pass metabolism in the GI tract and liver, OB_M is the portion of an absorbed nutraceutical that is still in an active state (and any other forms of metabolism) (Yao et al., 2015).

23.3.1 Determination of Bioactive Food Component Category

Plant-based foods are rich in various bioactive ingredients such as polyphenols, phytosterols, carotenoids, tocopherols, tocotrienols, organosulfur compounds (including isothiocyanates and diallyl sulfide compounds), soluble and insoluble fiber, and fructo-oligosaccharides (Abuajah, 2019). Polyphenols, the most abundant and widely distributed class of bioactive molecules, include flavonoids like catechins, flavins, and isoflavones, with nearly 8,000 different varieties. These compounds are found in vegetables, fruits, cereals, legumes, nuts, tea, wine, and other fruit- and vegetable-based beverages. The polyphenol content in foods can vary significantly, such as 590 to 1,500 mg/100 g dry matter in barley and millet, and 37 to 429 mg/100 g fruit in berries (Abuajah et al., 2015).

Organosulfur compounds, found in cruciferous vegetables like broccoli and allium vegetables like garlic, become bioactive only when the vegetable is cut, chewed, or crushed. Enzymes like myrosinase and allinase convert these compounds into health-promoting isothiocyanates and diallyl sulfides, respectively (Bhattacharya et al., 2022c). Phytosterols, plant equivalents of cholesterol, include beta-sitosterol, campesterol, and stigmasterol, which are found in high amounts in nuts, seeds, raw plant oils, and legumes. A lacto-vegetarian diet typically includes over 500 mg/day of unsaturated phytosterols compared to about 250 mg/day in a non-vegetarian diet. Plant stanols, the saturated end product of plant sterols like sitostanol, are naturally present in wood pulp, long oil, and soybean oil, contributing 150 to 400 mg in an average Western diet (Gupta, 2020).

Carotenoids, lipid-soluble plant pigments, include nonpolar bioactive carotenoids like beta-carotene and lycopene, and polar carotenoids like lutein. These compounds, found either unesterified or esterified to fatty acids in plant tissue, have their content significantly influenced by storage conditions. Vegetable oils, nuts, and cereal germ are also rich in tocopherols and tocotrienols, with RRR-alpha-tocopherol being the most bioactive and prevalent form in human tissues and blood (Edgar and Wang, 2017). These bioactive food ingredients collectively contribute to the health-promoting properties of plant-based foods, providing essential nutrients and protective compounds that support overall well-being.

23.3.2 Designing Food Matrix for Oral Consumption

The food matrix refers to the complex physical and chemical interactions between nutrients and non-nutrients within food, impacting the release, stability, accessibility, and digestion of food molecules. It significantly influences the digestion and absorption of food components in the GI system, as well as the microbial fermentation and absorption of byproduct metabolites in the colon. The ratio of nutrients absorbed in the colon to those released during digestion defines the food matrix, which affects the biotransformation and physiological responses of food components in the body. Bioavailability, the amount of nutrients absorbed, has become the standard for assessing the nutritional benefits of nutrients and bioactive compounds (Mendes et al., 2022). The food matrix can alter the bioactive ingredients in food, meaning that foods with similar chemical compositions can have different physicochemical and physiological effects. The bioavailability of hydrophobic bioactive pharmaceuticals and nutraceuticals taken orally can be limited by factors like improper release, low water solubility, digestion and metabolism in the GI tract, and low cellular permeability. Carefully designed encapsulating matrices can enhance a drug's bioavailability, solubilization, transport, metabolism, and absorption. Many bioactive substances in dietary supplements and medications are lipophilic with limited bioavailability due to various physical, chemical, or physiological processes, such as low intestinal permeability and enzymatic changes in the digestive system. The composition and structure of foods consumed with these substances significantly impact their bioavailability. Research has shown that complete foods produce different physiological responses than isolated nutrients due to the complexity of nutritional interactions and the dietary matrix (Premathilaka et al., 2022).

Certain foods have been fortified with phytosterols and phytostanols to lower low-density lipoprotein (LDL) cholesterol levels. Special food matrices are designed to enhance the bioaccessibility and bioavailability of specific bioactive components, categorized into functional foods and excipient foods. *Foods classified as functional*: These foods have a bioactive component that is encased in a natural or artificial food matrix. If a bioactive ingredient is soluble, it is added to processed foods as is; if not, it is encapsulated with a technology that is appropriate for the mode of nutrition delivery (McClements, 2015). *Excipient foods*: An excipient food is a natural or processed food that contains a bioactive component and is consumed together with another food. The make-up and/or the excipient food's structure are created in a way that will boost the bioavailability of the bioactive ingredient. According to in vitro experiments on carrots and tomatoes, mixed micelles that were soluble in intestinal fluids were generated when digestible lipids were added, increasing the bioaccessibility of carotenoid compounds. Sucrose monoesters and rhamnolipids are examples of surface-active molecules that can increase the bioavailability of some bioactive components (Yu et al., 2016).

23.3.3 Selection Criteria of Nanoparticle-Based Delivery Systems

The nanoencapsulation of organic bioactive molecules or nutraceuticals is now revolutionizing the pharma industry (Afzal et al., 2022). A pictorial illustration of the advantage of nano-based therapeutics over conventional ones is depicted in Figure 23.2. Because of changed pharmacokinetics and biodistribution, the encapsulation of bioactives in a suitable carrier matrix might increase their bioavailability. Due to the increase in drug localization to specific tissues, the therapeutic index of medications has been demonstrated to rise when utilizing controlled drug delivery systems (Manzari et al., 2021).

The WHO (World Health Organization) has started a worldwide plan to address the issues surrounding traditional medicine in response to the growing curiosity of scientists and researchers about these treatments (Bhattacharya et al., 2022a). Priority is given to recent advances in research on the nanoencapsulation of nutraceuticals,

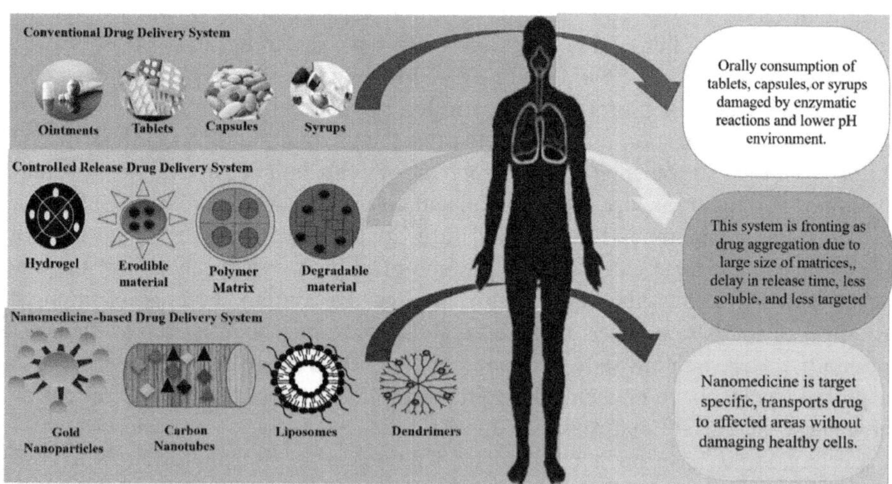

FIGURE 23.2 Advantage of nano-based therapeutics over conventional ones. (Adopted from Afzal et al. (2022) under the terms and conditions of the CC BY license granting unrestricted reproduction.)

aiming to increase their health benefits while removing any remaining restrictions. Following are several desired characteristics of nanoscale delivery system:

- They will first react differently in the GI system when reduced to the nanoscale compared to normal particle matter (Mohammadi et al., 2022).
- They cannot be predicted to be more harmful.
- To assure their safety, it is crucial to evaluate the possible toxicity.
- For the formulation of these delivery systems, food-grade materials must be used.
- These systems ought to be economically feasible, handy enough for real-world applications.
- The delivery system must maintain its functional properties while being physically and chemically resistant to environmental conditions.
- In the systemic circulation, the dose level should keep constant.
- It should be capable to facilitate lymphatic transport in the event of carrying a highly lipophilic molecule.
- Should be capable to lengthen the period of gastric retention (Afzal et al., 2022).

23.4 TYPES AND CHARACTERIZATION METHODS OF NANOPARTICLE-BASED DELIVERY SYSTEM

23.4.1 Different Types of Nanoparticle-Based Delivery Systems

23.4.1.1 Nanoemulsion

Nanoemulsions are isotropic dispersed systems of two immiscible liquids (water and oil). The spherical droplets that make up nanoemulsions are the dispersed phase, and the surrounding liquid is the continuous phase. The three types of nanoemulsions that can be produced are as follows: (i) water-in-oil (w/o) nanoemulsions (in the ongoing oil phase, water droplets are dispersed). The delivery of hydrophilic substances uses the w/o emulsions and (ii) oil-in-water (o/w) nanoemulsions (oil is disseminated in the continuous aqueous phase) (Singh et al., 2017). Hydrophobic active compounds can be delivered using these emulsion systems and (iii) bi-continuous nanoemulsions. Two immiscible liquids must be combined with an emulsifier to create a nanoemulsion. The dispersed and aqueous phase is composed of two immiscible liquids, one of which must be oily and the other of which must be aqueous in composition. A core-shell structure makes up the o/w and w/o nanoemulsion. For instance, in an o/w nanoemulsion system, the lipophilic core comprises nonpolar molecules, whereas the amphiphilic shell is formed of surface-active molecules (Aswathanarayan and Vittal, 2019).

23.4.1.1.1 Benefits of Nanoemulsion

- It could serve as a replacement for vesicles and liposomes.
- It increases the drug's bioavailability.
- Its nature makes it neither poisonous nor allergic.

- Tiny droplets in nanoemulsion have a greater surface area which helps to increase absorption.
- It facilitates lipophilic drug solubilization.

23.4.1.2 Lipid Nanoparticles (LNPs)

LNPs are used in pharmaceutical industries as promising delivery systems for a range of medicines. An adaptable platform for the delivery of nanomedicine is the liposome, an early version of LNPs. A diverse liposomal drug has been approved for usage and is now being used in clinical settings. The physical stabilities and the complexity of later generations of lipid nanocarriers, such as solid lipid nanoparticles (SLNs), nanostructured lipid carriers (NLCs), and cationic lipid-nucleic acid complexes, are improved. SLNs can be compared to nanoemulsions, with the exception that bioactive chemicals are enclosed in solid phases made entirely of fully crystallized lipids from the emulsion. NLCs, which are LNPs that contain both crystalline and liquid phases of lipid (partially solid matrix), can be created by mixing a variety of lipid molecules, such as solid lipid and carrier lipid (oil) (Müller et al., 2002).

23.4.1.2.1 Benefits of LNPs

- LNPs improve the chemical and physical stability of the bioactive molecules.
- They improved sustained release qualities, loading capacity, bioavailability, and appropriateness for large-scale operations.
- Utilizing SLNs has the advantage of providing a method to incorporate lipophilic chemicals into stable particles without the need for organic solvents.
- For unstable bioactives, particularly lipophilic chemicals, SLNs, and NLCs have shown promise as better delivery and storage platforms.

23.4.1.3 Polymeric NPs

Polymeric NPs are small particles having diameters ranging from 1 to 1,000 nm that can contain active chemicals that have been surface-adsorbed onto the polymeric core or are entrapped within them. Surfactants or emulsifiers surround the polymeric NPs, which are made of polymer matrices with molecules trapped inside. Various polymers, including alginic acid, gelatin, polylactic acid, chitosan, polylactide-co-glycolide, and polycaprolactone, are frequently employed to make these nanocarriers (Dhanjal et al., 2021). Polymeric NPs are a reliable carrier that can entrap, disperse, and adsorb active ingredients (Singh et al., 2022).

23.4.1.3.1 Benefits of Polymeric NPs

- Their capacity for controlled release,
- Ability to shield drugs and other molecules from the environment,
- Ability to increase bioavailability and therapeutic index, and
- Ability to combine therapy with imaging ('theranostics') and protection of drug molecules and their precise targeting.

23.4.1.4 Nanovesicles

Nanovesicles are versatile systems for the delivery and targeting agents of drugs, biomolecules, and contrast agents. Incorporating nanovesicles inside a hydrogel system is one potential strategy for avoiding repeated injections and extending the drug's release time. The ability of entrapping hydrophilic pharmaceuticals in the aqueous environment and lipophilic medications in their bilayers makes them a special carrier for drug delivery (Moghassemi and Hadjizadeh, 2014). The three primary categories of nanovesicles are 'polymersomes', 'liposomes', and 'niosomes'. Some other nanovesicles are 'ethosomes', 'transfersomes', and 'pharmacosomes' which are developed for vesicular delivery systems (Ishak et al., 2017).

23.4.1.4.1 Benefits of Nanovesicles

- Liposome increases the bilayer stability and fluidity of the membrane while lowering the permeability of water-soluble compounds through the membrane. But liposomes have lots of drawbacks, including toxicity, affordability, and pH stability difficulties (Bhardwaj et al., 2020).
- Niosomes have greater chemical stability, osmotic activity, and a longer shelf life than liposomes (Bhardwaj et al., 2020).
- Nanosized polymersomes have been developed as vehicles for several medical applications, such as prodrug delivery, gene therapy, and the delivery of imaging and other therapeutic probes to exact sites in the body.

23.4.1.5 Nanocrystals

A new perspective on enhanced drug research is provided by nanocrystal formulation. In a nanocrystal, a medication or bioactive is crystallized and encased in a surfactant or polymeric stabilizer. Hybrid nanocrystals provide an innovative and practical approach to enhance the solubility, dissolution rate, bioimaging capabilities, and bioavailability of medicines that are poorly water soluble (Zhang et al., 2022).

23.4.1.5.1 Benefits of Nanocrystals

The food industry gains benefit from nanocrystals which also improve formulation performance through increased saturation solubility and bioactive particle dissolution rates. Additionally, because of the high loading capacities of the nanocrystals, bioactives can be transported into cells with a higher rate of efficiency, allowing them to have the required therapeutic concentration for the intended pharmacological effects (Yetisgin et al., 2020).

Figure 23.3 illustrates various fields of therapeutic applications of nanotechnology in the biomedical domain.

23.4.2 Characterization Methods for Nanoparticle-Based Carriers

Characterizing biomolecular therapies using nano-based formulations requires a detailed analysis of their nanostructures, considering their articulation, establishment, evaluation, and biological transit (Mahmood et al., 2017). Researchers utilize several advanced techniques, each with its strengths, limitations, and potential future directions. Key techniques include *Dynamic Light Scattering (DLS):* This method evaluates the rotational and translational diffusion coefficients of NPs, correlating with their shape and size. The polydispersity index (PDI), a dimensionless measure derived from DLS, indicates the breadth of the nanoparticle size

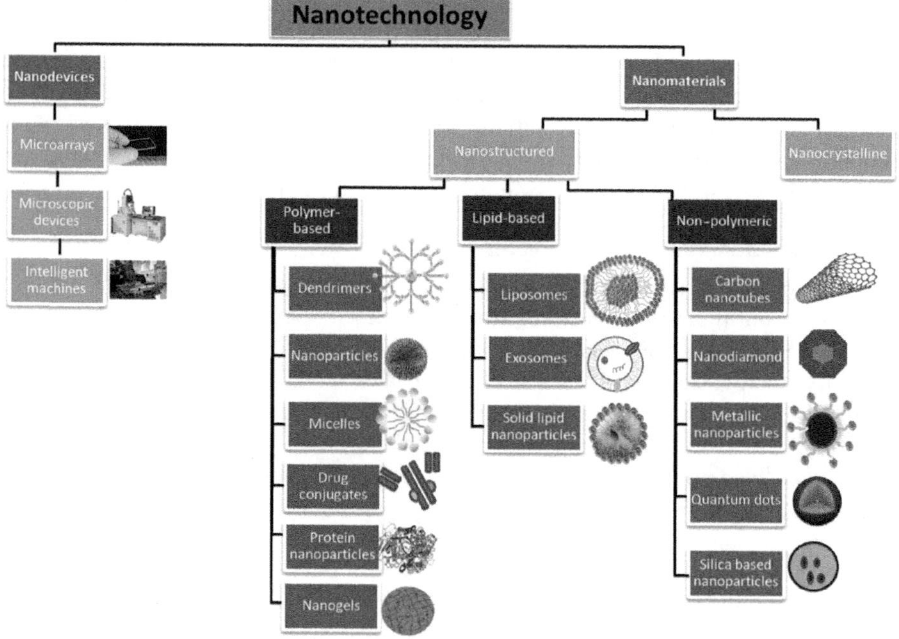

FIGURE 23.3 Various therapeutic applications of nanotechnology. (Adopted from Yetisgin et al. (2020) under CC-BY license granting unrestricted reproduction.)

distribution. However, DLS is limited when particles are dispersed in liquids. *Zeta Potential Analysis:* Using a zetasizer, this technique measures the electropotential state of NPs by assessing their electrophoretic mobility. The zeta potential, which indicates the electric charge at the double-layer boundary, helps determine formulation stability. A zeta potential greater than +30 mV or less than −30 mV suggests a high degree of stability, preventing particle agglomeration (Bhattacharya et al., 2019). Single Particle Inductively Coupled Plasma-Mass Spectrometry (ICP-MS): This technique performs elemental analysis of inorganic NPs at extremely low concentrations. It uses chromatograms to determine nanoparticle size and frequency of transient signals to ascertain particle concentration (Lee et al., 2019). *Tunable Resistive Pulse Sensing (TRPS):* TRPS precisely assesses nanoparticle concentration, size distribution, and size in the range of 40–10 nm. *UV-Visible Spectrophotometry:* This method characterizes NPs with plasmon resonance properties, such as gold and silver NPs, by examining their size, shape, concentration, and aggregation state using light interaction (Rocha et al., 2018). *Scanning Electron Microscopy (SEM):* SEM provides high-resolution images of bulk materials and solids with microstructured composition. It detects particles as small as 10–20 nm and offers magnification of up to 100,000x (Mourdikoudis et al., 2018). The newer field emission SEM (FESEM) offers even greater image quality with magnification of up to 300,000x. *Transmission Electron Microscopy (TEM):* TEM projects electrons through thin sample slices to produce two-dimensional images,

SI no.	Parameters need to be characterized	Characterization instrument/techniques
1	Size	TEM, XRD, DLS, NTA, SAXS, HRTEM, SEM, AFM, EXAFS, FMR, DCS, ICP-MS, UV-vis, MALDI, NMR, TRPS, EPLS, DCS, ICP-MS, superparamagnetic relaxometry, DTA,
2	Structure	TEM, HRTEM, AFM, EPLS, FMR, 3D-tomography
3	Elemental-chemical composition	XRD, XPS, ICP-MS, ICP-OES, SEM-EDX, NMR, MFM, LEIS
4	Crystal structure	XRD, EXAFS, HRTEM, electron diffraction, STEM
5	Ligand binding/mass/surface composition	XPS, FTIR, NMR, SIMS, FMR, TGA, SANS
6	Surface area and specific surface area	BET, liquid NMR
7	Surface charge	Zeta potential, EPM
8	Concentration	ICP-MS, UV-vis, RMM-MEMS, PTA, DCS, TRPS
9	Agglomeration state	Zeta potential, DLS, DCS, UV-vis, SEM, Cryo-TEM, TEM
10	Density	DCS, RMM-MEMS
11	3D visualization	3D-tomography, AFM, SEM
12	Dispersion of NP in matrices/supports	SEM, AFM, TEM
13	Structural defects	HRTEM, EBSD
14	Optical properties	UV-vis-NIR, PL, EELS-STEM
15	Magnetic properties	SQUID, VSM, Mössbauer, MFM, FMR, XMCD, magnetic susceptibility

FIGURE 23.4 Chart of important parameters of nanoformulations that needs to be determined and the corresponding characterization techniques. (Adopted from Mourdikoudis et al. (2018), licensed under a Creative Commons Attribution 3.0 license granting unrestricted reproduction.)

providing clearer views compared to optical microscopes. *Atomic Force Microscopy (AFM):* AFM generates high-resolution three-dimensional topographical images of samples, providing detailed surface characterization (Mahmood et al., 2017; Mourdikoudis et al., 2018). These techniques collectively contribute to a comprehensive understanding of nanoparticle-based formulations, enabling improvements in their stability, bioavailability, and overall effectiveness. A detailed chart, including various characterization techniques, is given in Figure 23.4.

23.5 GI BIOAVAILABILITY OF NANOCARRIERS

After oral administration, bioactive-loaded NPs interact with the intestinal mucosa and epithelial cells for absorption and then circulate systemically to organs, such as the heart, lungs, kidneys, spleen, liver, and brain. Metabolism involves the biotransformation of bioactives and NPs in tissues, with excretion handled by organs like the liver and kidneys. NPs face various obstacles from intake to excretion, including enzymes, low stomach pH, mucus, GI epithelium, blood components, the blood–brain barrier, liver metabolism, and bile excretion (Koshani and Jafari, 2019).

23.5.1 Ingestion

NPs are partially broken down by salivary enzymes with a pH range of 5–7, which results in the ingestion of those particles. NPs will remain in the stomach for 3–4 hours after entering through the esophagus, depending on whether the stomach is fasting or properly fed. The stomach's digestive enzymes and acidic pH will break down the proteins and carbs if glycolipid and protein are employed to produce the NPs, which will result in significant deterioration of the NPs. Following a 3–6 hours stay in the small intestine via the duodenum, the breakdown products and undigested NPs will go to the large intestine or colon. Along with carrier lipids, the bioaccessibility of encapsulated bioactives may also be influenced by the type of surfactant utilized to create the nanoparticle. According to a study, there was a favorable correlation between the amount of fat digestion in a simulated digestive system and with the surfactant's 'hydrophilic–lipophilic balance'. The bioaccessibility of nutraceuticals can also be influenced by nanoparticle size. For instance, it has been claimed that a nanoemulsion with smaller particles has increased bioaccessibility of β-carotene because they can speed up the production of mixed micelles during lipid digestion (Speranza et al., 2013).

23.5.2 Absorption

Most NPs and released bioactives are absorbed in the small intestine, which is lined with epithelial cells forming a mucosal layer to aid nutrient absorption and block harmful substances. Nanoparticle penetration depends on mucosal diffusion and gut epithelial membrane permeability. The mucosal layer is the first defense, and nanoparticle size influences diffusion speed; smaller particles diffuse faster, but 200 nm particles have shown a higher diffusion coefficient than 100 nm particles. Typically, NPs under 500 nm are halted by mucus. The mucosal layer's pore size (around 100 mm) affects diffusion, and factors like diet and exercise can alter mucus quantity, as seen in rats with reduced dietary fiber showing decreased mucosal thickness. Surface charge also impacts absorption: anionic NPs reach the epithelial surface, while cationic ones are confined in the mucosal layer. (Desai et al., 2016). After crossing the mucosal layer, NPs must pass the GI epithelium (enterocytes). Lipophilic supplements are absorbed by enterocytes and delivered to the lymphatic system via chylomicrons, lipid particles formed using lipid components from mixed micelles. Some bioactives remain trapped in non-digested NPs and might enter the body through the para-cellular pathway, a channel between epithelial cells linked by tight junctions. Certain polymers, like chitosan, can disrupt these tight junctions, aiding absorption. Another uptake pathway involves trans-cellular transport through M-cells in Peyer's patches, with subsequent release at the basolateral side of the intestinal epithelium. NPs can enter M-cells via endocytosis, influenced by size, surface charge, and surfactant coating (Liu et al., 2016). Figure 23.5 illustrates the absorption pathway of different nanoformulations (Subramanian, 2021).

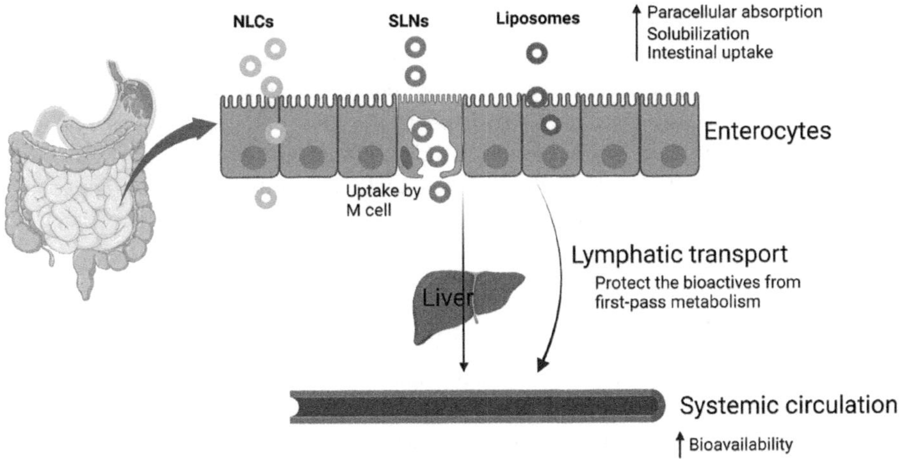

FIGURE 23.5 Absorption process of nanoformulations in GI tract. (Adopted from Subramanian (2021) under the terms and conditions of the CC BY license granting unrestricted reproduction.)

23.5.3 Distribution and Metabolism

If NPs resist local metabolism or breakdown in the digestive tract, they can pass through the GI epithelium and reach the blood and lymphatic systems. The gut-associated lymphoid tissue absorbs hydrophobic NPs and transports them to the lymphatic circulation, bypassing the liver and avoiding first-pass metabolism, which increases blood nutraceutical levels. Alternatively, NPs entering the via hepatic portal vein undergo processing before systemic distribution. Once in circulation, NPs are delivered to organs like heart, lungs, spleen, kidneys, liver, and brain, potentially interacting with blood components, such as platelets and plasma proteins, influencing their distribution and excretion (Mao et al., 2019).

The type of material used to create NPs significantly impacts their metabolism. Encapsulated bioactives in NPs gradually release and diffuse into target organs' cells or tissues. Natural barriers like the blood–brain and placental barriers restrict nanoparticle passage. Polymers like alginate and chitosan, used layer-by-layer, can stabilize bioactive release, and polymers sensitive to specific conditions can control release mechanisms. For instance, polyethylene glycol can enhance pH-stimulated lysozyme release (Bhattacharya et al., 2022c). The bioactives' fate depends on their release site. If absorbed in the colon, bioactives are transported to the liver or lymphatic system. Hydrophilic bioactives circulate more widely than hydrophobic ones. Bioactives follow water-soluble or fat-soluble pathways based on their properties, leading to diverse bioactivities depending on the organ's metabolism. For example, g-tocopherol, a vitamin E form, is effective in inhibiting cancer-related processes (Yao et al., 2020).

23.5.4 Excretion

NPs are excreted when they cannot pass through epithelial cells or when liver metabolism breaks them down. NPs can also avoid being absorbed by epithelial cells and mucus before entering the colon for disposal. Despite being able to pass through epithelial cells, they are still subject to liver's metabolism, which might cause them to re-enter the intestines and ultimately be expelled. If a hydrophilic nanoparticle's average size is less than 10 nm, the kidney may eliminate it through the urinary system (Ishak et al., 2017).

23.6 CONCLUSIONS

The food and pharmaceutical business has several uses for nanotechnology. Nanotechnology will provide the next generation of food items, with the promise of food that can change its color, flavor, or nutritional content to suit the preferences or health requirements of each individual. The use of nanotechnology will help to solve a number of problems that nutraceuticals are now facing. It holds enormous promise for lowering their dosage levels and improving and prolonging the stability of nutraceuticals. Bioactive substances will benefit from enhanced patient acceptance; superior characterization; and, most importantly, great repeatability of their therapeutic efficacy thanks to their formulation as nanomaterials products. There are several commercially produced nanosized nutraceutical items on the market. However, significant work needs to be done with nanonutraceuticals obtained from bioengineering, genetically modified, and tissue culture in order to demonstrate their efficacy in comparison to those derived from naturally produced sources.

ACKNOWLEDGMENTS

The authors like to thank Research and Development Laboratory of Department of Food Technology, Guru Nanak Institute of Technology, Kolkata, and JIS group for providing necessary infrastructural support.

REFERENCES

Abuajah, C.I., 2019. Functional components and medicinal properties of food. In: Mérillon, J.M., Ramawat, K.G. (eds) B*ioactive Molecules in Food. Reference Series in Phytochemistry*. Springer, Cham, pp. 1343–1376. https://doi.org/10.1007/978-3-319-78030-6_39

Abuajah, C.I., Ogbonna, A.C., Osuji, C.M., 2015. Functional components and medicinal properties of food: A review. *J. Food Sci. Technol.* 52, 2522–2529. https://doi.org/10.1007/s13197-014-1396-5

Afzal, O., Altamimi, A.S.A., Nadeem, M.S., Alzarea, S.I., Almalki, W.H., Tariq, A., Mubeen, B., Murtaza, B.N., Iftikhar, S., Riaz, N., Kazmi, I., 2022. Nanoparticles in drug delivery: From history to therapeutic applications. *Nanomaterials (Basel)* 12(24), 4494. https://doi.org/10.3390/nano12244494

Ali, A., Ahmad, U., Akhtar, J., Badruddeen, Khan, M.M., 2019. Engineered nano scale formulation strategies to augment efficiency of nutraceuticals. *J. Funct. Foods* 62, 103554. https://doi.org/10.1016/j.jff.2019.103554

Aswathanarayan, J.B., Vittal, R.R., 2019. Nanoemulsions and their potential applications in food industry. *Front. Sustain. Food Syst.* 3. https://doi.org/10.3389/fsufs.2019.00095

Bai, L., Huan, S., Zhu, Y., Chu, G., McClements, D.J., Rojas, O.J., 2021. Recent advances in food emulsions and engineering foodstuffs using plant-based nanocelluloses. *Annu. Rev. Food Sci. Technol.* 12, 383–406. https://doi.org/10.1146/annurev-food-061920-123242

Bhardwaj, P., Tripathi, P., Gupta, R., Pandey, S., 2020. Niosomes: A review on niosomal research in the last decade. *J. Drug Deliv. Sci. Technol.* 56, 101581. https://doi.org/10.1016/j.jddst.2020.101581

Bhattacharya, S., 2020. *Biological Production of Biopharmaceuticals and Purification Using Advanced Separation Technology*. Jadavpur Univerity. Kolkata.

Bhattacharya, S., Chakraborty, P., Sen, D., Bhattacharjee, C., 2022a. Kinetics of bactericidal potency with synergistic combination of allicin and selected antibiotics. *J. Biosci. Bioeng.* https://doi.org/10.1016/j.jbiosc.2022.02.007

Bhattacharya, S., Gupta, D., Sen, D., Bhattacharjee, C., 2021. Development of micellized antimicrobial thiosulfinate: A contemporary way of drug stability enhancement. In: *Lecture Notes in Bioengineering*, pp. 83–89. https://doi.org/10.1007/978-981-15-7409-2_8

Bhattacharya, S., Mazumder, A., Sen, D., Bhattacharjee, C., 2022b. Bioremediation of dye using mesophilic bacteria: Mechanism and parametric influence. In: *Dye Biodegradation, Mechanisms and Techniques: Recent Advances*, pp. 67–86. https://doi.org/10.1007/978-981-16-5932-4_3

Bhattacharya, S., Sen, D., Bhattacharjee, C., 2022c. Strategic development to stabilize bioactive diallyl thiosulfinate by pH responsive non ionic micelle carrier system. *Process Biochem.* 120, 64–73. https://doi.org/10.1016/j.procbio.2022.05.027

Bhattacharya, S., Sen, D., Bhattacharjee, C., 2019. In vitro antibacterial effect analysis of stabilized PEGylated allicin-containing extract from Allium sativum in conjugation with other antibiotics. *Process Biochem.* 87, 221–231. https://doi.org/10.1016/j.procbio.2019.09.025

Čižauskaitė, U., Jakubaitytė, G., Žitkevičius, V., Kasparavičienė, G., 2019. Natural ingredients-based gummy bear composition designed according to texture analysis and sensory evaluation in vivo. *Molecules* 24, 1442. https://doi.org/10.3390/molecules24071442

Desai, M.S., Seekatz, A.M., Koropatkin, N.M., Kamada, N., Hickey, C.A., Wolter, M., Pudlo, N.A., Kitamoto, S., Terrapon, N., Muller, A., Young, V.B., Henrissat, B., Wilmes, P., Stappenbeck, T.S., Núñez, G., Martens, E.C., 2016. A Dietary fiber-deprived gut microbiota degrades the colonic mucus barrier and enhances pathogen susceptibility. *Cell* 167, 1339–1353.e21. https://doi.org/10.1016/j.cell.2016.10.043

Dhanjal, D.S., Mehta, M., Chopra, C., Singh, R., Sharma, P., Chellappan, D.K., Tambuwala, M.M., Bakshi, H.A., Aljabali, A.A.A., Gupta, G., Nammi, S., Prasher, P., Dua, K., Satija, S., 2021. Novel controlled release pulmonary drug delivery systems: Current updates and challenges. In: *Modeling and Control of Drug Delivery Systems*. Elsevier, pp. 253–272. https://doi.org/10.1016/B978-0-12-821185-4.00001-4

Edgar, J.Y.C., Wang, H., 2017. Introduction for design of nanoparticle based drug delivery systems. *Curr. Pharm. Des.* 23. https://doi.org/10.2174/1381612822666161025154003

Gupta, E., 2020. β-Sitosterol: Predominant phytosterol of therapeutic potential. In: *Innovations in Food Technology*. Springer Singapore, Singapore, pp. 465–477. https://doi.org/10.1007/978-981-15-6121-4_32

Harman, C.L.G., Patel, M.A., Guldin, S., Davies, G.-L., 2019. Recent developments in Pickering emulsions for biomedical applications. *Curr. Opin. Colloid Interface Sci.* 39, 173–189. https://doi.org/10.1016/j.cocis.2019.01.017

Ishak, K.A., Mohamad Annuar, M.S., Ahmad, N., 2017. Nano-delivery systems for nutraceutical application. In: *Nanotechnology Applications in Food*. Elsevier, pp. 179–202. https://doi.org/10.1016/B978-0-12-811942-6.00009-1

Khalaf, A.T., Wei, Y., Alneamah, S.J.A., Al-Shawi, S.G., Kadir, S.Y.A., Zainol, J., Liu, X., 2021. What is new in the preventive and therapeutic role of dairy products as nutraceuticals and functional foods? *Biomed Res. Int.* 2021, 1–9. https://doi.org/10.1155/2021/8823222

Koshani, R., Jafari, S.M., 2019. Ultrasound-assisted preparation of different nanocarriers loaded with food bioactive ingredients. *Adv. Colloid Interface Sci.* 270, 123–146. https://doi.org/10.1016/j.cis.2019.06.005

Lee, K.W., Eakins, G.S., Carlsen, M.S., McLuckey, S.A., 2019. Increasing the upper mass/charge limit of a quadrupole ion trap for ion/ion reaction product analysis via waveform switching. *J. Am. Soc. Mass Spectrom.* 30, 1126–1132. https://doi.org/10.1007/s13361-019-02156-z

Levi, S., Rac, V., Manojlovi, V., Raki, V., Bugarski, B., Flock, T., Krzyczmonik, K.E., Nedovi, V., 2011. Limonene encapsulation in alginate/poly (vinyl alcohol). *Procedia Food Sci.* 1, 1816–1820. https://doi.org/10.1016/j.profoo.2011.09.266

Liem, D.G., Russell, C.G., 2019. The influence of taste liking on the consumption of nutrient rich and nutrient poor foods. *Front. Nutr.* 6. https://doi.org/10.3389/fnut.2019.00174

Liu, M., Zhang, J., Zhu, X., Shan, W., Li, L., Zhong, J., Zhang, Z., Huang, Y., 2016. Efficient mucus permeation and tight junction opening by dissociable "mucus-inert" agent coated trimethyl chitosan nanoparticles for oral insulin delivery. *J. Control. Release* 222, 67–77. https://doi.org/10.1016/j.jconrel.2015.12.008

MacDonald, R., Reitmeier, C., 2017. Nutrition and food access. In: *Understanding Food Systems. Elsevier*, pp. 227–285. https://doi.org/10.1016/B978-0-12-804445-2.00007-7

Mahmood, S., Mandal, U.K., Chatterjee, B., Taher, M., 2017. Advanced characterizations of nanoparticles for drug delivery: Investigating their properties through the techniques used in their evaluations. *Nanotechnol. Rev.* 6, 355–372. https://doi.org/10.1515/ntrev-2016-0050

Manzari, M.T., Shamay, Y., Kiguchi, H., Rosen, N., Scaltriti, M., Heller, D.A., 2021. Targeted drug delivery strategies for precision medicines. *Nat. Rev. Mater.* 6, 351–370. https://doi.org/10.1038/s41578-020-00269-6

Mao, Y., Feng, S., Li, S., Zhao, Q., Di, D., Liu, Y., Wang, S., 2019. Chylomicron-pretended nano-xself-assembling vehicle to promote lymphatic transport and GALTs target of oral drugs. *Biomaterials* 188, 173–186. https://doi.org/10.1016/j.biomaterials.2018.10.012

Mazumder, A., Bhattacharya, S., Bhattacharjee, C., 2020. Role of nano-photocatalysis in heavy metal detoxification. In: *Nanophotocatalysis and Environmental Applications: Detoxification and Disinfection*, pp. 1–33. https://doi.org/10.1007/978-3-030-12619-3_1

McClements, D.J., 2015. *Food Emulsions*. CRC Press. https://doi.org/10.1201/b18868

Mendes, V., Niforou, A., Naska, A., 2022. Appraising diet–disease associations to be used in risk assessment, including an insight in nutritional epidemiology. *EFSA J.* 20. https://doi.org/10.2903/j.efsa.2022.e200411

Moghassemi, S., Hadjizadeh, A., 2014. Nano-niosomes as nanoscale drug delivery systems: An illustrated review. *J. Control. Release* 185, 22–36. https://doi.org/10.1016/j.jconrel.2014.04.015

Mohammadi, Z.B., Zhang, F., Kharazmi, M.S., Jafari, S.M., 2022. Nano-biocatalysts for food applications; immobilized enzymes within different nanostructures. *Crit. Rev. Food Sci. Nutr.* 1–19. https://doi.org/10.1080/10408398.2022.2092719

Mourdikoudis, S., Pallares, R.M., Thanh, N.T.K., 2018. Characterization techniques for nanoparticles: Comparison and complementarity upon studying nanoparticle properties. *Nanoscale* 10, 12871–12934. https://doi.org/10.1039/C8NR02278J

Müller, R.H., Radtke, M., Wissing, S.A., 2002. Solid lipid nanoparticles (SLN) and nanostructured lipid carriers (NLC) in cosmetic and dermatological preparations. *Adv. Drug Deliv. Rev.* 54, S131–S155. https://doi.org/10.1016/S0169-409X(02)00118-7

Premathilaka, R., Rashidinejad, A., Golding, M., Singh, J., 2022. Oral delivery of hydrophobic flavonoids and their incorporation into functional foods: Opportunities and challenges. *Food Hydrocoll.* 128, 107567. https://doi.org/10.1016/j.foodhyd.2022.107567

Riseh, R.S., Tamanadar, E., Pour, M.M., Thakur, V.K., 2022. Novel approaches for encapsulation of plant probiotic bacteria with sustainable polymer gums: Application in the management of pests and diseases. *Adv. Polym. Technol.* 2022, 1–10. https://doi.org/10.1155/2022/4419409

Rocha, F.S., Gomes, A.J., Lunardi, C.N., Kaliaguine, S., Patience, G.S., 2018. Experimental methods in chemical engineering: Ultraviolet visible spectroscopy-UV-Vis. *Can. J. Chem. Eng.* 96, 2512–2517. https://doi.org/10.1002/cjce.23344

Singh, A.R., Desu, P.K., Nakkala, R.K., Kondi, V., Devi, S., Alam, M.S., Hamid, H., Athawale, R.B., Kesharwani, P., 2022. Nanotechnology-based approaches applied to nutraceuticals. *Drug Deliv. Transl. Res.* 12, 485–499. https://doi.org/10.1007/s13346-021-00960-3

Singh, Y., Meher, J.G., Raval, K., Khan, F.A., Chaurasia, M., Jain, N.K., Chourasia, M.K., 2017. Nanoemulsion: Concepts, development and applications in drug delivery. *J. Control. Release* 252, 28–49. https://doi.org/10.1016/j.jconrel.2017.03.008

Speranza, A., Corradini, M.G., Hartman, T.G., Ribnicky, D., Oren, A., Rogers, M.A., 2013. Influence of emulsifier structure on lipid bioaccessibility in oil–water nanoemulsions. *J. Agric. Food Chem.* 61, 6505–6515. https://doi.org/10.1021/jf401548r

Subramanian, P., 2021. Lipid-based nanocarrier system for the effective delivery of nutraceuticals. *Molecules* 26, 5510. https://doi.org/10.3390/molecules26185510

Tundisi, L.L., Ataide, J.A., Costa, J.S.R., Coêlho, D. de F., Liszbinski, R.B., Lopes, A.M., Oliveira-Nascimento, L., de Jesus, M.B., Jozala, A.F., Ehrhardt, C., Mazzola, P.G., 2023. Nanotechnology as a tool to overcome macromolecules delivery issues. *Colloids Surfaces B Biointerfaces* 222, 113043. https://doi.org/10.1016/j.colsurfb.2022.113043

Vinarov, Z., Abrahamsson, B., Artursson, P., Batchelor, H., Berben, P., Bernkop-Schnürch, A., Butler, J., Ceulemans, J., Davies, N., Dupont, D., Flaten, G.E., Fotaki, N., Griffin, B.T., Jannin, V., Keemink, J., Kesisoglou, F., Koziolek, M., Kuentz, M., Mackie, A., Meléndez-Martínez, A.J., McAllister, M., Müllertz, A., O'Driscoll, C.M., Parrott, N., Paszkowska, J., Pavek, P., Porter, C.J.H., Reppas, C., Stillhart, C., Sugano, K., Toader, E., Valentová, K., Vertzoni, M., De Wildt, S.N., Wilson, C.G., Augustijns, P., 2021. Current challenges and future perspectives in oral absorption research: An opinion of the UNGAP network. *Adv. Drug Deliv. Rev.* 171, 289–331. https://doi.org/10.1016/j.addr.2021.02.001

Yao, M., Li, Z., Julian McClements, D., Tang, Z., Xiao, H., 2020. Design of nanoemulsion-based delivery systems to enhance intestinal lymphatic transport of lipophilic food bioactives: Influence of oil type. *Food Chem.* 317, 126229. https://doi.org/10.1016/j.foodchem.2020.126229

Yao, M., McClements, D.J., Xiao, H., 2015. Improving oral bioavailability of nutraceuticals by engineered nanoparticle-based delivery systems. *Curr. Opin. Food Sci.* 2, 14–19. https://doi.org/10.1016/j.cofs.2014.12.005

Yetisgin, A.A., Cetinel, S., Zuvin, M., Kosar, A., Kutlu, O., 2020. Therapeutic nanoparticles and their targeted delivery applications. *Molecules* 25, 2193. https://doi.org/10.3390/molecules25092193

Yu, X., Trase, I., Ren, M., Duval, K., Guo, X., Chen, Z., 2016. Design of nanoparticle-based carriers for targeted drug delivery. *J. Nanomater.* 2016, 1087250. https://doi.org/10.1155/2016/1087250

Zabot, G.L., Schaefer Rodrigues, F., Polano Ody, L., Vinícius Tres, M., Herrera, E., Palacin, H., Córdova-Ramos, J.S., Best, I., Olivera-Montenegro, L., 2022. Encapsulation of bioactive compounds for food and agricultural applications. *Polymers*. 14, 4194. https://doi.org/10.3390/polym14194194

Zhang, X., Guan, J., Mao, S., 2022. Applications of hybrid nanocrystals in drug delivery. In: *Hybrid Nanomaterials for Drug Delivery*. Elsevier, pp. 53–83. https://doi.org/10.1016/B978-0-323-85754-3.00014-9

24 Augmentation of Nanorobots in the Field of Biomedicine

Gayatri Sahini, Vivek Kaushik, Ajaya Kumar Behera, and Suvendu Manna

24.1 INTRODUCTION

24.1.1 What are Nanobots?

Nanorobotics, a sub-division of nanotechnology, includes the production of machines and robots in micro- and nanoscale. Nanorobots, also known as nanobots or nanomachines, are tiny robotic devices designed and engineered at the nanoscale (typically ranging from 1 to 100 nm) to perform specific tasks at the atomic, molecular, or cellular level. These nanobots are also considered technological bacteria or viruses, as they can be programmed in order to perform the tasks at the atomic level. At times, the devices or the machines that interacted with the nanoscaled objects or were used in nanoassembly and nanomanipulation are considered nanorobots (Thiruchelvi et al., 2020). DNA and functional proteins, such as contractile proteins, antibodies, and enzymes, are the materials that are frequently used and have been thoroughly studied for the purpose of creating and producing nanobots (Ganguly et al., 2023). These tiny creatures are usually capable of absorbing ultrasonic vibrations and converting them into electric power, which is further used as a form of energy to keep them working. Based on the design and structure, nanobots are majorly classified into helices, nanorods, and DNA nanobots.

Helices: Magnetic helical micro- and nanorobots can perform 3D navigation in various liquids with sub-micrometer precision under low-strength rotating magnetic fields (<10 mT). Since magnetic fields with low strengths are harmless to cells and tissues, magnetic helical micro/nanorobots are promising tools for biomedical applications, such as minimally invasive surgery, cell manipulation and analysis, and targeted therapy. Magnetic helical micro/nanorobots are controlled and tuned by changing the magnetic fields manually. Automatic control should be integrated to facilitate the control of these devices (kianfar, 2021; Qiu & Nelson, 2015).

Nanorods: Cylindrical rods containing different metal segments. These are also called swimmer nanobots. Ultrasound waves help in the movement of these nanorods, which help in mimicking the action of particular enzymes, targeted drug delivery, detection, and treatment of cancer cells and may also act as 2D swimmers. Though

DOI: 10.1201/9781003432661-24

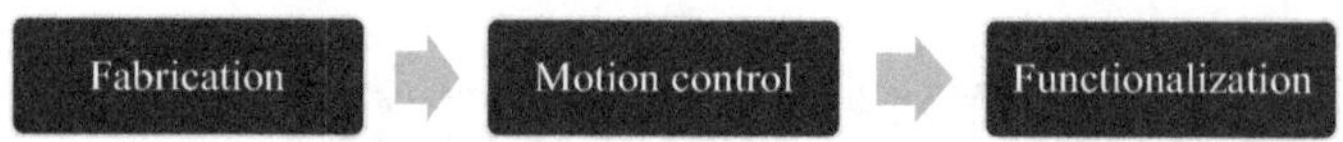

FIGURE 24.1 General operation of nanobots.

the usual nanorods are cylindrical, there are some nanorods that are V-shaped, nano fishes, and hybrid between helices and nanorods.

DNA nanobots: Consist of deoxyribonucleic acid molecules, thus using DNA as construction material for nanosized devices. Sometimes, they are based on DNA origami, where DNA molecules are folded to create patterns and shapes (Arvidsson & Hansen, 2020). Landscapes, cages (icosahedral/hexagonal), nanocapsules, and tubular nanobot are some kinds of DNA nanobots. These can play a major role as drug cargos and carry payloads with increased specificity.

Based on the function, nanobots are classified as assemblers and self-replicators. Assemblers are the nanobots, which resemble normal cells and have the ability to assemble the molecules through various (chemical, physical, and biological) mechanisms to form precisely large parts. Self-assembly occurs at all scales, from atoms and molecules to mesoscopic and macroscopic objects. And it is an important way to form components into the desired system structures (Wei et al., 2021). Self-replicators are basically assemblers that can self-replicate themselves in times of need faster (Figure 24.1).

24.2 COMMON METHODS FOR NANOBOTS ASSEMBLY

In general, there are various mechanisms involved for the assembly and functionalization of different helices based on the material used and the medium they're supposed to act in. A variety of approaches have been investigated for the synthesis of noble metal nanorods, in particular gold and silver particles. These can mainly be classified as electrochemical, photochemical, seed-mediated, or based on a rigid template. Among these, the method based on the seed-mediated growth process has been the most widely used, especially for gold nanorods (GNRs) (Mannelli & Marco, 2010). DNA nanorobots can be programmed with a combination of several unique features, such as tissue penetration, site targeting, stimuli responsiveness, and cargo loading, which makes them ideal candidates as biomedical robots for precision medicine (Hu, 2021). The main components that are needed for a nanobot are payload, microcamera, electrodes, laser, ultrasonic signal generators, and swimming tails. Assembling all these components either manually or through self-assemble to formerly assembled parts of a nanobot completes the nanobot and aids in proper, errorless functioning of it (Manjunath & Kishore, 2014).

24.3 USES OF NANOBOTS IN VARIOUS SECTORS

Various sectors, such as the medical industry, agricultural industry, and electronic sector have escalated demand for nanobots. In the biomedical sector, the nanobots are again classified into respirocytes, microbivores, and clottocytes. Each of them has its own significance. The primary medical applications of reciprocates would include lung disorders, enhancement of cardiovascular/neurovascular procedures, tumor therapies and diagnostics, prevention of asphyxia, artificial breathing, and a variety of sports, veterinary and battlefield transfusable blood substitution, and partial treatment for anaemia (Thiruchelvi et al., 2020). Microbivores are the nanorobots, which function as artificial white blood cells and are also known as nanorobotic phagocytes. The main function of microbivore is to absorb and digest the pathogens in the bloodstream by the process of phagocytosis. They can also be used to clear respiratory or cerebrospinal bacterial infection or infections in urinary fluids and synovial fluids. The theoretically designed clottocyte describes an artificial mechanical platelet or clottocyte that would complete hemostasis in approximately 1 second. The major risk associated with the clottocytes is that the additional activity of the mechanical platelets could trigger the disseminated intravascular coagulation, resulting in multiple microthrombi (Wei et al., 2021). There are many other predicted theories where nanobots can be used to reverse the aging process by maintaining the enzyme production and functioning of organs. In agricultural and environmental sectors, the nanobots are used for water purification, air filtration, pest control, and nutrient delivery. Food safety and quality control management in the food industry can also be done with the help of nanobots.

24.4 USES OF NANOBOTS IN VARIOUS BIOMEDICAL SECTORS

In the upcoming era of personalized precision medicine, the remarkable advancements in nanorobotics have a vision into the various mechanisms leading life activities and have significantly expanded the field of medical robotics. This has remarkably shown an emerging and promising way to advance the level of diagnosis and treatment (Li et al., 2021b). At the vanguard of transdisciplinary research are nanobots, one of the most promising uses of nanomedicines. Through the site-specific and target-oriented administration of precise medications, nanotechnology provides several advantages in the treatment of chronic human illnesses. Chemotherapeutic agents, biological agents, immunotherapeutic agents, and other exceptional uses of nanomedicine have been observed recently in the treatment of a wide range of illnesses (Patra et al., 2018). The various sectors include precision medicine, targeted delivery, hypothermia, photoablation therapy, bioimaging, and biosensing.

24.5 TARGETED DRUG DELIVERY

Drug delivery might be revolutionized by nanobots since they can precisely administer medications to certain human regions or cells. They can be set up to release medications at a certain time or place, which can help minimize adverse effects and increase the effectiveness of medications. The blood–brain barrier presents a major obstacle to medication administration, but nanobots can also be utilized to overcome it. They may be made to specifically target and deliver medications to particular cells or tissues, such as cancer cells (Lau et al., 2019; J. Sun et al., 2019). Current nanodevices and nanobiocomponents that are useful in target drug delivery include nanopores, which can be pore-forming proteins or can be present in a synthetic material such as silicon or graphene. A nanopore can be employed as a single-molecule detector if it is present in an electrically insulating membrane. Industrial filtration, anthrax detection, and DNA sequencing are just a few of the many uses for nanopores (Iqbal & Bashir, 2011). An established method called "molecular imprinting" involves a combination of functionalized monomers interacting reversibly with a target molecule only through noncovalent forces, which is usually done through nanobots. Clinical applications for molecularly imprinted polymers may include controlled drug release, drug monitoring devices, rapid biochemical separations and assays, recognition components in biosensors and chemosensors, and biological and receptor mimics such as synthetic antibodies (plastibodies) or biomimicking enzymes (plastizymes) (Denis et al., 2021). Quantum bots can be coupled with biomolecules to create sensitive, long-lasting probes that are up to 1,000 times brighter than traditional dyes for the purpose of identifying particular compounds used to track biological processes and in numerous biological tests and events by concurrently labeling every biological component (such as distinct DNA sequences or proteins) with color-specific nanodots. Many other devices, such as nanotubes, fullerenes, dendrimers, and bio-nonrobotic devices such as DNA tweezers, Rotaxanes, and Catenanes, also play a crucial role in targeted drug delivery (Hussan Reza et al., 2011).

Drug delivery could be revolutionized by nanobots because they can precisely deliver medications to particular body tissues or cells. Here are a few ways that nanobots can be used to deliver drugs on demand. Passive targeting: Depending on their size, shape, and surface characteristics, nanobots can be made to gather in particular tissues or organs (Gupta, 2023). Active targeting: By attaching ligands or antibodies to particular receptors on the surface of target cells, nanobots can be made functional. Vascular targeting: To enhance medication delivery to tumors, nanobots can be engineered to specifically target the endothelial cells that encircle blood vessels in tumors. Targeting the slightly acidic microenvironment of tumors: It is possible to create nanobots that will release medication in reaction to the slightly acidic environment of tumors. Temperature specificity: Medication can be programmed into nanobots so they will release medication when the temperature changes. Nuclear targeting: Certain medications may work better if nanobots are made to specifically target the nucleus of cells (Zhang et al., 2022).

The use of nanocarriers formulated with solid lipid nanoparticles (NPs), crystal NPs, liposomes, micelles, superparamagnetic iron oxide NPs, and dendrimers, along with gold, silver, cadmium sulfide, and titanium dioxide polymeric NPs, has significantly increased the efficacy of these natural products. Novel natural biomaterials have been in high demand due to their low toxicity, biodegradability, biocompatibility, and easy availability (Patra et al., 2018).

Although targeted medicine delivery has shown considerable promise for nanobots, there are a number of drawbacks to its application. The possibility that healthy cells and tissues could be harmed by nanobots is one of the primary worries. Furthermore, little is known about how long-term exposure to nanobots would affect the human body (Patra et al., 2018). Several obstacles must be overcome when using large-sized materials for drug administration, including in vivo instability, poor solubility, poor bioavailability, poor absorption in the body, problems with target-specific distribution, tonic efficacy, and likely side effects. The short lifespan of biobots,

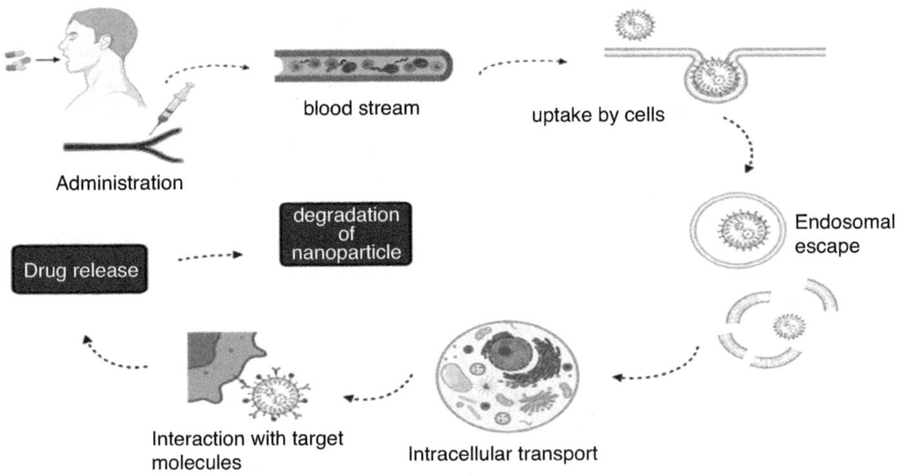

FIGURE 24.2 Nanorobots for healthcare.

their inability to perceive intelligently, and the lack of imaging methods that allow real-time tracking of nanobots are just a few of the numerous obstacles that scientists in this field still need to overcome (Hamid & Manzoor, 2021). Notwithstanding these obstacles, the application of nanotechnology in medication delivery has the promise of revolutionizing the management of a number of illnesses, including diabetes, cancer, neurodegenerative disorders, vascular diseases, and more (Hamid & Manzoor, 2021) (Figure 24.2).

24.6 BIOSENSORS

A biosensor is a chemical detection device that combines a biological element with a physicochemical detector. The International Union of Pure and Applied Chemistry (IUPAC) defines a biological sensor as a device that detects chemical compounds using a precise biochemical mechanism arbitrated by the immune system, isolated enzymes, organelles, or tissues via the sensing of optical, thermal, or electrical signals (Ramesh et al., 2022). Biosensors have various advantages, including simplicity of utilization, scalability, and a straightforward production procedure (Ramesh et al., 2022). Because of their high specific surface area, which allows for the immobilization of a greater number of bioreceptor units and the ability to operate as a transduction element (Holzinger et al., 2014), nanomaterials are suitable for biosensing applications.

Biosensor consists of three segments, namely, sensor, transducer, and electrical circuit, and works on the principle of signal transduction and biorecognition of elements. All the biological materials, including enzyme, antibody, nucleic acid, hormone, organelle, or whole cell can be used as sensors or detectors in a device. But the desired bioreceptor is usually a specific deactivated enzyme. Biosensors are classified as follows based on the sensor device and biological material:

(i) Biosensors based on electrochemistry, (ii) biosensors for calorimetric/thermal sensing, (iii) biosensors based on light, (iv) biosensors based on piezoelectric technology, and (v) biosensors with resonant properties. Biomaterials are used as biosensing platforms, resulting in instruments with a high degree of specificity and sensitivity, quick detection, portability, economy, and ease of use. Because of their unique characteristics, such as environmentally conscious manufacturing techniques, biocompatibility, biodegradability, and biopolymer-based nanomaterials are being considered as excellent candidates for biosensor development among biomaterials (Scala-Benuzzi et al., 2023).

There are some biosensors that mimic the human touch, taste, smell, hearing, and sight. The e-skins should, however, have the following characteristics: they need to be flexible, elastic, self-healing, and capable of sensing temperature, pressure (not just contact), and strain. With recent advances in nanomaterials and self-healing polymers, it is now possible to create e-skins that outperform their organic counterparts, particularly in terms of spatial resolution and heat sensitivity (Hammock et al., 2013). Electronic tongues (e-tongues) typically feature an array of sensing units with detection principles based mostly on electrochemical approaches and spectroscopy of impedance. E-noses help detect the smell based on vapor sensing. Their specific electrical responses to the odorant receptor ligands allowed them to distinguish between fresh and decaying fish scents (Murugathas et al., 2019).

The goal-specific molecules or cells are the focus of the nanobots' particular interactions, which include attaching to them and signaling their detection (Ramesh et al., 2022). The nanobots' sensing agents can be triggered to deliver a payload—possibly a medication for treatment of the targeted cell (Malik et al., 2013; Ponmozhi et al., 2012). A series of atoms make up the response mechanism of nanobots, which respond cohesively to external energy (Katiyar et al., 2022). Nanobot sensors are able to identify certain signals or circumstances, such as the existence of a particular kind of substance or molecule, and relay this data to the system of control (Ramesh et al., 2022).

Two possible risks have been brought to light by nanorobots: (i) the use of UV light and toxic compounds in nanobots, and (ii) the possible loss of propulsion and targeting control (Arvidsson & Hansen, 2020).

Electrochemical biosensors are among the biosensors with the most limitations. These include the expensive nature of the biomolecules, their high susceptibility to various environmental conditions like temperature, pH, oxygen content, and devitalizers, their lower long-term stability, their complicated immobilization process, and their instability toward specific chemicals (Ramesh et al., 2022).

24.7 BIOIMAGING

The study of non-invasive real-time biological process visualization is known as bioimaging. Bioimaging aims to get data regarding the three-dimensional structure of the seen specimen from outside, without physical intervention while causing the least amount of disruption to life processes. Observing subcellular structures, complete cells, tissues, and even entire multicellular creatures are all included in the field of bioimaging. It employs a variety of imaging sources, including light, fluorescence, electrons, ultrasound, X-rays, magnetic resonance, and positrons (Ho & Hutmacher, 2006). Another imaging target that may be widely monitored, 3D imaging, even in the clinical environment, utilizing single-photon emission computed tomography (SPECT), is inflammation, which always occurs in conjunction with tissue regeneration (Basu et al., 2009). To label or view the target substrates, cells, or organs correlating to the imaging modalities, a variety of materials are needed. Thus, these imaging modalities are effective and valuable tools in stem cell injection-based and 3D scaffold-based regenerative medicine (Kircher et al., 2011).

In vivo optical imaging tools have gained popularity, and green fluorescent protein (GFP) transgenic animals or GFP-positive cells are now commercially accessible, but the depth margin is less than 1 cm, which results in less defined results (Yamaoka, 2014). MRI is another highly used technique, as it produces images with really high spatial resolution. As the cells are invisible, a cell staining agent is required, and the most commonly used one is superparamagnetic iron oxide (SPIO). The sensitivity of detection of SPIO particles is higher than that of other contrast agents. Using SPIO, a homing characteristic of stem cells generated from adipose tissue toward cerebral infarctions was described. Through the use of coculturing, cells that were targeted were often tagged with SPIO (Srinivas et al., 2010). It has been discovered that internalized SPIO particles have the ability to leak out of cells and stay there even in the event of cell death, indicating that cell viability tracking cannot be achieved via SPIO imaging (Yamaoka, 2014). The primary goal of cell monitoring is to observe only viable cells, which can't be done using 19F or SPIO labeling. Recently, an efficient intracellular delivery mechanism and a technique for monitoring cells that are alive using a water-soluble contrast ant were developed (Tachibana et al., 2014). Gd-DOTA (1,4,7,10-tetraazacyclododecane-N, N0, N00, N000-tetraacetic acid) was introduced into cells by electrophoretic technology using water-soluble polymers (Shin et al., 2012).

Gold NPs (GNPs), silica NPs, magnetic NPs, quantum dots, carbon nanotubes, fullerenes, and graphene have been used for imaging applications (Rani et al., 2019). A new work titled "DNA nanotechnology-empowered nanoscopic imaging of biomolecules" emphasizes the benefits of DNA nanostructures in bridging bioimaging bottlenecks (Li et al., 2021a).

A potential technology for biomedical uses, such as bioimaging, is nanobots. Nevertheless, there are a few restrictions on the application of nanobots in bioimaging. A primary obstacle is controlling the nanobots' velocity and targeting, which may be difficult given the intricate surroundings of biological systems. The usage of UV light and toxic elements in nanorobots, which may be harmful to the environment and human health, is another drawback (Arvidsson & Hansen, 2020).

24.8 TISSUE ENGINEERING

The multidisciplinary discipline of tissue engineering uses concepts from biology and engineering to create biological replacements that can replace, preserve, enhance, or restore various biological tissue types. Replacement or repair of bone, cartilage, arteries, veins, the bladder, muscles, skin, and other tissues are just a few of the many uses for tissue engineering. It has also been used in attempts to use cells in artificial support systems—like artificial pancreas or bio-artificial liver—to carry out particular biochemical tasks. Scientific developments in stem cells, biomaterials, growth and differentiation components, and biomimetic conditions have made it possible to create new or better tissues in the lab by combining cells, biologically active molecules, and engineered extracellular matrices (scaffolds) (Caddeo et al., 2017).

The following are the primary uses of nanomaterials in dentistry: (i) antibacterial agents to prevent oral infections; (ii) nanofillers to enhance or repair the mechanical characteristics and biological functions of materials utilized in periodontal therapy; (iii) novel implant coatings; and (iv) tooth paste and personal hygiene products. PLGA is a synthetic aliphatic polyester that exhibits exceptional mechanical qualities, a highly tuneable breakdown rate, and remarkable biocompatibility. It is produced from PLA and PGA (Sun et al., 2017). Furthermore, due to its biological compatibility, it has been employed in studies concerning the management of periodontal disease (Elangovan & Karimbux, 2010). Currently, periodontal medication administration, alveolar bone protection, bacterial infection suppression, tissue regeneration guidance, and cement formation are the main uses of PLGA-based materials in dental tissue engineering (Serino et al., 2003).

Besides dentistry, nanobots and nanomaterials also play an intriguing role in wound healing. The physiological processes of wound healing, which include hemostasis, inflammation, proliferation, and remodeling/maturation, are sensitive (Dreifke et al., 2015). Acute wounds are characterized by a break or puncture in the epidermis that heals quickly. Because chronic wounds typically develop in conjunction with other illnesses like obesity and diabetes, they are typically difficult to cure in the near term (Bodnar, 2015). Angiogenesis plays a crucial role in the process of wound healing. In addition to supplying enough blood flow, nourishment, oxygen, and other elements, the vascular formation can hasten wound healing and serve as the foundation for the development of granulation tissue. The responsiveness of implanted components, the ensuing immune response, the possible toxicity, the influence on fertility and even the impact on embryonic development, etc., all need to be carefully examined when using these nanomaterials in tissue engineering for the replacement of damaged organs (Zheng et al., 2021).

24.9 USAGE OF NANOBOTS IN TREATING DIFFERENT HEALTH CONDITIONS

24.9.1 Cancer

By permitting the exact targeting of cancerous cells and ensuring the passage of medications precisely to the tumor site, nanobots hold the potential to completely transform the way that cancer is treated. Therapeutic treatments, such as radiation or chemotherapy medications, can be delivered specifically to the location of the tumor because they can be trained to identify and adhere to cancer cells. Early cancer cell detection with nanobots paves the way for an earlier diagnosis and course of therapy. They may be made to identify certain biomarkers linked to cancer cells and be used to track the disease's development in real-time (Kong et al., 2023). Usage of proper nanomaterials, fabrication of a significant core, and designing a proper pathway are really crucial for nanobots in treating cancer, be it malignant or benign.

Medical nanorobots have a significant advantage over traditional nanomaterials in that they are very good at targeting, a feature that is mostly due to the complex sensors that are built into their architecture. Thanks to these sensors, nanorobots can detect even the smallest changes in the body, including changes in temperature, pH, or the presence of certain biomolecules, like proteins, enzymes, or other biological markers (Wang et al., 2022).

Active power systems are installed on medical nanorobots, enabling them to use external power sources, including magnetic forces, ultrasound, or near-infrared light. They can also take advantage of the natural flow of biological media, such as blood, to move throughout the body (Grifantini, 2019). This active propulsion feature greatly enhances their mobility and navigation, enabling them to effectively approach certain objectives and carry out their assigned tasks with exceptional accuracy (Singh et al., 2019). On the other hand, typical nanomaterials travel through biological systems by passive mechanisms like diffusion or convection rather than active power systems (Kashyap et al., 2021). When compared to their nanorobot counterparts, these passive transport techniques inherently limit the mobility and capability of nanocarriers, making them less effective and adaptable in some medication delivery applications. Due to their dual roles as a dose booster in radiation and as a carrier of anticancer drugs in chemotherapy, GNPs are widely employed. The majority of GNPs employed in the investigations were found in the cytoplasm of the cells (Yang et al., 2014).

There are many ways where nanobots come in hand in treating cancer. Some of them are as follows: Drug delivery: By delivering medications straight to cancer cells, nanobots can reduce the adverse impacts of chemotherapy and other therapies (Kong et al., 2023). Targeted therapy: The nanobots can be programmed to identify and attach to cancer cells, enabling the delivery of therapeutic agents like chemotherapy medications or radiation promptly to the tumor site. Nanobots can also be used for tumor sensing and diagnosis, recognizing particular markers that correspond to cancer cells and monitoring the disease's progression in real-time. Minimally invasive surgery: By using nanobots to carry out this type of procedure, tumors may be removed without causing harm to healthy tissue. Additional all-encompassing therapies: By interrupting the blood flow to tumors, nanobots can reduce their size.

Versatile protease nanosensors, which respond to the cancer cell microenvironment, generate a colorimetric signal that can be tracked through urine. In a study involving collected urine samples from mouse models with colorectal cancer, it was observed that mice affected by tumors exhibited a 13-fold signal increase in comparison to their healthy counterparts. Additionally, the development of innovative imaging agents with enhanced sensitivity and specificity has the potential to enhance early detection (Zhang et al., 2019).

24.9.2 Hematology

While surgeries, which have enjoyed a high success rate in the past, have become more viable and are routinely conducted to access infected internal regions that cannot be treated externally, there are still regions in the body that remain physically inaccessible to doctors. One persistent challenge is the presence of internal blood clots, which can sometimes be located in areas too deep within the body to be reached effectively, such as deep arteries or veins and narrow internal sections of the brain or lungs. The integration of nanorobotics is being explored as a solution for addressing the issue of internal blood clots. The approach involves the development of fleets of nanobots within the blood stream, serving as carriers for delivering medications to locations that are challenging to access for conventional physical treatment. This not only simplifies the procedure but also holds the potential for significantly enhanced efficiency, precision, and reduced invasiveness in comparison to presently available techniques (Malhotra & Shahdadpuri, 2020).

Nanobots help in removing the clot by precise targeting, minimal invasion, efficient, reduced side effects, improved outcomes, faster treatment, and the need for non – invasive monitoring (Saadeh & Vyas, 2014). Respirocytes are tiny devices that function at the molecular level and may be thought of as nanorobots. There is a chance that respirocytes can be utilized in an emergency to replace platelets. Respirocytes will also have an impact on the treatment of coronary heart disease. Additionally, current research indicates that respirocytes have the capacity to carry 200 times more respiratory gas molecules than do naturally occurring red blood cells in the same amount. Additionally, clottocytes—a kind of nanobot may be utilized to stop bleeding by acting as artificial platelets. Clottocytes are an exact replica of natural platelets that have a propensity to create a fiber-like mesh resistor in order to halt bleed (Krummenacker & Lewis, 1995). The capacity of clottocytes to be a thousand times more effective than an equivalent quantity of normal platelets (Viswanathan et al., 2019).

They offer a multitude of advantages compared to conventional drug delivery methods. Nanobots are exceptionally precise and specific, resulting in fewer side effects as they release medications in a controlled fashion. They also reduce the potential for surgical errors. Computer – regulated drug administration and the heightened pace of drug action represent additional exceptional qualities. The primary drawback lies in the high cost of designing nanobots, along with the considerable complexities involved in their development. The most challenging hurdle is related to the power supply. In order for the nanobots to circumvent the body's immune response, additional is required (Viswanathan et al., 2019).

24.9.3 Cardiovascular Diseases

According to a 2017 WHO report, CVD was the leading cause of death worldwide in 2015, resulting in 17.7 million deaths. By 2030, estimates indicate that number will rise to 23.6 million (Rehman et al., 2021). Heart disease is one of the leading causes of death and morbidity in the world today. Since NPs have unique properties such as size, shape, aspect ratio, surface charge, and surface area, they are becoming more and more significant in controlling stem cell activity. NPs have the potential to improve stem cell retention following transplantation, track the stem cells in vivo for extended monitoring, and allow gene transfer in stem cells with regard to cardiac illness. Using NPs to treat peripheral vascular disease has several benefits, such as enabling stem cell therapy, simulating the extracellular matrix, and providing a secure, non-viral gene delivery mechanism (Sun et al., 2020).

The use of molecular imaging for cardiovascular disease diagnosis has gained increasing prominence in recent years. Alongside the continual advancement of diverse imaging techniques, novel contrast agents play a pivotal role in enabling real – time, rapid, high – sensitivity, and high – resolution diagnostics (Chandarana et al., 2018). In comparison to traditional contrast agents, nanocontrast agents offer the following benefits:

- In vivo stabilization, regulable distribution, and prolonging the half – life of contrast agents or drugs.
- Controllable physical and chemical properties and imaging performance.
- Specific identification of certain biomolecules.
- Ability of multimodal imaging realization.
- Values in individualized diagnosis and therapy are expected to be realized.

The use of nanocarrier as an efficient, precise, and controllable intercellular drug delivery method offers distinct advantages in the diagnosis and treatment of cardiovascular diseases. It effectively addresses issues related to targeting, localized drug delivery, controlled and sustained release, as well as toxicity reduction as it advances toward multifunctional and integrated diagnostic and therapeutic approaches. With ongoing innovation in nanotechnology and in – depth investigation into the molecular pathological mechanisms of CVDs, the application of nanodrug development systems (NDDSs) will be further promoted, providing new techniques and methods for clinical diagnosis and therapy (Deng et al., 2020; Chopra et al., 2022). Advancement in medical technology and therapies for CVDs have made substantial progress, with the goal of enhancing the quality of life and extending lifespan (Chandarana et al., 2018). There is a pressing need to discover improved approaches for CVD treatment, considering that an estimated mere 15% of the current practice guidelines are substantiated by high – quality evidence (Chandarana et al., 2018; Chopra et al., 2022).

25.10 CONCLUSIONS

The field of nanorobotics has great promise for the development of biological fields, including pharmacology, hematology, cancer, and many more. Their minuscule size facilitates access to areas that are inaccessible to conventional machinery. The creation of these extremely useful microorganisms for information processing, signaling, and sensing might lead to significant advances in medicine. They are employed in electronic devices, aerospace, and defense in addition to biological applications. The use of nanobots in the hematology department extends from blood clotting to oxygen transportation. Respirocytes are believed to be 200 times more efficient than red blood cells (RBCs) since they function as fake RBCs and aid in the transfer of gasses throughout the bloodstream until the patient is stabilized. Clottocytes are the cells that have 10,000 times the effectiveness of platelets. More specifically, they may be used for everything from a little cut to a major hemorrhage.

However, in the field of oncology, these nanobots aid in the prognosis of the illness by early tumor identification. These nanobots have an integrated communication system that allows them to convey the data they've collected and react to acoustic cues. Because they have chemotic sensors on their surfaces', targeted treatment is also an option in this situation. The pharmaceutical industry can benefit from the development and application of biochips, immune NPs, and nanosensors. Numerous cutting-edge pharmaceutical forms, such as nanoliposomes and nanotubes, improve the efficacy of drug delivery. Lastly, nanorobots have a significant impact on the development of therapy, medication administration, and prognostic strategies. Conflicts, however, are more likely to arise when creating a dynamic model for algorithm control and the appropriate operation of materials that may be dangerous for humans.

REFERENCES

Arvidsson, R., & Hansen, S. F. (2020). Environmental and health risks of nanorobots: An early review. *Environmental Science: Nano*, *7*(10), 2875–2886. https://doi.org/10.1039/D0EN00570C

Basu, S., Zhuang, H., Torigian, D. A., Rosenbaum, J., Chen, W., & Alavi, A. (2009). Functional imaging of inflammatory diseases using nuclear medicine techniques. *Seminars in Nuclear Medicine*, *39*(2), 124–145. https://doi.org/10.1053/j.semnuclmed.2008.10.006

Bodnar, R. J. (2015). Chemokine regulation of angiogenesis during wound healing. *Advances in Wound Care*, *4*(11), 641–650. https://doi.org/10.1089/wound.2014.0594

Caddeo, S., Boffito, M., & Sartori, S. (2017). Tissue engineering approaches in the design of healthy and pathological in vitro tissue models. *Frontiers in Bioengineering and Biotechnology*, *5*. https://doi.org/10.3389/fbioe.2017.00040

Chandarana, M., Curtis, A., & Hoskins, C. (2018). The use of nanotechnology in cardiovascular disease. *Applied Nanoscience*, *8*(7), 1607–1619. https://doi.org/10.1007/s13204-018-0856-z

Chopra, H., Bibi, S., Mishra, A. K., Tirth, V., Yerramsetty, S. V., Murali, S. V., Ahmad, S. U., Mohanta, Y. K., Attia, M. S., Algahtani, A., Islam, F., Hayee, A., Islam, S., Baig, A. A., & Emran, T. Bin. (2022). Nanomaterials: A promising therapeutic approach for cardiovascular diseases. *Journal of Nanomaterials*, *2022*, 4155729. https://doi.org/10.1155/2022/4155729

Deng, Y., Zhang, X., Shen, H., He, Q., Wu, Z., Liao, W., & Yuan, M. (2020). Application of the nano-drug delivery system in treatment of cardiovascular diseases. *Frontiers in Bioengineering and Biotechnology*, *7*. https://doi.org/10.3389/fbioe.2019.00489

Denis, M., Gindre, D., & Felpin, F.-X. (2021). Ultra-fast covalent molecular printing on cellulose paper by photo-strain-triggered click ligation: UV LED versus laser irradiations. *Journal of Materials Science*, *56*(8), 5006–5014. https://doi.org/10.1007/s10853-020-05585-4

Dreifke, M. B., Jayasuriya, A. A., & Jayasuriya, A. C. (2015). Current wound healing procedures and potential care. *Materials Science and Engineering: C*, *48*, 651–662. https://doi.org/10.1016/j.msec.2014.12.068

Elangovan, S., & Karimbux, N. (2010). Review paper: DNA delivery strategies to promote periodontal regeneration. *Journal of Biomaterials Applications*, *25*(1), 3–18. https://doi.org/10.1177/0885328210366490

Ganguly, K., Dutta, S. D., Patel, D. K., Patil, T. V., Luthfikasari, R., & Lim, K.-T. (2023). Biomolecule-based nanorobot for targeted delivery of therapeutics. In *Nanorobotics and Nanodiagnostics in Integrative Biology and Biomedicine* (pp. 35–52). Springer International Publishing. https://doi.org/10.1007/978-3-031-16084-4_3

Grifantini, K. (2019). The state of nanorobotics in medicine. *IEEE Pulse*, *10*(5), 13–17. https://doi.org/10.1109/MPULS.2019.2937150

Gupta, P. K. (2023). Nano-based drug delivery systems. In *Nanotoxicology in Nanobiomedicine* (pp. 91–110). Springer International Publishing. https://doi.org/10.1007/978-3-031-24287-8_6

Hamid, R., & Manzoor, I. (2021). Nanomedicines: Nano based drug delivery systems challenges and opportunities. In *Alternative Medicine - Update*. IntechOpen. https://doi.org/10.5772/intechopen.94353

Hammock, M. L., Chortos, A., Tee, B. C. - K., Tok, J. B. - H., & Bao, Z. (2013). 25th anniversary article: The evolution of electronic skin (E-skin): A brief history, design considerations, and recent progress. *Advanced Materials*, *25*(42), 5997–6038. https://doi.org/10.1002/adma.201302240

Ho, S. T., & Hutmacher, D. W. (2006). A comparison of micro CT with other techniques used in the characterization of scaffolds. *Biomaterials*, *27*(8), 1362–1376. https://doi.org/10.1016/j.biomaterials.2005.08.035

Holzinger, M., Le Goff, A., & Cosnier, S. (2014). Nanomaterials for biosensing applications: A review. *Frontiers in Chemistry*, *2*. https://doi.org/10.3389/fchem.2014.00063

Hu, Y. (2021). Self-assembly of DNA molecules: Towards DNA nanorobots for biomedical applications. *Cyborg and Bionic Systems,* 2021, 9807520.

Hussan Reza, K., Asiwarya, G., Radhika, G., & Bardalai, D (2011). Nanorobots: The future trend of drug delivery and therapeutics. *International Journal of Pharmaceutical Sciences Review and Research*, 10(1), 60–68.

Iqbal, S. M., & Bashir, R. (Eds.). (2011). *Nanopores*. Springer US. https://doi.org/10.1007/978-1-4419-8252-0

Kashyap, D., Tuli, H. S., Yerer, M. B., Sharma, A., Sak, K., Srivastava, S., Pandey, A., Garg, V. K., Sethi, G., & Bishayee, A. (2021). Natural product-based nanoformulations for cancer therapy: Opportunities and challenges. *Seminars in Cancer Biology*, *69*, 5–23. https://doi.org/10.1016/j.semcancer.2019.08.014

Katiyar, N. K., Goel, G., & Goel, S. (2022). Nanomaterials based biosensing: Methods and principle of detection In *Advanced Micro-and Nano-manufacturing Technologies: Applications in Biochemical and Biomedical Engineering* (pp. 1–27). https://doi.org/10.1007/978-981-16-3645-5_1

kianfar, E. (2021). Magnetic nanoparticles in targeted drug delivery: A review. *Journal of Superconductivity and Novel Magnetism*, *34*(7), 1709–1735. https://doi.org/10.1007/s10948-021-05932-9

Kircher, M. F., Gambhir, S. S., & Grimm, J. (2011). Noninvasive cell-tracking methods. *Nature Reviews Clinical Oncology*, *8*(11), 677–688. https://doi.org/10.1038/nrclinonc.2011.141

Kong, X., Gao, P., Wang, J., Fang, Y., & Hwang, K. C. (2023). Advances of medical nanorobots for future cancer treatments. *Journal of Hematology & Oncology*, *16*(1), 74. https://doi.org/10.1186/s13045-023-01463-z

Krummenacker, M., & Lewis, J. (Eds.). (1995). *Prospects in Nanotechnology: Toward Molecular Manufacturing*. John Wiley & Sons, Inc. Hoboken, New Jersey.

Lau, F.-L. A., Büther, F., Geyer, R., & Fischer, S. (2019). Computation of decision problems within messages in DNA-tile-based molecular nanonetworks. *Nano Communication Networks*, *21*, 100245. https://doi.org/10.1016/j.nancom.2019.05.002

Li, F., Li, J., Dong, B., Wang, F., Fan, C., & Zuo, X. (2021a). DNA nanotechnology-empowered nanoscopic imaging of biomolecules. *Chemical Society Reviews*, *50*(9), 5650–5667. https://doi.org/10.1039/D0CS01281E

Li, M., Xi, N., Wang, Y., & Liu, L. (2021b). Progress in nanorobotics for advancing biomedicine. *IEEE Transactions on Biomedical Engineering*, *68*(1), 130–147. https://doi.org/10.1109/TBME.2020.2990380

Malhotra, P., & Shahdadpuri, N. (2020). Nano-robotic based thrombolysis: Dissolving blood clots using nanobots. In *2020 IEEE 17th India Council International Conference (INDICON)* (pp. 1–4). https://doi.org/10.1109/INDICON49873.2020.9342510

Malik, P., Katyal, V., Malik, V., Asatkar, A., Inwati, G., & Mukherjee, T. K. (2013). Nanobiosensors: Concepts and variations. *ISRN Nanomaterials*, 2013, 327435. https://doi.org/10.1155/2013/327435

Manjunath, A., & Kishore, V. (2014). The promising future in medicine: Nanorobots. *Biomedical Science and Engineering*, 2(2), 42–47.

Mannelli, I., & Marco, M. P. (2010). Recent advances in analytical and bioanalysis applications of noble metal nanorods. *Analytical and Bioanalytical Chemistry*, 398, 2451–2469.

Murugathas, T., Zheng, H. Y., Colbert, D., Kralicek, A. V., Carraher, C., & Plank, N. O. V. (2019). Biosensing with Insect odorant receptor nanodiscs and carbon nanotube field-effect transistors. *ACS Applied Materials & Interfaces*, *11*(9), 9530–9538. https://doi.org/10.1021/acsami.8b19433

Patra, J. K., Das, G., Fraceto, L. F., Campos, E. V. R., Rodriguez-Torres, M. del P., Acosta-Torres, L. S., Diaz-Torres, L. A., Grillo, R., Swamy, M. K., Sharma, S., Habtemariam, S., & Shin, H.-S. (2018). Nano based drug delivery systems: Recent developments and future prospects. *Journal of Nanobiotechnology*, *16*(1), 71. https://doi.org/10.1186/s12951-018-0392-8

Ponmozhi, J., Frias, C., Marques, T., & Frazão, O. (2012). Smart sensors/actuators for biomedical applications: Review. *Measurement*, *45*(7), 1675–1688. https://doi.org/10.1016/j.measurement.2012.02.006

Qiu, F., & Nelson, B. J. (2015). Magnetic helical micro- and nanorobots: Toward their biomedical applications. *Engineering*, *1*(1), 021–026. https://doi.org/10.15302/J-ENG-2015005

Ramesh, M., Janani, R., Deepa, C., & Rajeshkumar, L. (2022). Nanotechnology-enabled biosensors: A review of fundamentals, design principles, materials, and applications. *Biosensors*, *13*(1), 40. https://doi.org/10.3390/bios13010040

Rani, R., Sethi, K., & Singh, G. (2019). *Nanomaterials and Their Applications in Bioimaging* (pp. 429–450). https://doi.org/10.1007/978-3-030-16379-2_15

Rehman, S., Rehman, E., Ikram, M., & Jianglin, Z. (2021). Cardiovascular disease (CVD): Assessment, prediction and policy implications. *BMC Public Health*, *21*(1), 1299. https://doi.org/10.1186/s12889-021-11334-2

Saadeh, Y., & Vyas, D. (2014). Nanorobotic applications in medicine: Current proposals and designs. *American Journal of Robotic Surgery*, *1*(1), 4–11.

Scala-Benuzzi, M. L., Piguillem Palacios, S. V., Takara, E. A., & Fernández-Baldo, M. A. (2023). Biomaterials and biopolymers for the development of biosensors. In *Biomaterials-Based Sensors* (pp. 3–24). Springer Nature, Singapore. https://doi.org/10.1007/978-981-19-8501-0_1

Serino, G., Biancu, S., Iezzi, G., & Piattelli, A. (2003). Ridge preservation following tooth extraction using a polylactide and polyglycolide sponge as space filler: A clinical and histological study in humans. *Clinical Oral Implants Research*, *14*(5), 651–658. https://doi.org/10.1034/j.1600-0501.2003.00970.x

Shin, C., Lee, W., Woo, J. S., Park, E.-A., Kim, P., Song, H. B., & Kim, H. S. (2012). *In vitro* MRI and characterization of rat mesenchymal stem cells transduced with ferritin as MR reporter gene. *Journal of the Korean Society of Magnetic Resonance in Medicine*, *16*(1), 47. https://doi.org/10.13104/jksmrm.2012.16.1.47

Singh, A. V., Ansari, M. H. D., Laux, P., & Luch, A. (2019). Micro-nanorobots: Important considerations when developing novel drug delivery platforms. *Expert Opinion on Drug Delivery*, *16*(11), 1259–1275. https://doi.org/10.1080/17425247.2019.1676228

Srinivas, M., Aarntzen, E. H. J. G., Bulte, J. W. M., Oyen, W. J., Heerschap, A., de Vries, I. J. M., & Figdor, C. G. (2010). Imaging of cellular therapies. *Advanced Drug Delivery Reviews*, *62*(11), 1080–1093. https://doi.org/10.1016/j.addr.2010.08.009

Sun, J., Mathesh, M., Li, W., & Wilson, D. A. (2019). Enzyme-powered nanomotors with controlled size for biomedical applications. *ACS Nano*, *13*(9), 10191–10200. https://doi.org/10.1021/acsnano.9b03358

Sun, X., Xu, C., Wu, G., Ye, Q., & Wang, C. (2017). Poly(lactic-co-glycolic acid): Applications and future prospects for periodontal tissue regeneration. *Polymers*, *9*(12), 189. https://doi.org/10.3390/polym9060189

Sun, Y., Lu, Y., Yin, L., & Liu, Z. (2020). The roles of nanoparticles in stem cell-based therapy for cardiovascular disease. *Frontiers in Bioengineering and Biotechnology*, *8*. https://doi.org/10.3389/fbioe.2020.00947

Tachibana, Y., Enmi, J., Agudelo, C. A., Iida, H., & Yamaoka, T. (2014). Long-term/bioinert labeling of rat mesenchymal stem cells with PVA-Gd conjugates and MRI Monitoring of the labeled cell survival after intramuscular transplantation. *Bioconjugate Chemistry*, *25*(7), 1243–1251. https://doi.org/10.1021/bc400463t

Thiruchelvi, R., Sikdar, E., Das, A., & Rajakumari, K. (2020). Nanobots in today's world. *Research Journal of Pharmacy and Technology*, *13*(4), 2033. https://doi.org/10.5958/0974-360X.2020.00366.2

Viswanathan, S. M., Rajan, A. R., & Rajan, R. (2019). Nanobots in medical field: A critical overview. *International Journal of Engineering Research & Technology (IJERT)*, *8*(12). https://doi.org/10.17577/IJERTV8IS120023

Wang, J., Dong, Y., Ma, P., Wang, Y., Zhang, F., Cai, B., Chen, P., & Liu, B. (2022). Intelligent micro-/nanorobots for cancer theragnostic. *Advanced Materials*, *34*(52). https://doi.org/10.1002/adma.202201051

Wei, F., Zhong, T., Zhan, Z., & Yao, L. (2021). Self-assembled micro-nanorobots: From assembly mechanisms to applications. *ChemNanoMat*, *7*(3), 238–252.

Yamaoka, T. (2014). Bioimaging materials. In *Encyclopedia of Polymeric Nanomaterials* (pp. 1–6). Springer, Berlin, Heidelberg. https://doi.org/10.1007/978-3-642-36199-9_283-1

Yang, C., Neshatian, M., & van Prooijen, M. (2014). Cancer nanotechnology: Enhanced therapeutic response using peptide-modified gold nanoparticles. *Journal of Nanoscience and Nanotechnology*, *14*(7), 4813–4819. https://doi.org/10.1166/jnn.2014.9280

Zhang, D., Liu, S., Guan, J., & Mou, F. (2022). "Motile-targeting" drug delivery platforms based on micro/nanorobots for tumor therapy. *Frontiers in Bioengineering and Biotechnology*, *10*. https://doi.org/10.3389/fbioe.2022.1002171

Zhang, Y., Li, M., Gao, X., Chen, Y., & Liu, T. (2019). Nanotechnology in cancer diagnosis: Progress, challenges and opportunities. *Journal of Hematology & Oncology*, *12*(1), 137. https://doi.org/10.1186/s13045-019-0833-3

Zheng, X., Zhang, P., Fu, Z., Meng, S., Dai, L., & Yang, H. (2021). Applications of nanomaterials in tissue engineering. *RSC Advances*, *11*(31), 19041–19058. https://doi.org/10.1039/D1RA01849C

Index

For Product Safety Concerns and Information please contact our EU representative GPSR@taylorandfrancis.com Taylor & Francis Verlag GmbH, Kaufingerstraße 24, 80331 München, Germany

Batch number: 10397790

Printed by Printforce, the Netherlands